HEALTHY INSPIRATION

MASSAGE

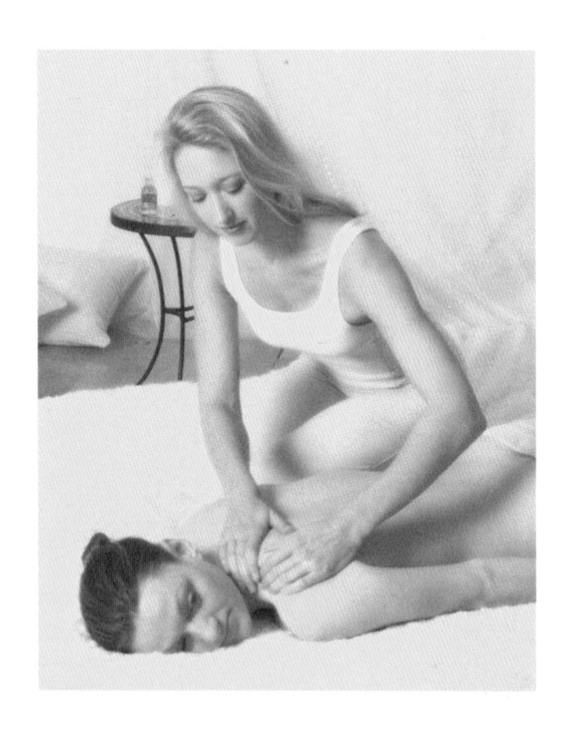

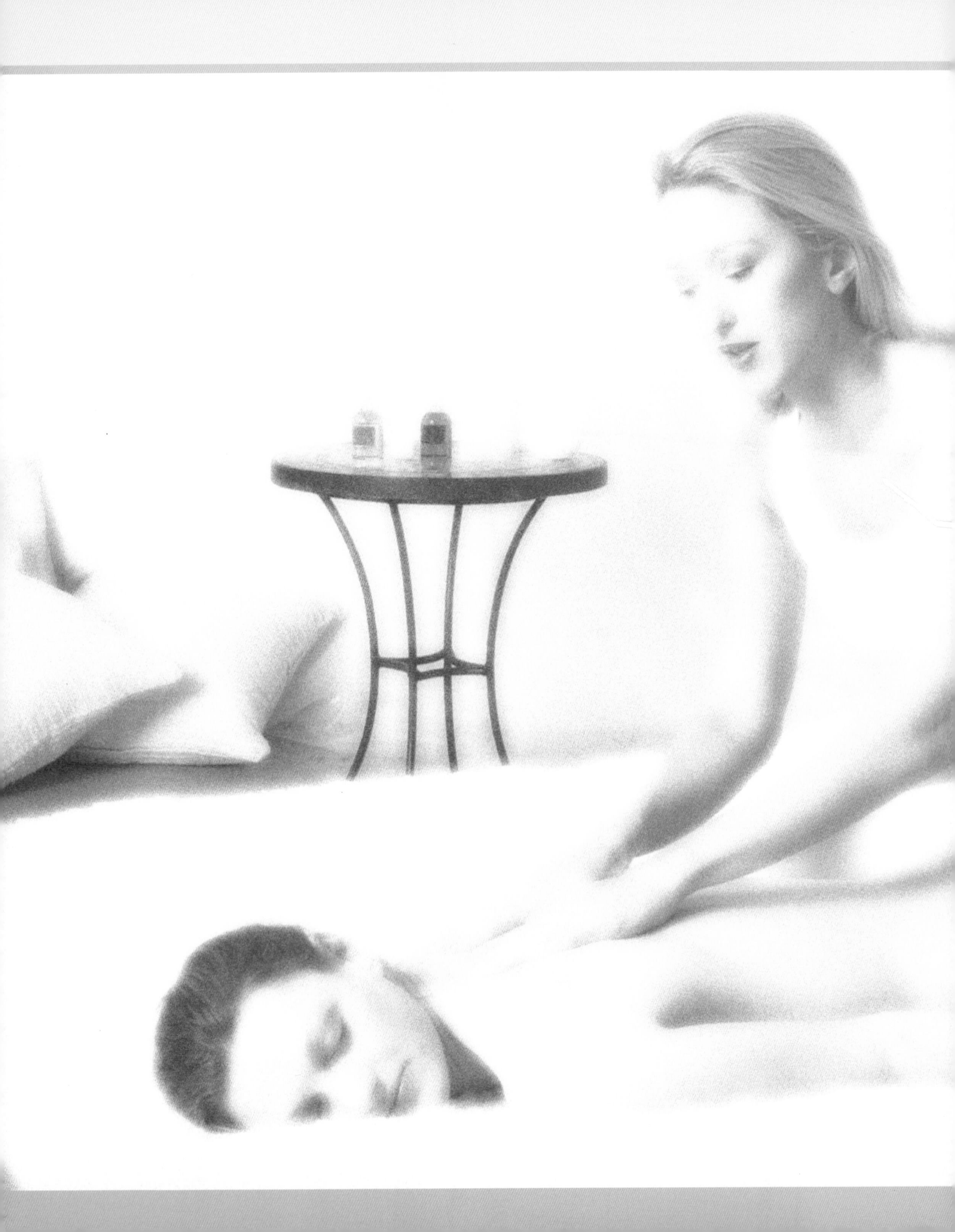

HEALTHY INSPIRATION

MASSAGE

Caron Bosler

Published by SILVERDALE BOOKS
An imprint of Bookmart Ltd
Registered number 2372865
Trading as Bookmart Ltd
Blaby Road
Wigston
Leicester LE18 4SE

D&S Books Ltd
Kerswell,
Parkham Ash, Bideford
Devon, England
EX39 5PR

e-mail us at:- enquiries@d-sbooks.co.uk

This edition printed 2005

ISBN 1-84509-273-2

DS0117. Healthy inspirations - Massage

Creative Director: Sarah King
Editor: Anna Southgate
Project editor: Judith Millidge
Designer: Debbie Fisher
Photographer: Paul Forrester

Fonts: Rotis Sans Serif and Vag Rounded

Printed in China

1 3 5 7 9 10 8 6 4 2

Contents

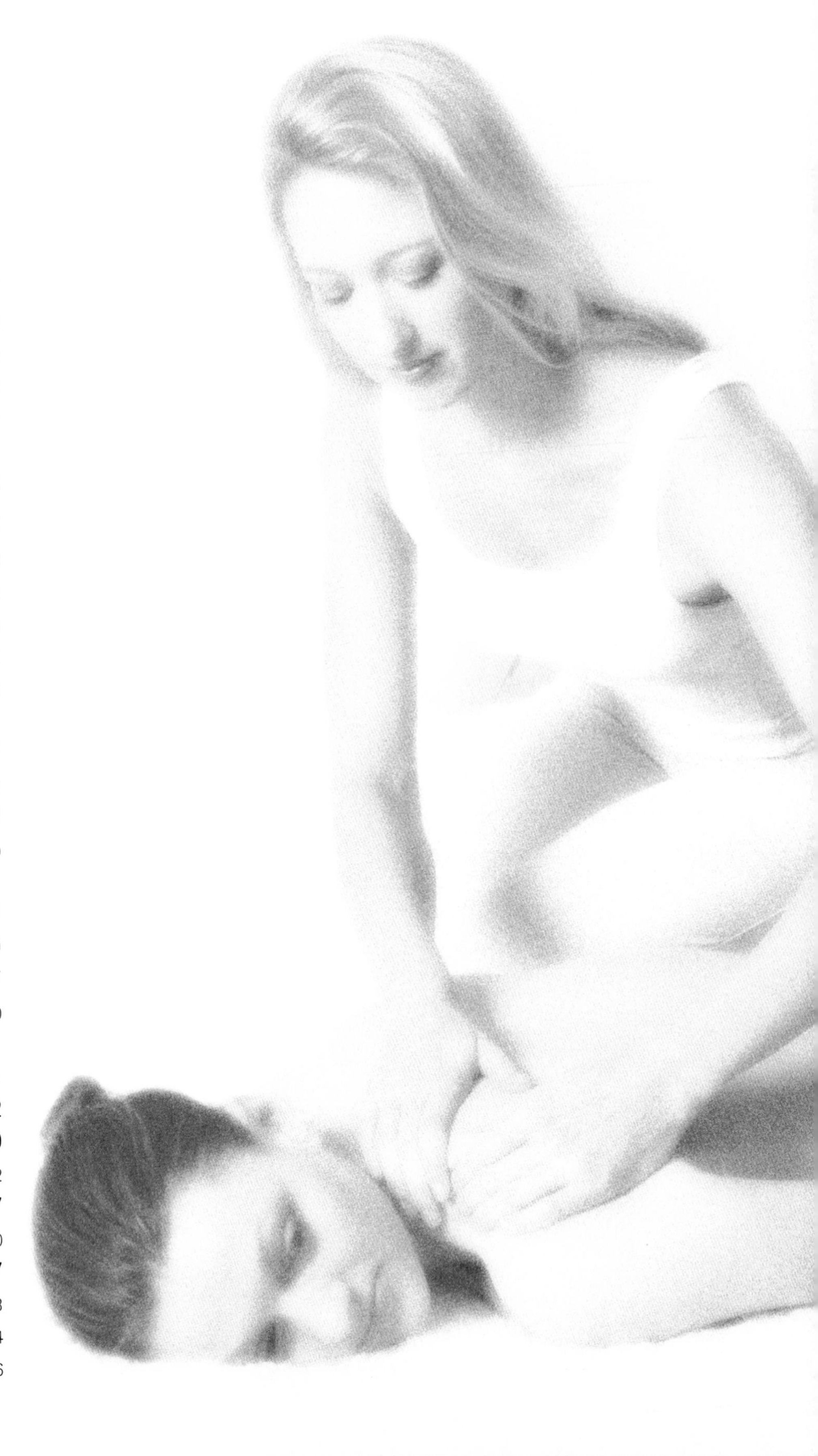

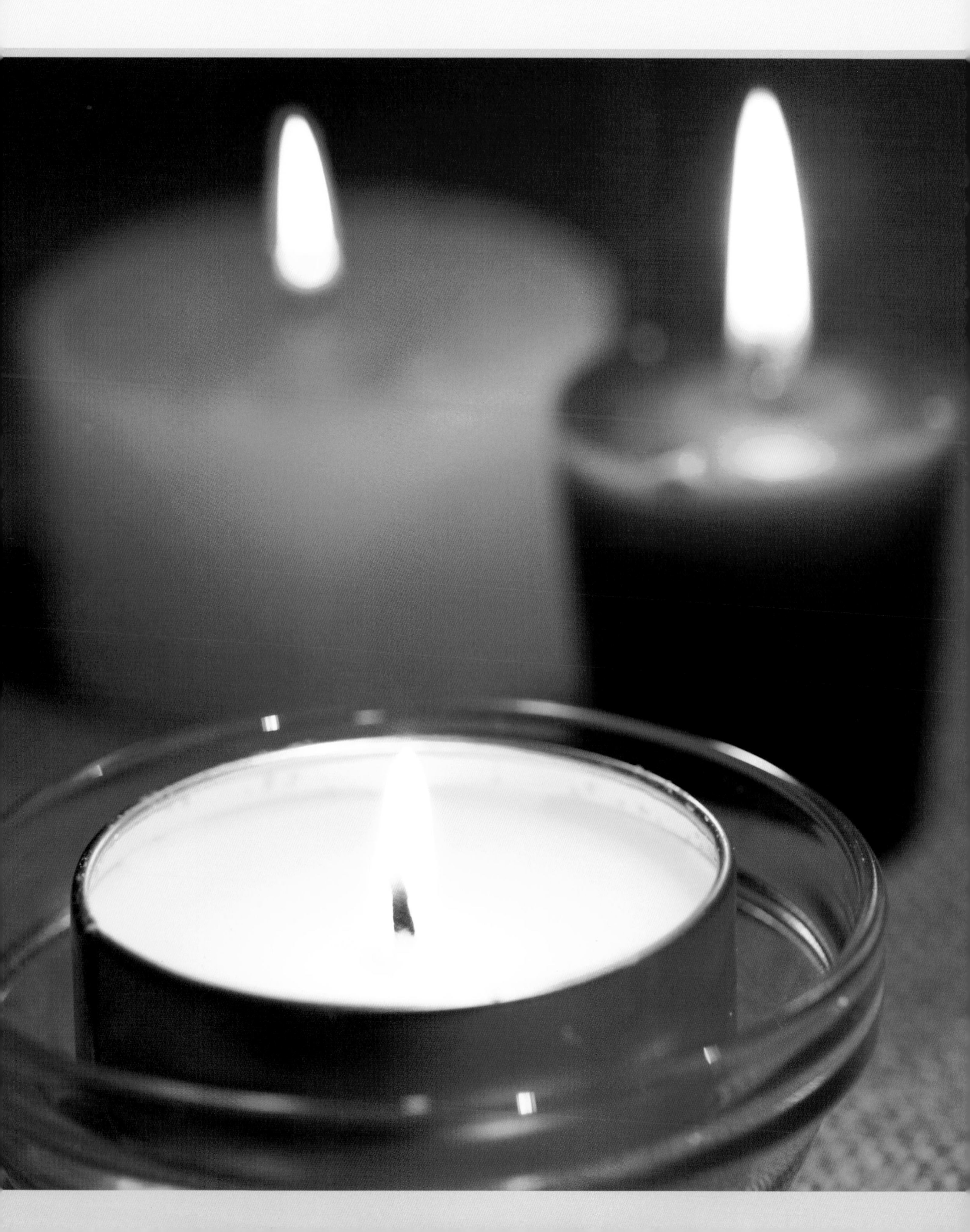

Introduction

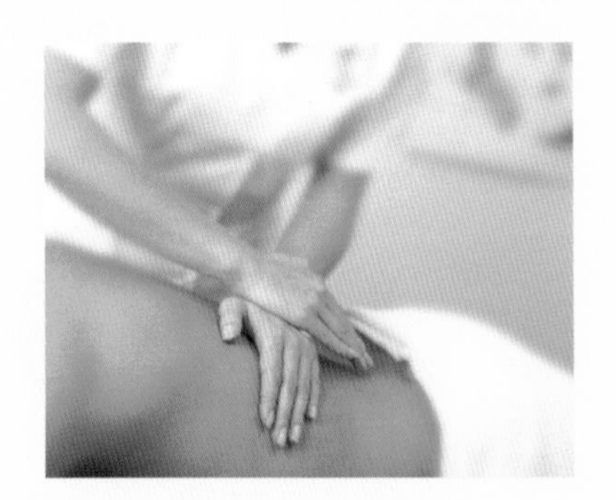

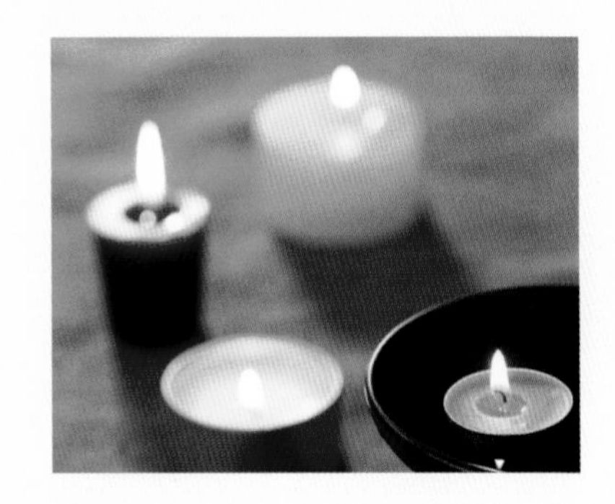

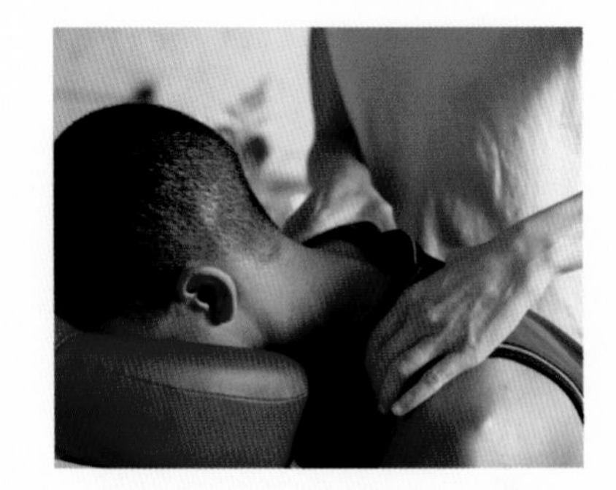

Touch and massage

Touch is the most natural form of communication, and is instinctive to us all. Touch is nurturing, comforting and healing. When we express love or caring we hug and hold each other. When we are upset emotionally, we want to be held. When we are hurt physically, our natural instinct is to hold or rub the area in pain. Touch transcends words; it comforts and relaxes both our physical and emotional bodies.

What is massage?

Massage is a holistic therapy that uses touch as a means to bring balance to the body. Releasing tension and toxins built up in the muscle tissue enables the body to become more relaxed and function more efficiently. Using pressure created through specific sequences, a massage can be either relaxing or stimulating. Massage releases muscle tension while relaxing the mind.

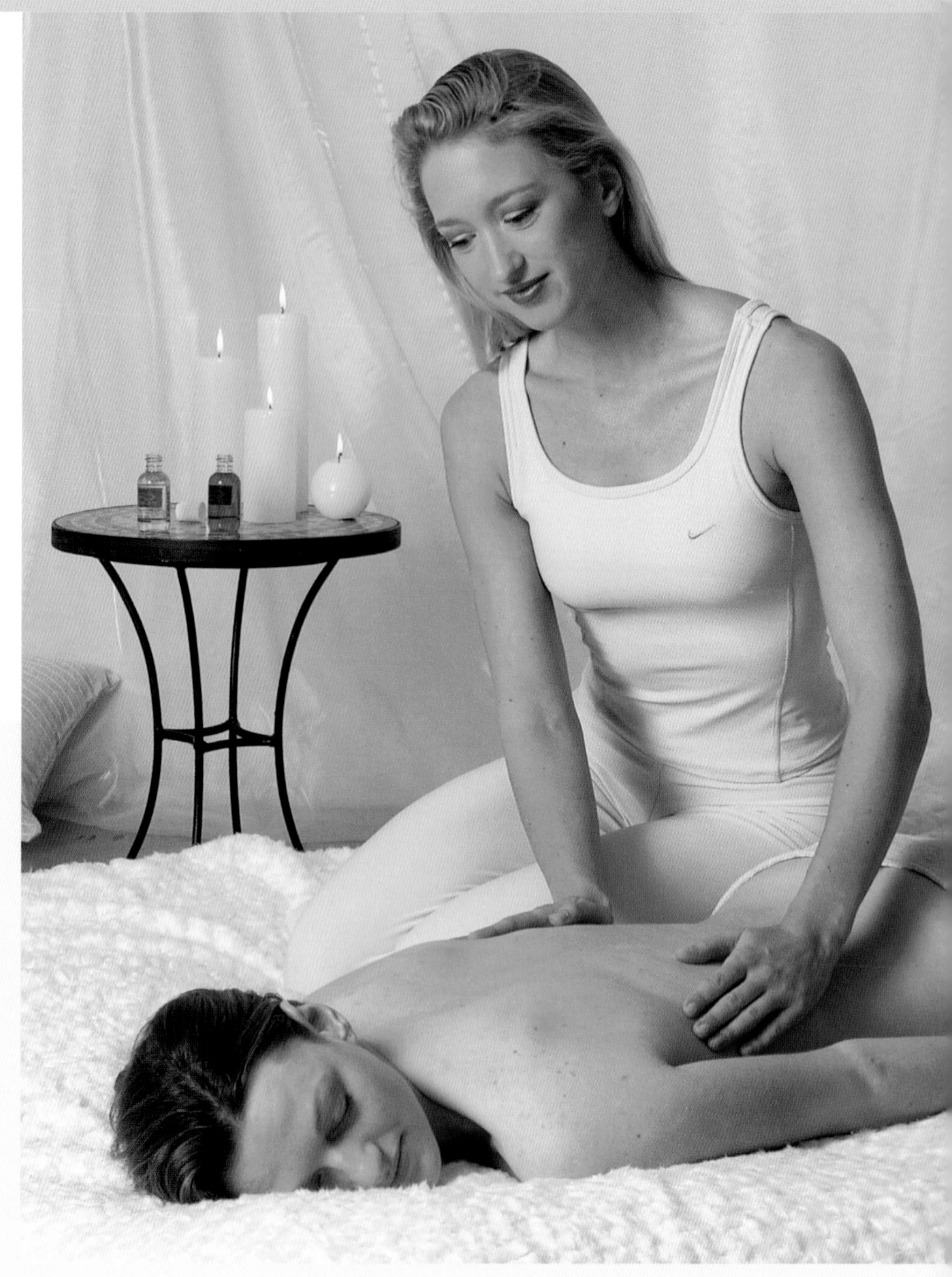

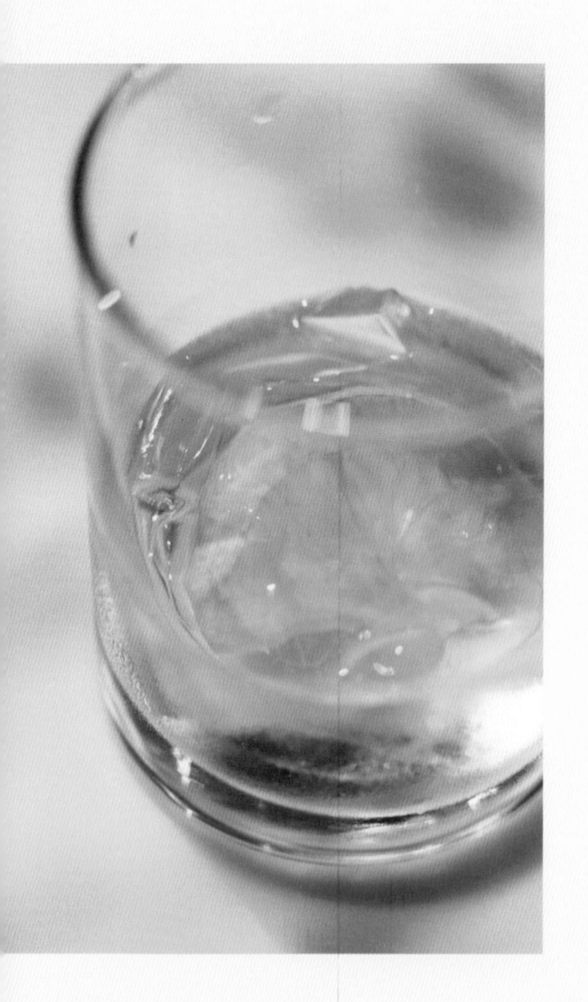

How does massage work?

Massage is designed to release muscle tension. Muscles naturally produce a toxin called lactic acid. When lactic acid builds up, muscles become tight and cellular processes slow down. When this happens, the speed at which cells absorb and remove fats, energy, oxygen and carbon dioxide is affected. Massage breaks down lactic acid build-up so muscles can function more efficiently. When lactic acid is broken down, it is released into the blood stream and is flushed out of the body through the urinary tract. Because massage releases this toxin into the blood stream, it is necessary to drink lots of water after receiving a massage. This will help to flush out the toxins and return the body to an optimum state of health.

The history of massage

The word massage has its roots in many different languages: in Latin massa means to touch or knead; in Greek massein means to knead; in Sanskrit makeh means to press; in Arabic mass means to feel or touch; and in French masser means to rub.

We can find evidence of the use of massage deeply rooted in Eastern practices. The Chinese are generally credited with creating the first form of massage in 3000 BCE. They used specific sequences for relaxation and health. In the sixth century, the Japanese started to manipulate energy within the body. This has developed into Shiatsu. Shiatsu uses pressure on specific points in the body to maintain optimum health. India, also, has a long history of massage as part of Ayurvedic medicine, which is still widely popular today.

In ancient Greece massage was integral to health. Hippocrates, a Greek physician and the 'father of medicine', called massage anatripsis. He wrote that massage can bind a joint that is too loose, and loosen a joint that is too rigid. In ancient Rome gladiators received massages before and after combat. Julius Caesar is said to have received daily massages to treat neuralgia. It is thought that he received pinching, an extreme form of massage, but massage none the less.

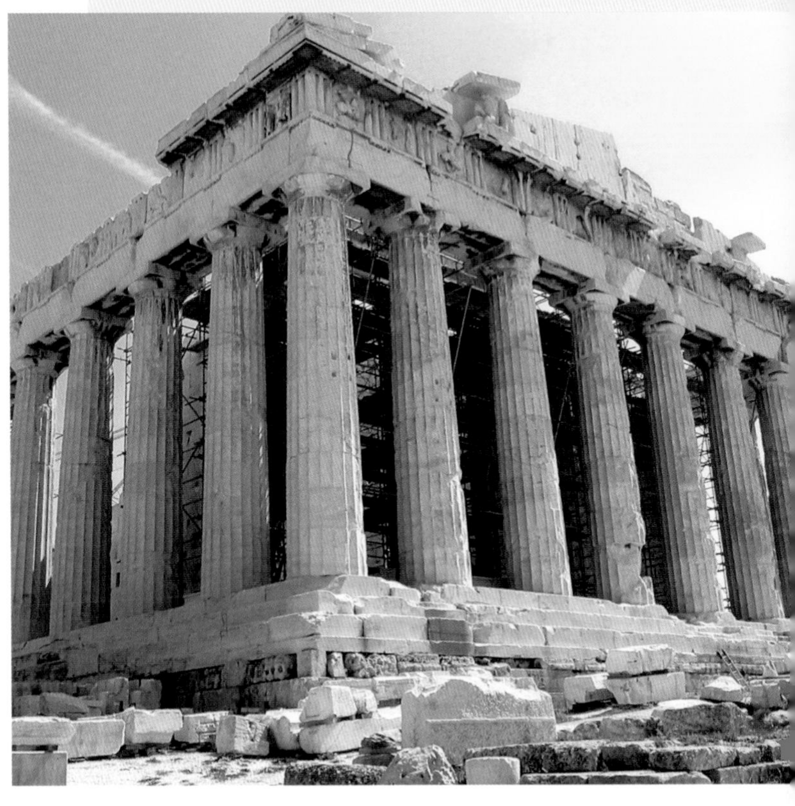

▲ Massage was important in Ancient Greek medicine.

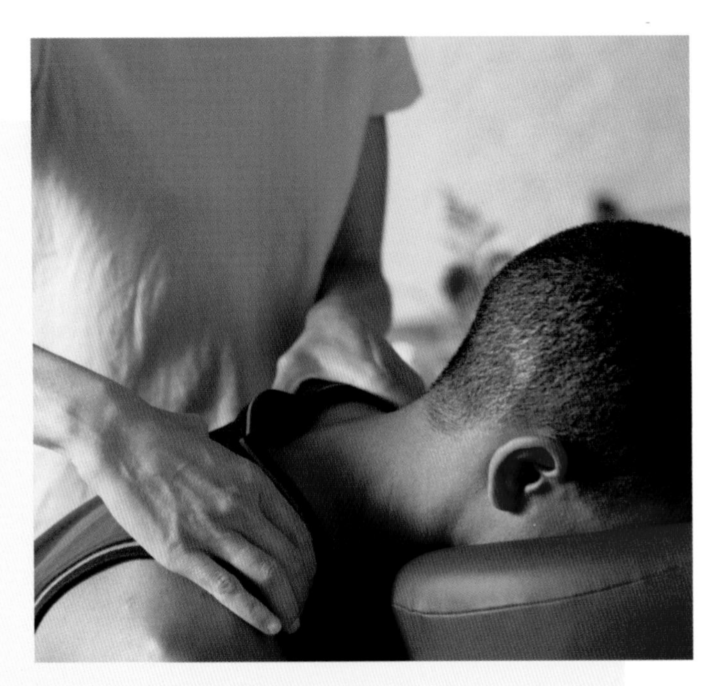

▲ Massage aids relaxation by releasing tension and stress.

Throughout the Middle Ages massage was repressed because it was believed that pleasures of the flesh were sinful. The most widely known form of massage practised in the West was begun by the Swedish doctor, poet and educator, Per Henrik Ling (1776–1839) in the 19th century. Ling originally studied divinity, and then went travelling. He returned to Sweden in 1804 and taught the arts. In 1805 he became fencing master at Lund University. In 1813 he established the Royal Gymnastics Central Institute, with massage as part of the curriculum. Ling believed in the body's natural ability to heal itself. He based his system on physiology, gymnastics and techniques borrowed from China, Egypt, Greece and Rome.

During World War II, patients suffering from nerve injury or shell shock were treated with massage. St Thomas's hospital in London had a department of massage until 1934, when electrical techniques began to be favoured over manual ones.

Massage lost credibility when the sex trade industry began to use it as a way to attract clients without gaining the attention of the authorities. Strict industry standards and licensing of practitioners has helped to raise the image of massage and promote its practice.

Anatomy

It is important to have a basic understanding of muscles and how they function in order to give a good massage. Spending a few moments learning where the main muscles are located will help you to visualise the reactions taking place beneath the skin. Also, if your partner has an injury it is important to know where the injury is located and if it is contraindicated or not.

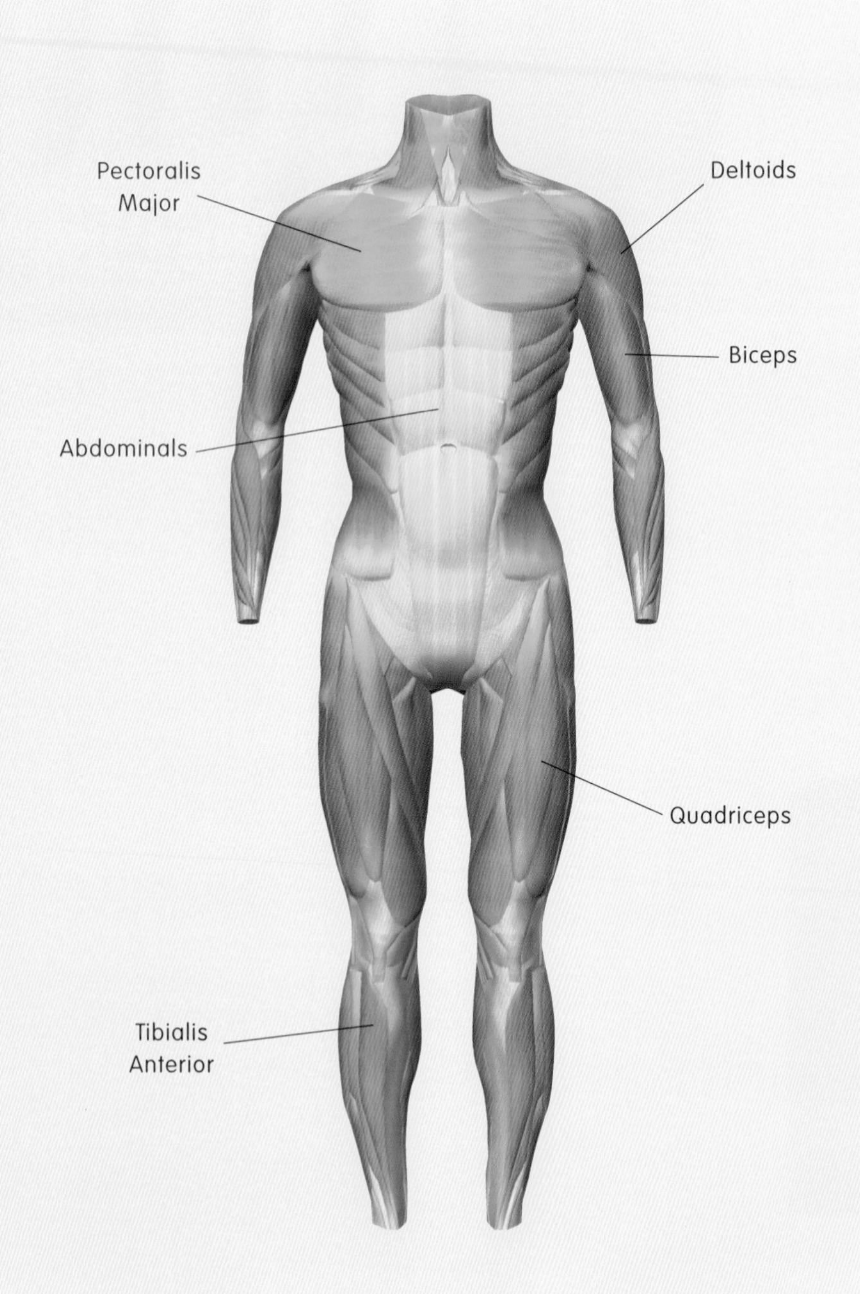

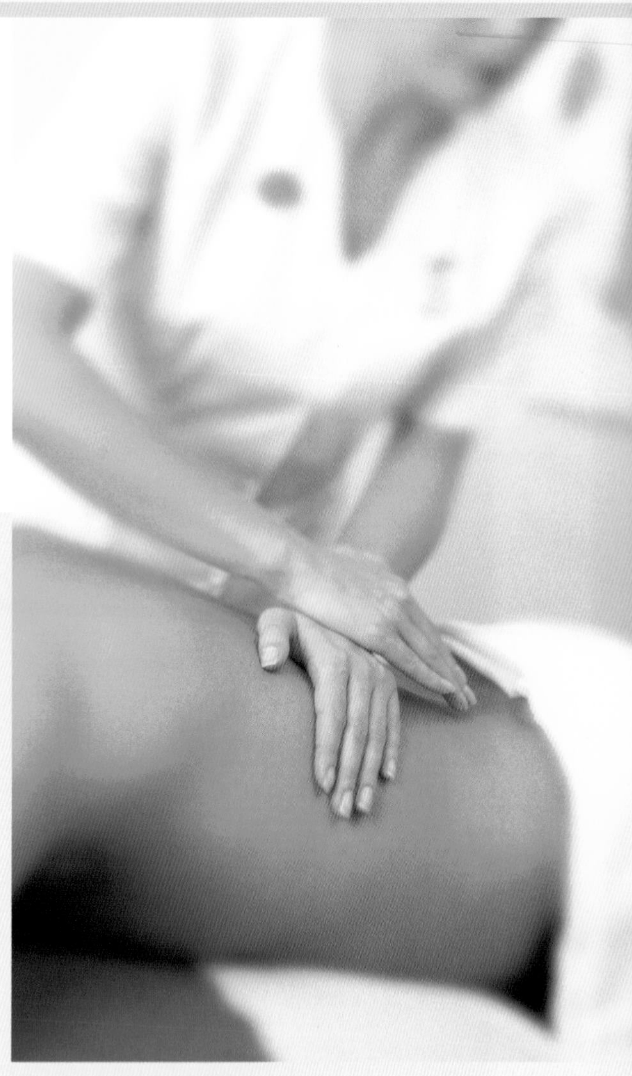

▲ Massage releases muscle tension. A good masseur will have a basic understanding of anatomy.

There are three types of muscle: cardiac, smooth and skeletal. Cardiac muscle is only found in the heart. Smooth muscle is involuntary, which means we do not have conscious control over it. It is found in organs like the stomach and walls of the intestines. Skeletal muscle is voluntary muscle and we do have conscious control over it. Voluntary muscle is found in places like the arms and legs. Voluntary muscle is surrounded by a thick fibrous material called fascia. Fascia becomes thicker at either end of a muscle and forms a tendon, which attaches to bone. In order to describe movement in the body, these tendons are called either origin or insertion. The origin is the tendon that attaches to the bone that does not move. The insertion is the tendon that attaches to the bone that is moving.

Muscles generally work in groups for efficient movement. The muscles that contract are called synergists. The muscles that work in opposition and relax to allow the other muscles to contract are called antagonists. Depending on the movement required, a muscle can act as either a synergist or an antagonist. For example, the quadriceps can flex the hip (synergist) while the hamstring relaxes (antagonist), or the hamstring can extend the hip (synergist) while the quadriceps relaxes (antagonist).

Muscle consists of bundles of fibres. These fibres overlap and are called actin and myosin. Muscle contraction takes place when actin and myosin slide across each other to contract the muscle. To visualise this action, lace the fingers of your hands together so that the fingers barely cross in front of you. This is what the fibres in the muscles look like at rest. Then, slowly slide the fingers together so that there are no spaces between your fingers. This is what the actin and myosin look like when they are contracted.

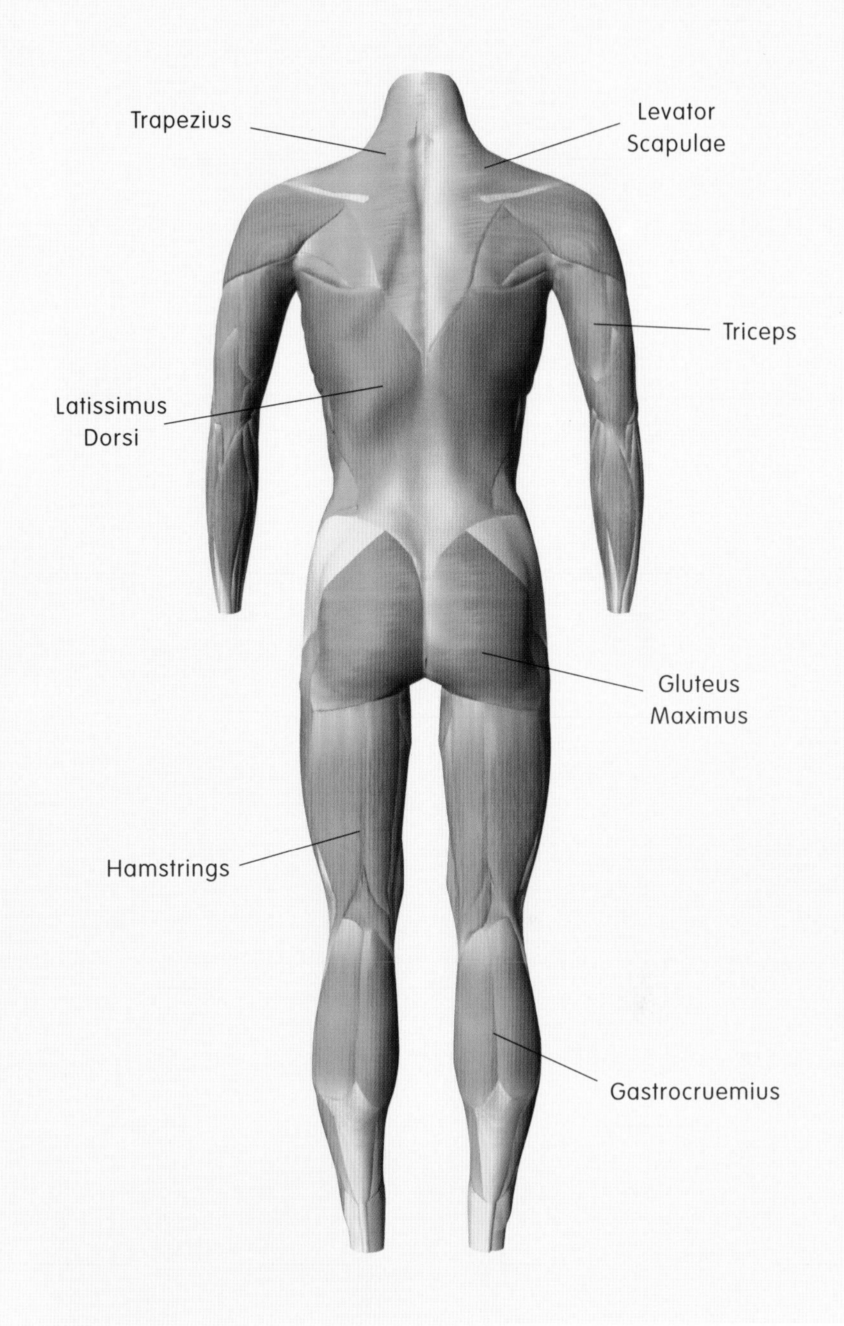

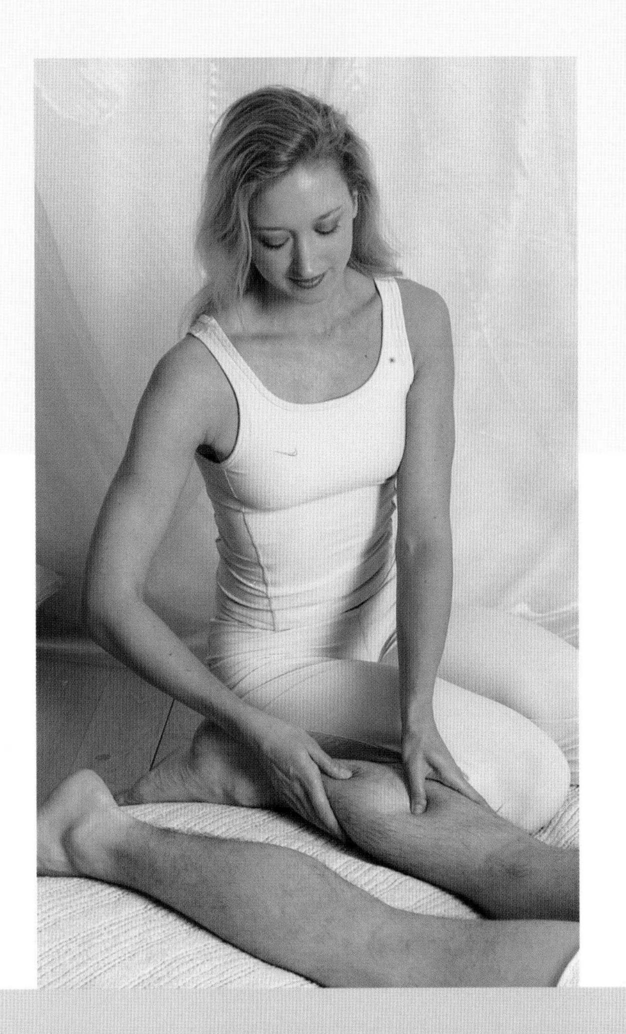

In order for muscles to function efficiently, they must have enough oxygen and nutrients. Cells in the muscle fibres produce waste, in the form of carbon dioxide, lactic acid and urea that must be expelled in order for muscles to function smoothly. A small amount of lactic acid in the muscle is completely normal. But when lactic acid builds up, muscles feel tense and knotted. The strokes in massage are designed to break up the lactic acid and release it into the blood stream so that the muscles can function more effectively.

◀ By working deeply into the belly of a muscle, massage can release lactic acid build-up to make the muscle function more efficiently.

The effects of massage

Massage affects us both psychologically and physiologically. Psychologically, it relaxes the mind and body and increases positive, happy feelings. Physiologically, it has a direct or indirect effect on all the systems of the body.

The most obvious effect massage has is on our skin. The skin is a living organ; its dead cells rise to the surface and are constantly being replaced by new cells underneath. This process is known as desquamation. Sliding the hands across the skin during massage removes dead skin cells, helping new cells rise to the surface. This process also brings blood to the surface, increasing colour and improving circulation. Massage also improves elasticity in skin by encouraging the natural production of oil called sebum, which helps to lubricate the skin and prevent dryness.

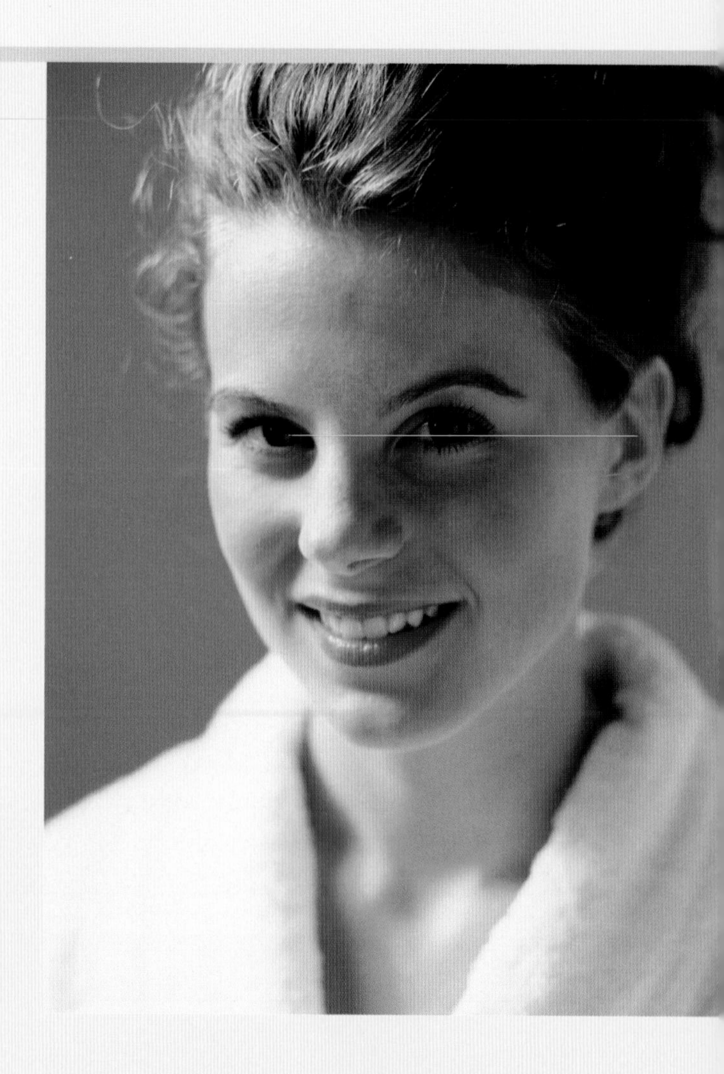

Massage affects the muscular system in many ways: it breaks down sections of lactic acid, thus increasing the speed of cell functions; it alleviates pain in muscles by breaking down the knots that cause stiffness; and it improves flexibility and range of movement.

Massage improves the circulatory system by aiding the flow of blood around the body. Massage strokes work in harmony with the body's natural circulation. Massage helps blood to carry oxygen and nutrients to the organs, and waste and carbon dioxide away. Massage can help lower high blood pressure by reducing the tension that causes it.

The lymphatic system removes waste products that cannot be removed through the circulatory system. It is an interesting system because it has no pump to circulate the lymph. Massage is extremely beneficial in helping the lymph to circulate around the body. Because massage works in harmony with the direction in which blood flows around the body, it is able to push the lymph towards the lymph nodes, aiding drainage. Massage can also help in the reduction of swelling, cellulite and lumpiness.

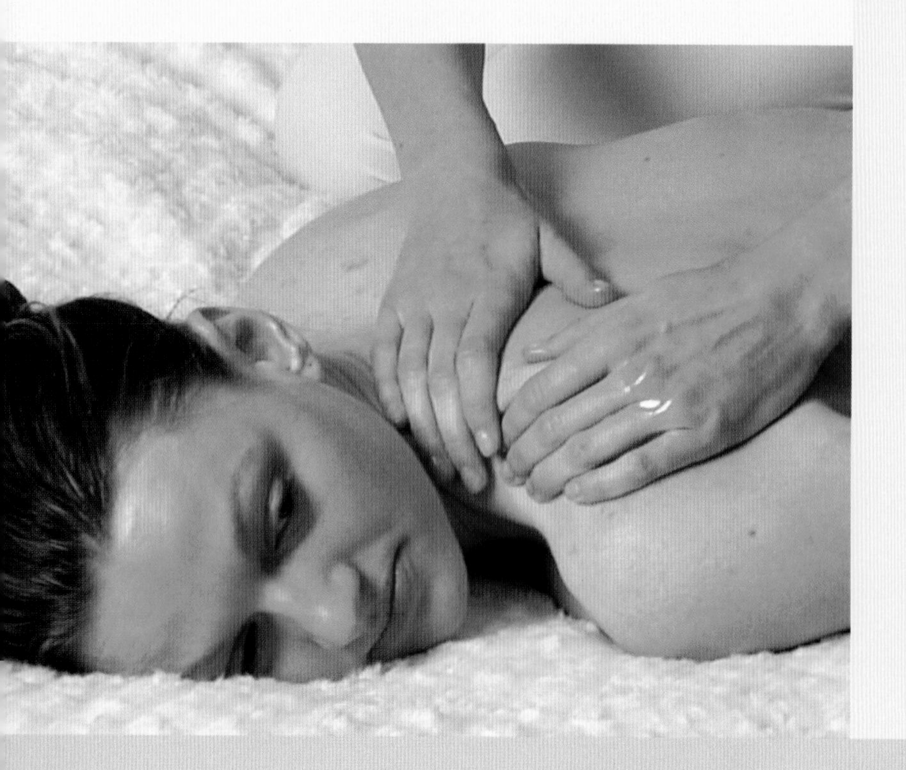

◄ Massage has a beneficial effect on all the systems of the body.

Massage has a positive effect on the respiratory system. When we are relaxed, we can breathe more easily and deeply. Oxygen can be absorbed and carbon dioxide removed in greater volumes. The main muscles involved in respiration, the diaphragm and intercostal muscles, are relaxed in a massage, enabling deeper breathing.

Massage affects the urinary system by encouraging waste removal. It activates the kidneys and reduces fluid retention.

The reproductive system can be affected by massage in that it can reduce period pains.

The effects on the nervous system will depend on the type of massage. A stimulating massage will invigorate the nervous system, while a relaxing massage will calm it down. A stimulating massage can also reduce fatigue and lethargy. Soothing strokes can help ease the nerves of someone who is stressed or tense.

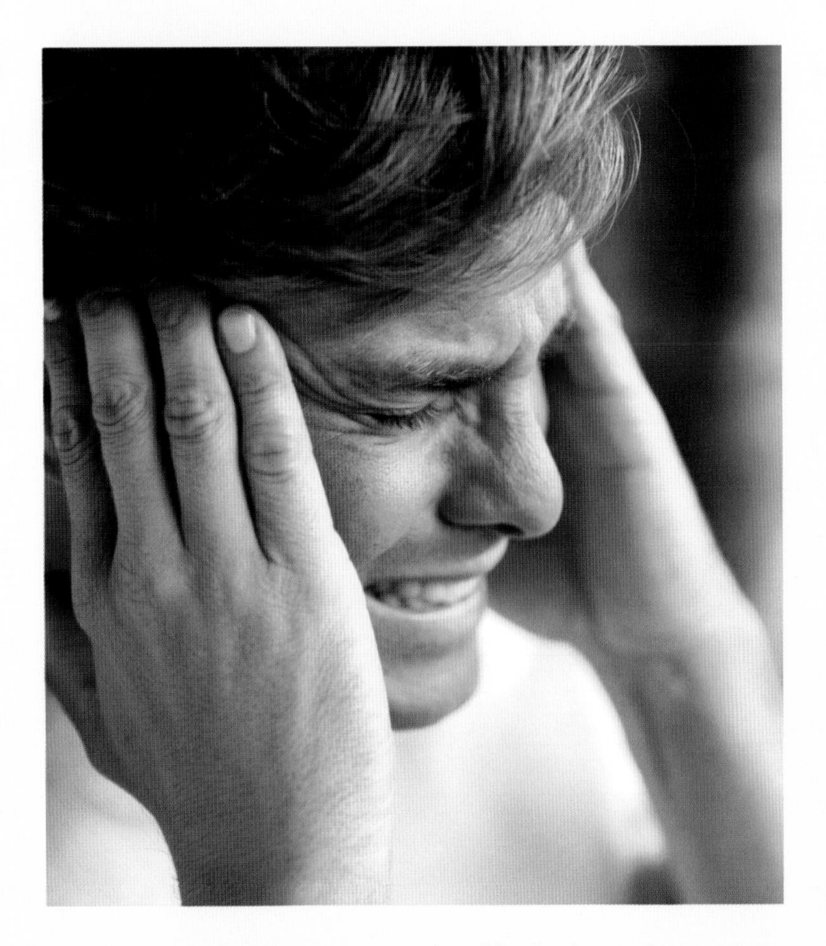

▲ Massage aids relaxation in mind and body, thus reducing stress.

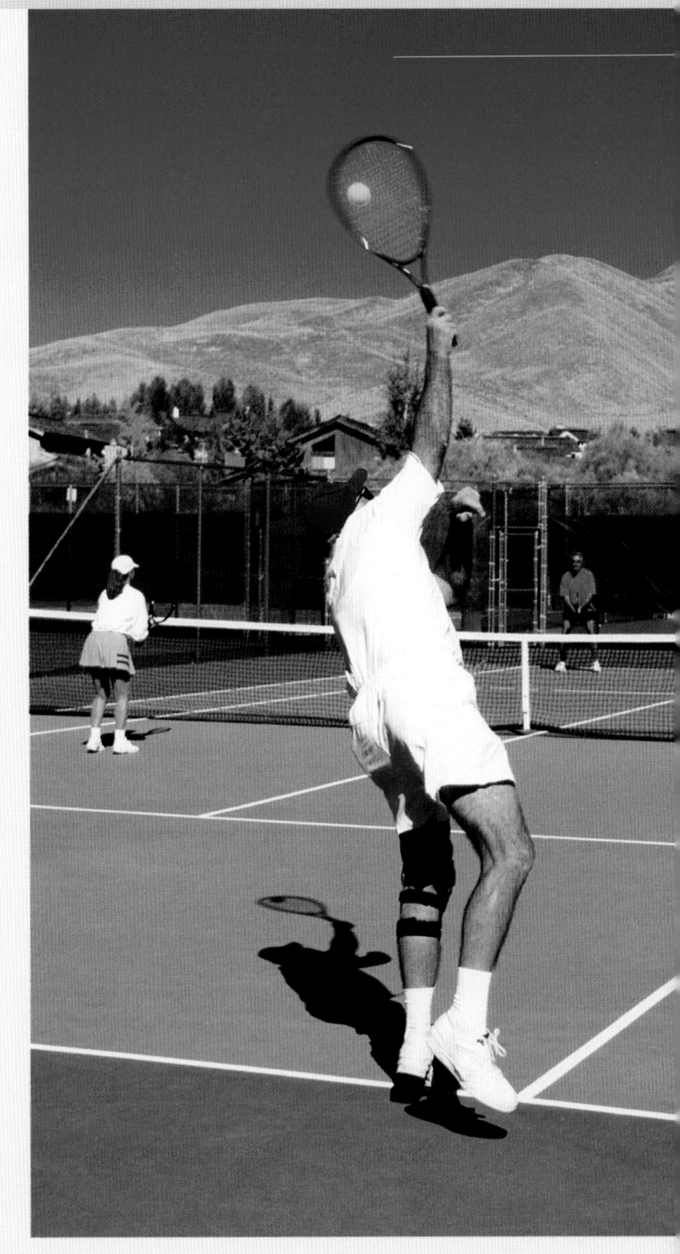

▲ Massage increases the range of motion by alleviating tension in joints.

The skeletal system is affected indirectly. Because the muscles are more relaxed, they cause less undue strain on the bones and joints. Mobility can increase with massage and posture may improve. Massage can relax tight muscles and strengthen loose tissue, thus changing the tensions created on the skeletal system.

Massage affects digestion by helping with both indigestion and constipation. Because massage improves circulation, it speeds up nutrients getting to the cells.

Contraindications

Massage is one of the safest forms of holistic therapy. However, there are certain instances when one should be cautious, or not massage at all. This list should be used as a general guideline. If in doubt, always consult a doctor.

Illnesses

It is common sense not to massage a person who is sick. Not only could they be contagious, but you could spread the infection around their body. This works both ways! If you are feeling ill, you can easily contaminate the person you are working on. Never massage a person when you are under the weather. When dealing with cancer or serious illness, always consult a doctor. If your partner has cancer, never massage directly over the tumour. Massage can be very beneficial for cancer patients, but make sure you do not work directly on the area affected.

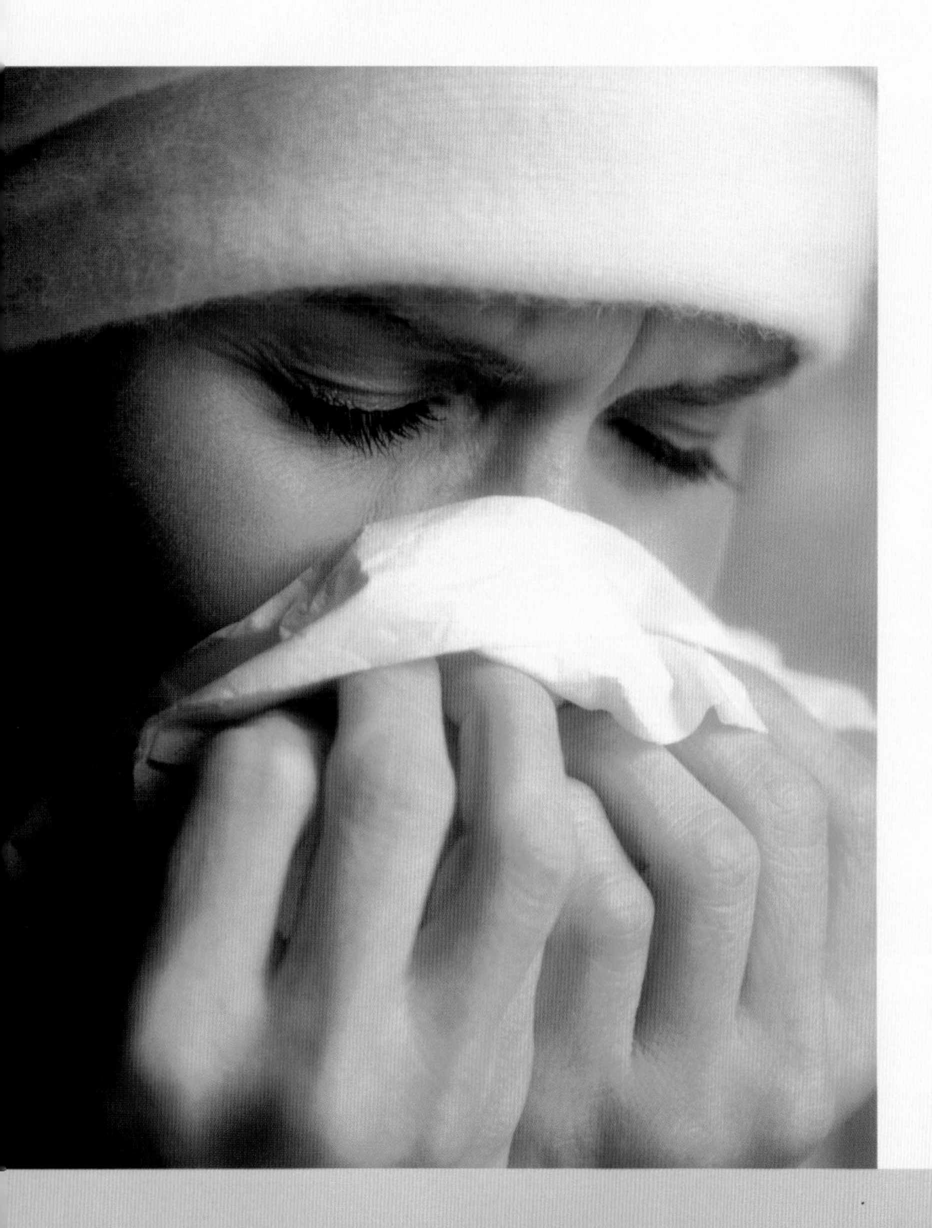

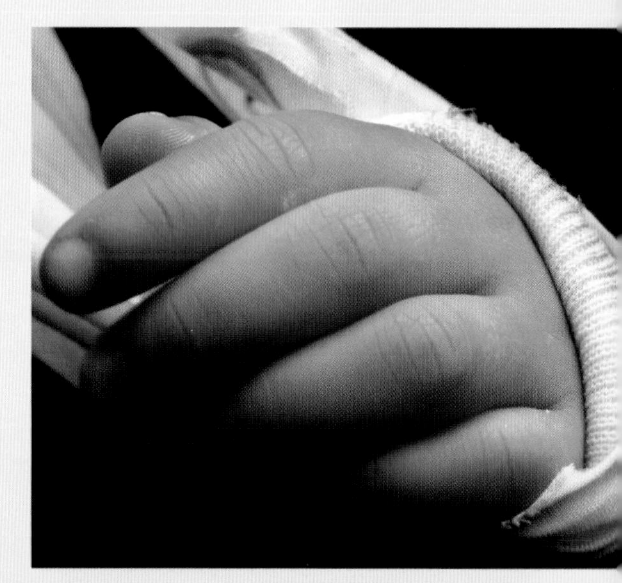

▲ A broken arm would be a localised contraindictation. Massage the rest of the body but avoid the injury.

Injuries

Recent injuries are a local contraindication. This means that you can massage everywhere on the body except over the injury. Never massage on swellings, open cuts, abrasions, bruises or broken bones.

Varicose veins

Do not massage directly on varicose veins as this can put pressure on already fragile veins and cause more damage. Lightly stroke the veins going upwards towards the heart. This is very calming and relaxing without causing damage. Also, never massage below varicose veins. For example, if you find varicose veins on the back of the knee, do not massage the calf. This can put added pressure on the veins, causing more damage than good.

◀ If either you or your partner are under the weather, it is better not to massage.

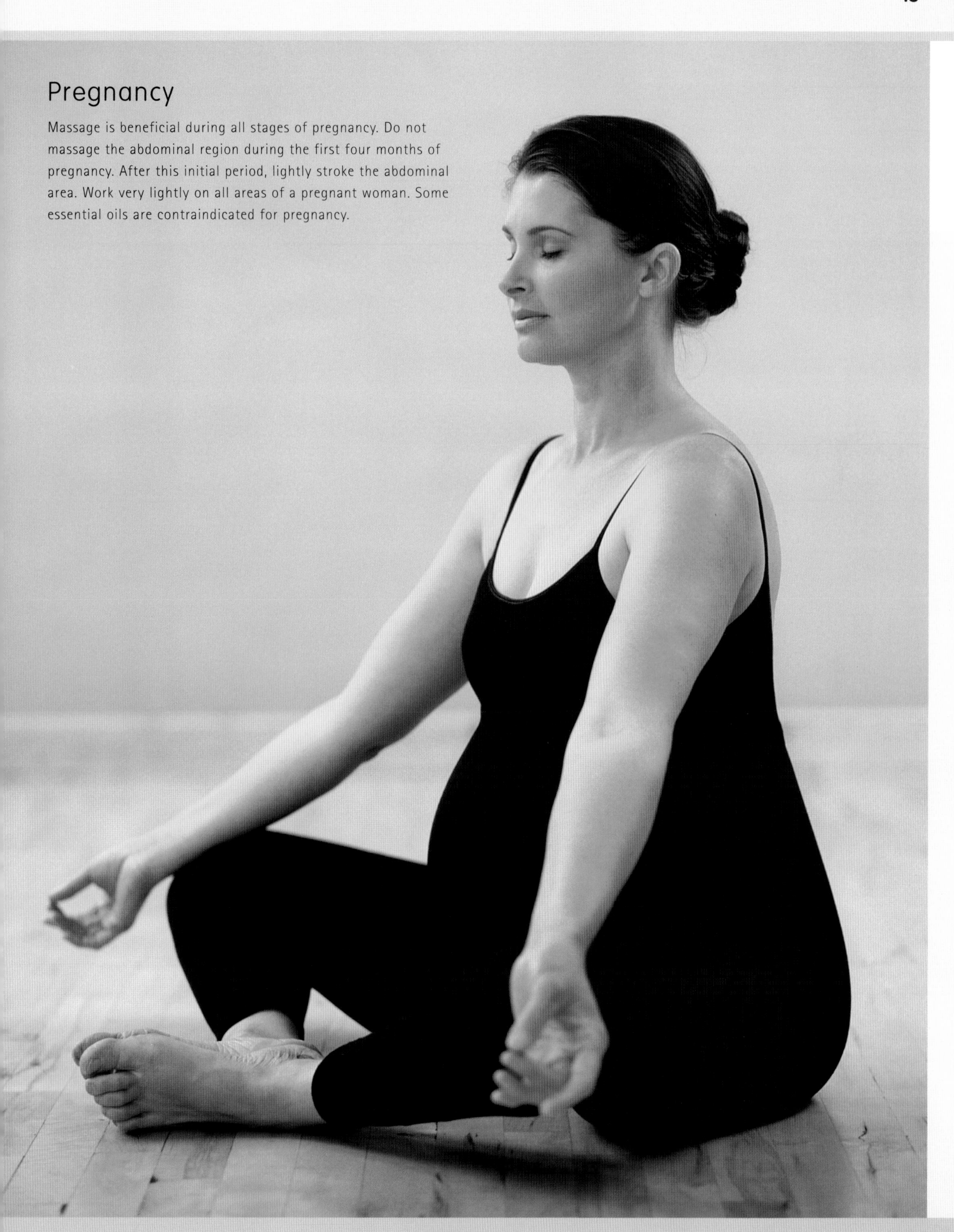

Pregnancy

Massage is beneficial during all stages of pregnancy. Do not massage the abdominal region during the first four months of pregnancy. After this initial period, lightly stroke the abdominal area. Work very lightly on all areas of a pregnant woman. Some essential oils are contraindicated for pregnancy.

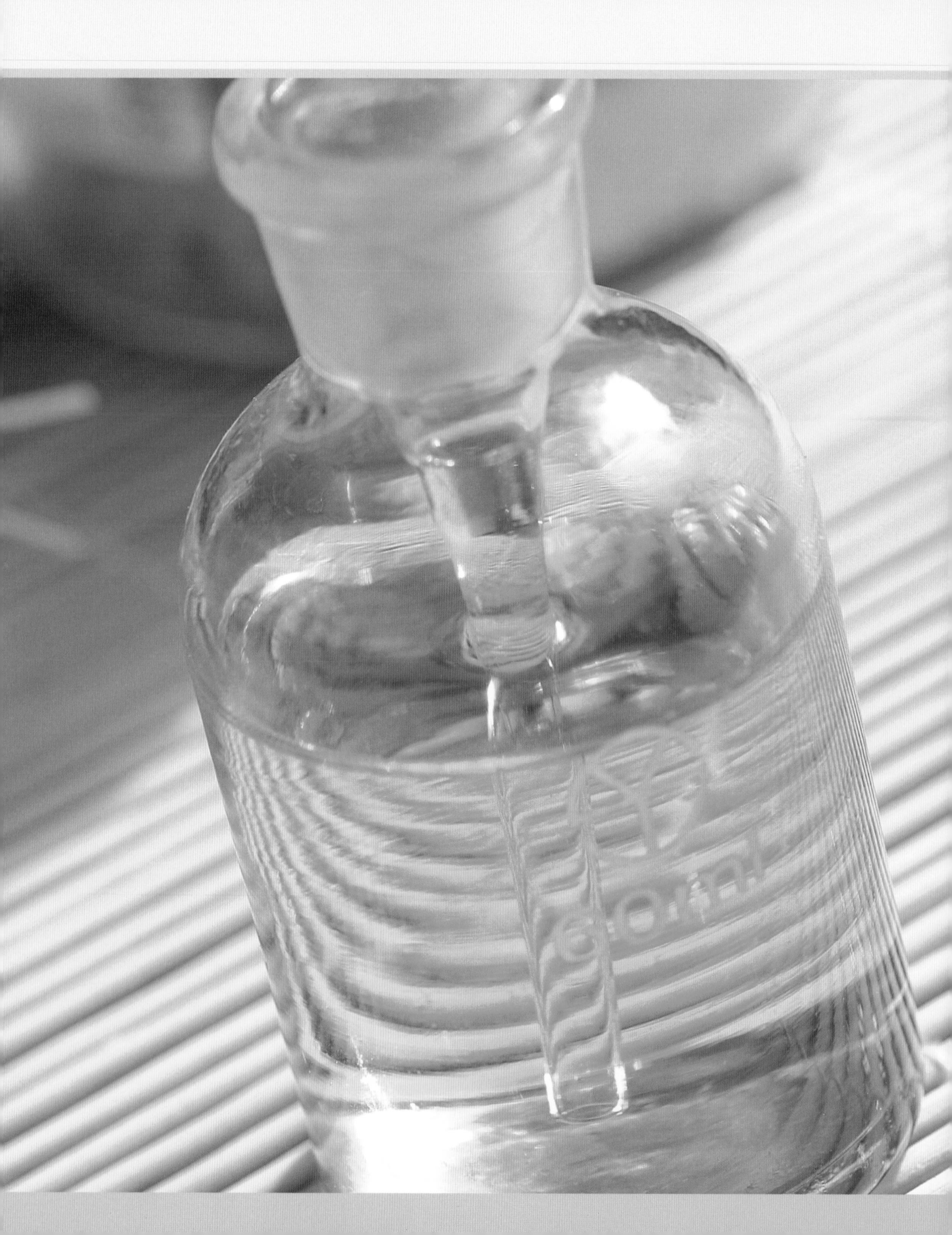

Massage mediums

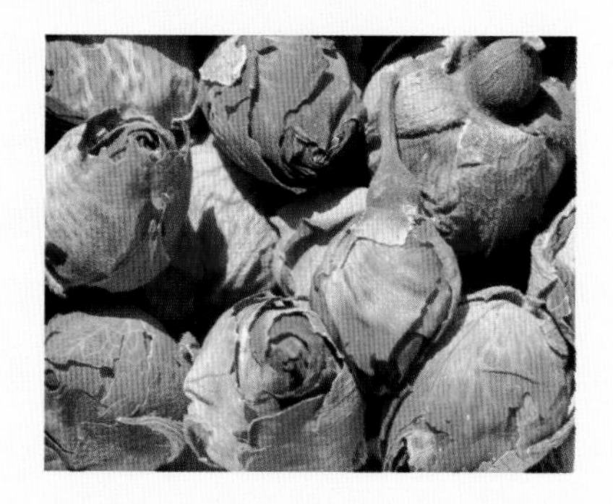

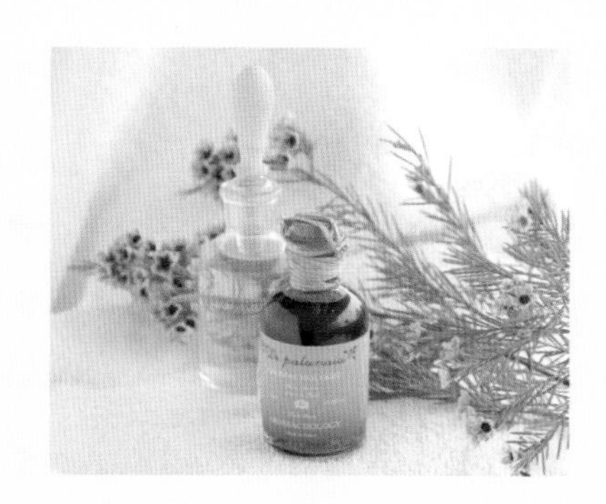

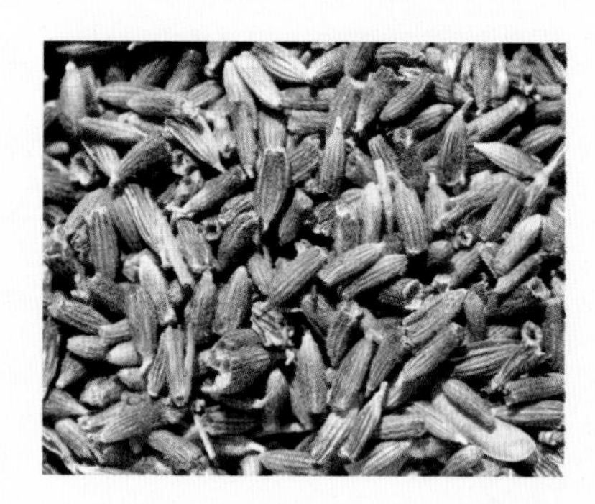

The most common massage medium used is oil. Lotion and talc may also be used, but I find they are not as effective. Oil is a great lubricant that enables the hands to glide along the skin without getting stuck, pulling, stretching or causing friction. All you really need for a massage is a small bottle of your favourite oil! There are many types of oils, however, so choosing one can seem daunting. Start off with a few that seem interesting to you; you can always add to your collection later.

About oils

Buying essential oils can be an overwhelming experience as the choice is extremely wide. Read through this section first so that you have an idea of what you want. It is probably best to start out with one or two base oils and three or four essential oils. This is a small investment and will give you plenty of opportunity to mix and match them to create a blend that is right for you.

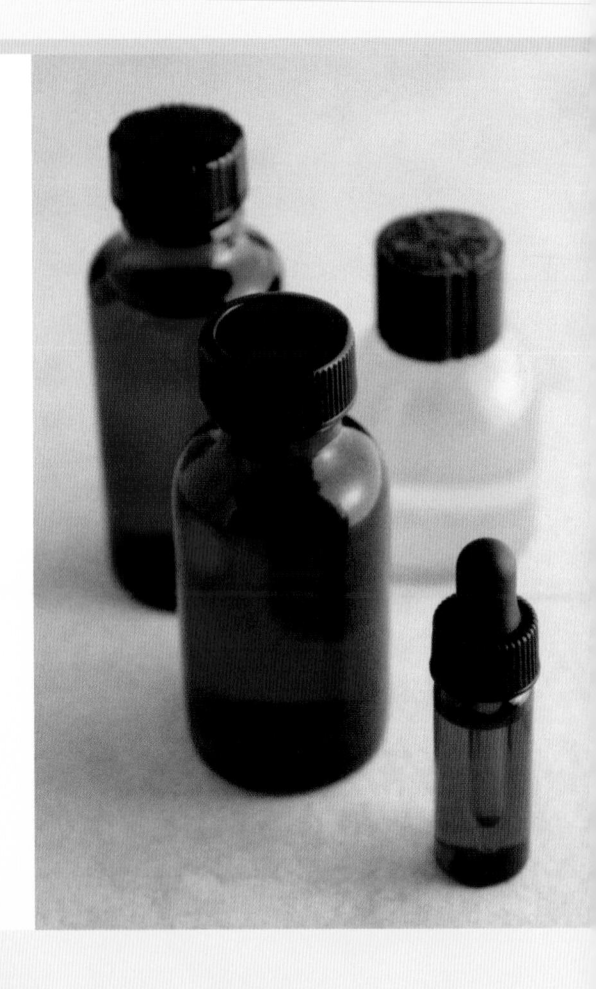

A base, or carrier oil is generally made from a vegetable, a seed or a nut. Always try to choose oil that is cold-pressed, unrefined or additive-free; the more processed the oil, the less effective it is.

I find sweet almond oil or grapeseed oil best for a whole body massage because they are light and excellent lubricants. You can add other base oils to these for their beneficial qualities. For example, 5–10% wheatgerm can be added to any blend to help preserve it, or try adding 5–10% avocado oil for its high nutrient quality.

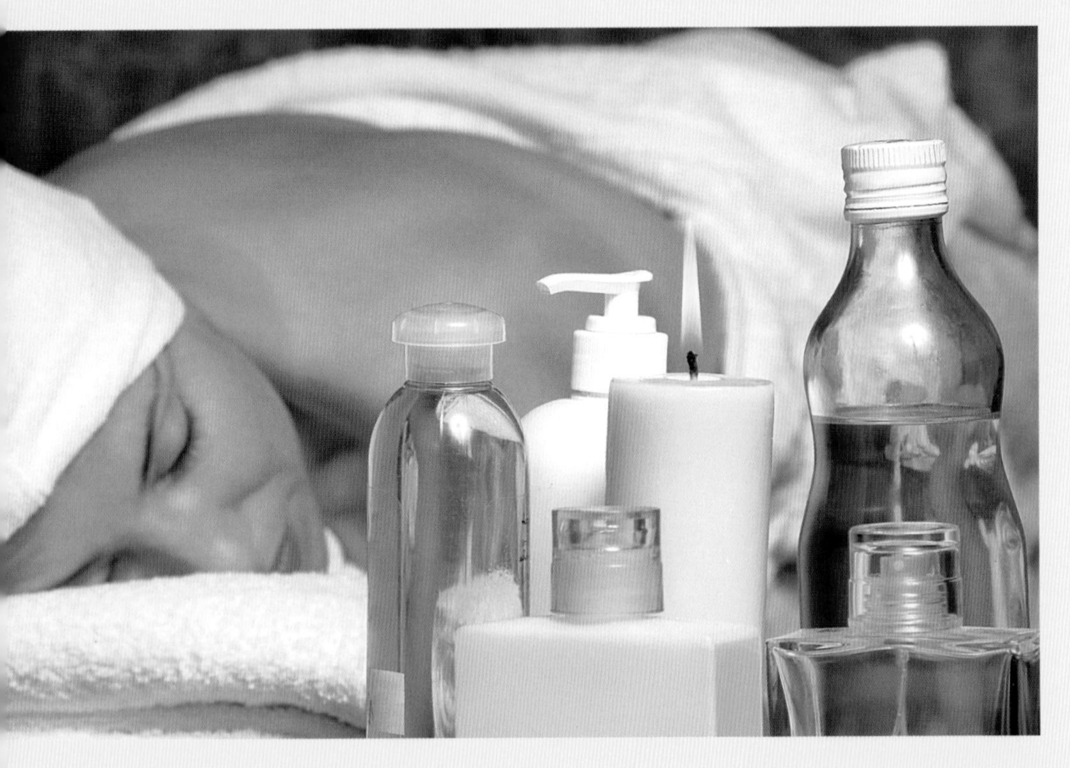

All base oils can act as a carrier for essential oils. Essential oils are not necessary for massage, but can enhance its quality.

Aromatherapy is the use of essential oils to bring the body back into harmony. Essential oil contain the essence, its life force, the quality and spirit of the plant that they are extracted from. The properties of the plants are extracted by various methods, and can affect the body's physical, mental and emotional states. Essential oils should never be ingested, and as a rule of thumb, always dilute them before they come into contact with the skin.

The pages that follow contain a list and description of base and essential oils that can be both fun and effective to use in a massage. Always check for allergies before using any oil on a person – dab a little on the inside of the elbow. Nut and wheat allergies are quite common and will affect your choice.

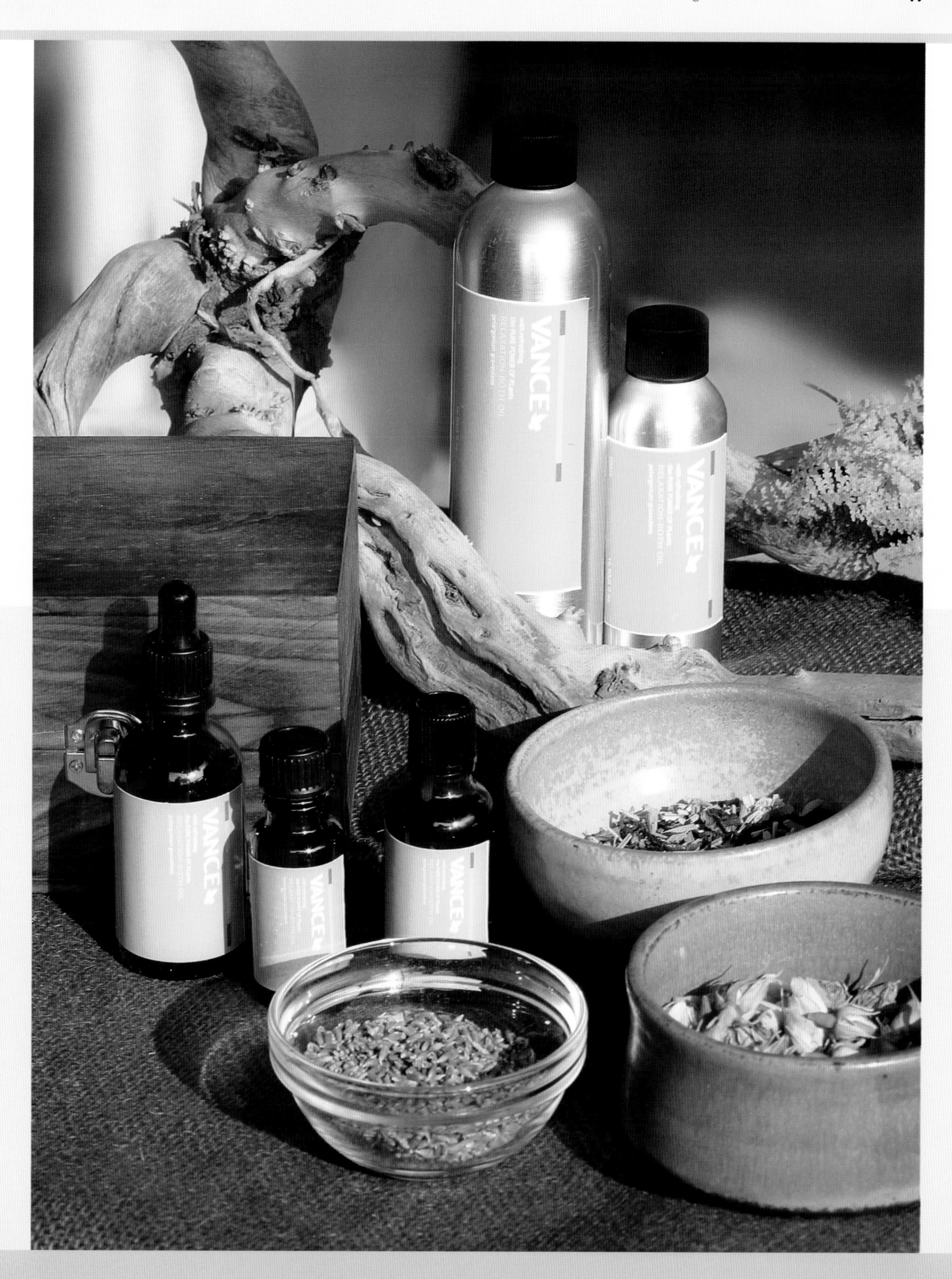
VANCE

Base (carrier) oils

▶ Calendula officinalis (Calendula)

This infused oil is used as an anti-inflammatory and for healing. It is excellent for skin problems such as eczema, bruises, rashes, sunburn and chapped, cracked skin. Add 5–10% to base oil.

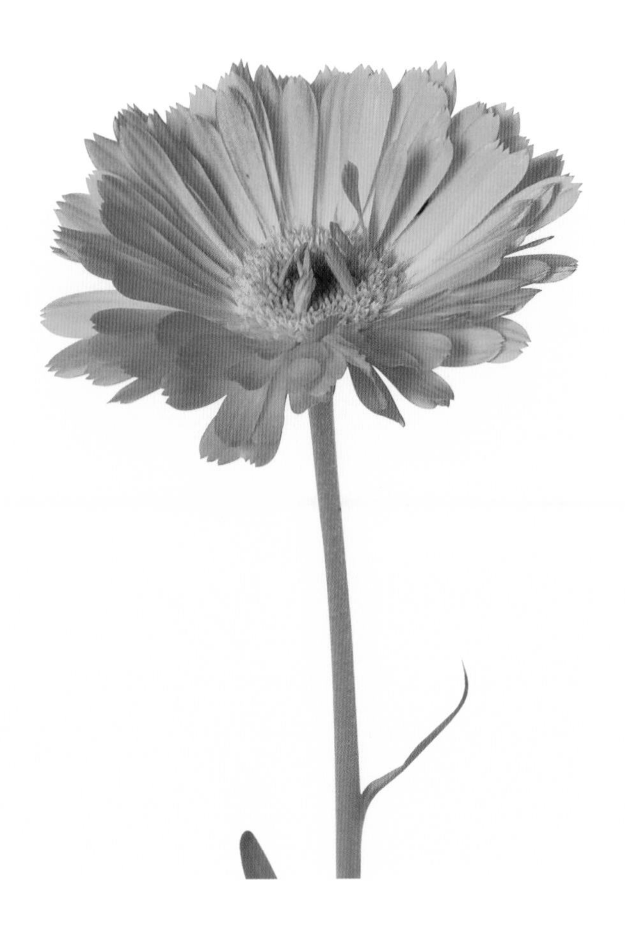

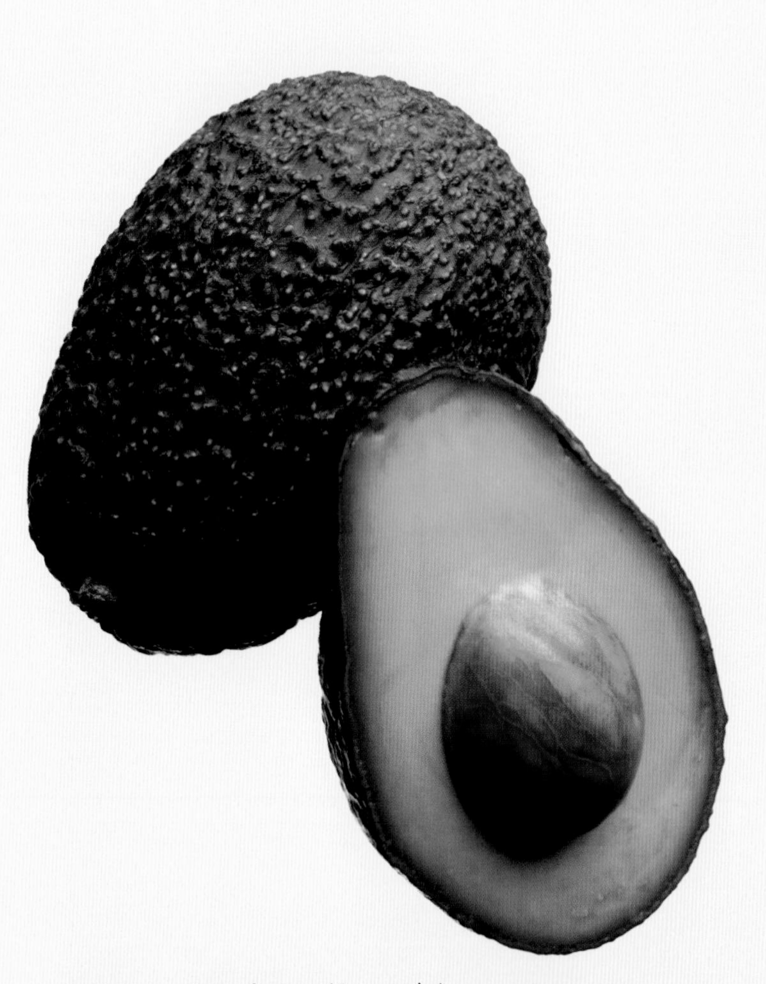

▲ Prunus Americana (Avocado)

This highly penetrative oil has a high vitamin content of A, B and D. Because of its rich, thick and sticky nature, only a tiny amount should be added to carrier oil. This easily absorbable oil contains a strong odour. It is good for dry, dehydrated or wrinkled skin.

▼ Macadamia integrifolia (Macadamia)

This oil is made from the macadamia nut. It is good for both oily and dry, wrinkled skin.

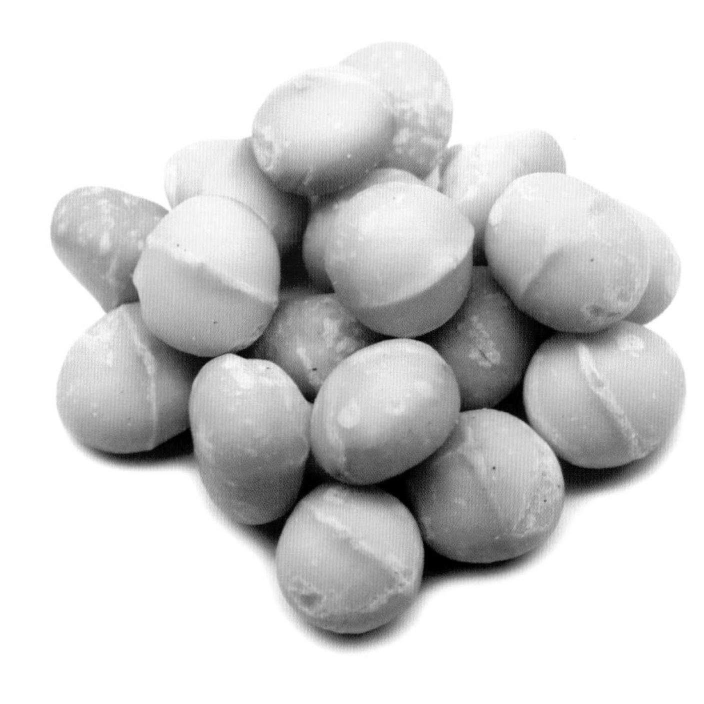

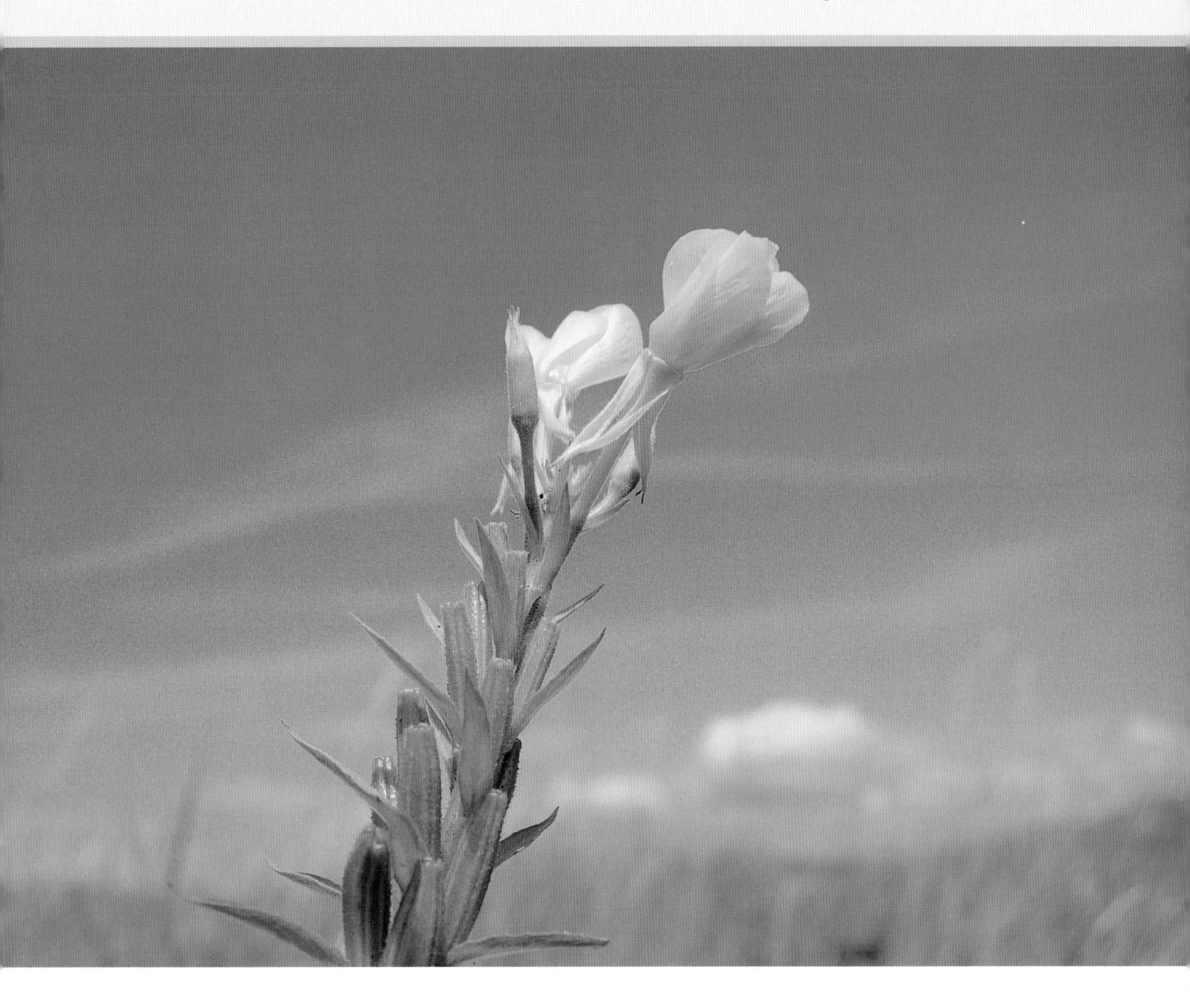

▲ Oenorthera biennis (Evening primrose)

This expensive oil is great for treating dry skin conditions such as eczema and dandruff. It also affects PMT, MS, heart disease and psoriasis. Add 5–10% to base oil.

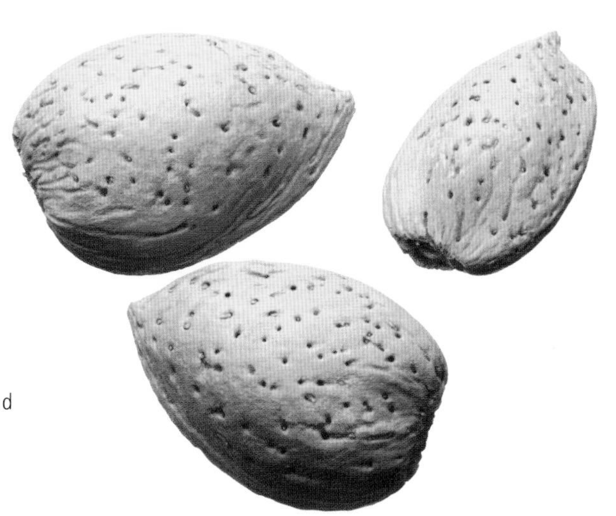

► Prunus amygdalis (Sweet almond)

This nourishing, light oil comes from the sweet almond nut. It is the most popular base oil because it is good for all skin types, and is inexpensive. It contains vitamins A, B1, B2 and B6, and can be used on its own or in a blend for a whole body massage.

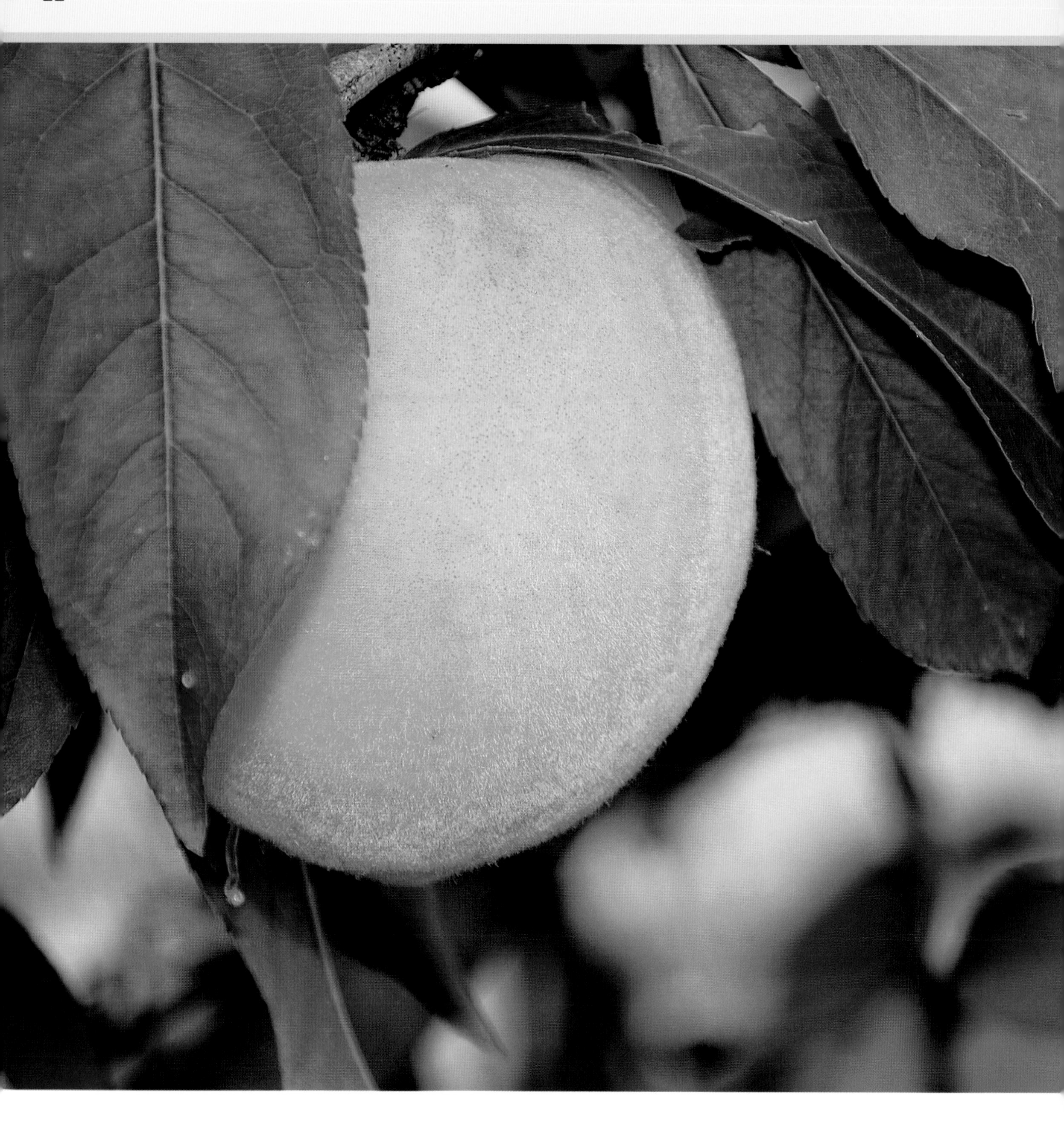

▲ **Prunus persica** (Peach kernel)

This light, rich oil is made from peach stones. It is good for all skin types, especially sensitive, dry and mature skin. It is also good for the face and contains vitamins A, B1, B2 and B6. It is expensive but can be used on its own or in a blend.

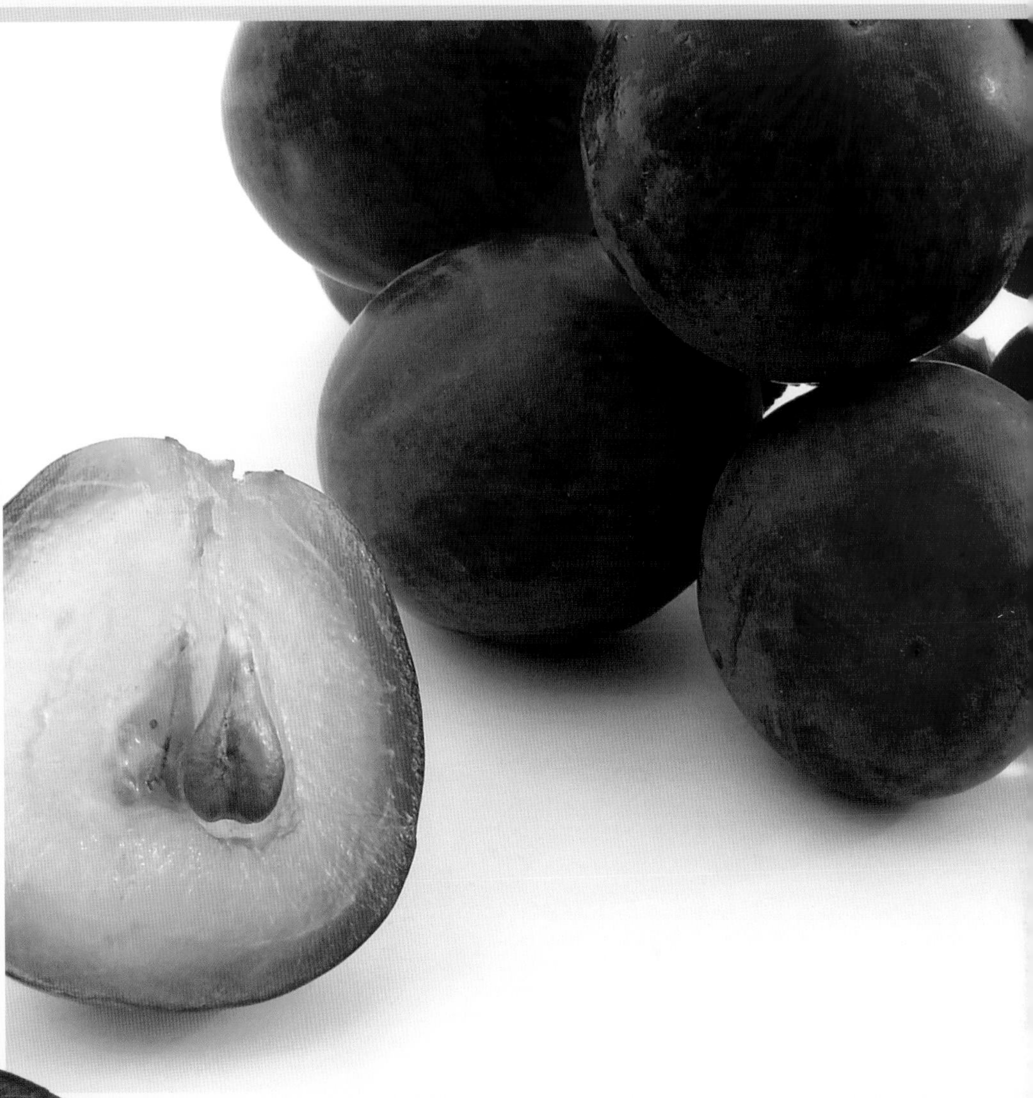

Triticum vulgare
(Wheatgerm)

This vitamin-rich oil is good for reducing scar tissue and stretch marks. It contains vitamin E and is good for dry skin. Adding 5–10% wheatgerm to any blend will preserve it. Because the oil is thick and sticky, it is not recommended for use on its own. Do not use it if you have a wheat allergy.

▼ Prunus armenica
(Apricot kernel)

This light oil is excellent for the face. It is used for all skin types and treats dry, sensitive, inflamed and mature skin. It can be used on its own or in a blend.

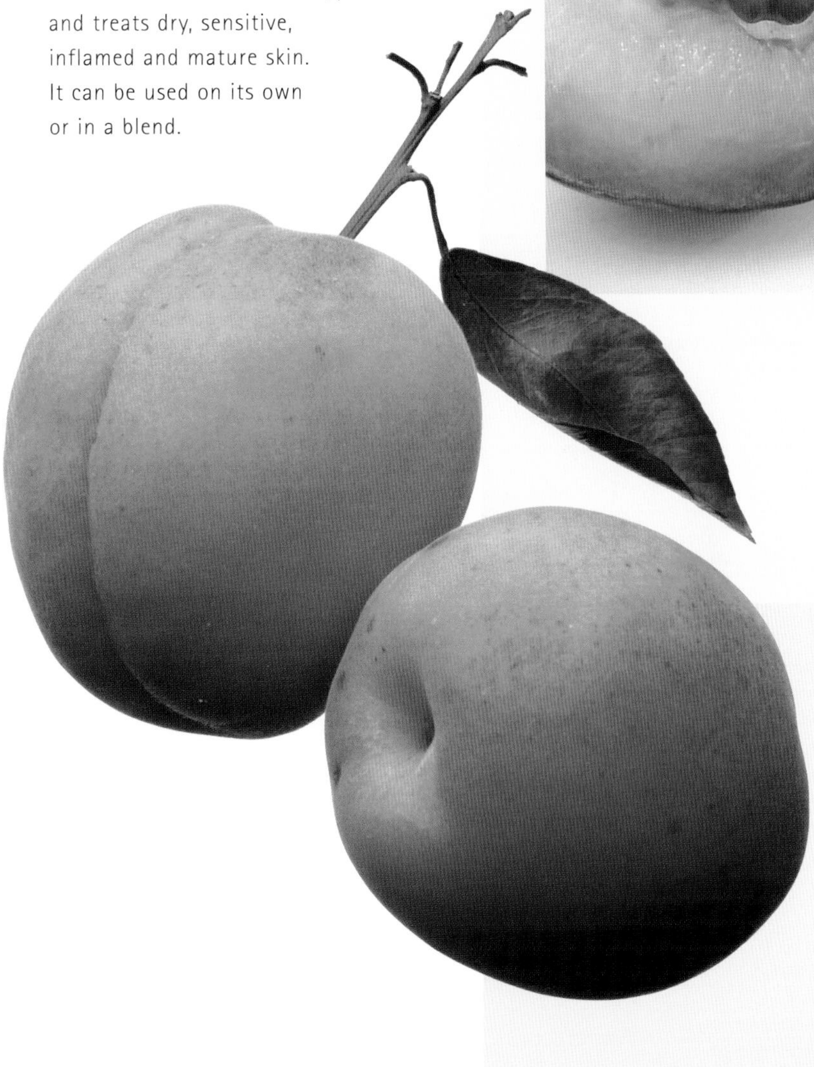

▲ Vitis vinifera (Grapeseed)

This smooth, light oil is also inexpensive and made from the seeds of grapes. It contains vitamin E, and is almost odourless. This oil is good for a full body massage and can be used alone or in a blend.

Simmondsia chinensis (Jojoba)

This oil is actually a liquid vegetable wax. Its smooth, rich texture is good for all skin types. Because the chemical structure is similar to that of the skin's natural sebum, it is excellent for massaging the face. It can be used on its own, but is usually blended because it is expensive.

Essential oils

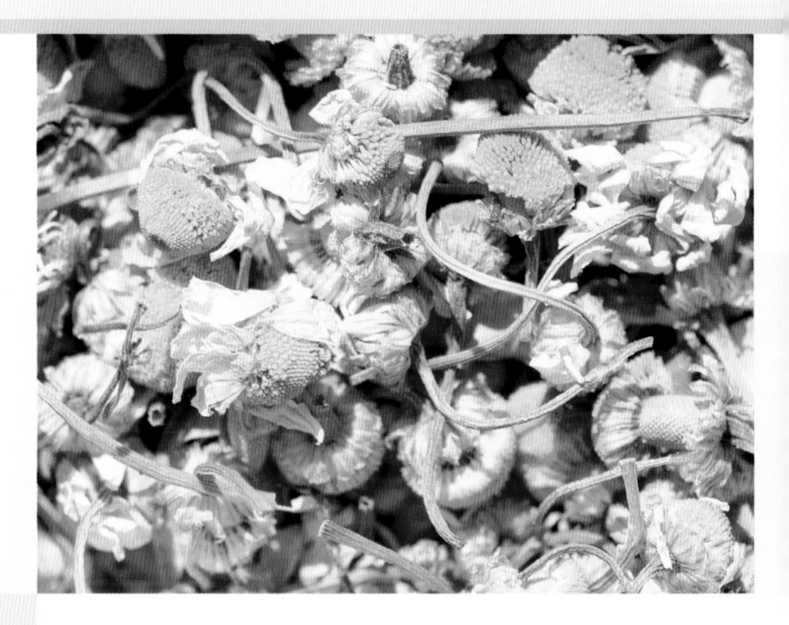

▶ **Anthemis nobilis** (Camomile)

Camomile is calming and good for all age groups: children, the frail and the elderly all react well to it. It aids teeth problems, period pains, indigestion, nausea, stress and depression. It helps many skin conditions, such as eczema, psoriasis, ulcers, bruises and acne. Do not take it while pregnant.

▶ **Salvia sclarea** (Clary sage)

Clary sage is a euphoric, relaxing tonic. It balances the hormones and eases fluid retention and painful cramping. It reduces inflammation, spasms and muscle fatigue. It is also good for depression and menstruation problems. Do not use during pregnancy, or before or after drinking alcohol.

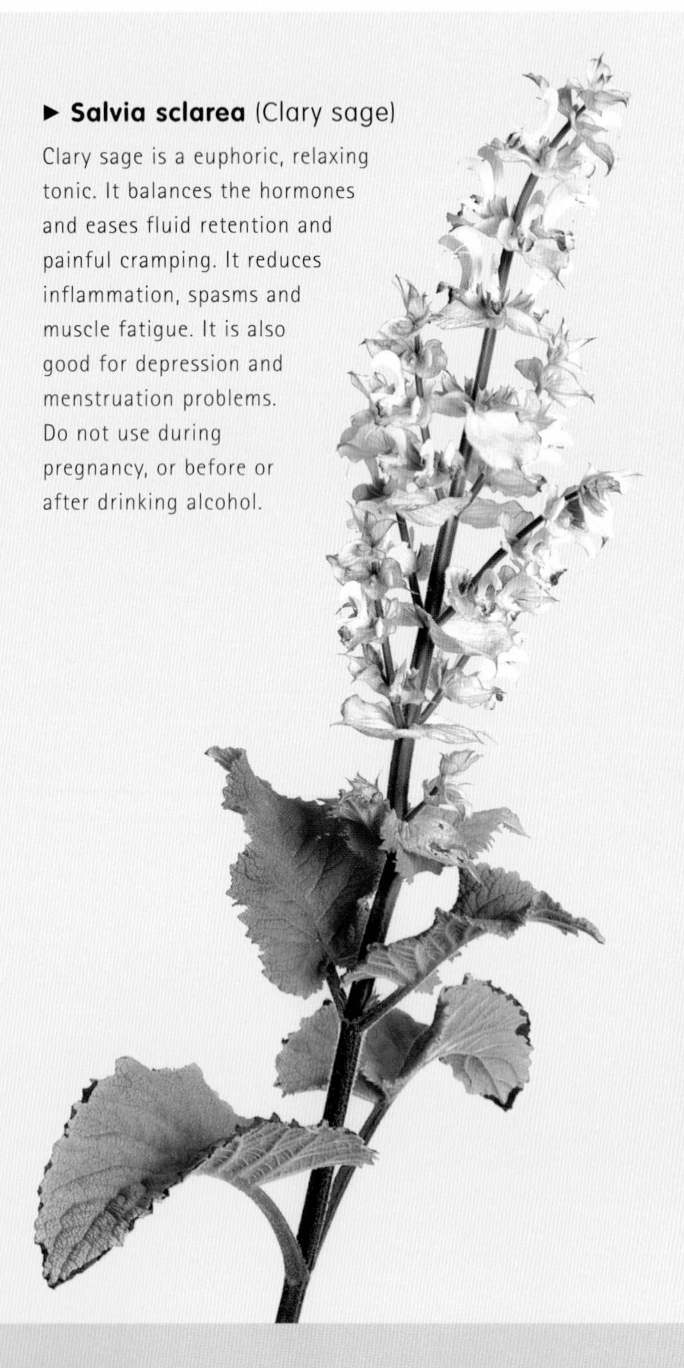

Melissa officinalis (Melissa)

Melissa is energising and uplifting, while easing stress-related conditions and shock. It soothes allergic reactions, reduces high blood pressure, anxiety and depression. Because it aids menstruation, it should not be used during pregnancy.

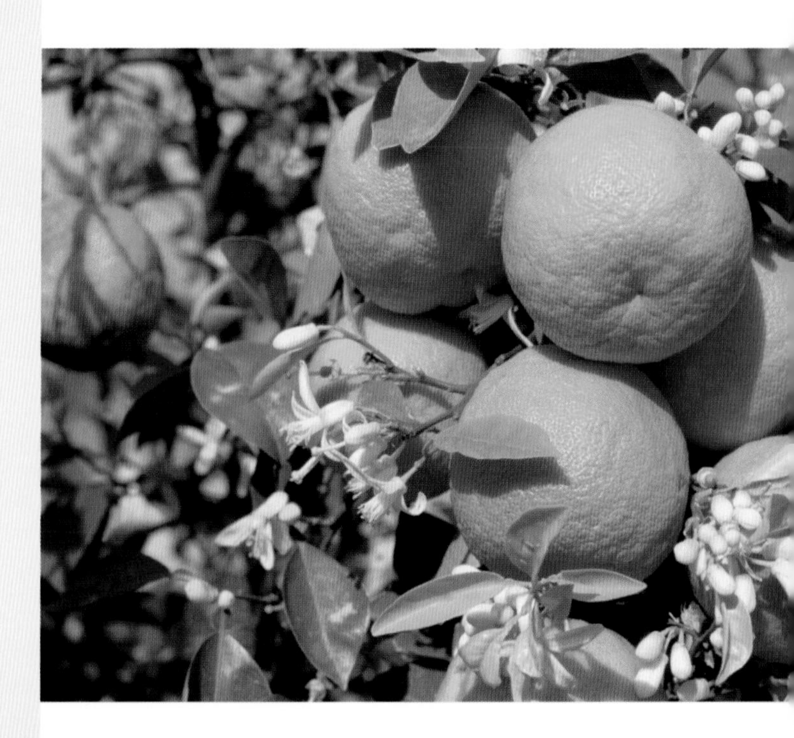

▲ **Citrus aurantium** (Neroli)

Neroli is great for boosting confidence and self-esteem. Because it creates a feeling of being alert while being relaxed, it is good for situations where one needs to be on good form. It helps in dealing with shock, nervous diarrhoea, insomnia, depression, scarring and stretch marks.

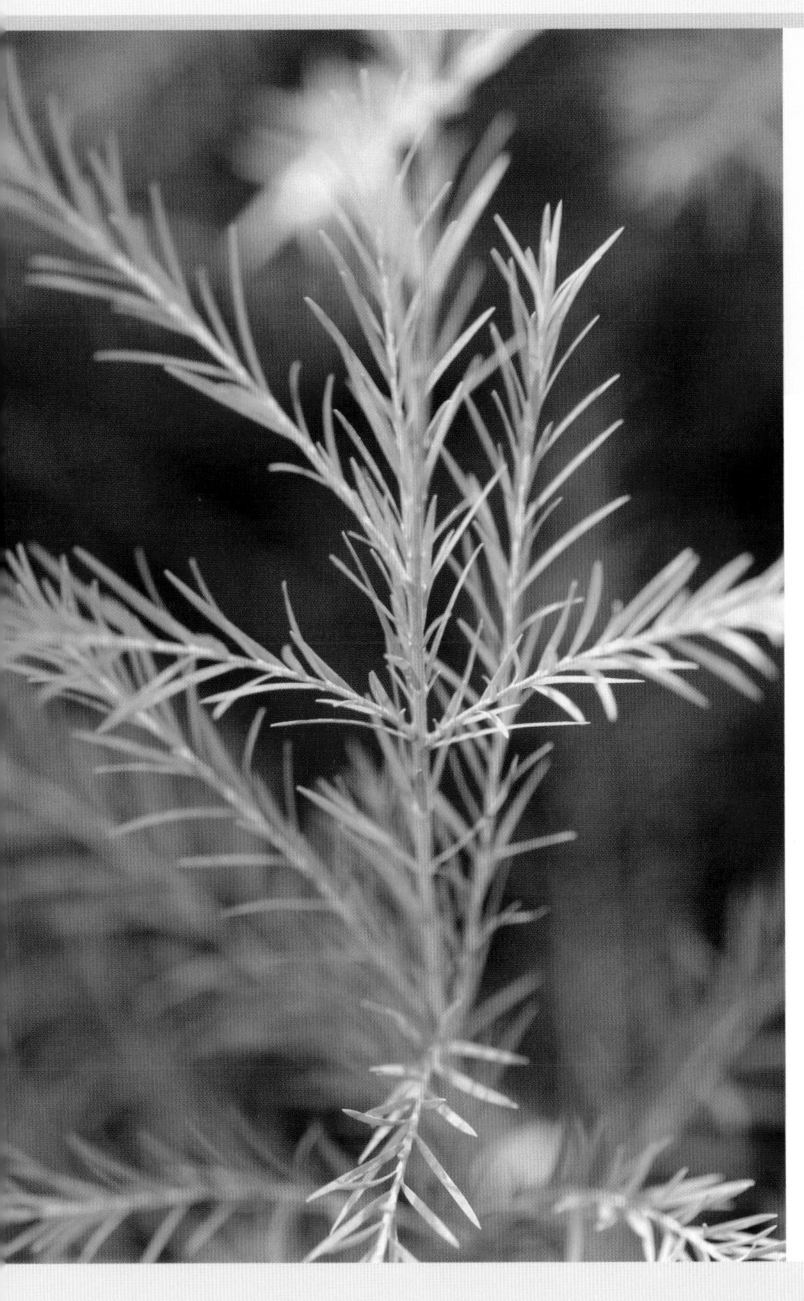

Citrus Bergamia (Bergamot)

Bergamot is the strongest anti-depressant oil on the market; it is extremely uplifting and good for stress and depression. It relieves digestion, cold and flu symptoms and inflammation. It also alleviates bad breath, sore throats and vaginal infections. Because bergamot increases sensitivity to ultraviolet light, do not it use before going into the sun or onto a sun bed.

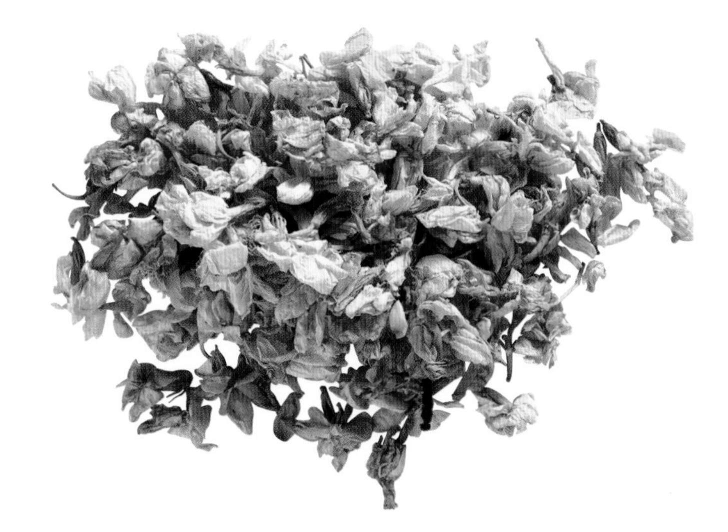

▲ **Jasminum officinale** (Jasmine)

Jasmine improves confidence and optimism. It is an anti-inflammatory that combats depression. It is good for the end of pregnancy because it strengthens uterine contractions (and thus cannot be used in the initial stages of pregnancy). It helps heel scar tissue, reduces stretch marks and increases elasticity. It also helps with male sexual problems by strengthening the male sexual organs.

▲ **Melaleuca alternifolia** (Tea tree)

Tea tree oil is the best oil for first aid; it fights infection, and helps preparation or recovery from an operation. It is great for sores, spots, acne, athletes foot, blisters, burns, sunburn, dandruff and itching.

► **Citrus paradisi** (Grapefruit)

Grapefruit combats depression, lethargy and fatigue. It is uplifting and refreshing while balancing mood swings. It boosts the immune system, helping to fight infection. It helps cellulite, acts as a mild diuretic and reduces water retention. It aids weight loss, poor digestion and hangovers. It is good before and after exercise.

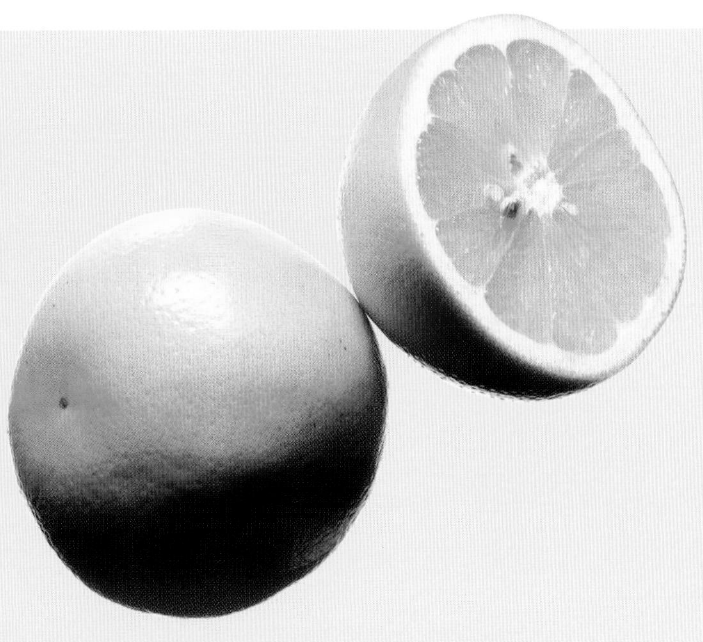

Cananga odorata (Ylang Ylang)

Ylang ylang is an aphrodisiac with sedating qualities. It reduces high blood pressure, impotency, stress, panic and depression. It balances the skin and is useful for both oily and dry skin.

Boswellia carterii (Frankincense)

Frankincense is emotionally balancing and uplifting. It clears the mind, comforts and uplifts. It smoothes wrinkles, eases cystitis, nephritis and genital infections and helps asthma, bronchitis, coughs and catarrh.

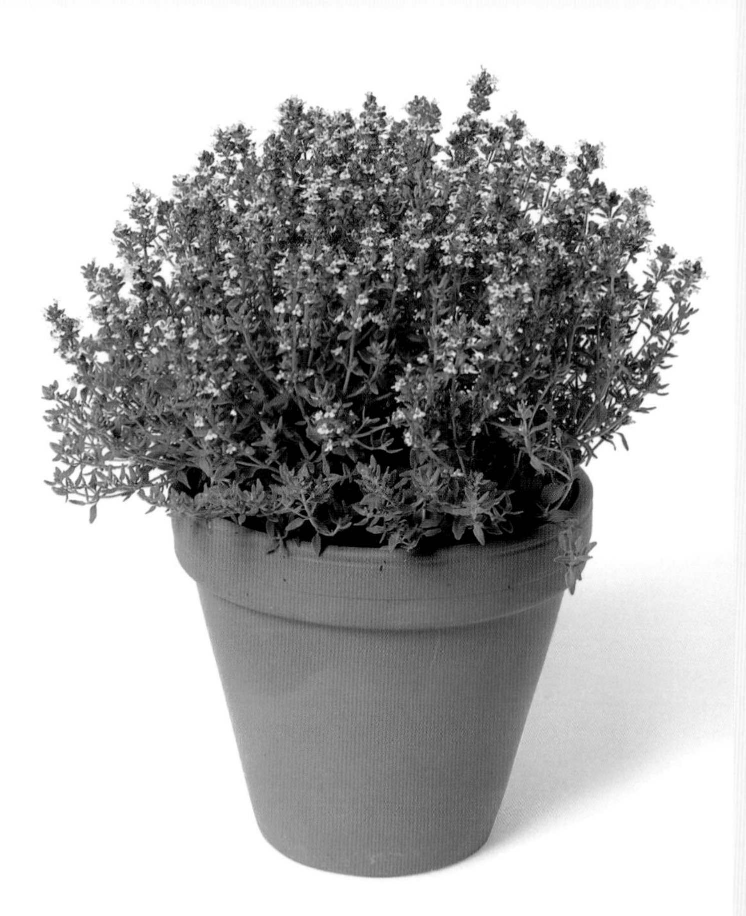

▲ **Thymus vulgaris** (Thyme)

Thyme is stimulating and good for respiratory infections. It aids memory, concentration, arthritis, nerves and cystitis. It should not be used on children under two years old or during pregnancy.

▼ **Lavendula offinalis** (Lavender)

Lavender is the most versatile oil and best all-rounder. It balances emotions, relieves aches and pains, headaches, tension and shock. It is good for burns, scars, insect bites, stings, sunburn, wounds, dermatitis, psoriasis, bronchitis, laryngitis, nausea, vomiting, cramps and lowering high blood pressure.

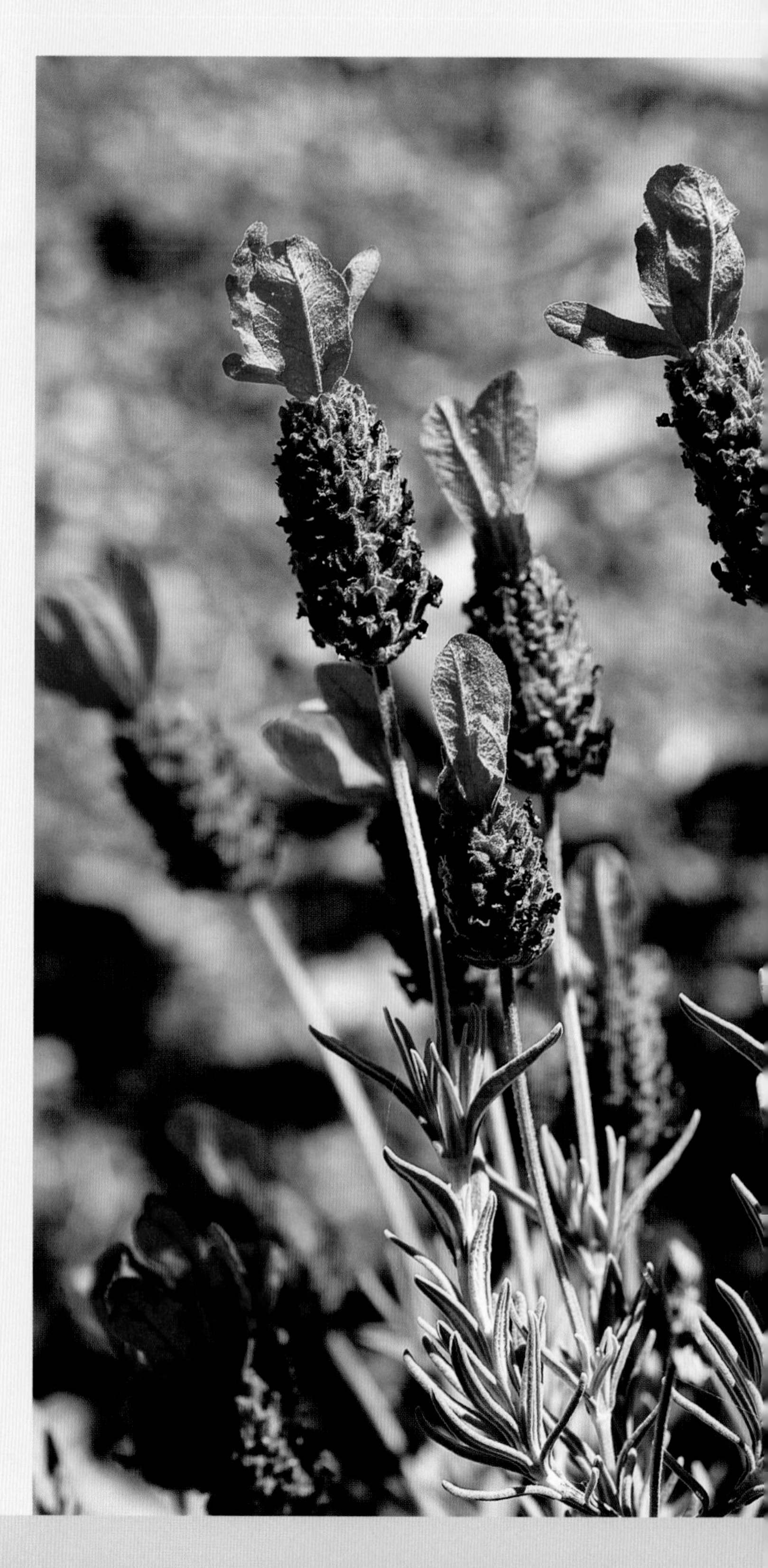

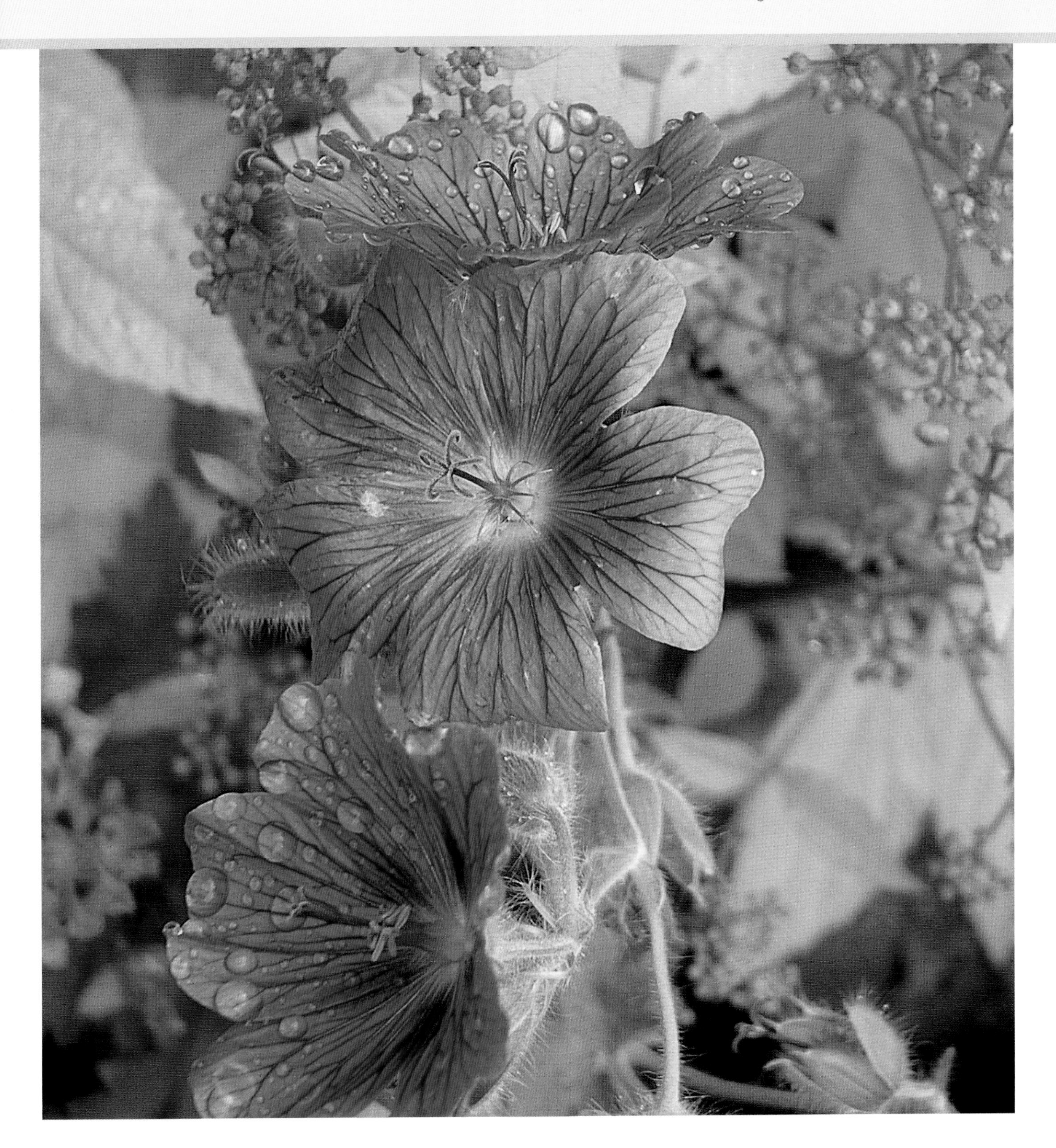

▲ **Pelargonium graveolens** (Geranium)

Geranium balances both the mind and the body. It is a tonic, relieving anxiety, depression and stress, while uplifting the spirit. It is beneficial for the circular and lymphatic systems, as well as all skin types. It is good for PMT, menopausal hot flushes, vaginal dryness and irregular periods. It is excellent for cellulite and water retention. It is also an anti-inflammatory and a good deodorant.

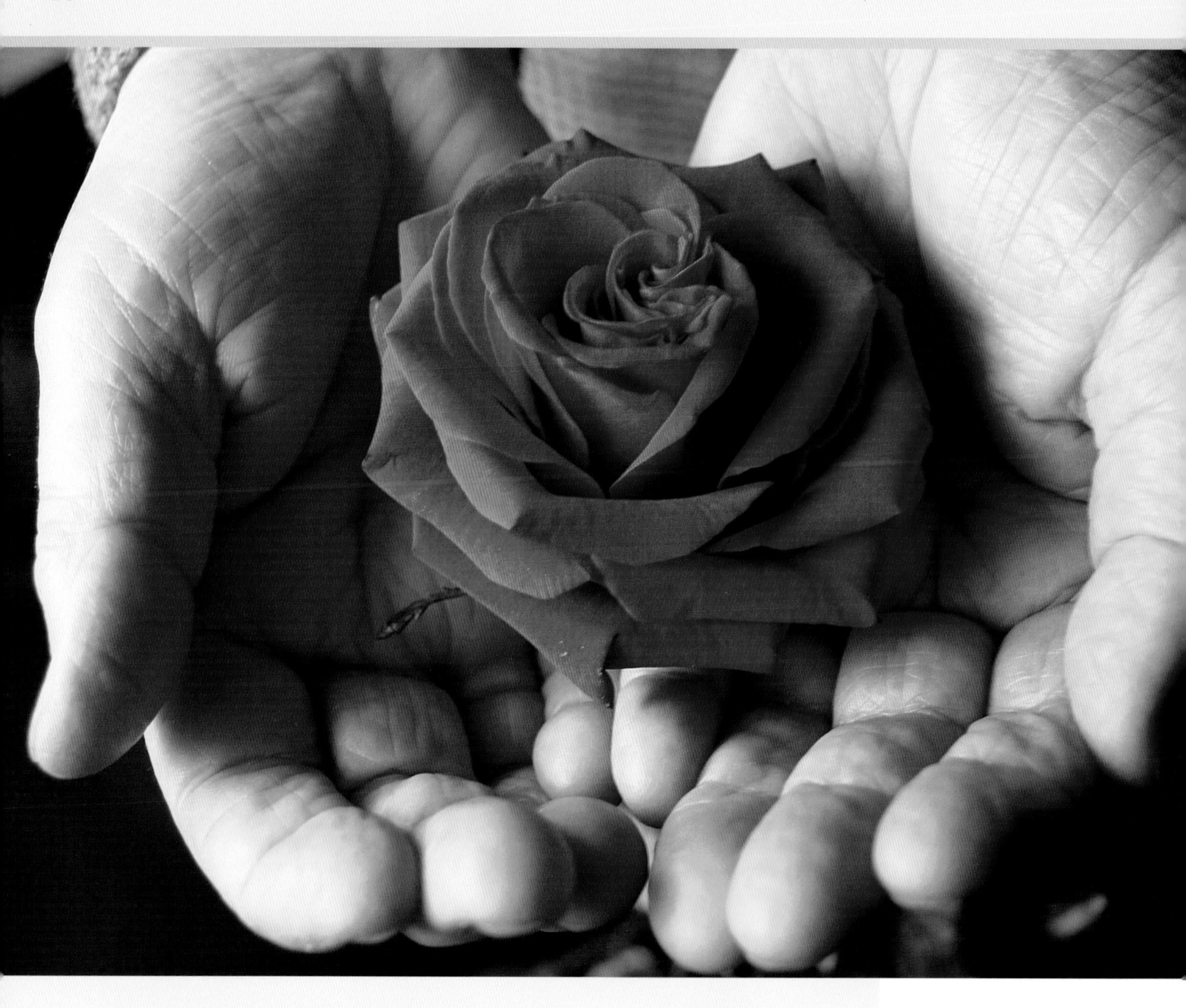

Pogostemon patchouli (Patchouli)

Patchouli is both a stimulant and a sedative. If used in small amounts it stimulates the nervous and digestive systems. Used in large amounts it is relaxing and soothing. It helps cell growth, scar tissue and dry skin. It aids weight loss and peristalsis. It also helps lethargy, anxiety and water retention.

► **Citrus reticulate** (Mandarin)

Mandarin is uplifting for the soul and soothing for the nerves. It is a mild diuretic and aids cellulite. It is good for scar tissue, stretch marks, digestion and wind. It is safe to use after the first trimester of pregnancy.

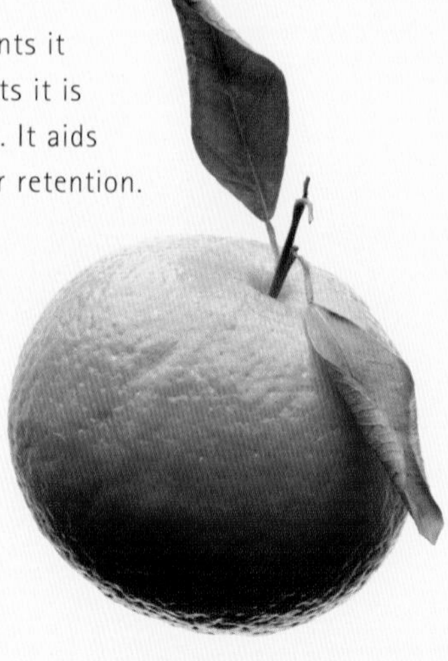

▲ **Rosa centifolia** (Rose)

Rose is an aphrodisiac that stimulates positive emotions while combating depression. It is good for nervous tension, stress, insomnia, inflammation, dry skin, menstrual problems, uterine disorders and semen production. Two drops on the hairline make a wonderful perfume!
Avoid during pregnancy.

▼ Rosemarinus officinalis (Rosemary)

Rosemary is another great all-rounder. It aids problems with circulation, infection, arthritis, rheumatism, bursitis, memory, fatigue, lethargy, headaches, migraines, vertigo, flu, cold, sinusitis and chest infections. Because it improves low blood pressure, it should not be used by people with high blood pressure. It should also be avoided by epileptics and during pregnancy. It acts as a good hair tonic.

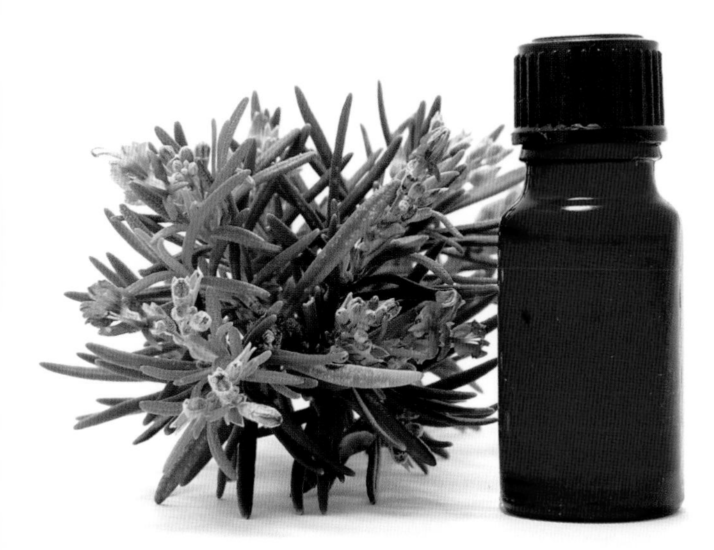

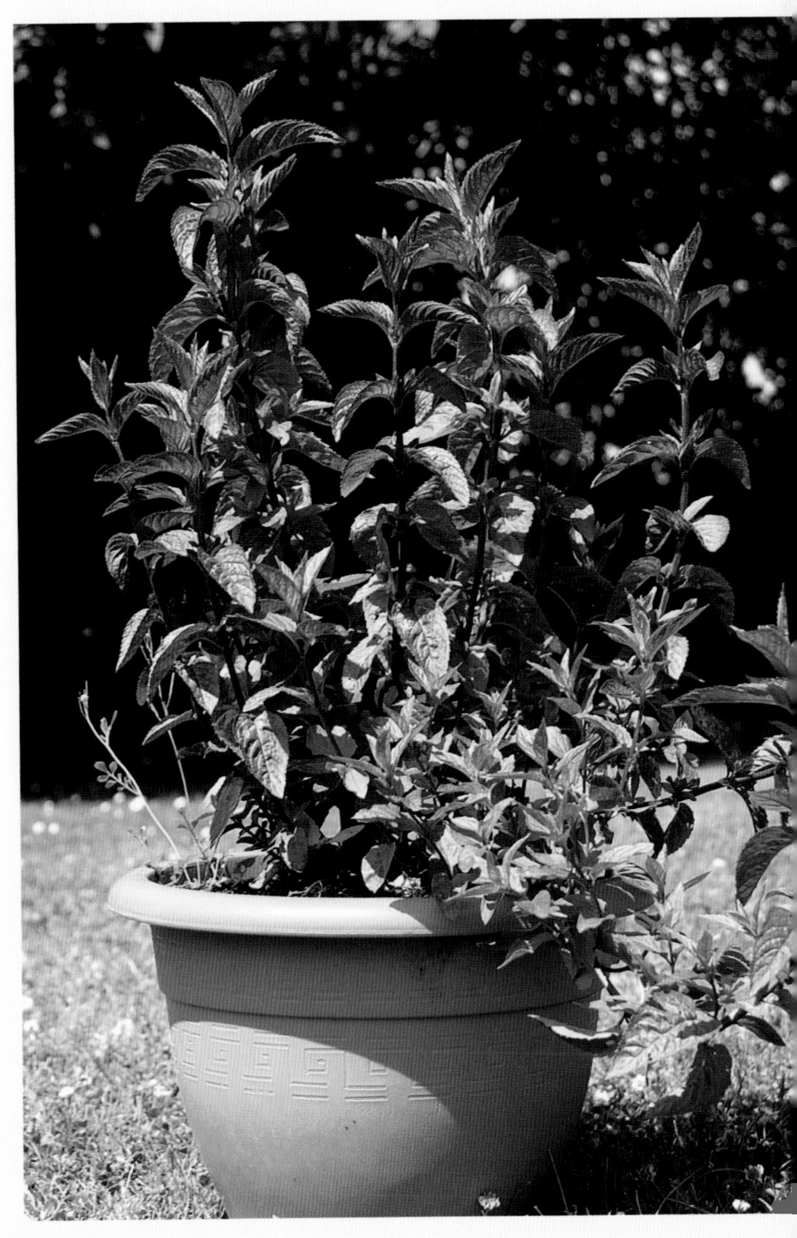

▼ Citrus limonum (Lemon)

Lemon lifts the emotions while stimulating the body's systems. It is great for varicose veins, broken capillaries, boils, warts, circulation, ulcers, indigestion, flatulence and acidity. It lowers high blood pressure and slows external bleeding, such as nosebleeds. It may cause sensitivity to sunlight.

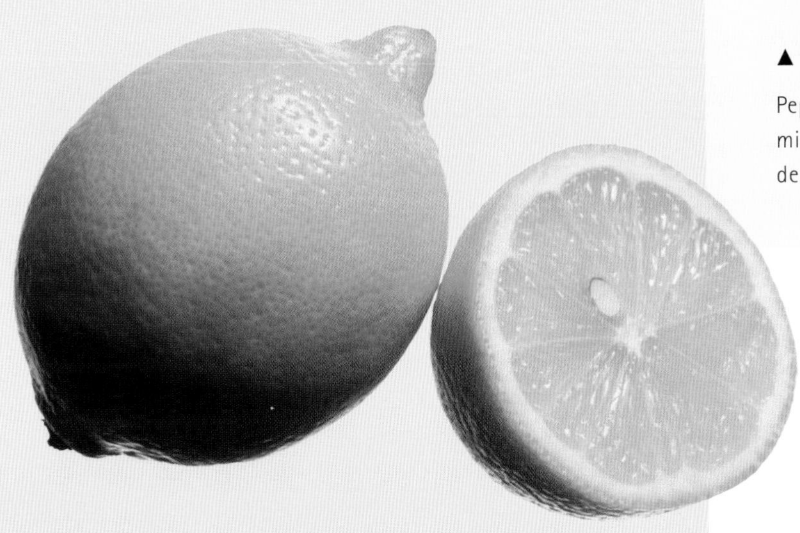

▲ Mentha piperita (Peppermint)

Peppermint heightens the senses, clearing and refreshing the mind. It cools sunburns and hot flushes. It is good for headaches, depression, flatulence, digestion, nausea, asthma and toothache.

Santalum album (Sandalwood)

Sandalwood is a very relaxing oil that calms the nerves and alleviates respiratory infections. It soothes cystitis, diarrhoea, varicose veins, depression and dry, irritated skin.

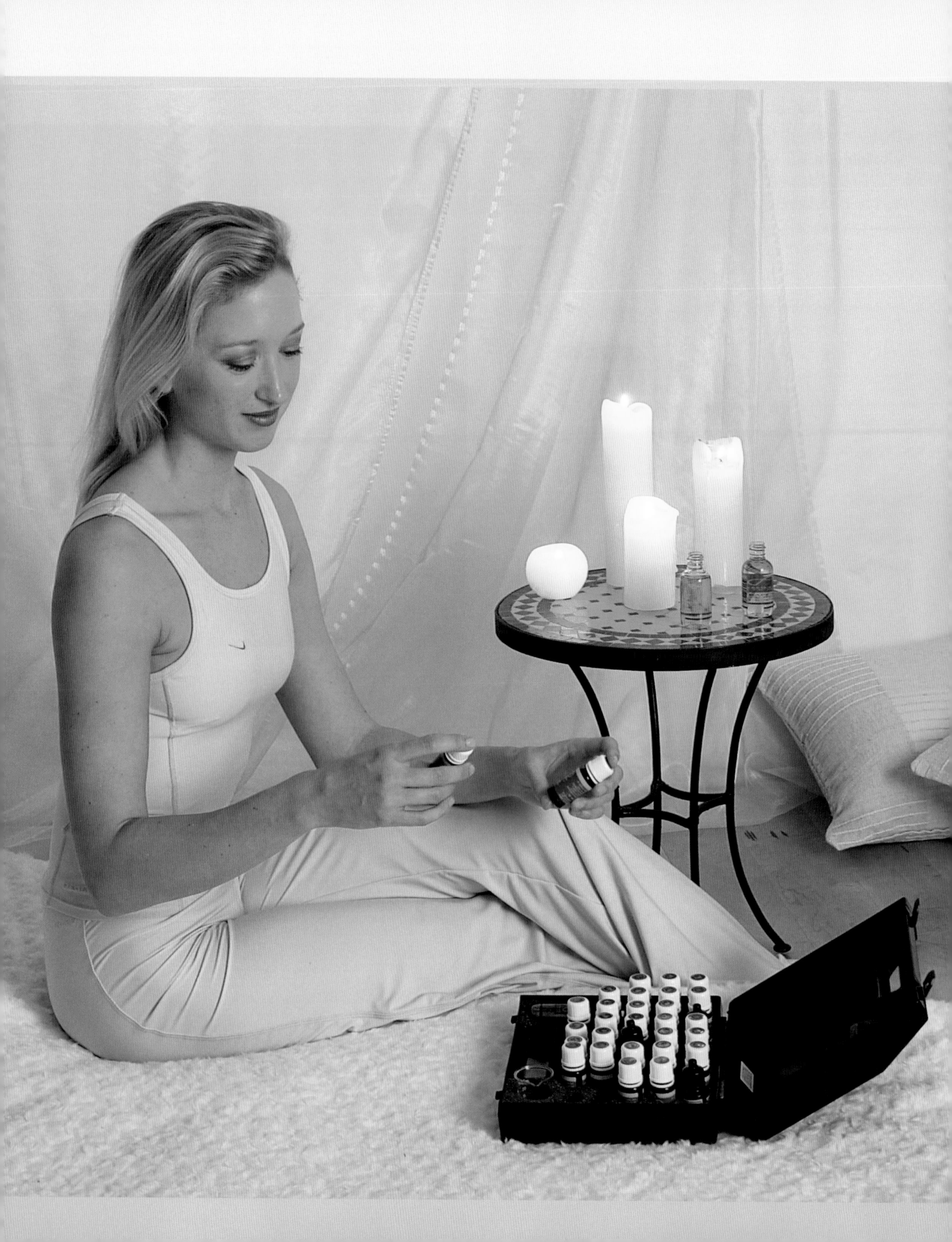

How to use essential oils

Amount of oil to use

The amount of oil you use on each area depends on the size of the area you are covering. Obviously, you would use less oil on the foot than you would to cover the whole back. Pour a small amount of oil into your hand anywhere between the size of a pea and the size of a wine-bottle top.

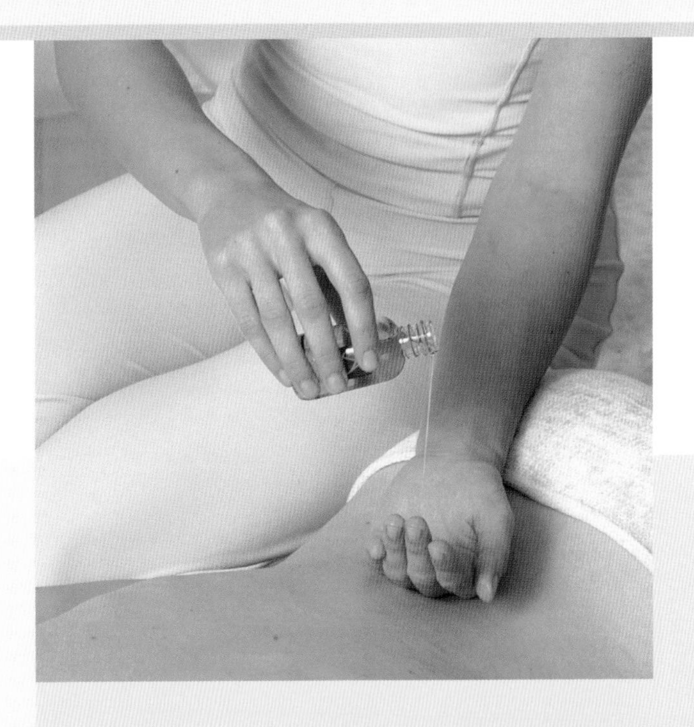

1 As a general rule, always dilute essential oils before they come into contact with the skin.

2 Add no more than 8 drops of essential oils to carrier oil for a massage. One massage uses about 35ml of base oil. If a person is large or has a lot of body hair, adjust accordingly.

3 Until you become familiar with the essential oils and their smells, only blend two together for a massage.

Care of essential oils

Keep all essential oils in dark containers in a cool, dry place. Some oils react with light and their properties change, making them less beneficial. Keeping essential oils in a hot place is equally damaging.

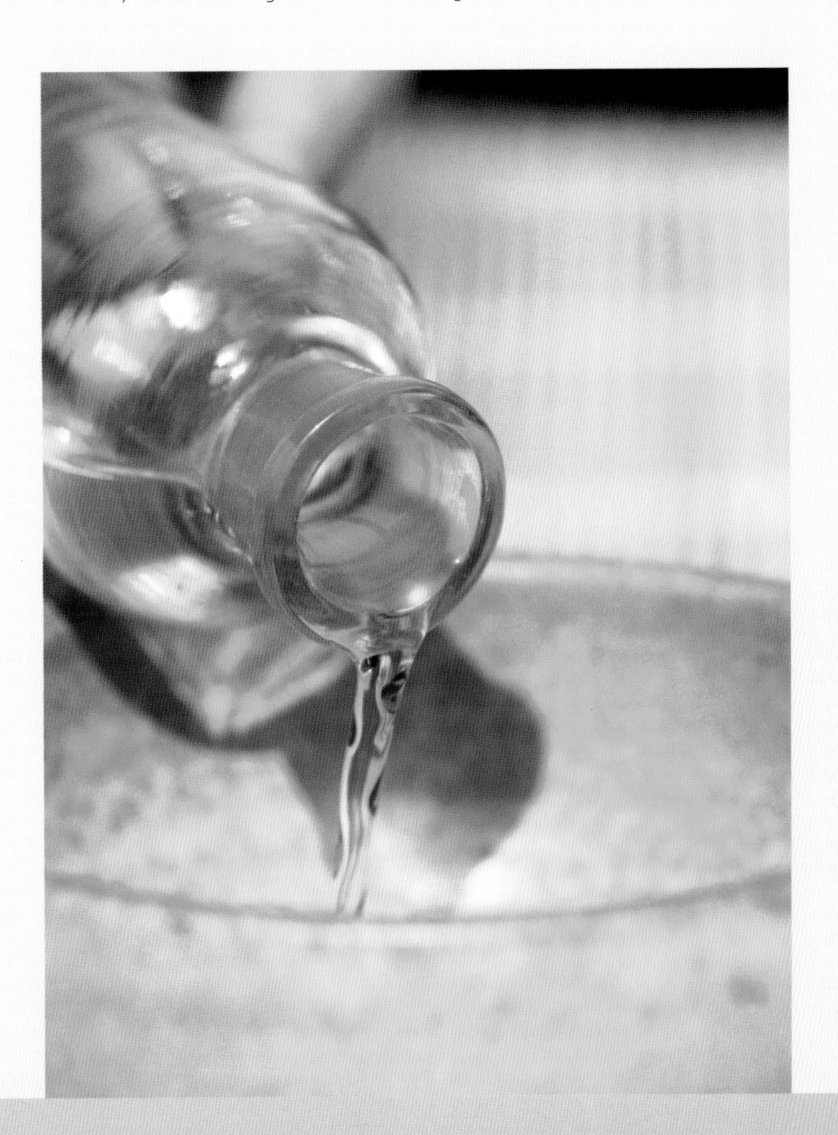

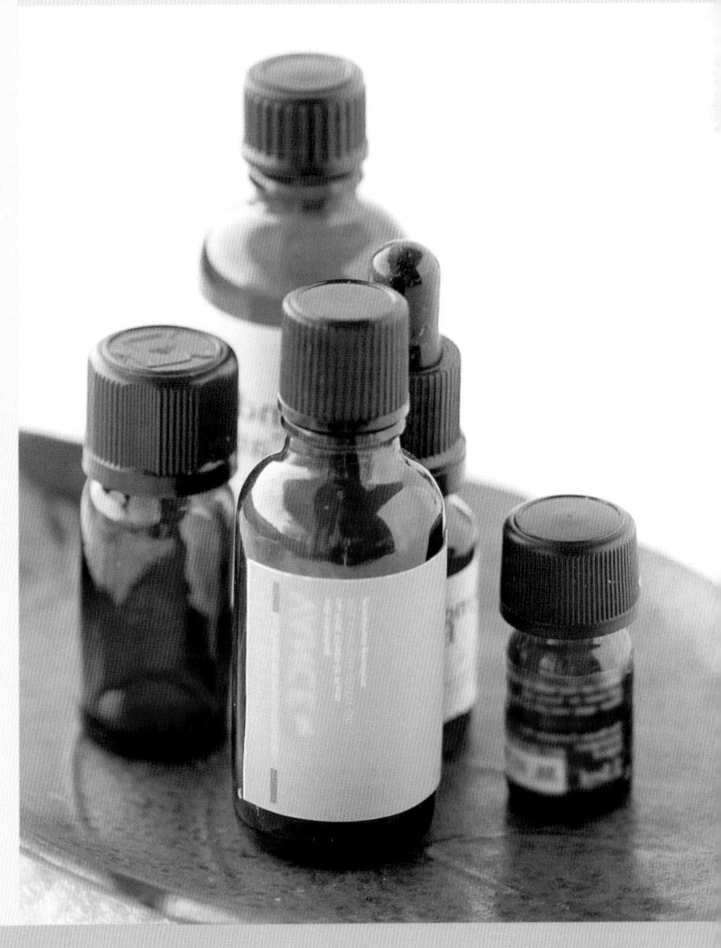

Oil blends

Blending essential oils is an art form. Until you become more familiar with your collection of oils, do not blend more than two at a time. If you are unsure how the essential oils might smell once blended, hold your choices under your nose together. Make a small circle with your wrist and waft the combined aroma of the oils to your nose. Another way to test the compatibility of essential oils is to take two strips of paper and place a drop of oil on each one. Again, inhale the aromas at the same time to see how well they blend together.

If you really like a particular blend, remember to make a note of how you created it so that you can enjoy it again.

Add a total of 8 drops essential oil to 35ml of carrier oil.

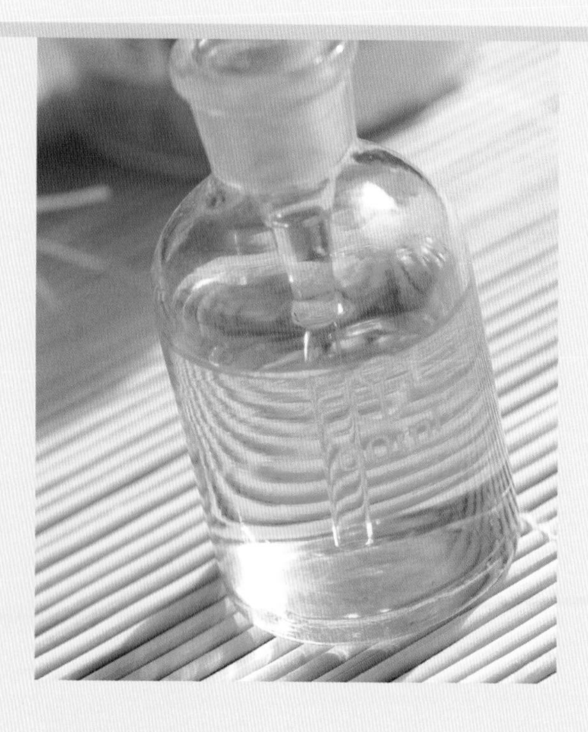

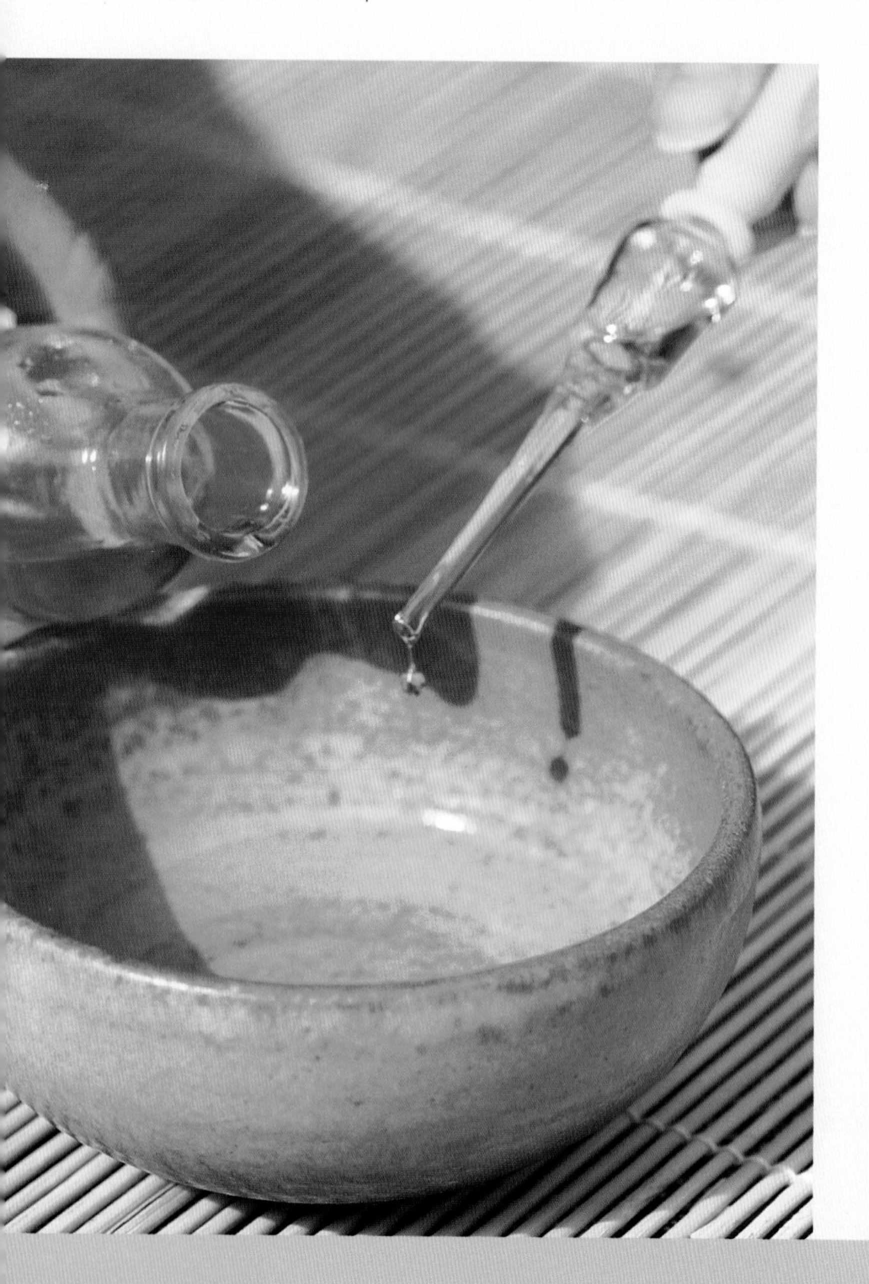

Aches and pains oil

Juniper 2 drops
Jasmine 3 drops
Marjoram 3 drops

Antidepressant oil

Frankincense 3 drops
Lavender 3 drops
Bergamot 2 drops

Anxiety oil

Mandarin 2 drops
Melissa 3 drops
Ylang Ylang 3 drops

Relaxing oil

Bergamot 3 drops
Geranium 3 drops
Sandalwood 2 drops

Sensual oil

Rosemary 2 drops
Rose 3 drops
Jasmine 3 drops

Uplifting oil

Grapefruit 2 drops
Lavender 3 drops
Jasmine 3 drops

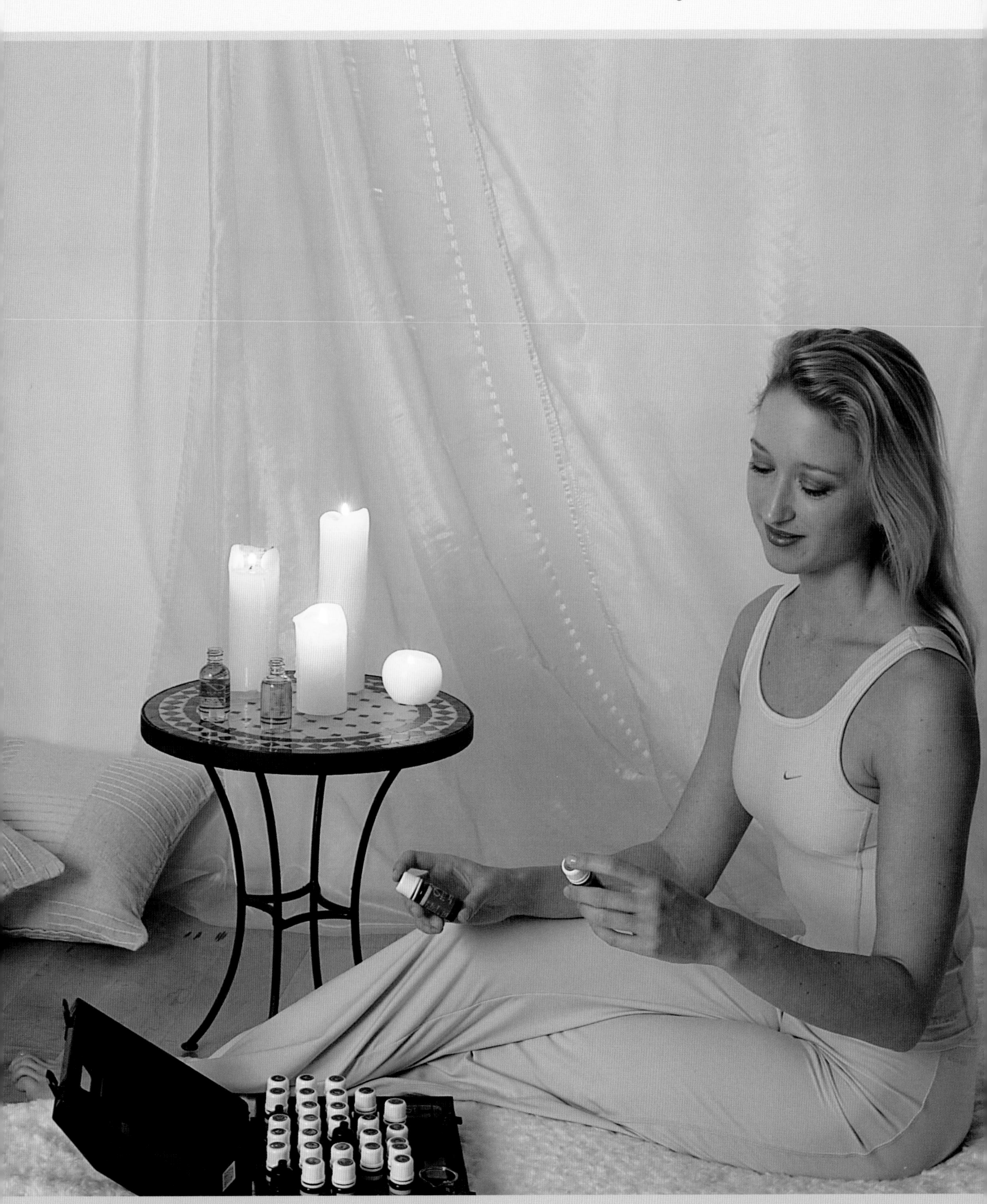

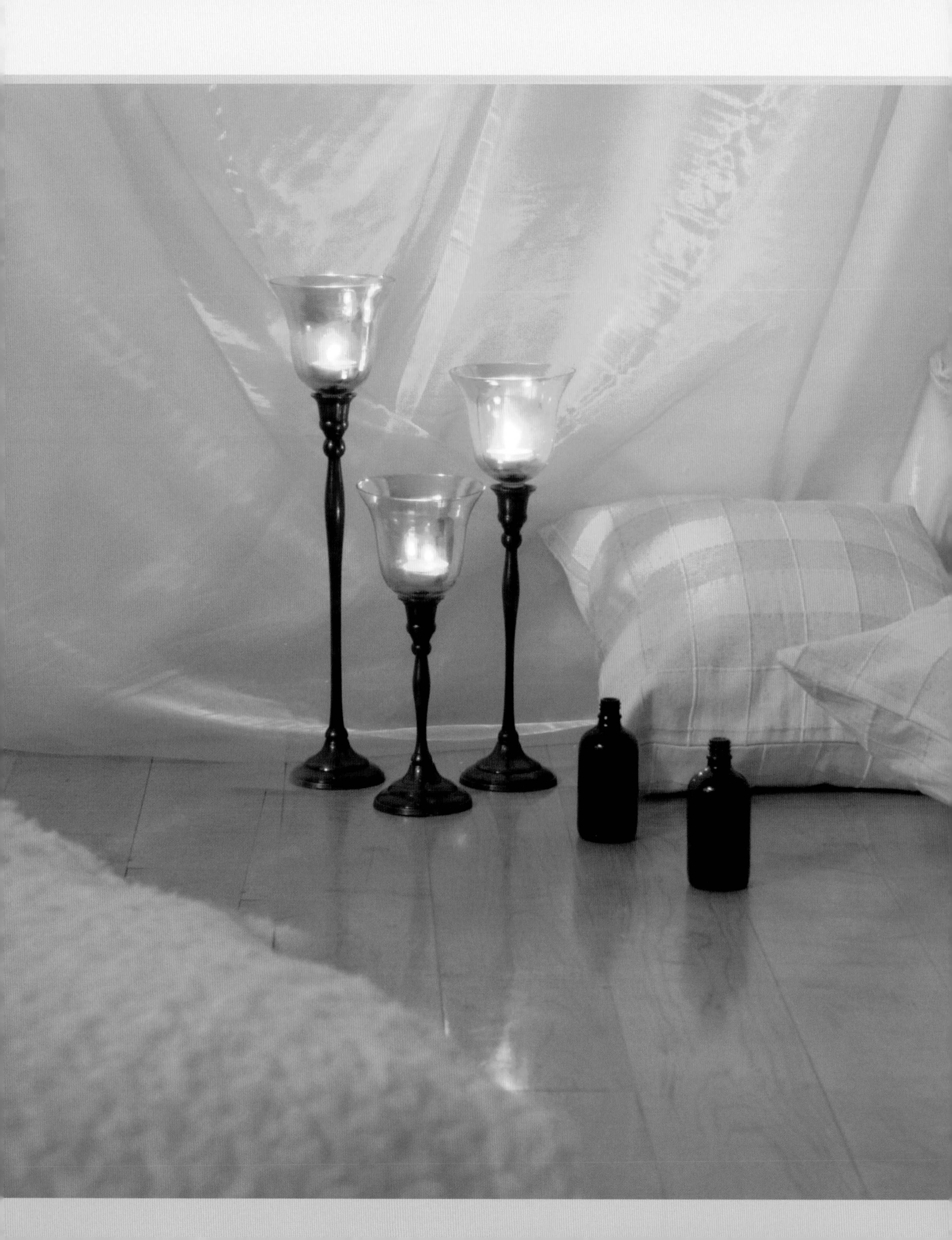

Preparation for massage

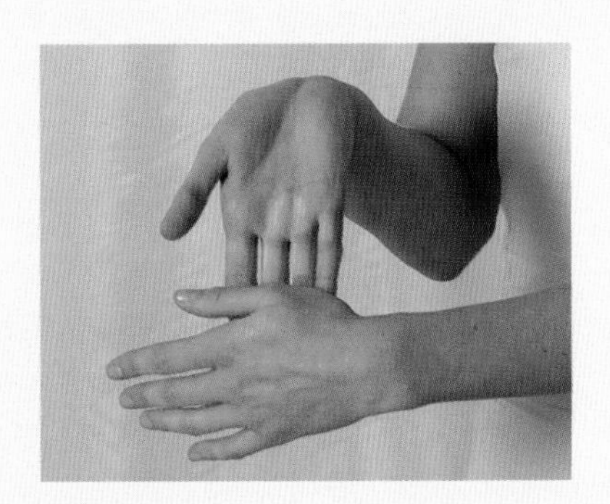

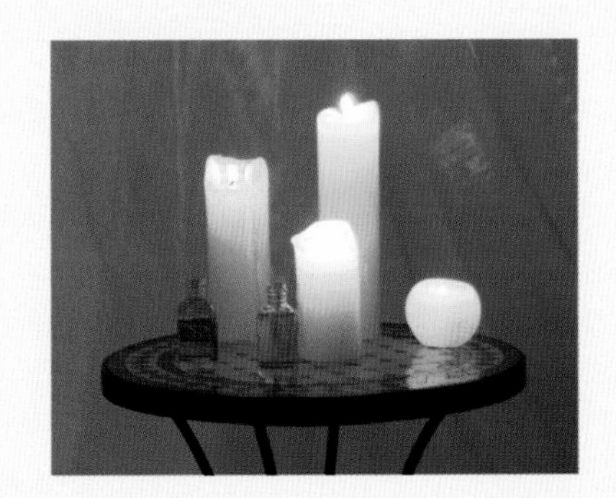

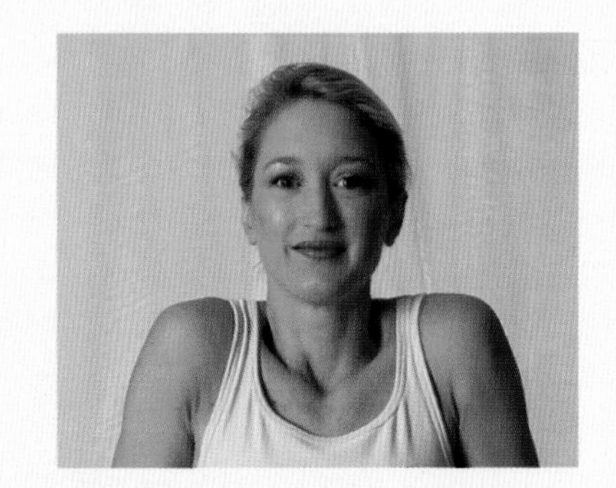

Whether you are working on the floor or on a bed, it is important to create a relaxing atmosphere. Make sure you unplug or turn off all phones, so that you are not disturbed. You can create a relaxing mood by putting on some meditative music. Creating a beautiful atmosphere can be as simple as lighting a candle. Instead of bright overhead lights, try turning on a small lamp. Have plenty of large, freshly laundered towels. Also, have the oils you have chosen to work with in a bowl readily at hand. You do not want to leave your partner to get supplies, once you have made initial contact.

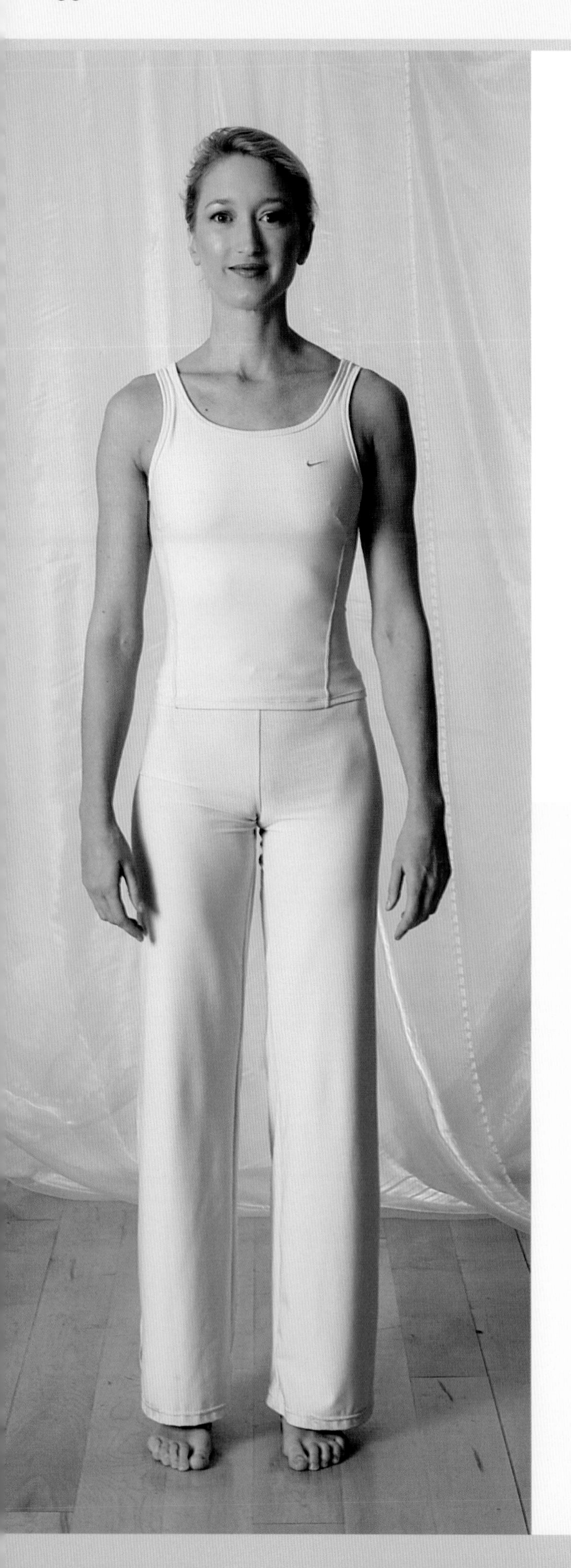

Preparing yourself

Time

It is extremely important that you allow yourself plenty of time before and after a massage. You will need time to set up the room, change your clothes, create the atmosphere and lay out the fresh towels and oils. After a massage give your partner time to get up slowly, get dressed and talk about the experience. Imagine how it would feel to be rushed out of the room after a massage – all the good would be undone. A massage is an experience that should be pleasant and relaxing from the moment you arrive until the moment you leave.

Clothes and hygiene

Make sure you take off all your jewellery, as it might scratch your partner or get in the way. Do not wear any strong perfumes or deodorants, as your partner could be allergic to them. Wear loose, comfortable clothing that you can move easily in. Make sure that you cut your nails or they could cause extreme discomfort for your partner. Your nails should be short enough so that you cannot feel them when you press against the tip of the finger. Always wash your hands before and after a massage, preferably with an anti-bacterial soap.

Centring

It is important that you are relaxed and centred before you give a massage. To centre yourself, stand with your feet hip width apart and your arms relaxed down by your sides. Close your eyes. Take a couple of moments to relax, and focus on your breathing. Feel the rise and fall of your stomach as you inhale and exhale. When you feel relaxed and comfortable, slowly open your eyes.

Focus

The quality of the massage will be enhanced if you focus your mind on it at all times. Think about the muscles you are working on and feel the reaction to your touch. The body holds all of our emotions, fears, anxiety and stress. Imagine a dialogue between you and the muscles you are working on. What is the muscle saying? How does it feel? Is it tense? Relaxed? Knotted? Loose? The massage will be less effective if you are thinking of your day ahead or the shopping you need to do.

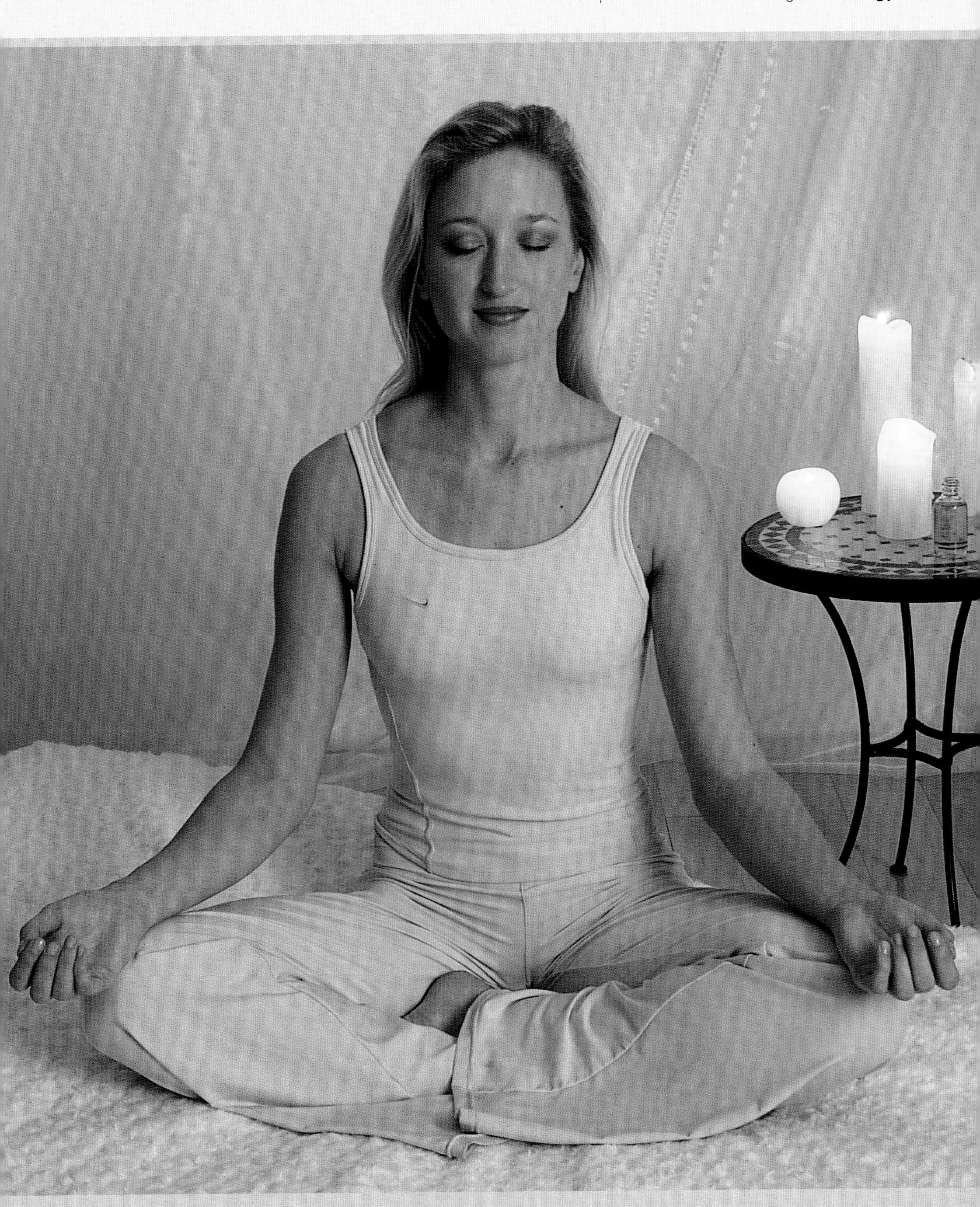

Position

Whenever you give a massage, try to make sure you are in a comfortable position that is not causing you undue strain. If you have a massage table, your knees should be bent and your upper body long and tall. Your weight should shift onto your front leg as you carry out long, sweeping motions. As much as possible, you need to use your whole body weight behind the movements. This takes the pressure off your fingers and means that you will not get fatigued as quickly.

If you do not have a massage table, it is possible to improvise using a futon or folded blankets on the floor. Make sure there is enough padding so that your partner can lie down comfortably. However, you need to be able to move freely around them while remaining on the blanket. Here are some comfortable positions for giving a massage on the floor. Experiment to discover which ones feel best on your body. You want to make sure you do not feel pressure in your back while giving a massage. You should position yourself however you feel most comfortable.

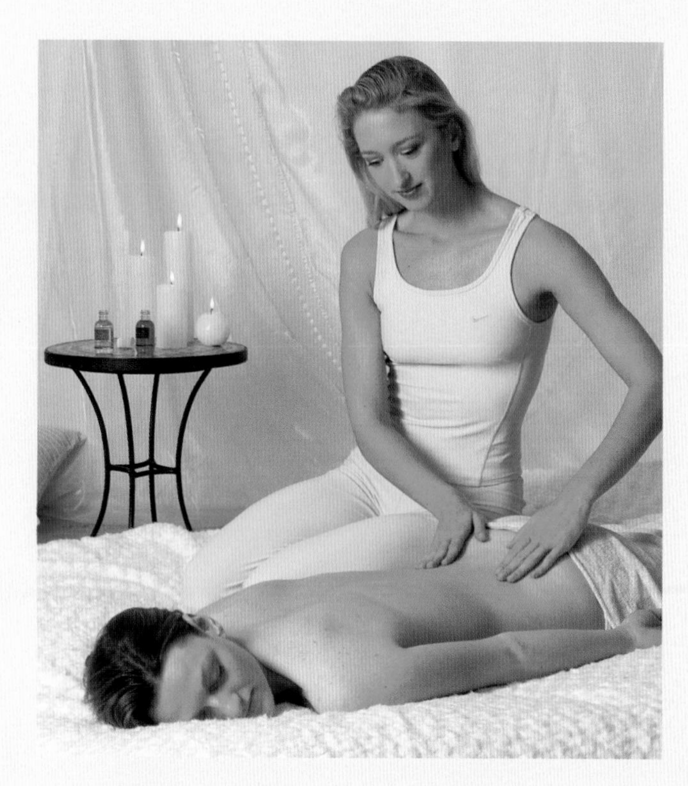

Kneeling: Bend your knees and sit on your heels. This position is usually great because you can lift up off your heels or relax back depending upon the stroke.

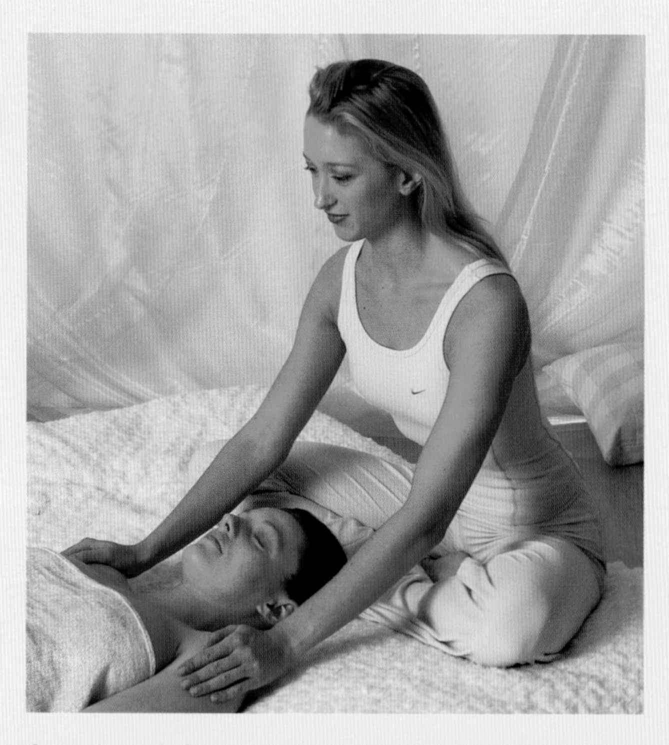

Cross-legged: Sit on your buttocks with your ankles crossed and your knees bent. This position is very comfortable when working on the feet or on the head.

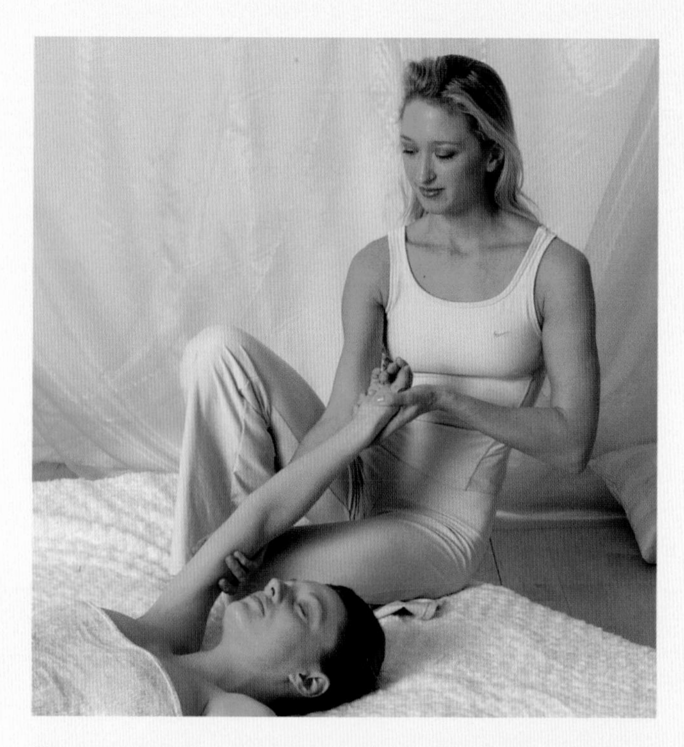

On one knee: If you are on the right side of your partner, sit on your left heel with your right leg bent and your right foot flat on the floor. This is a comfortable position when working on the back or on the legs.

Preparing your partner

Being massaged should be a wonderful experience. Let your partner know what is about to happen, especially if they have never experienced a massage before. Explain that you are going to leave the room and when you do you would like them to undress down to their undergarments. (No bras for the ladies.) Ask them to lie down underneath the towels on their stomach. They may feel vulnerable, so you want to maintain their modesty. Only uncover the area you are working on. Make sure that your partner feels safe and secure at all times.

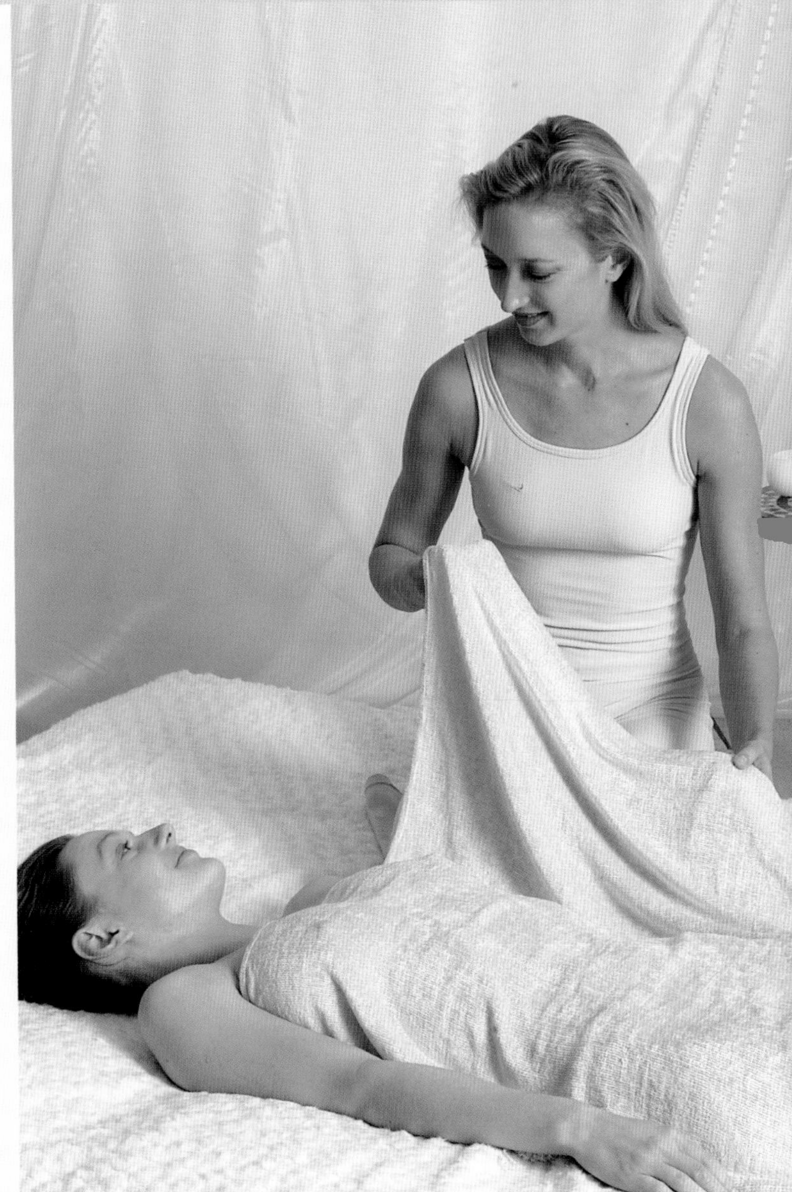

▲ Cover your partner with large freshly laundered towels. Make sure that they stay warm throughout the entire massage.

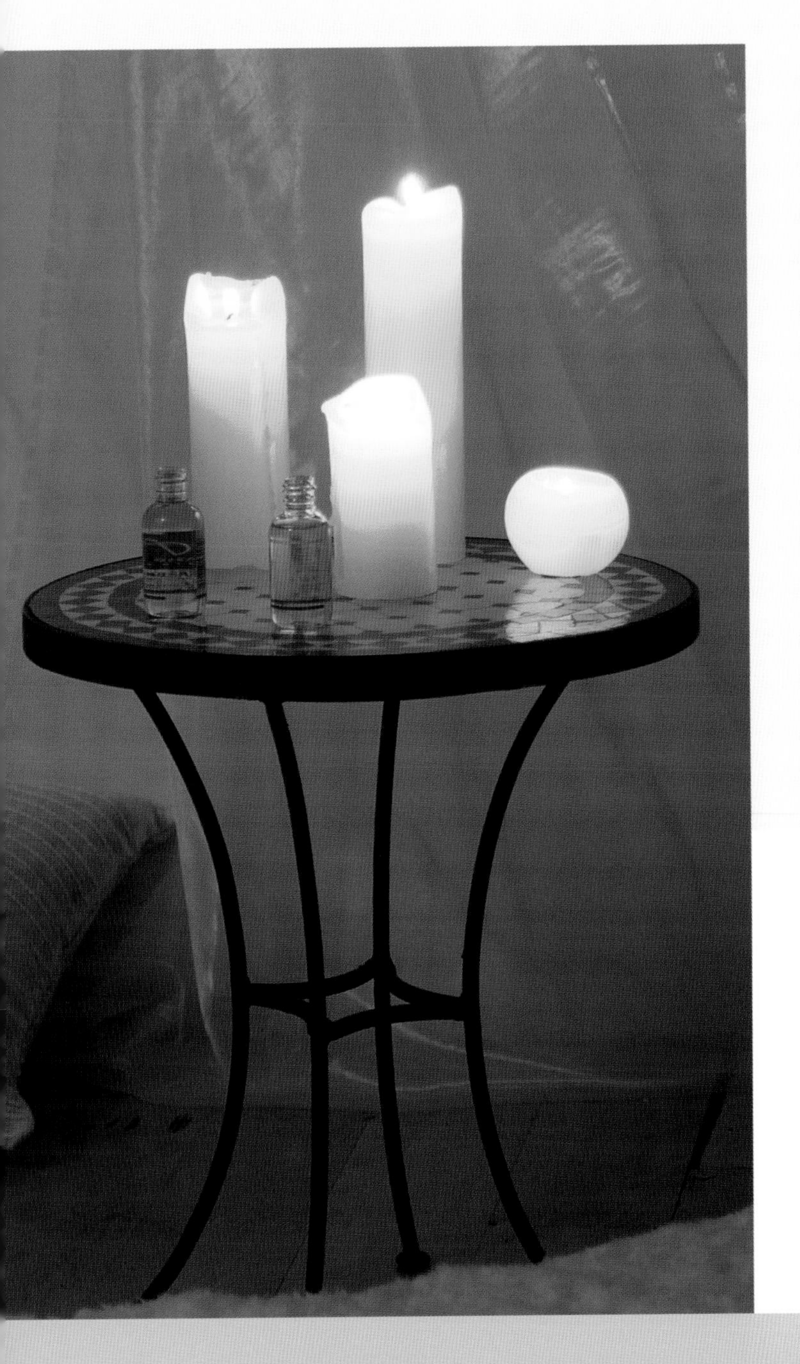

For the purposes of clarity while photographing the different techniques used throughout this book, we have left both legs or both arms uncovered on the model. This is not normally done during a massage. Please make sure that your partner is covered, with only the limb you are working on exposed. Your partner might get cold during the massage, so please have some extra towels ready nearby just in case.

Before starting

There are some simple stretches you can do to prepare yourself for giving a massage that will relax your muscles and raise your energy.

Neck rolls

1 Stand with your feet hip width apart and your knees soft. Think of energy going to the top of your head and down through your feet.

2 Inhale as you turn your head to look over the left shoulder.

3 Exhale and slowly roll the head down to the right, thinking of your chin touching your chest as you move.

4 Inhale as you look over your right shoulder.

Exhale and slowly roll the head back down to the left, thinking of your chin touching your chest as you move.

Repeat 3-4 times.

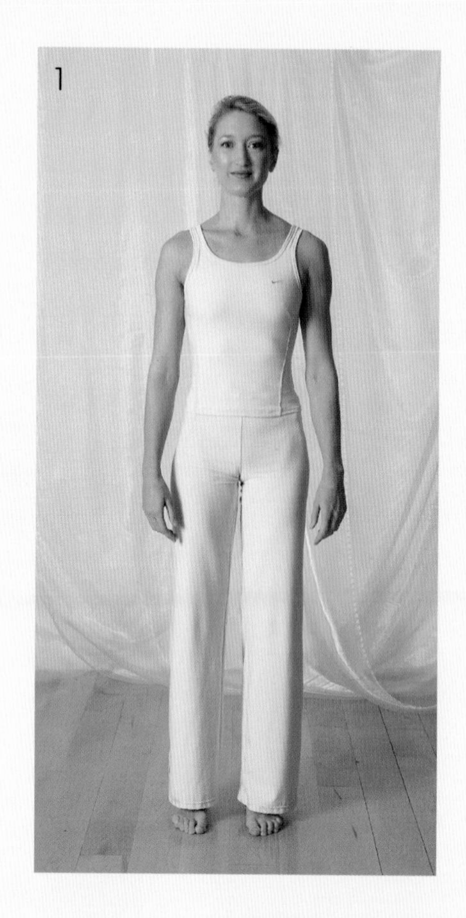
1

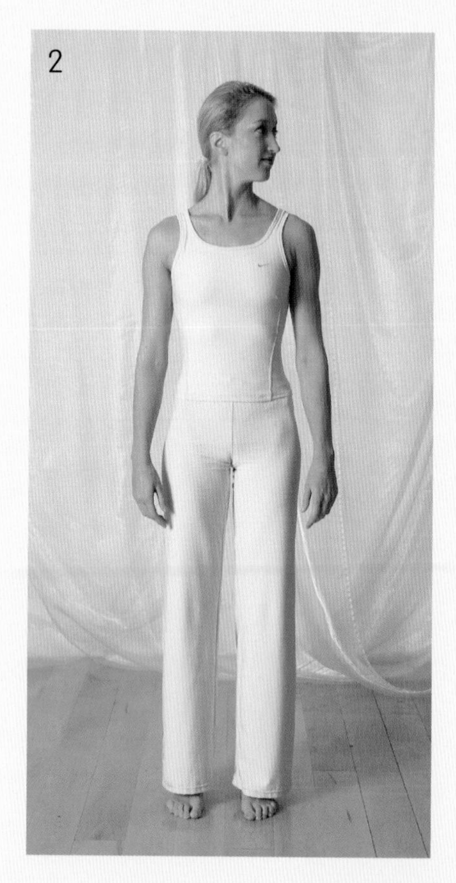
2

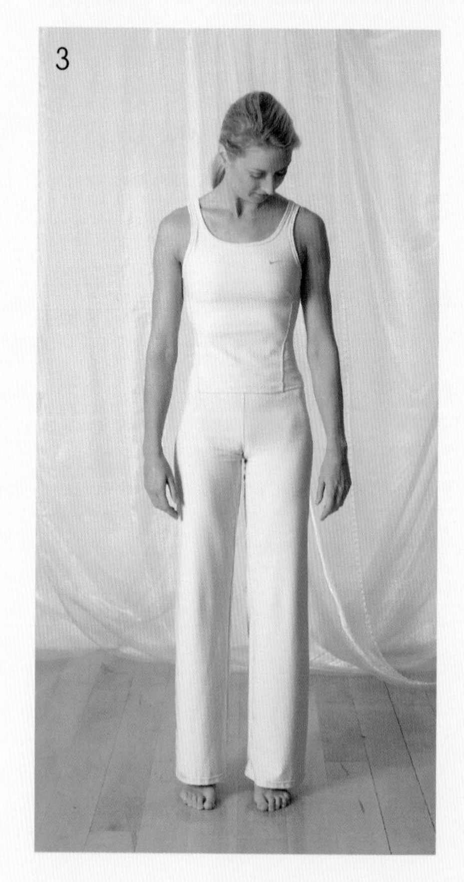
3

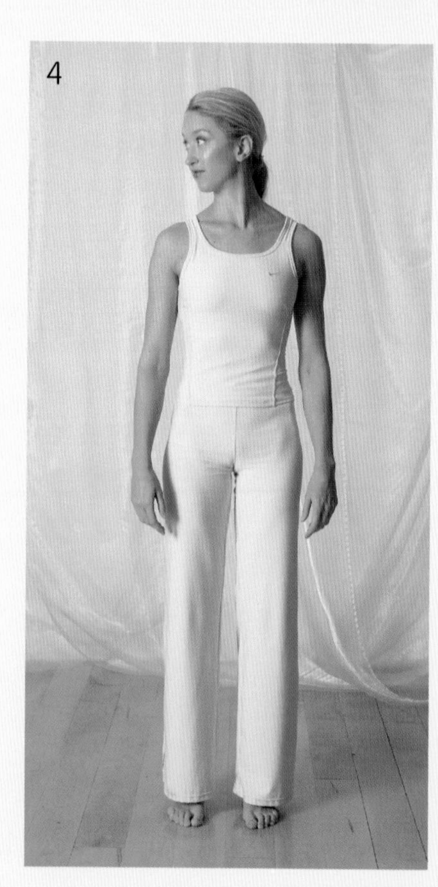
4

Shoulder circles

1 Continue standing with your feet hip width apart and your knees soft.

2 Inhale as you roll your shoulders forwards.

3 Raise your shoulders up to your ears.

4 Exhale and roll the shoulders back, keeping your ribs closed.

Repeat 3 times in this direction.

Reverse, ensuring that you inhale as you roll the shoulders back and exhale as you bring the shoulders forward.

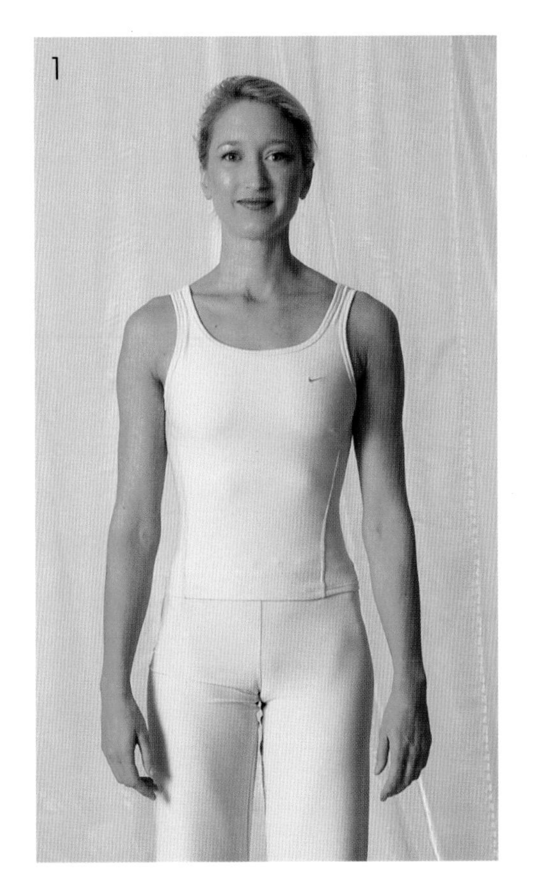
1

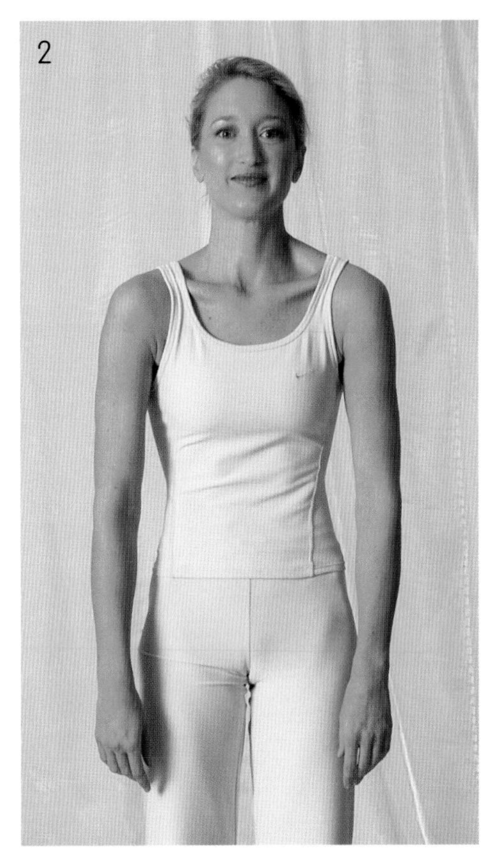
2

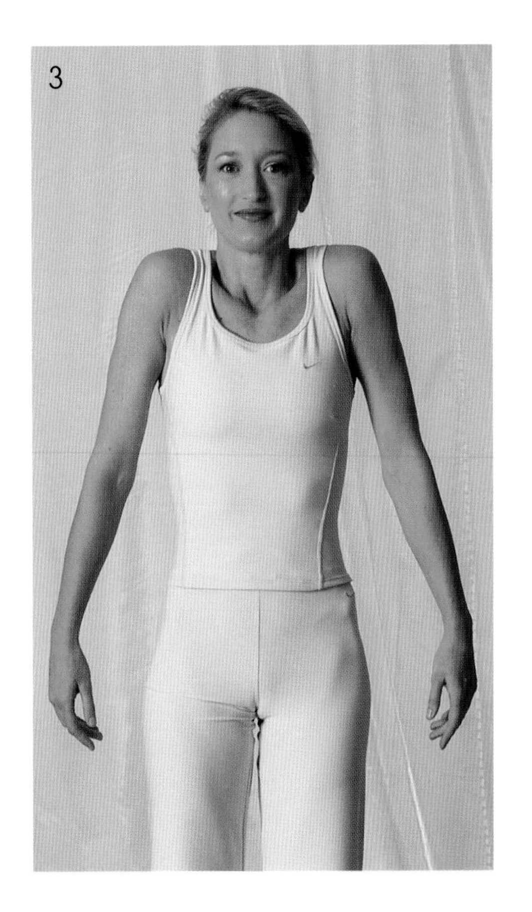
3

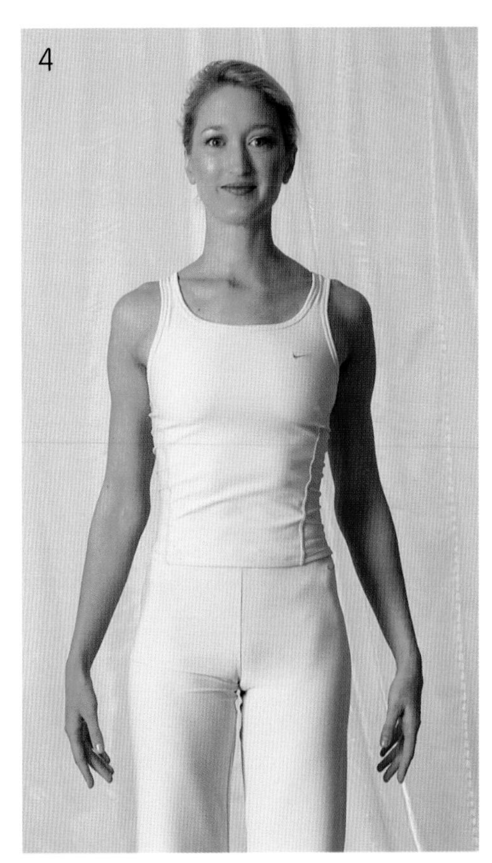
4

Hand circles

This exercise can also be done sitting or standing. Circle the hands around the wrist.

Repeat in the other direction.

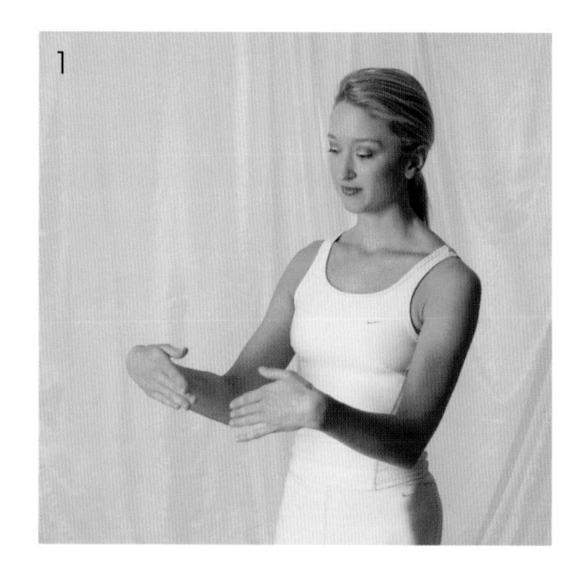

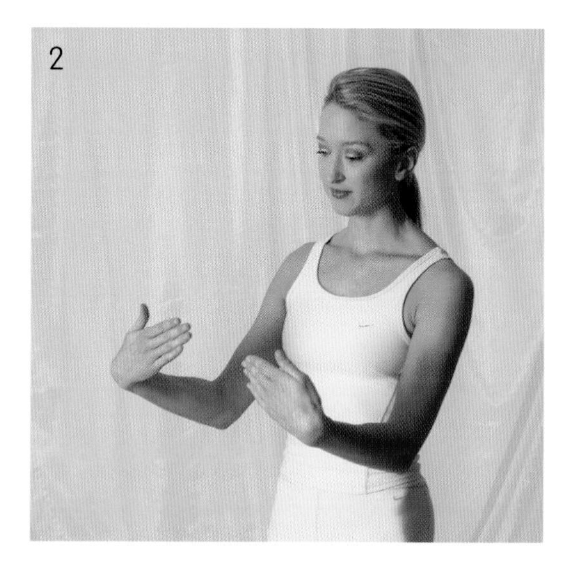

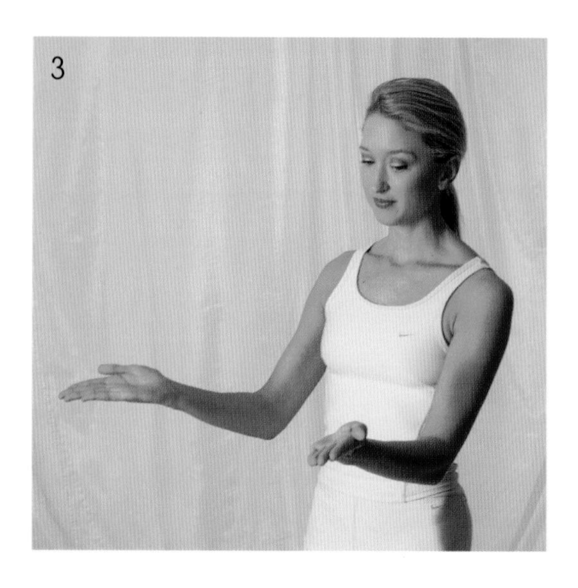

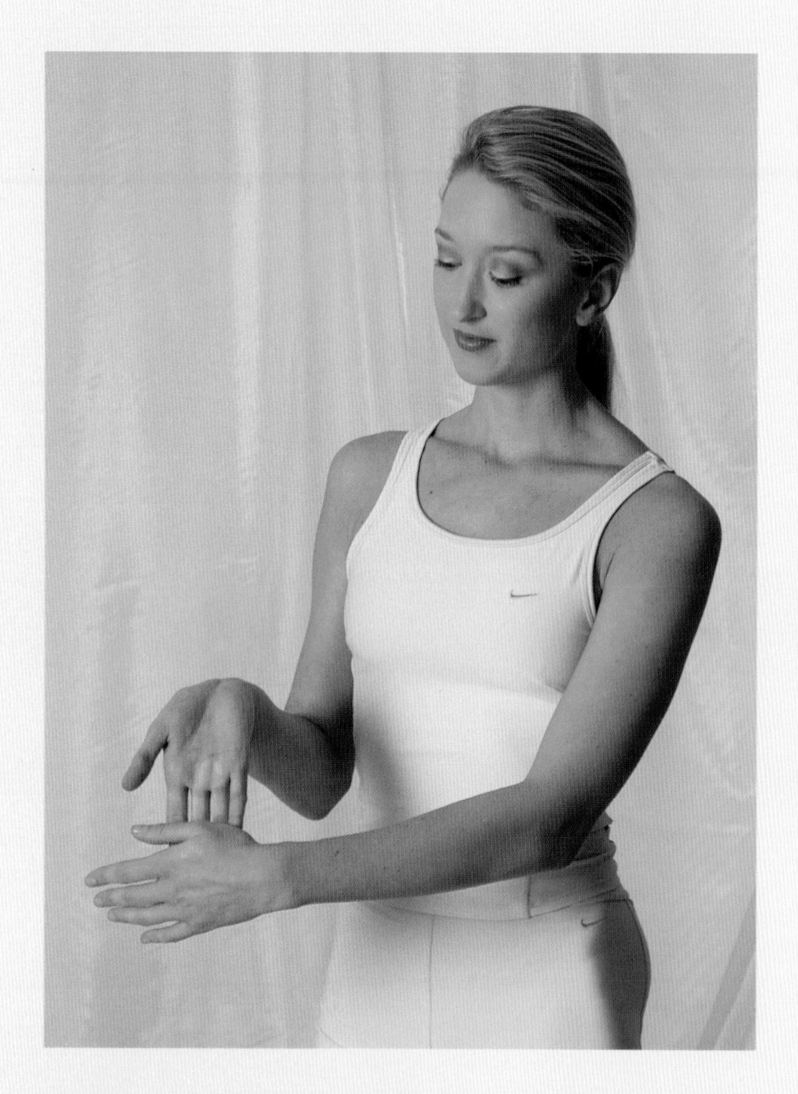

Hand stretches

This exercise can be done sitting or standing. Place the palm of one hand on the fingertips of the other. Stretch the fingers back towards the wrist.

Repeat to the other side.

Shaking the hands

Continue sitting or standing. Shake the hands vigorously, and think about releasing any tension.

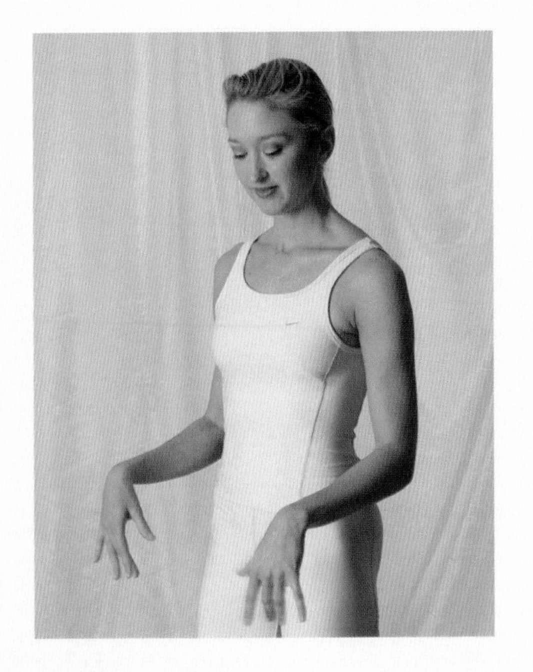

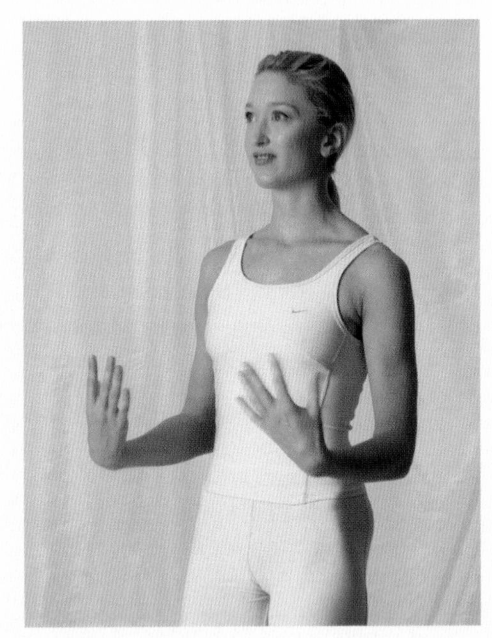

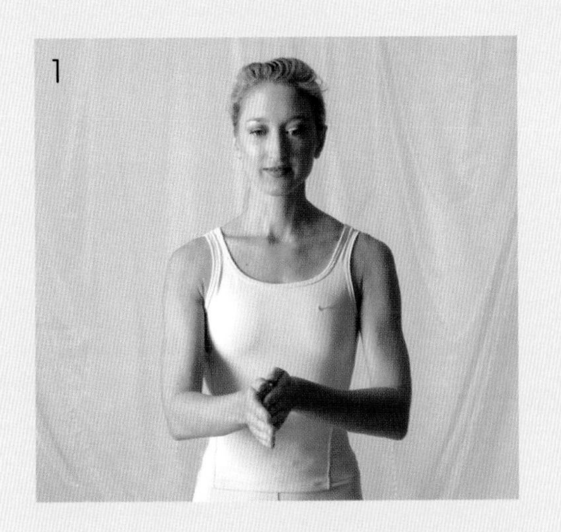

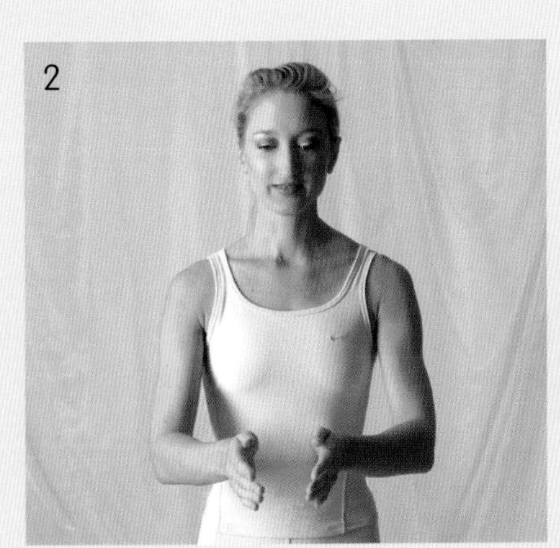

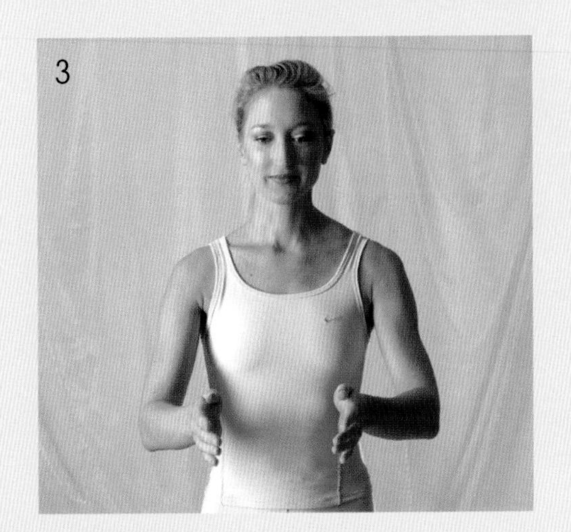

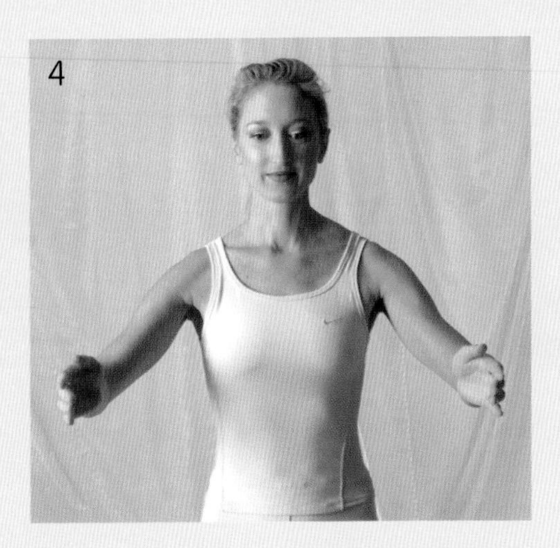

Friction with the hands

1 Rub your hands quickly together.

2 Slowly separate the hands until they are 23 cm apart. Try to feel the heat between the hands.

3 Separate the hands a few more centimetres. See if you can still feel the energy between the hands.

4 Gradually see how far you can separate the hands without losing the connection between them.

Ball of energy

In a massage there is a natural transference of energy and hands naturally give off heat. The next three exercises are fun ways to feel the energy created by your hands or your partner's hands.

1 Bring your hands about 5 cm apart with the palms facing each other. Try to feel the energy between the hands.

2 Slowly move the hands back and forth trying to play with the energy between them.

3 Circle the hands around each other trying to form a ball of energy.

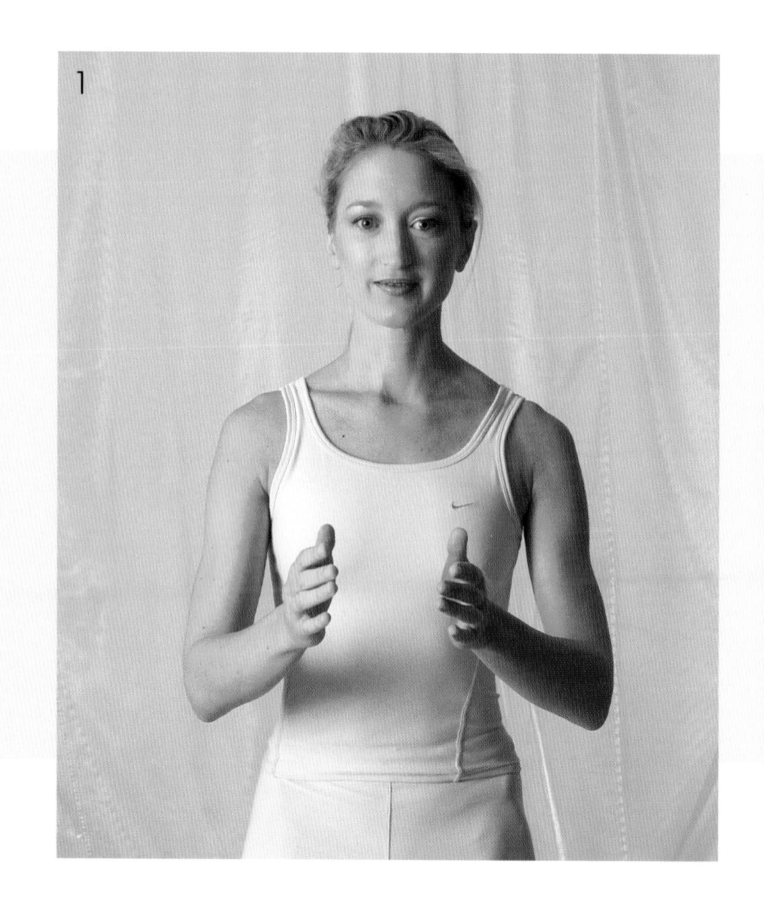
1

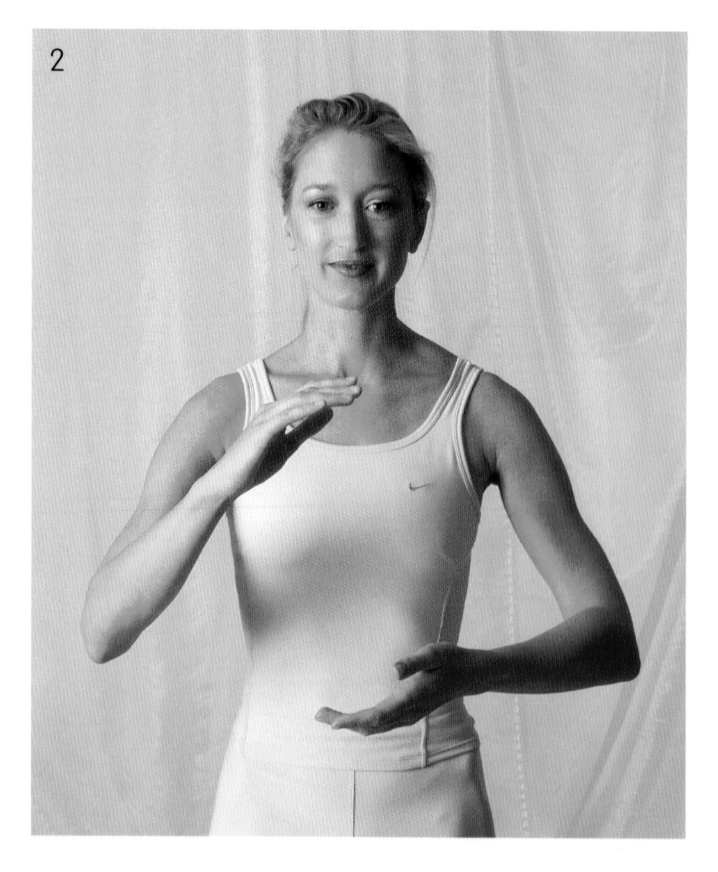
2

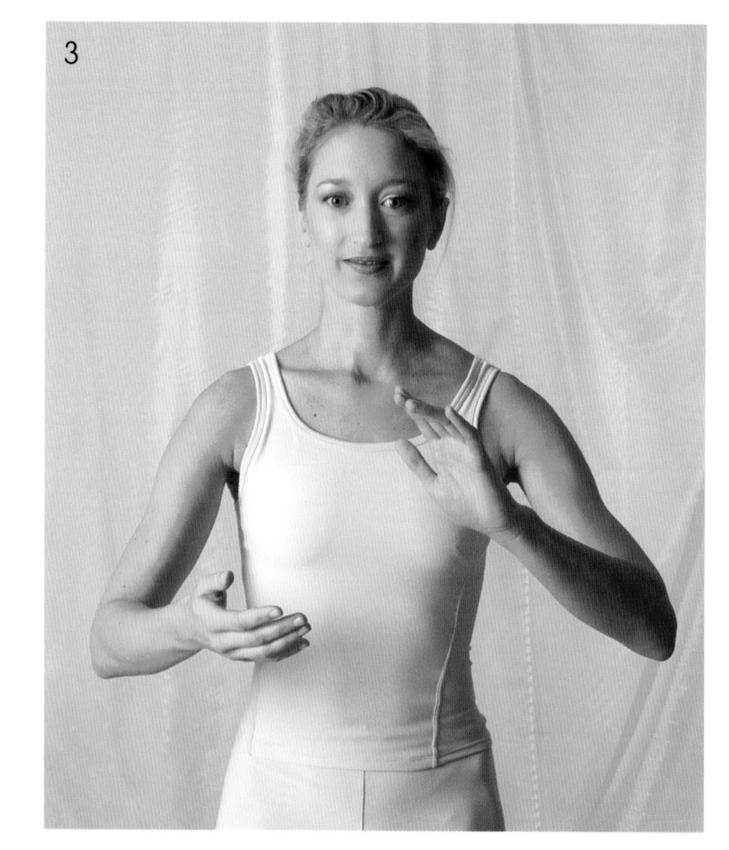
3

Connecting to your partner

Part of giving a massage is connecting to the person you are with. Here are some exercises to help relaxation and to connect the energies between you for an optimum massage.

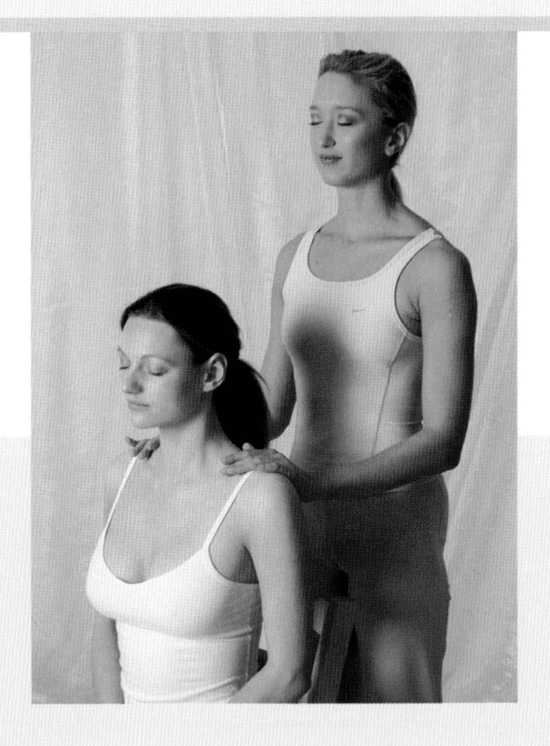

Hands on shoulders

Ask your partner to sit on a chair in front of you. Stand behind them and place your hands on their shoulders. Close your eyes and ask your partner to do the same. Feel the energy passing between the palms of your hands and your partner's shoulders.

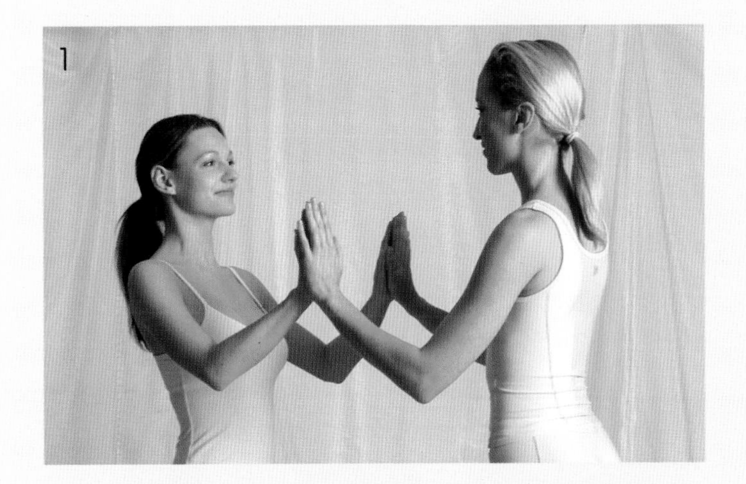

1

Partner work

1 Stand or sit facing your partner with the palms of your hands touching each other. Feel the heat given off by your hands touching.

2 Move your palms 23 cm apart. See if you can still feel the energy between you and your partner.

3 Separate the hands a few more centimetres. Try to retain the connection between you.

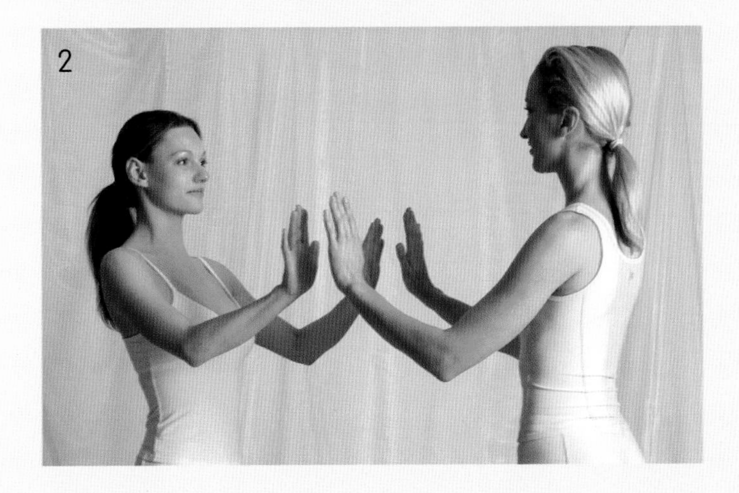

2

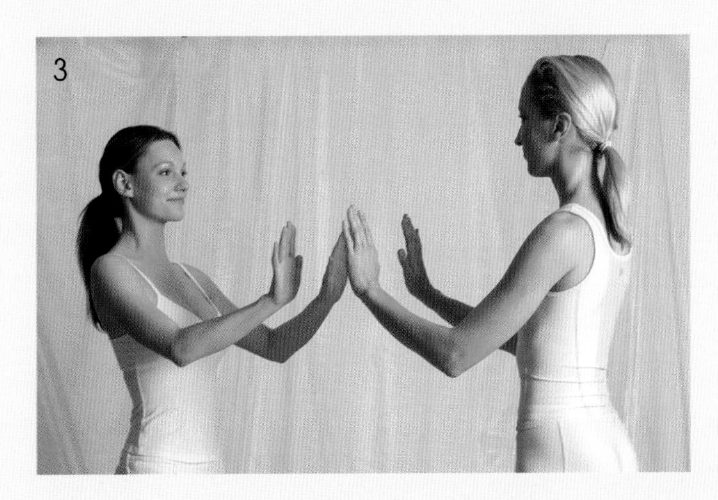

3

How to use this book

This book is divided into three sections (followed by another on advanced massage) . Each section contains a series of strokes and then shows you how to use them when giving a massage. Read about each stroke and then practise it. Once you are familiar with the movements, try to connect the strokes so that the transition is smooth from one to another. These massages are just to give you a starting point. Combine the strokes in any way you feel comfortable. Each massage has a reference guide at the end. Once you are familiar with the strokes this acts as an easy reminder page.

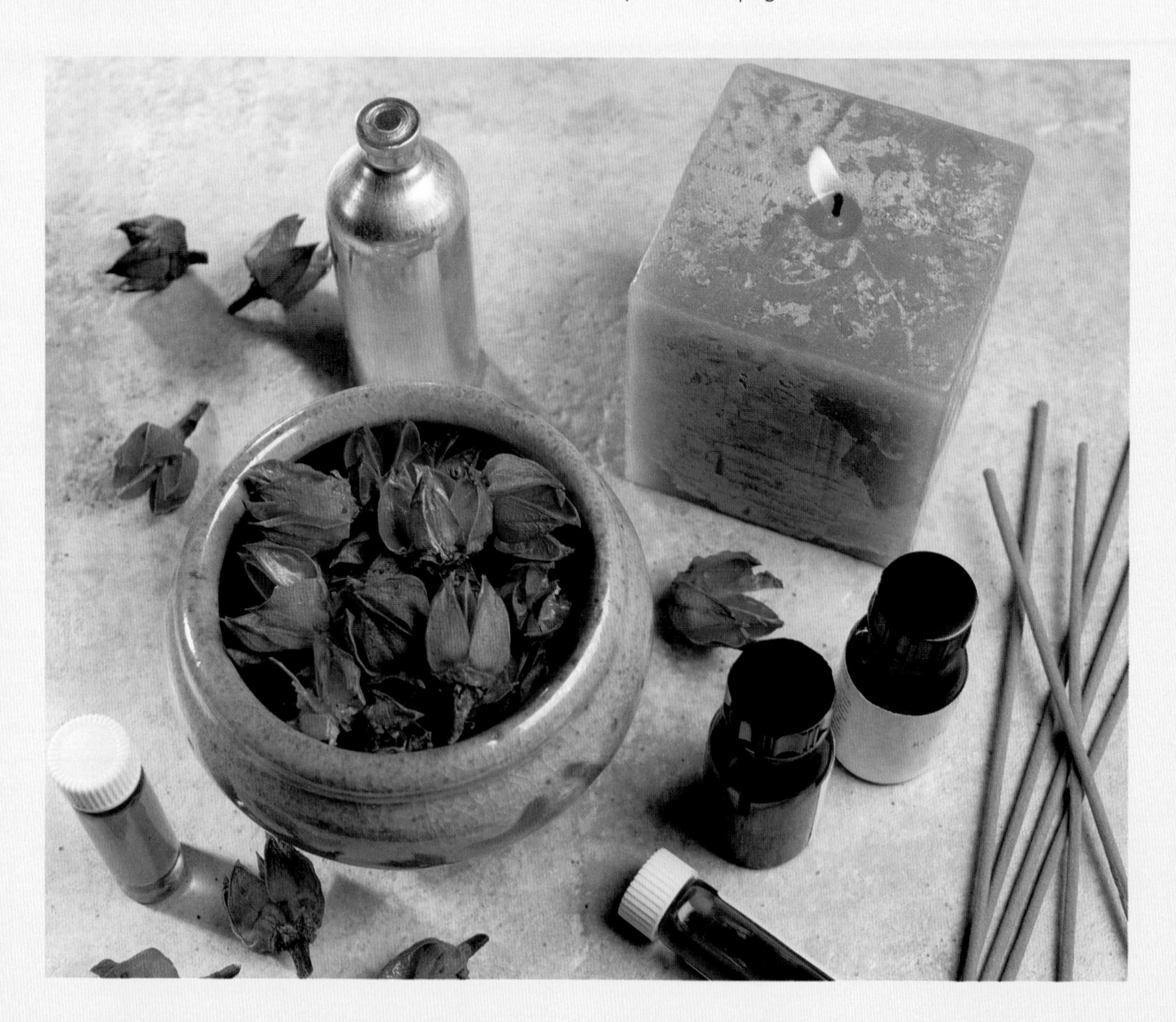

Basic techniques

This section looks at the basic strokes of massage, and then guides you through a relaxing massage based on these strokes.

There are many different strokes you can use when giving a massage. Start with the basic strokes. Read about each one and then practise it. Once you get familiar with the movements, try to connect different strokes so that they transition smoothly from one to another. When the whole hand is making contact with the body, make sure you apply pressure firmly and evenly throughout the palm and fingers.

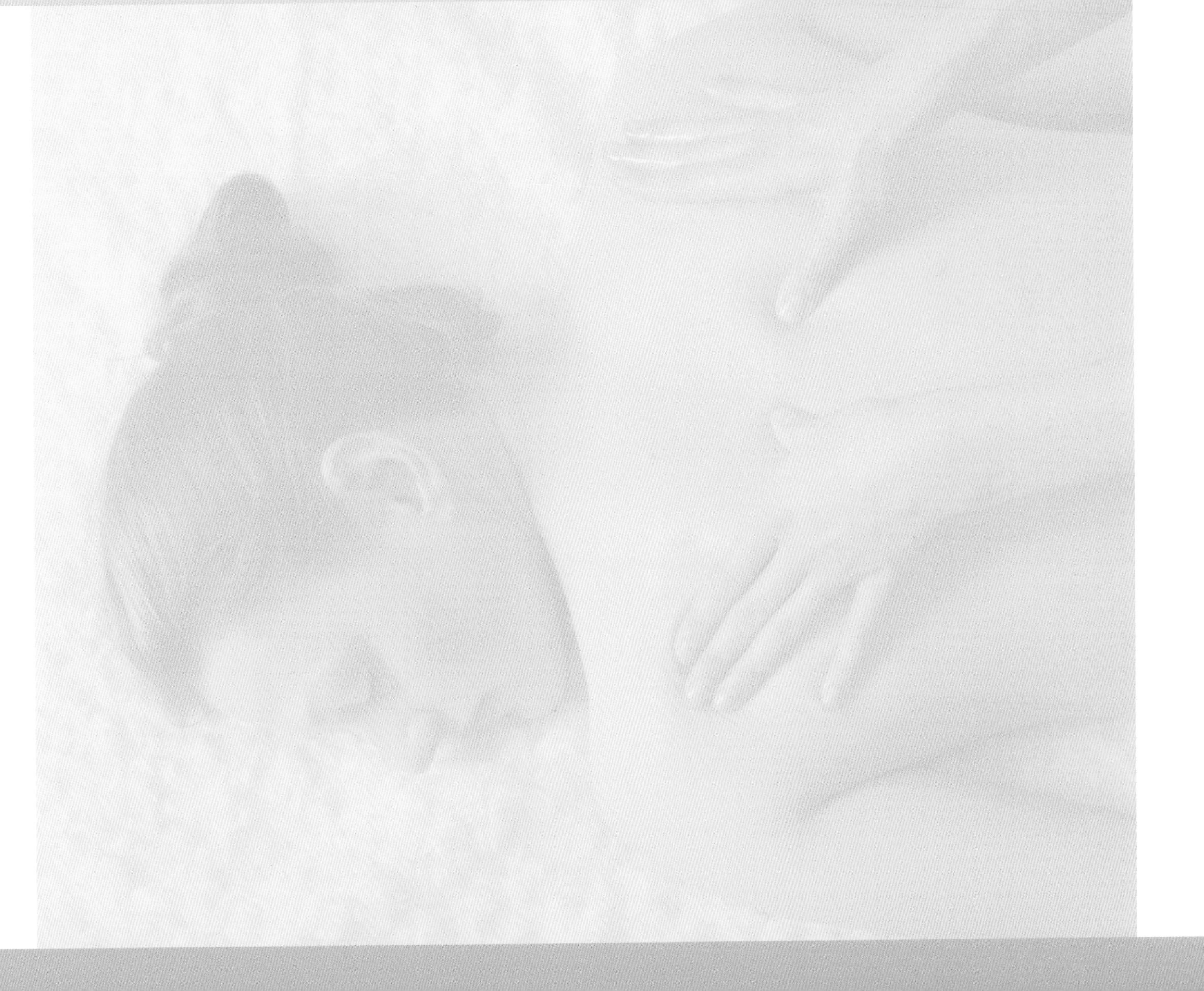

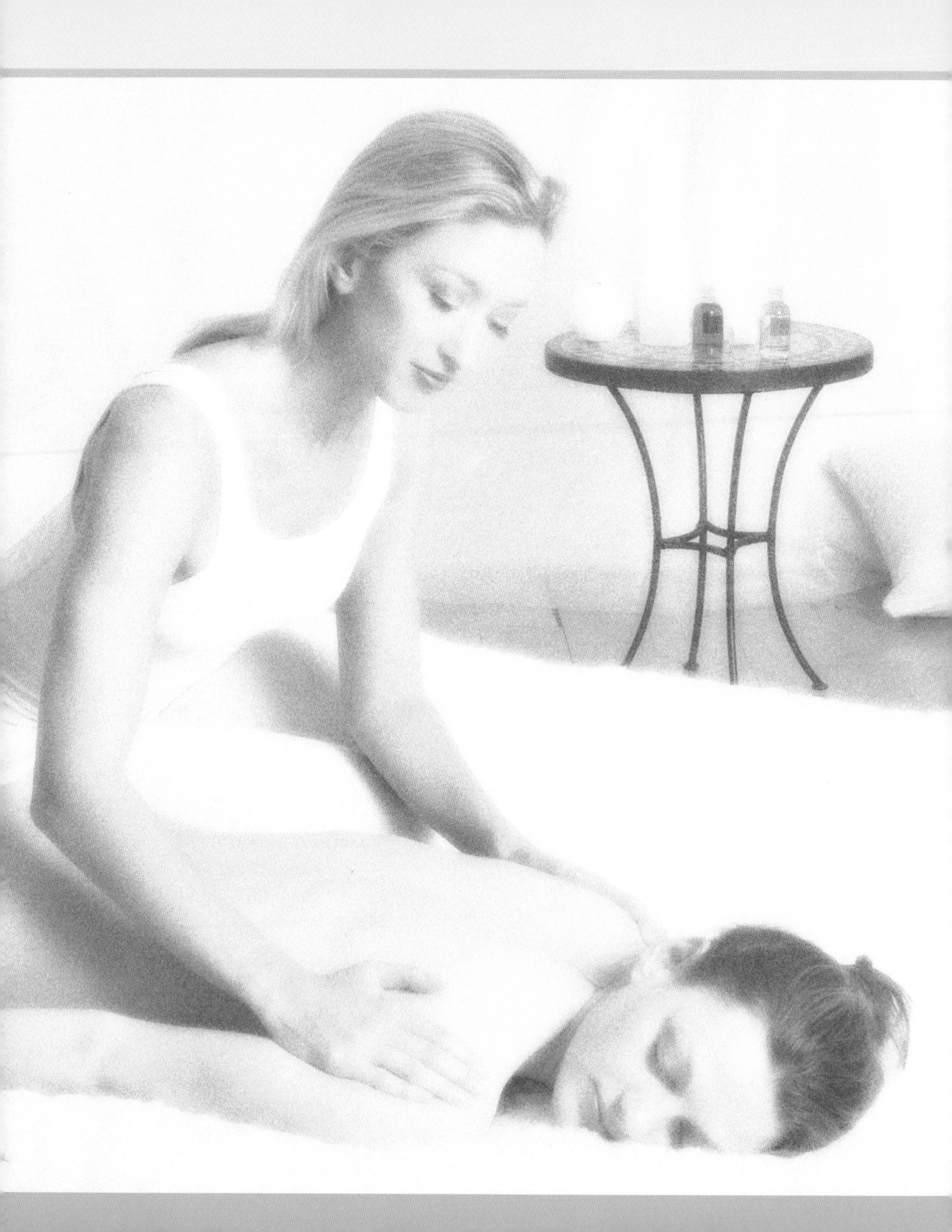

Strokes

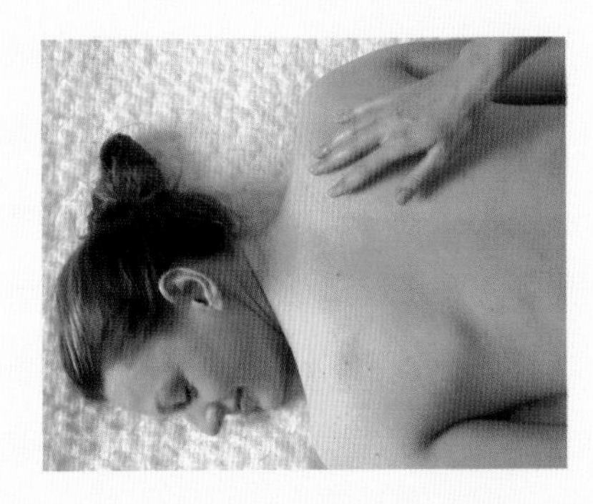

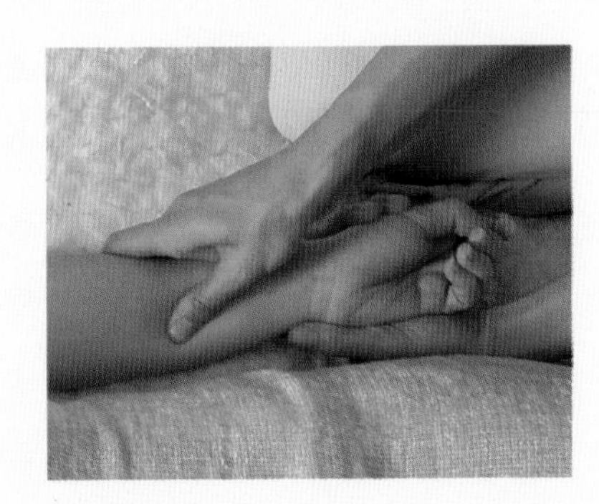

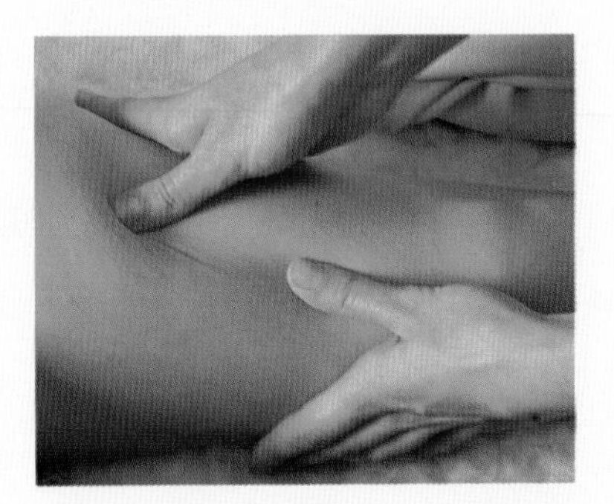

The techniques on the following pages are excellent basic strokes that you will find yourself returning to many times. They can be used on most parts of the body and are relaxing and soothing. Do not forget to assess the pressure you use when learning these techniques. Ask your partner if the pressure is too hard or too light, and adjust your movements accordingly.

Effleurage

Effleurage is the primary stroke in massage. It is derived from the French word effleurer, meaning to stroke. The stroke is used to initiate the massage, spread the oil and connect strokes throughout the massage. On initial contact, use light strokes, trying to sense if there are any areas of tightness or tension. Let the hands mould themselves to the contour of the body, gradually pressing more deeply as they go towards the heart and more lightly as they return. Make sure the whole hand has continuous contact with the body at all times.

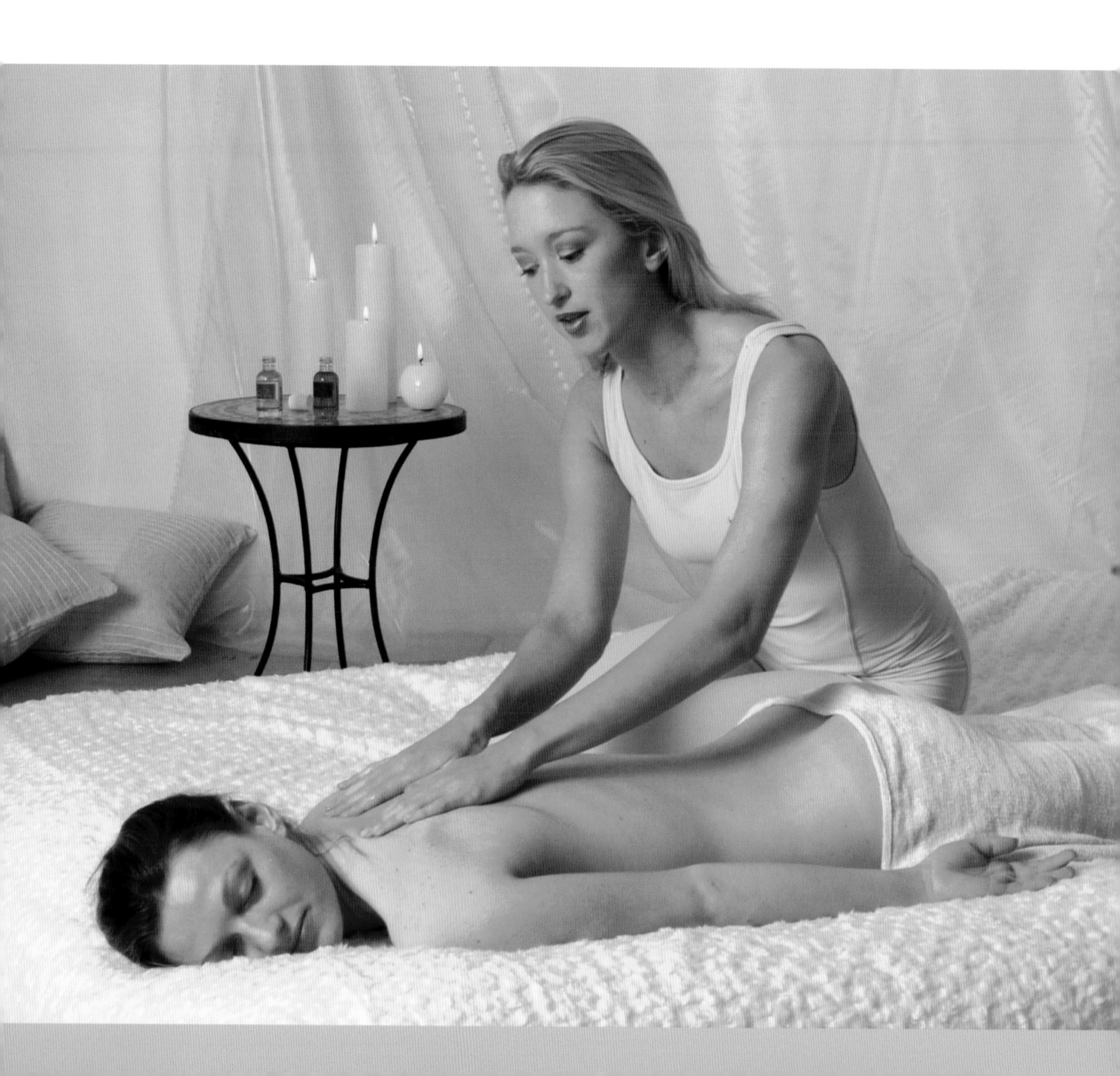

Basic effleurage

To the back

1 Place the hands on either side of the base of the spine with your fingers towards the head and your thumbs about 5 cm apart.

2 Pressing evenly through the hands, glide them along the spine.

3 Then glide across the neck.

4 Then the shoulders and lightly down the outside of the back.

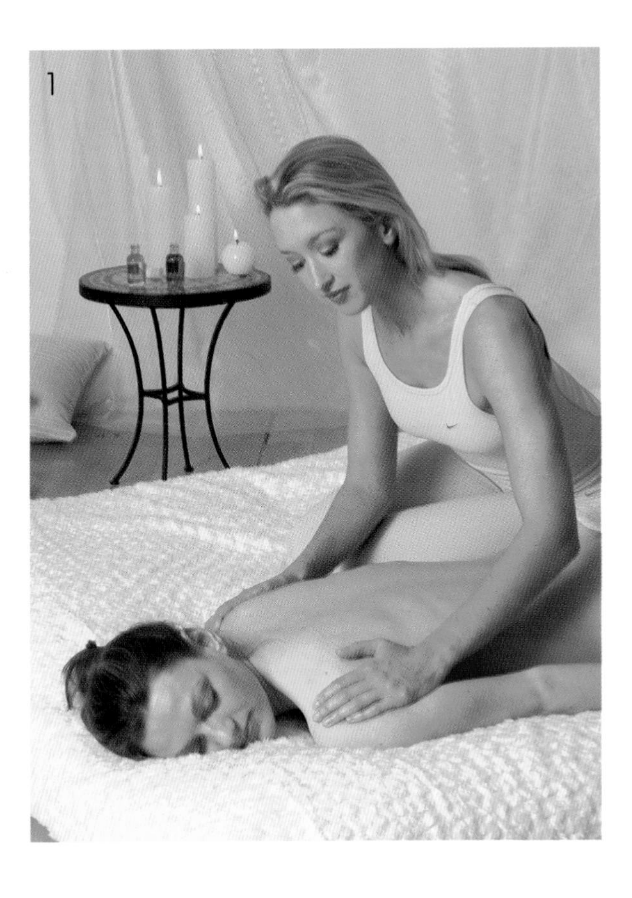
1

Note: Keep one continuous motion the whole time, gradually working deeper towards the heart, and lighter away.

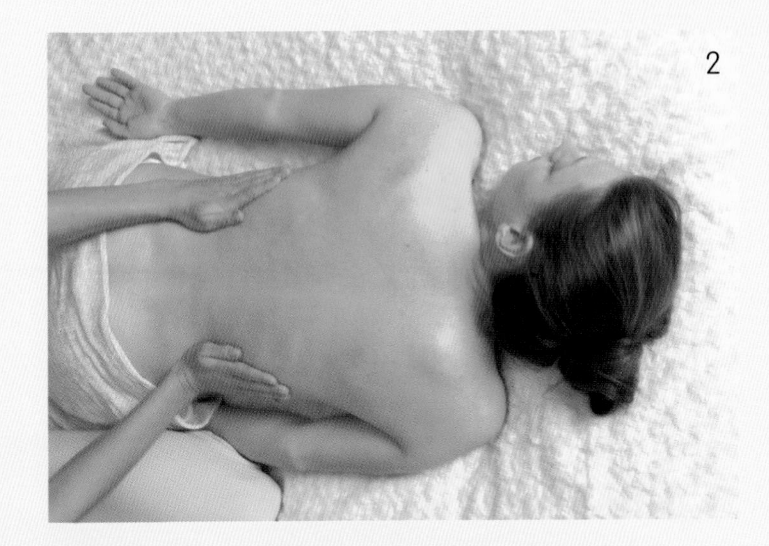
2

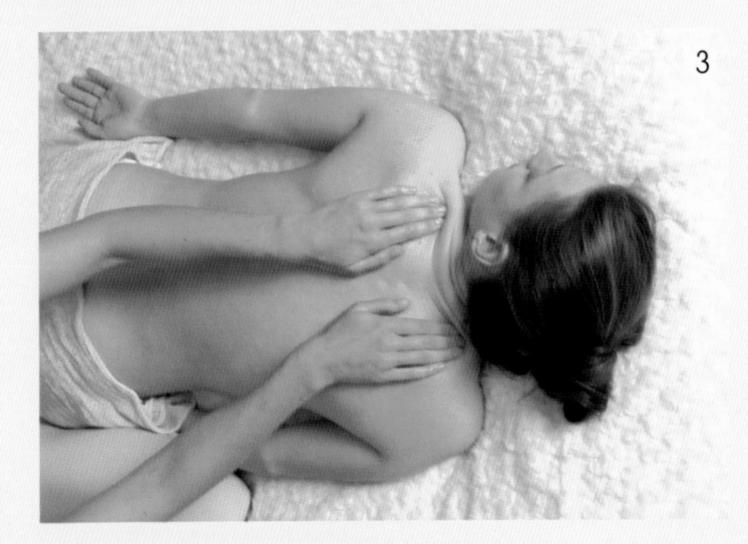
3

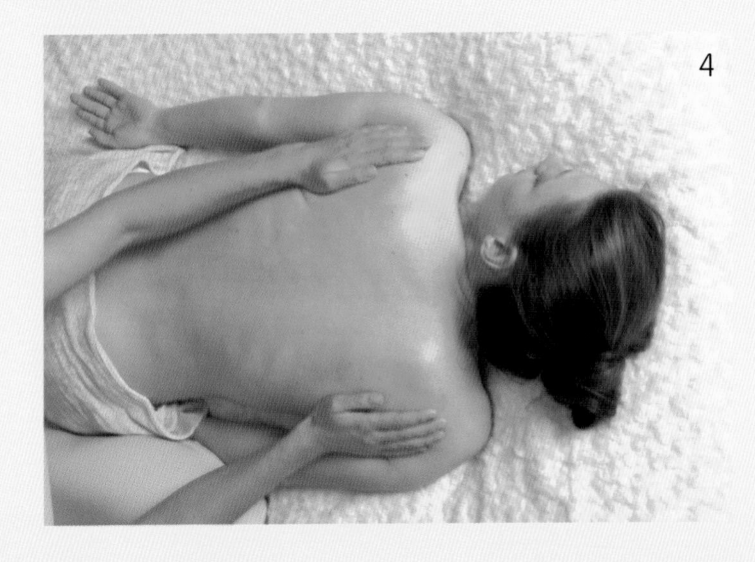
4

To the legs

1 Start with both hands on the ankle with your thumbs together and the fingertips towards your partner's head.

2 With even pressure, slide the hands up towards the hip, avoiding the back (or front) of the knee.

3 Lightly bring the hands back along the slides of the leg, keeping contact with the whole hand.

Smoothly repeat with long, continuous strokes.

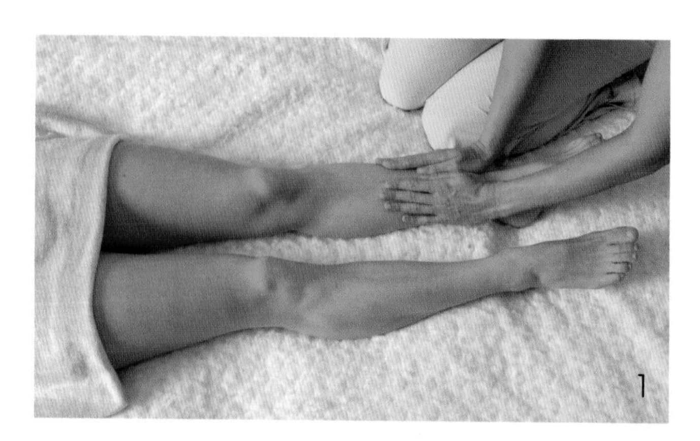
1

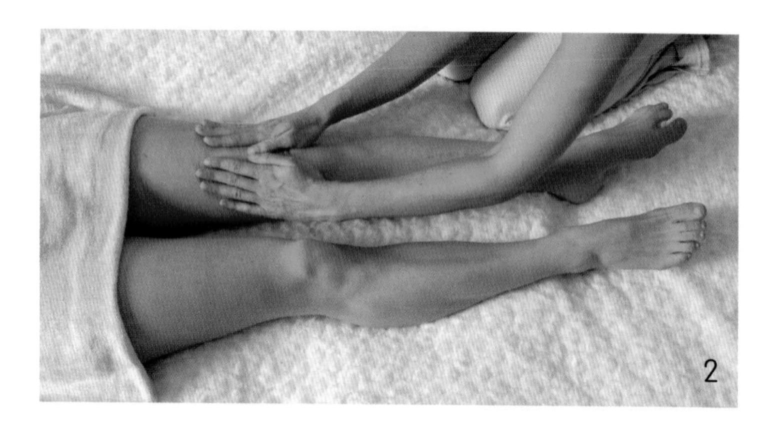
2

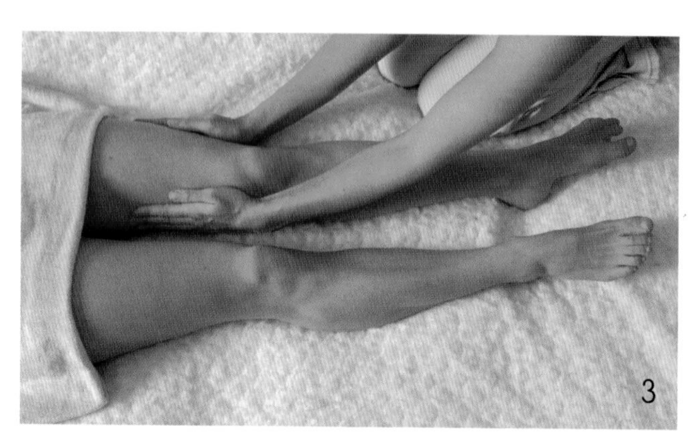
3

To the arms

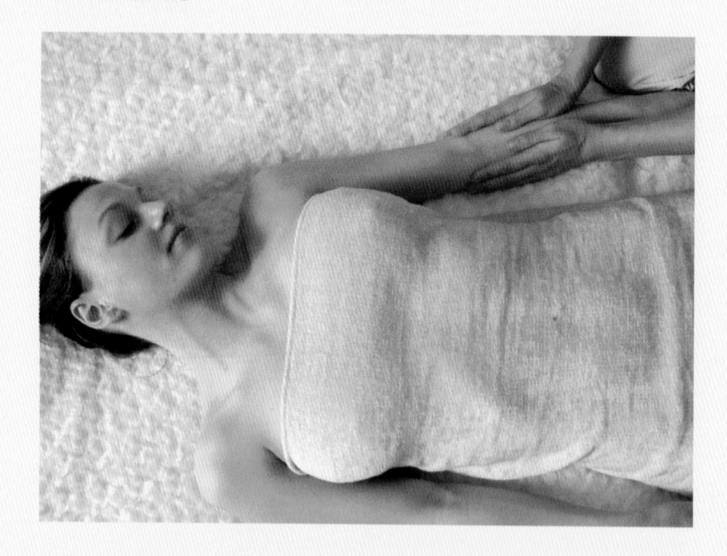

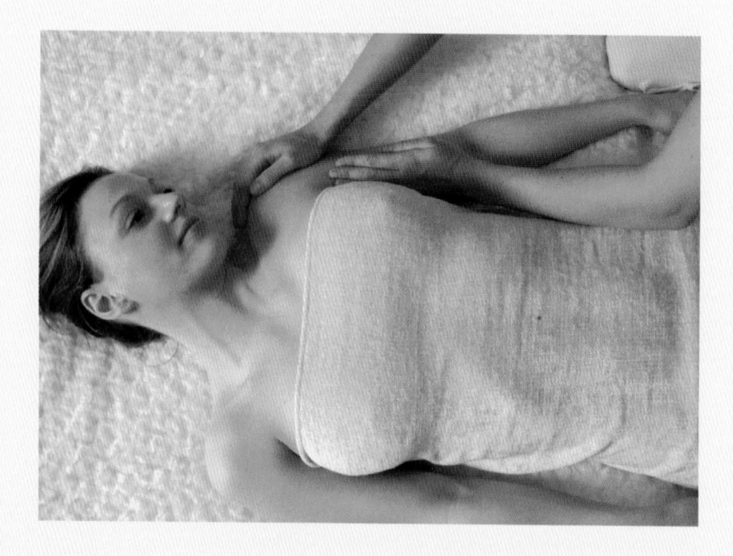

1 Start with the hands on your partner's wrist, the fingertips towards their shoulder. Glide the hands up to the shoulder, being careful not to put pressure on the elbow joint.

2 Slide the hands back along the outside of the arm.

Alternating effleurage

Effleurage is a great stroke both before and after you have worked deeply into an area of the body. It helps to flush the toxins out of the area and acts as a smooth transition between strokes.

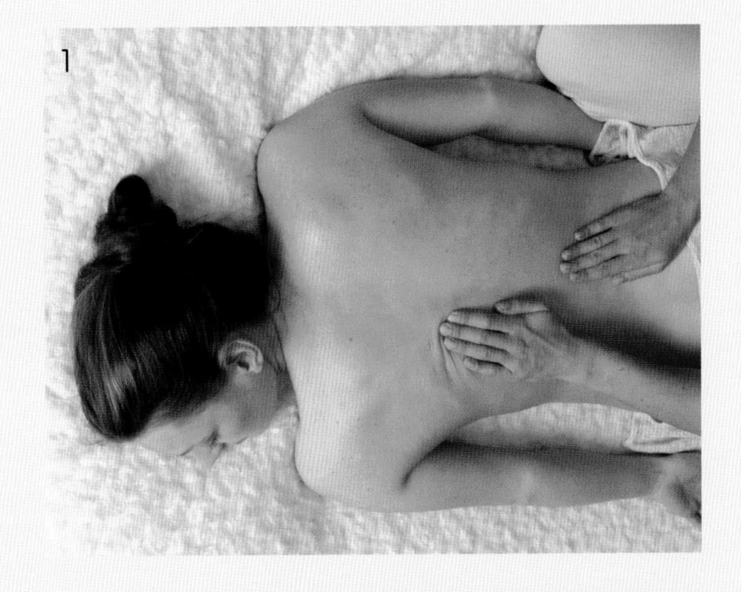

To the back

1 Start with the palms at the base of the spine and the fingertips towards the head. Glide the left hand up the left side of the spine to the base of the neck.

2 Mould the hand to the contour of the body as you press your left hand towards their left shoulder.

3 As the left hand is sliding down the left side of the body, start gliding the right hand up the right side of the spine and towards the right shoulder.

4 Keep alternating hands, pressing firmly up the side of the spine, and gently down the outside of the back.

Note: never put pressure straight onto the spine.

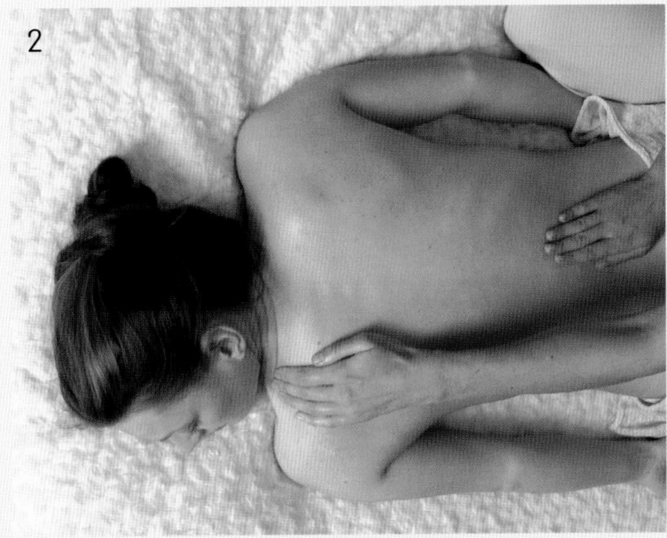

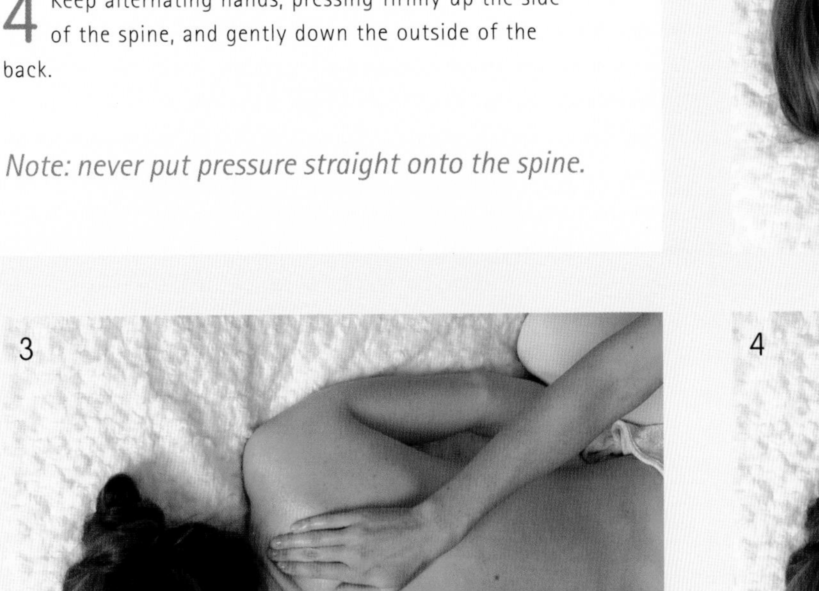

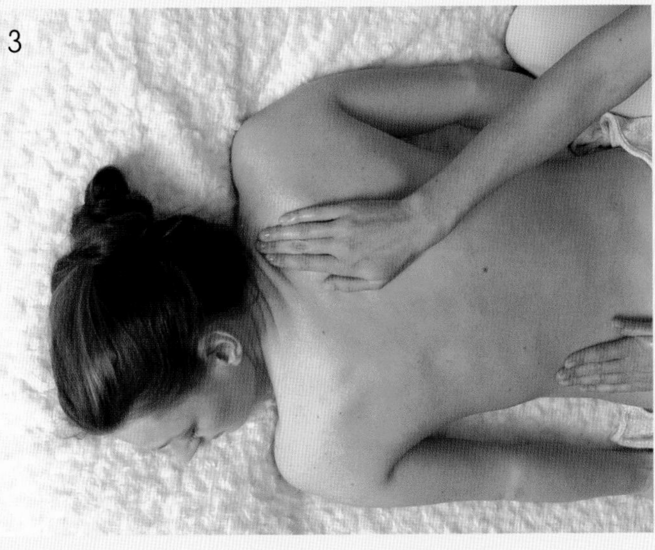

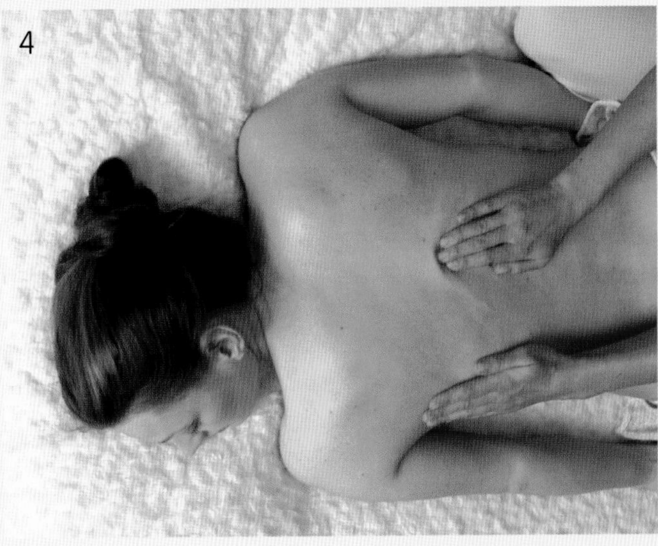

To the legs

Start with both hands at the ankle, the fingertips towards the hip. Glide the left hand along the contours of the leg, avoiding the back (or front) of the knee. Lightly slide the right hand down the outside of the leg. When the right hand almost returns to the ankle, start sliding the left hand up the leg.

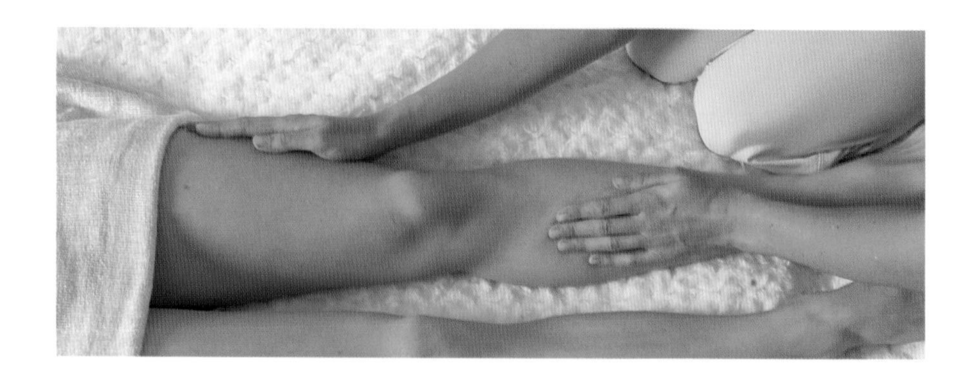

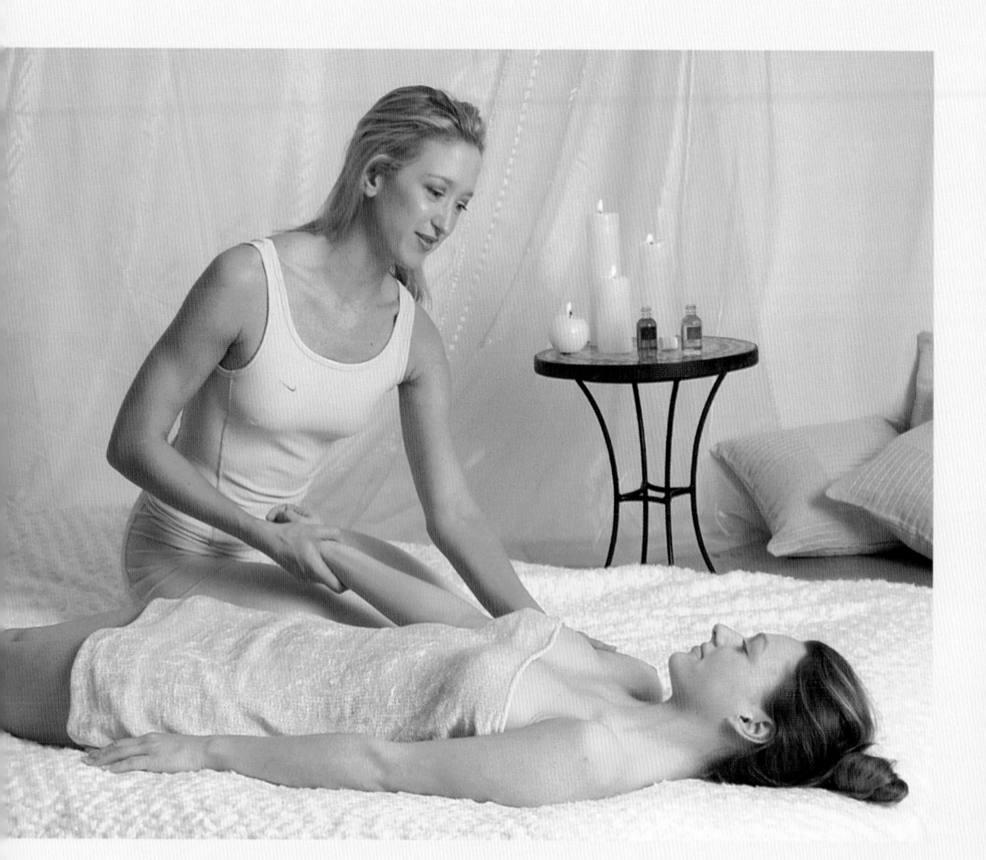

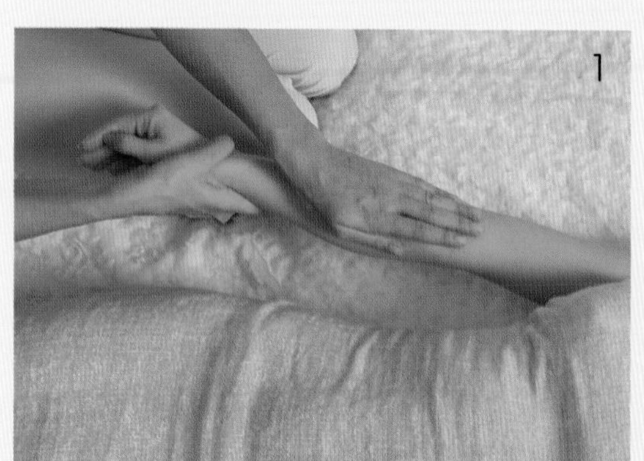

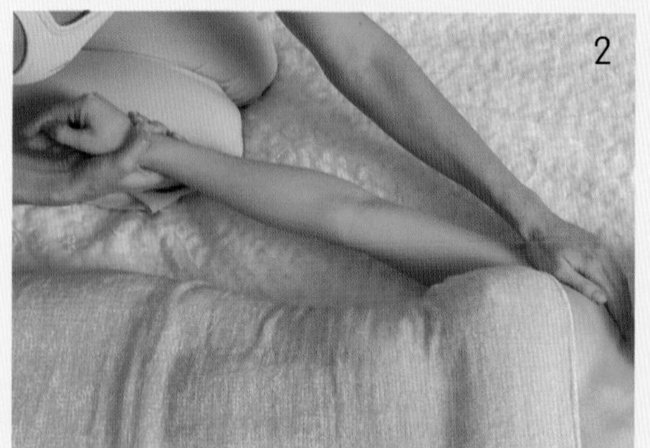

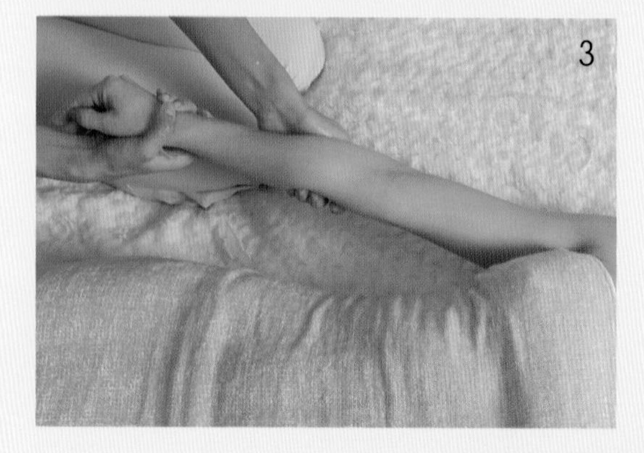

To the arms

1 Start with both hands at the right wrist. Hold the wrist lightly with your right hand. Gently press the left hand up towards the shoulder, avoiding the elbow joint.

2 Circle the shoulder with the hand.

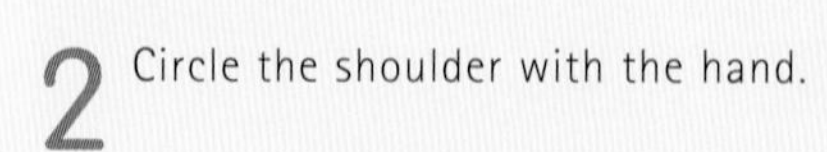

3 Then slide it down the back of the arm.

Repeat with the left hand.

Kneading

The best image for this stroke is to think of kneading dough. Kneading squeezes the toxins out of the muscles and brings the blood to the surface of the skin. It is relaxing and soothing due to the rhythm and flow created through the movement. Kneading can be performed on any of the fleshy areas of the body.

To the back

1 Start at the side of your partner. Reach over to the opposite side with your fingertips facing down and your thumbs and elbows out. Pick up some of the flesh along the waist in one hand. As you gently squeeze it, bring the flesh towards the other hand and release.

2 As you release, grab the flesh with your opposite hand and repeat. Think of passing the dough between the hands with smooth, rhythmic strokes. The pressure is more localised on the squeeze and more sweeping on the release.

Note: try to get your body weight shifting from side to side with the movement. This will alleviate the pressure on the hands.

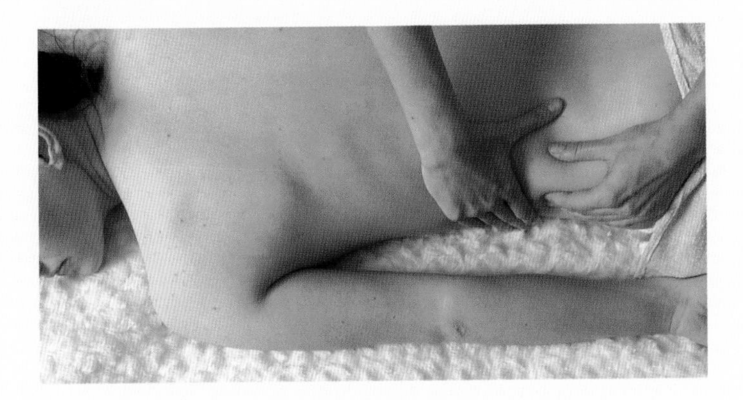

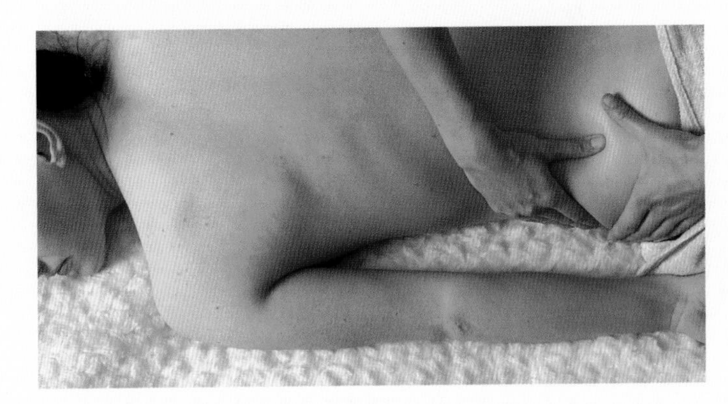

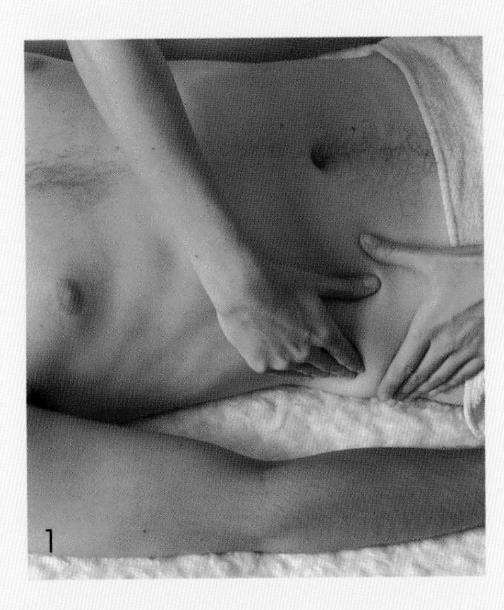
1

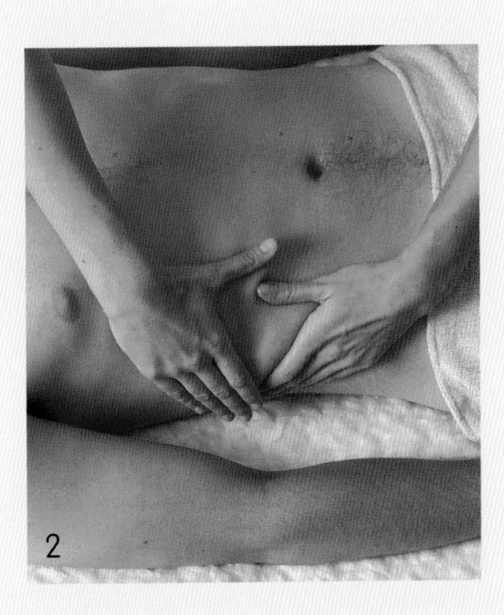
2

To the stomach

1 The stomach is a very sensitive area. Kneel on the opposite side of the area you are working on. Place the hands lightly on the other side of the waist with the fingers facing down and the thumbs and elbows out. Pick up some of the skin and slide it across to the other hand.

2 As you release the skin, start picking it up with the opposite hand. Work very gently as you slide the hands back and forth along the sides of the body.

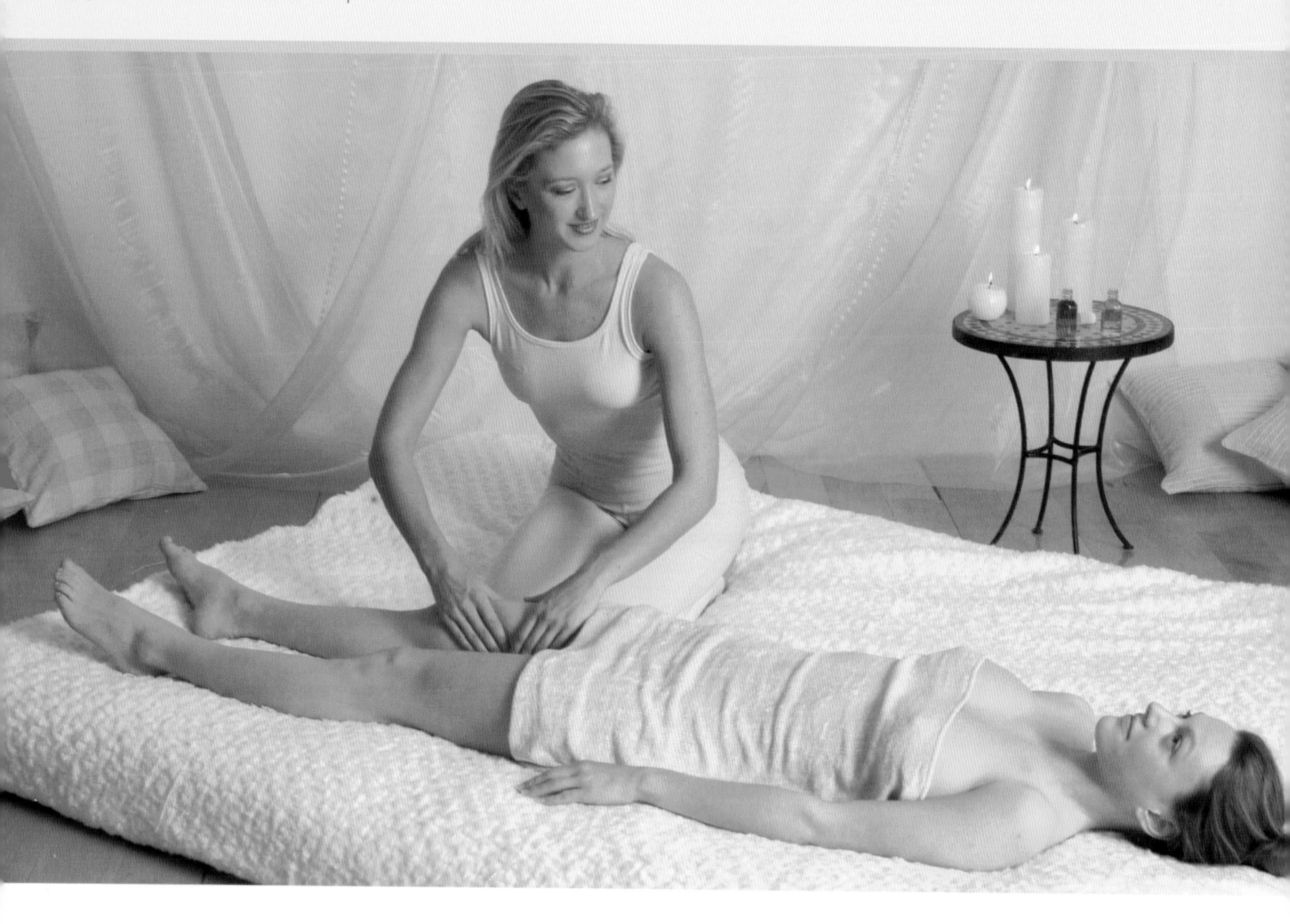

To the thigh or calf

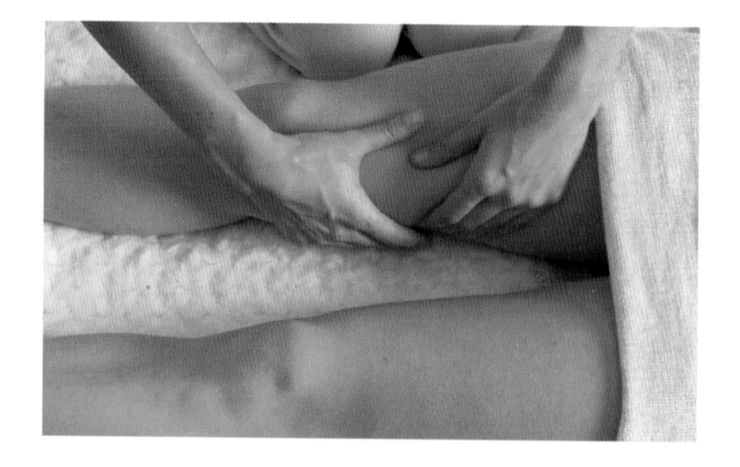

1 Start facing the top of the thigh. Place the hands on the inner thigh with the fingertips facing down and the thumbs and elbows out. Think of moving the thigh muscles back and forth between your hands as you shift your weight back and forth.

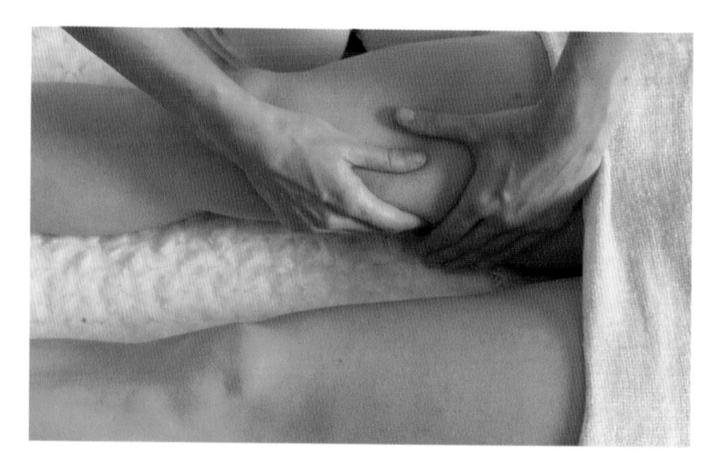

2 As you move the flesh to the right, shift your weight to the right. As you move to the left, shift your weight back to the left.

Wringing

This movement lifts the muscle away from the bone. It squeezes out the toxins in a similar fashion to wringing out a towel. It should be performed on large, fleshy areas, but can also be performed lightly on the arms.

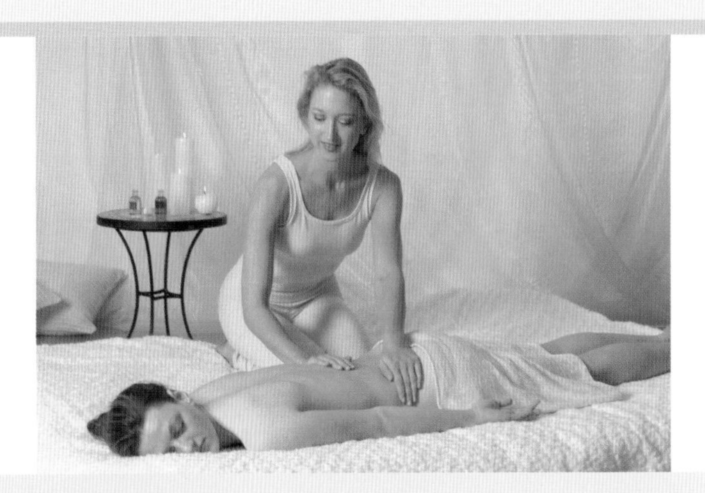

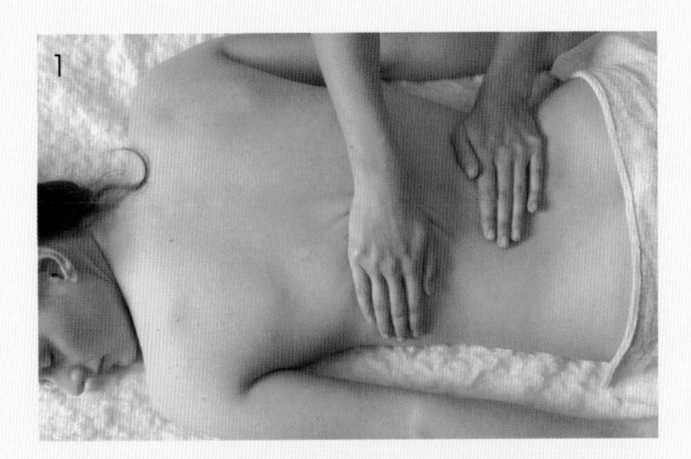

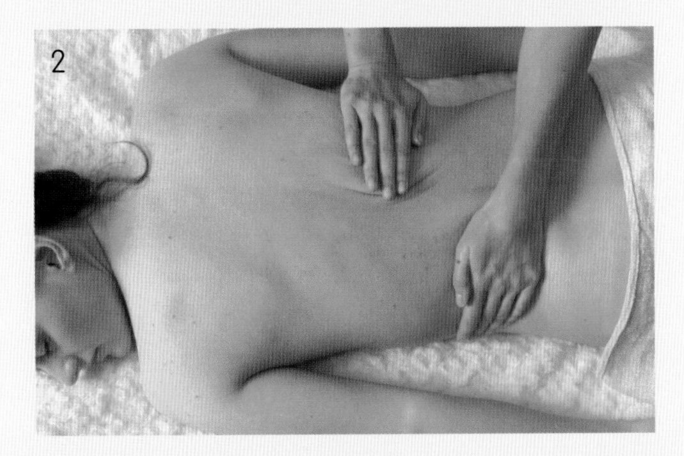

To the back

1 Place the hands on either side of the back with your fingertips facing away from you. Press in and lift the muscle up as you slide the hands across the back in opposite directions. You want the hands to be 58 cm apart so that the muscles gently twist without creating a burning sensation.

2 Continue sliding the hands in opposite directions to the other side. The pressure is in towards the muscle as you are lifting up, and relaxing as you bring the hands back down.

To the leg

1 Start with both hands on opposite sides of the leg and the fingers facing away from you. Pick up the muscles as your hands glide in opposite directions over the leg. Make sure your hands are sufficiently apart so that the flesh moves but there is no discomfort.

2 The hands should end up on the opposite side from the one they started on.

Repeat several times.

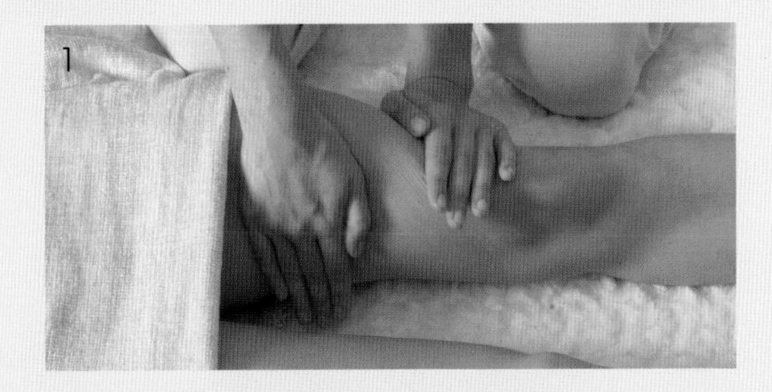

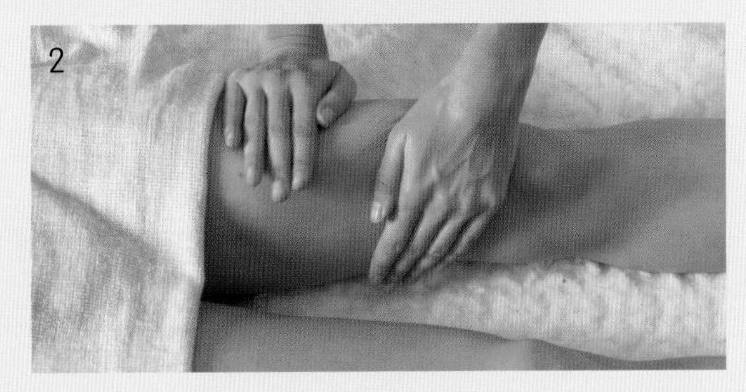

Note: this stroke should be performed on the front and back of the thigh and the calf. The shin does not have enough flesh for this stroke to be beneficial.

Friction

Friction penetrates the muscles more deeply, breaking up lactic acid and releasing toxins. Friction is performed with the pads of the thumbs in small circles. This stroke can get quite tiring; it is easier if you keep the thumb joint stable and move the whole arm in a circular motion. This puts less pressure on the thumbs and allows deeper penetration.

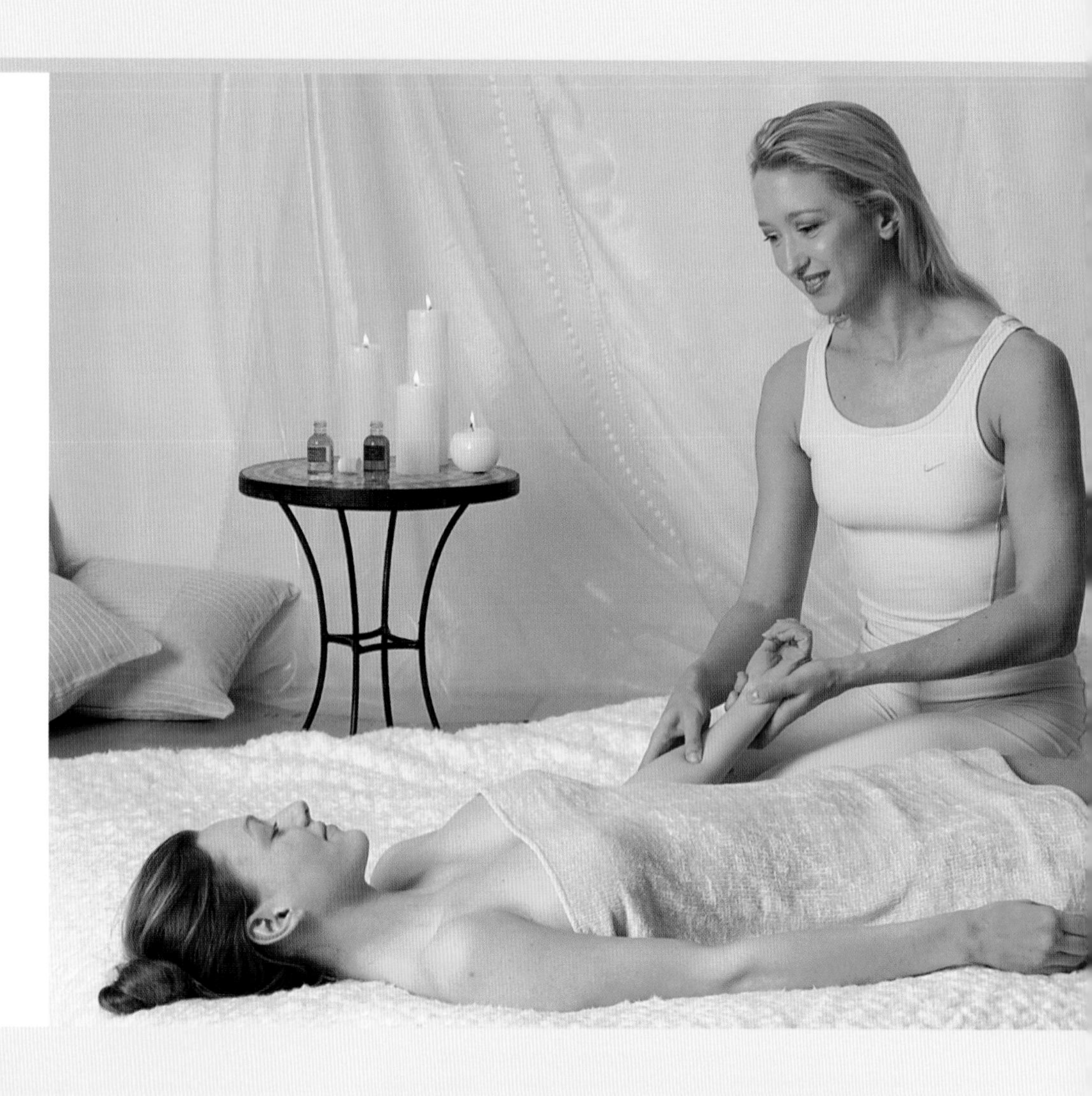

To the back

Start at the base of the spine with the thumbs on either side. Lock the thumb joint and use your whole arm to make small circles up either side of the spine towards the neck.

When the thumbs reach the neck, relax the hands and slide the whole hand along the neck towards the shoulders. Glide the hands down the outside of the body towards the hips.

Circle the hands to the original position and repeat 3 times.

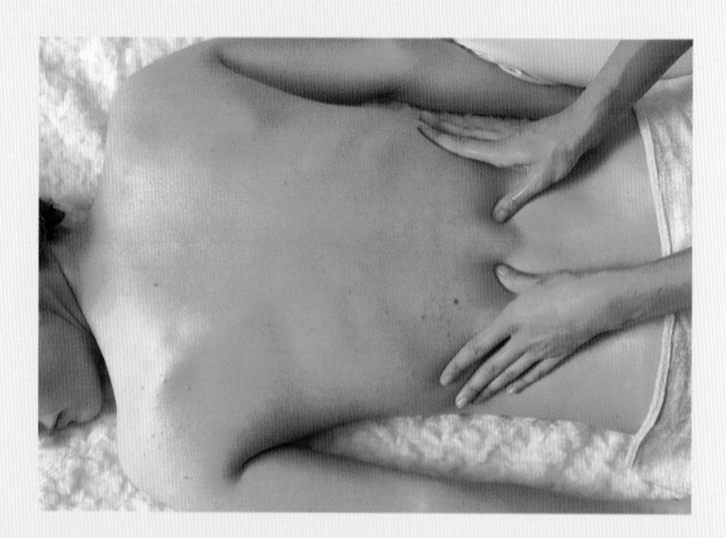

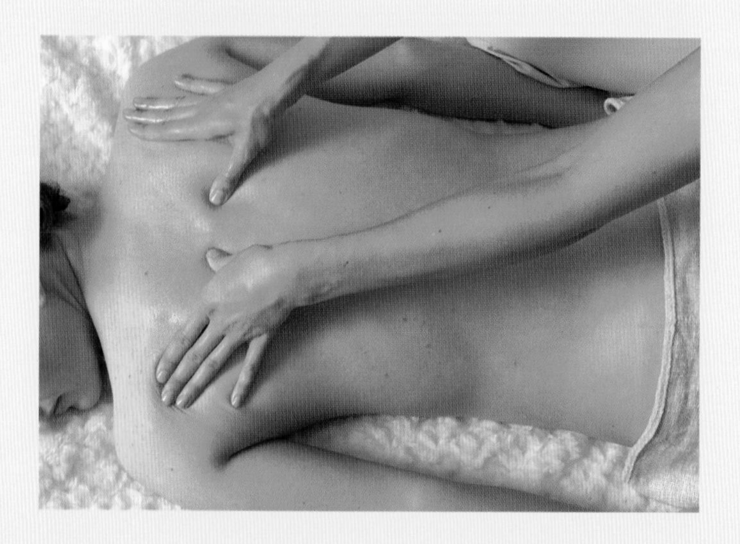

Note: many people hold tension in their lower backs. This stroke is great for breaking up tight muscles.

To the legs

Start with the thumbs just above the knee and the fingers relaxed to the sides. Make small, circular sweeping motions with the thumbs across the whole thigh area. Work deeply, trying to break up any tense areas.
Repeat to the calf, making sure you do not press on the back of the knee.

Note: do not stay on one area for too long or it can feel sore and overworked.

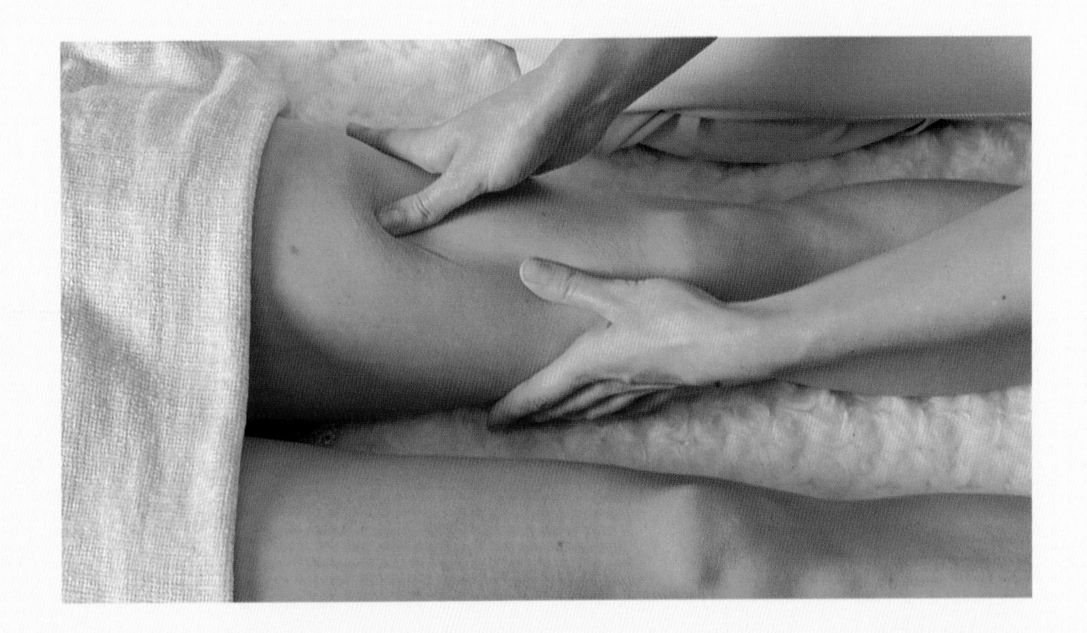

To the arms

Start with the hands at the wrists. Circle the thumbs up towards the elbows, making sure you cover the whole forearm with the thumbs. Work the thumbs up the inside of the arm, then turn the palm over and repeat to the other side of the arm.

Repeat the same circular motion to the top of the arm. Place the thumbs on the top of the arm with your fingers underneath. Massage the underneath side of the arm with the fingers while the thumbs circle the top.

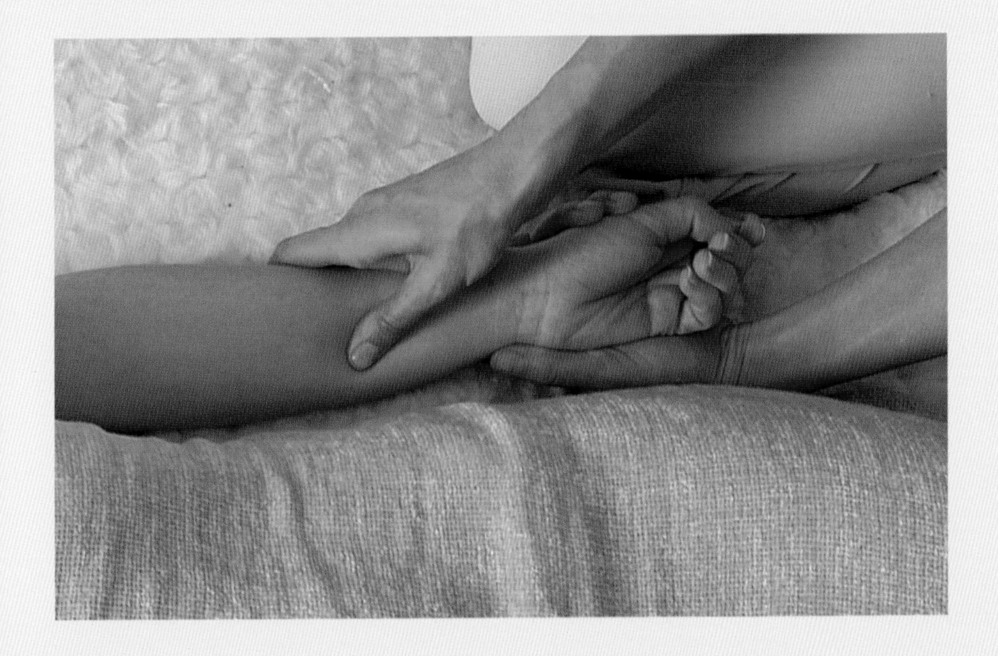

Tight knots

Friction is ideal for any localised areas of tension. Place the thumbs over the knot or tension. Make small circling motions with first one thumb, and then the other. Slowly work deeper into the area trying to break up the tension.

Note: this stroke should produce a tangible release of tension.
Do not stay on the area too long, as this can create soreness.

Feather stroking

This stroke is performed at the very end of each section of the body. It is the finishing touch before you pull the towel over that part and move on.

This stroke is performed moving away from the heart. Imagine your fingertips are light feathers, just barely touching the surface of the skin. Lightly drag the fingertips of one hand down the section you are working on. As that hand gets to the end, start the other hand lightly stroking down the body. Repeat three to four times.

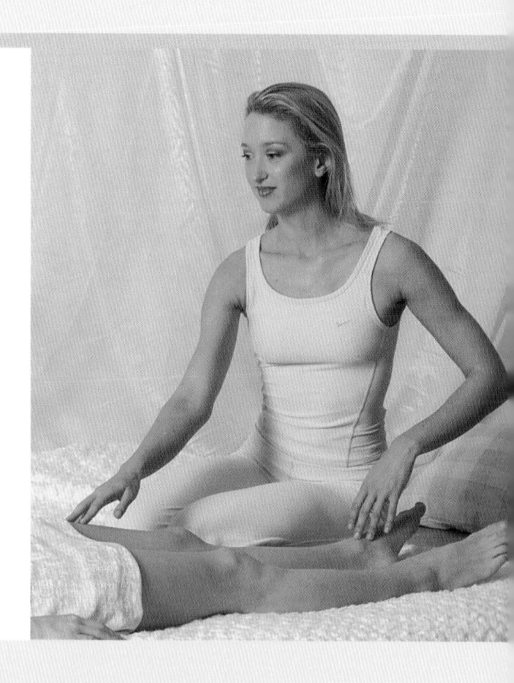

To the back

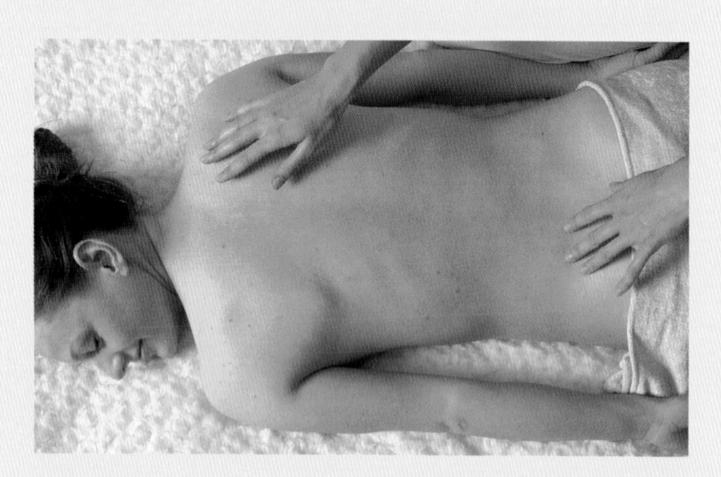

1 Start with the fingertips at the top of the shoulders. Stroke one hand lightly down the back like a cat. The fingertips should barely brush the back.

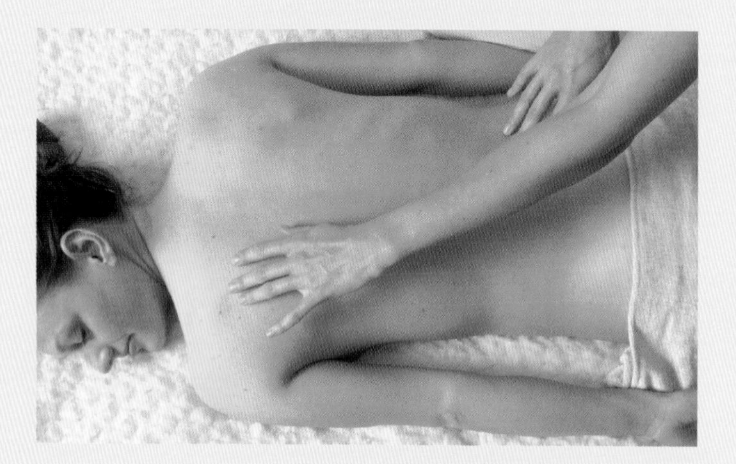

2 As one hand gets to the base of the spine, stroke the other hand down the back.

To the arms

Start with the fingertips of one hand at the shoulder. Slide the fingers down the arm, moulding to the contours of the arm. As the hand gets to the wrist, start the opposite hand moving down the arm.

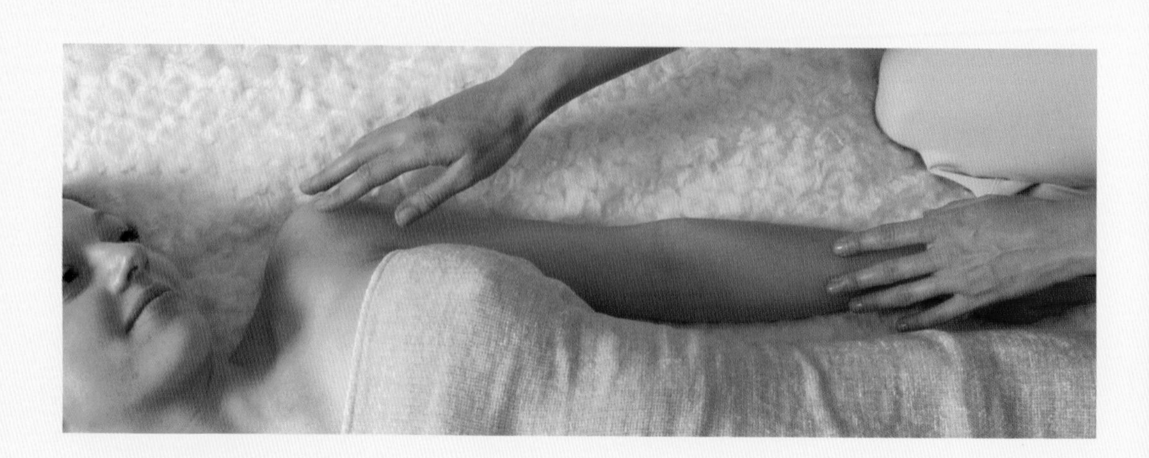

To the legs

Start with one hand at the top of the leg near the hip joint. Lightly caress the fingers down the leg. As one hand gets to the ankle, start the other hand gently gliding down the leg.

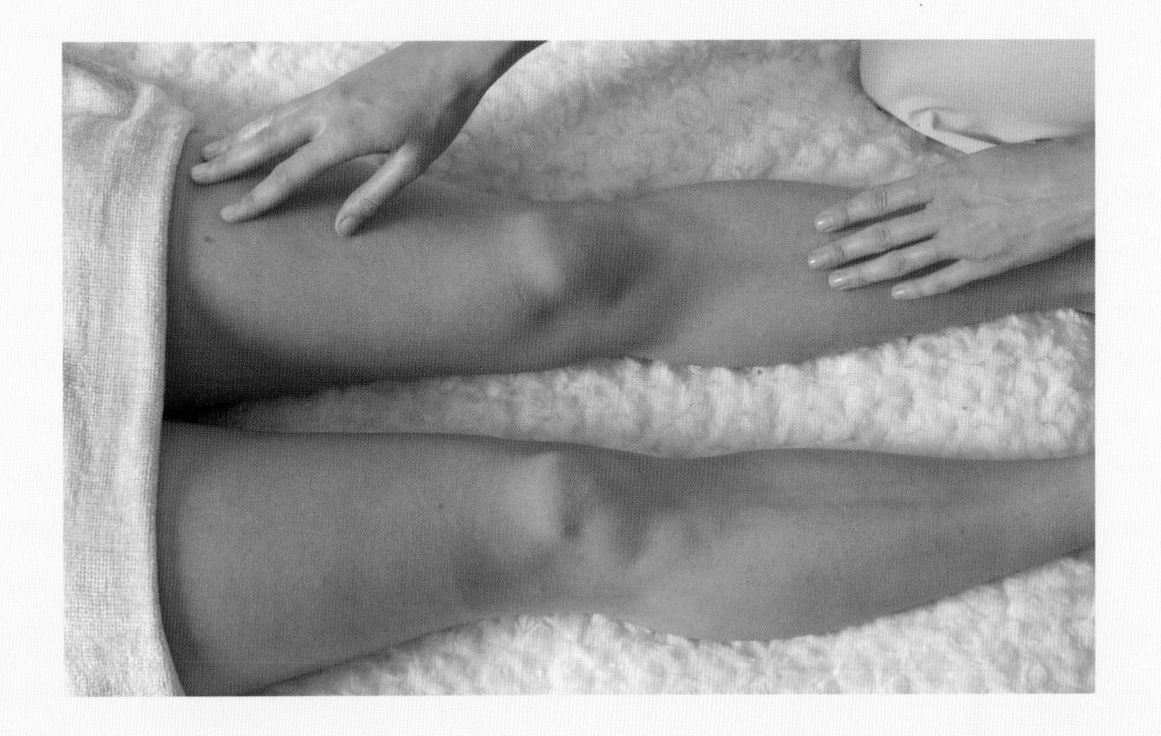

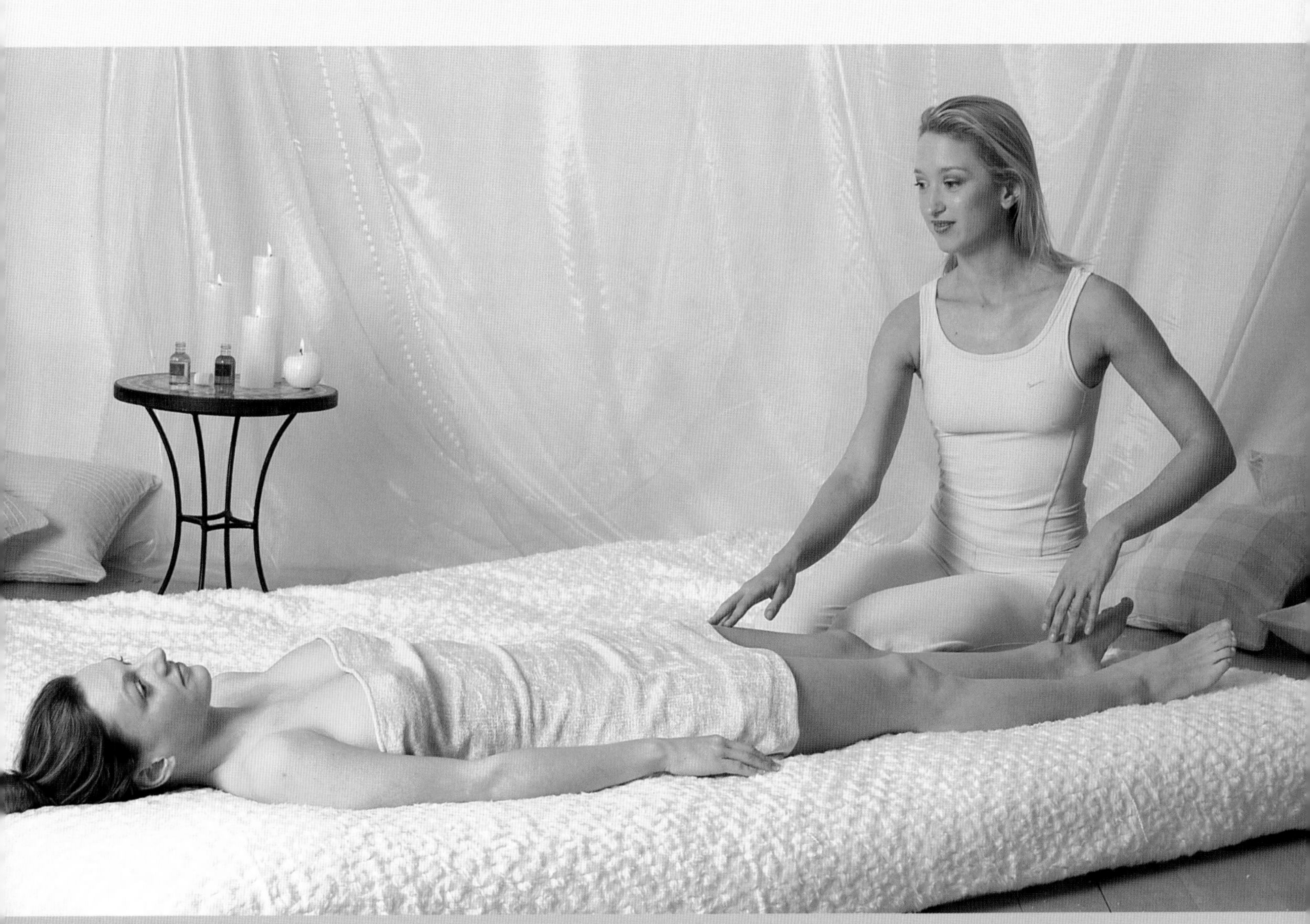

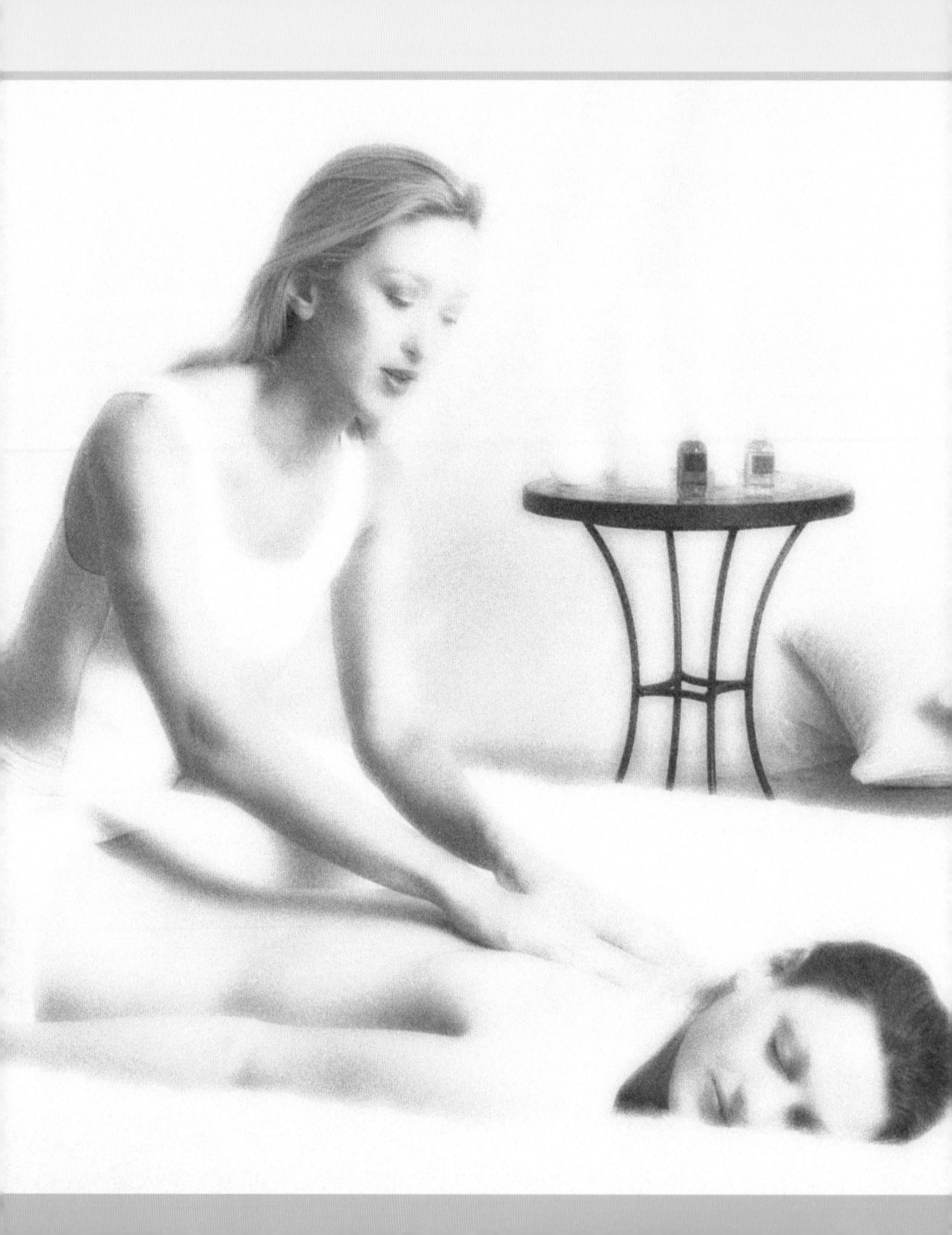

Relaxing massage

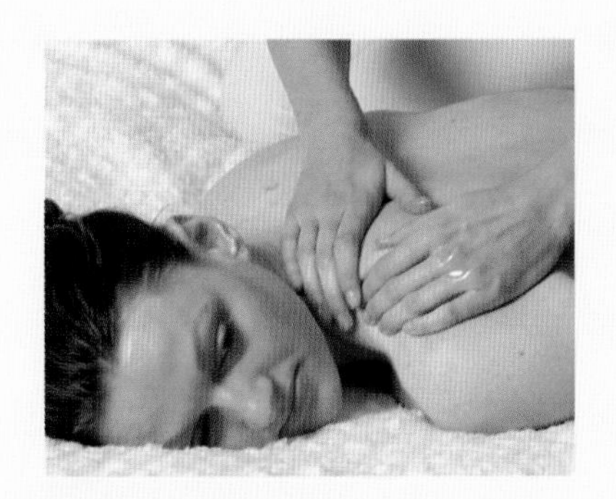

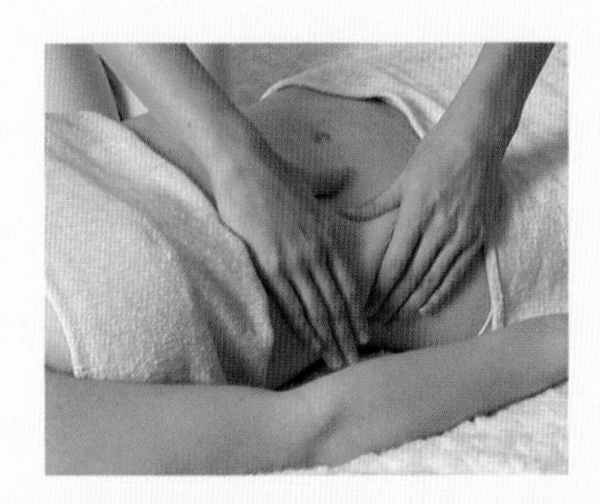

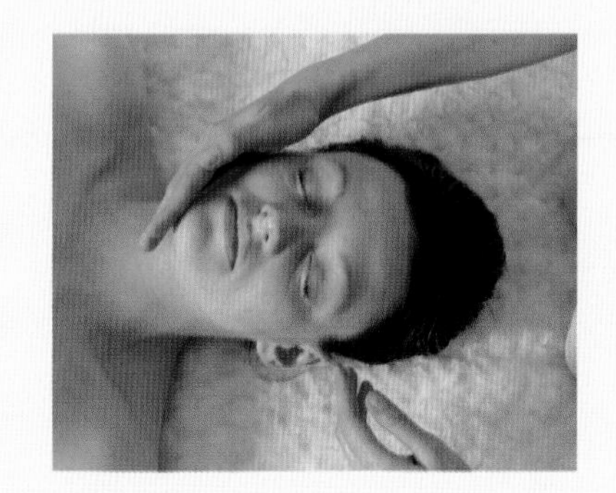

This series is designed to start out with simple strokes first, slowly working towards the more complicated movements. Work first on getting comfortable with the strokes. Then work on the flow between the movements, trying to make the transitions smooth and seamless. Start out with a light pressure and then gradually build up to deeper pressure. Ask your partner how it feels and adjust the pressure accordingly.

Start and end the massage with your partner completely covered in the towels except for their head. Only uncover the areas you are working on so that the person stays warm. If you are using essential oils, this also helps prevent the oils from evaporating.

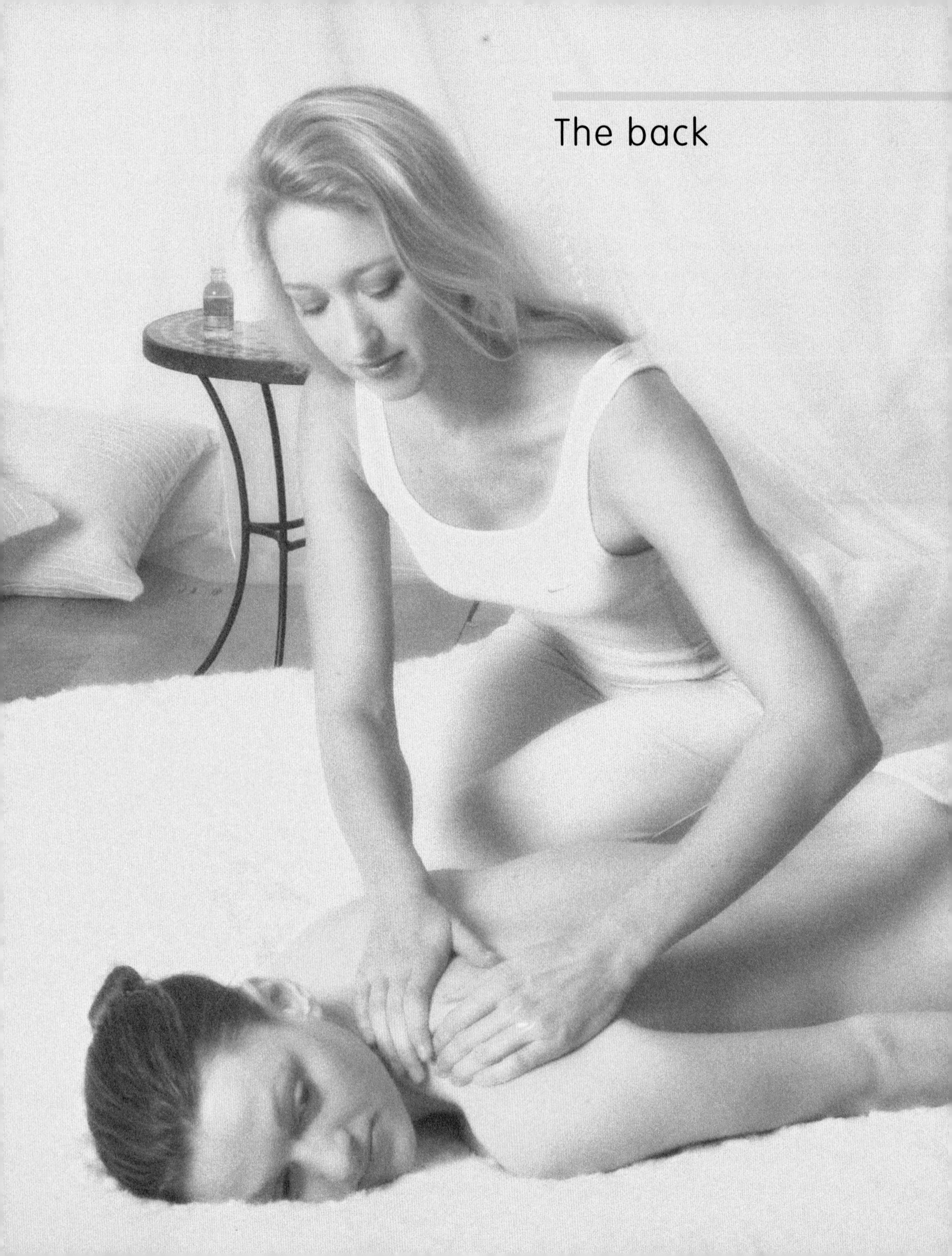

The back

Start to the side of your partner. Slowly place one hand between the shoulder blades and the other on the base of the spine over the towel. This helps you to connect to your partner and lets your partner know the massage has begun.

1 **Spreading the oil:** Fold back the towel so the back is exposed down to the top of the buttocks. Pour a small amount of oil into one hand.

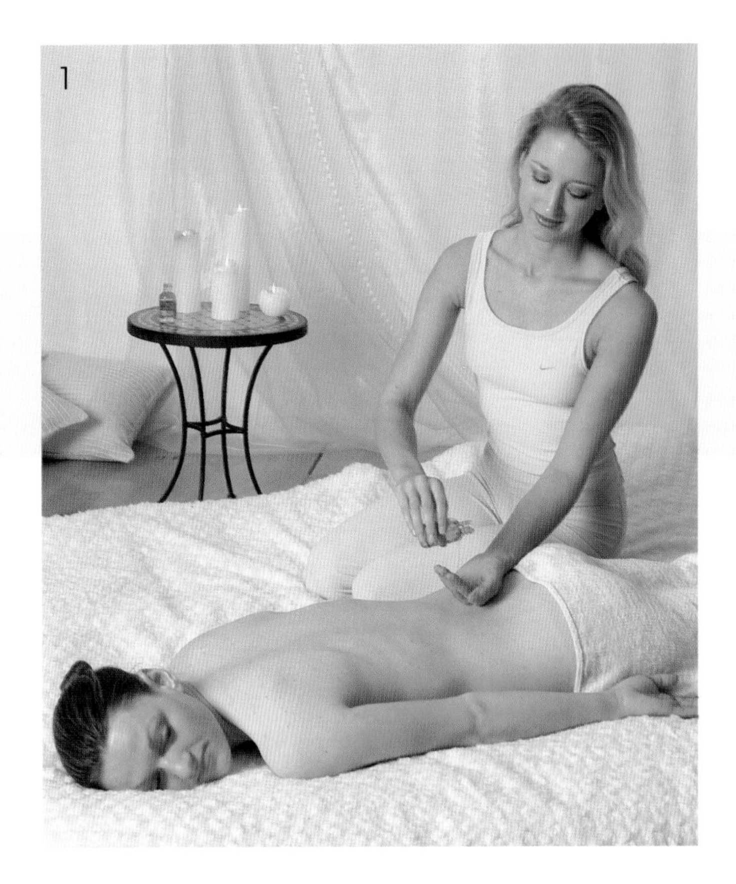
1

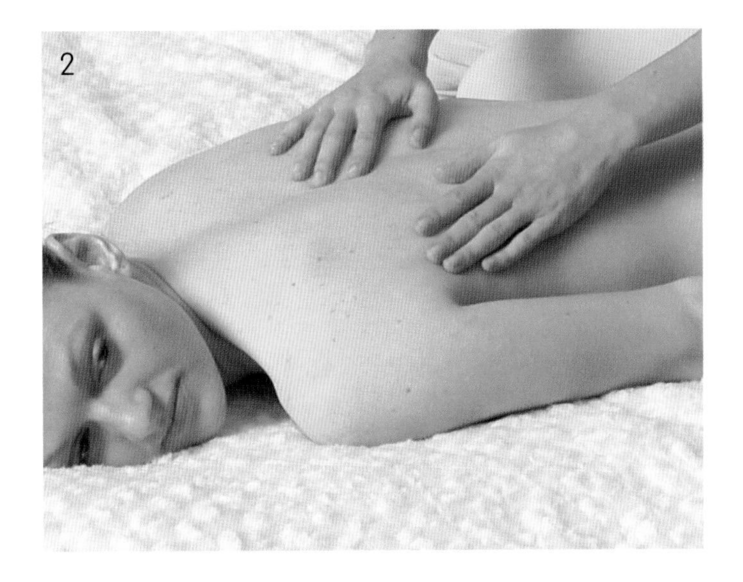
2

2 Rub the oil between your hands to warm it before it touches your partner. Never pour oil directly onto the skin as it might be cold and will not feel pleasant! Spread the oil evenly up the back.

3 **Basic effleurage:** Kneel at the side of your partner, facing their head. Place both hands at the base of the spine, thumbs together and fingers facing your partner's head. Gently glide the hands up either side of the spine to the nape of the neck. Slide the hands in opposite directions out along the shoulders and lightly back down the outside of the back towards the pelvis. Bring the hands together at the base of the spine to start again. The pressure should gradually deepen on the way up the back, and remain light on the way down. Let the hands mould to the contour of the back feeling for any tension or stiffness. Repeat this stroke 3 times.

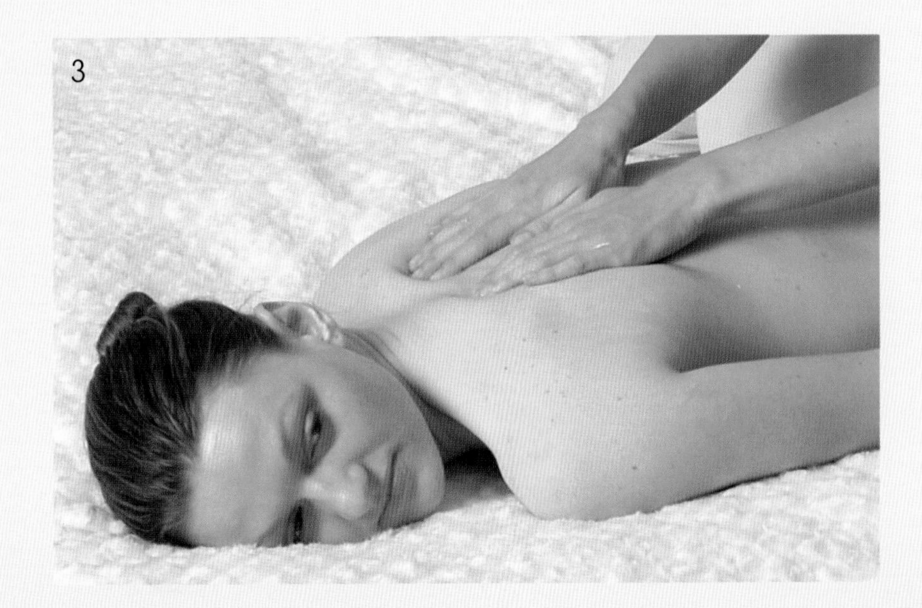
3

4 Kneading to the sides: Kneel facing the side of your partner. Reach your hands to the opposite side with the fingers facing down and the elbows and thumbs slightly out. Think of kneading dough as you pick up the flesh with one hand, gently squeeze it as you bring it towards the opposite hand and release. As you release the flesh, pick it up with the opposite hand and repeat. Move your body weight with the movement to ease the stress on your arms. Knead for about 30 seconds and repeat to the opposite side.

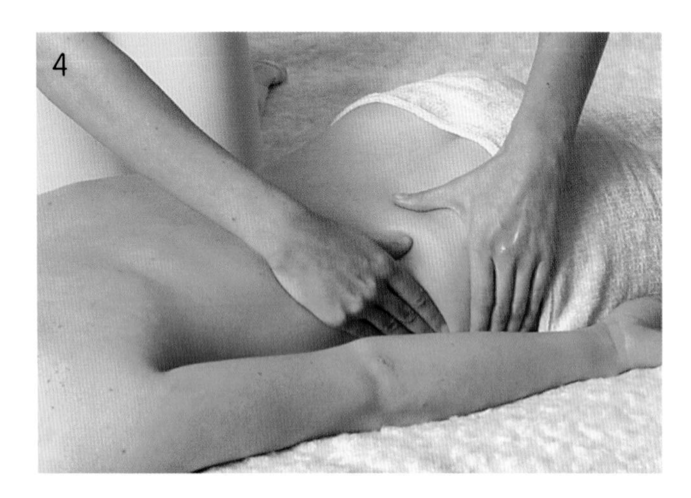

5 Friction up the spine: Kneel near your partner's hips, facing their head. Place the thumbs on either side of the base of the spine and lock the thumb joint. Making small circles from the arm, work the thumbs into the fleshy part of the muscle on either side of the spine all the way up to the nape of the neck. Flatten the hand as you slide along the top of the shoulders to the outside of the back and back to the base of the spine. Make sure the pressure is strong on the way up and light as you slide across and down. Repeat 3 times.

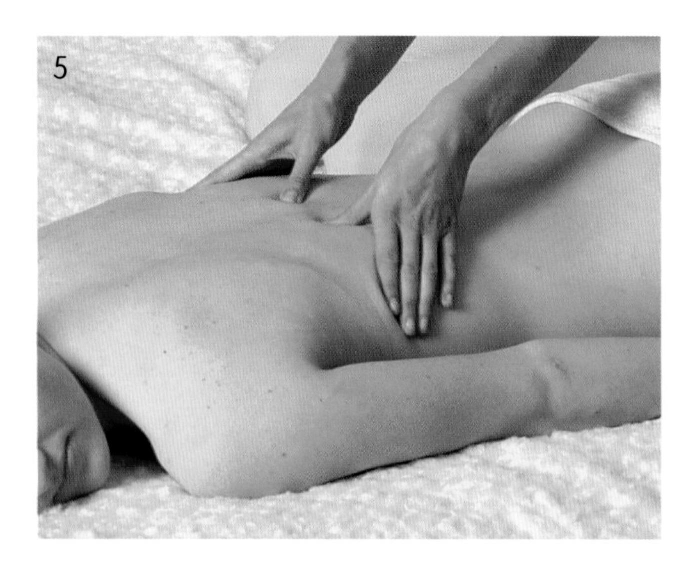

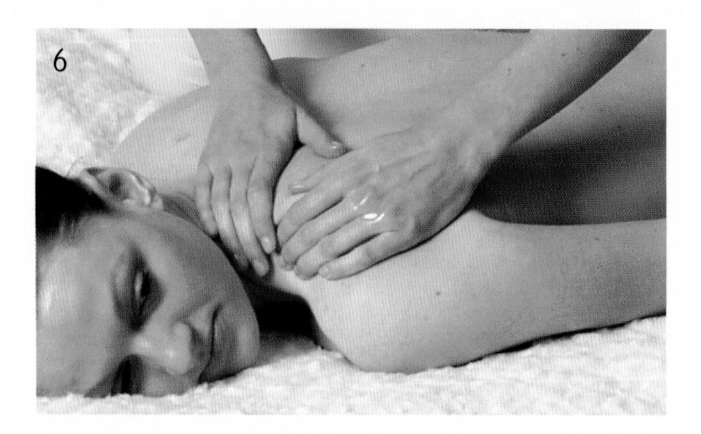

6 Kneading to the shoulders and neck: Place both hands on one shoulder. Pick up the flesh with one hand. Gently squeeze the flesh as you slide it towards your other hand. Release it as you pick the flesh up with the opposite hand. Repeat for about 30 seconds with smooth, continuous movements. This area of the body is usually tight. Work lightly, and slowly increase the pressure. Repeat to the opposite side. Knead the back of the neck with one hand. Place the thumb on one side on the neck and the fingers on the other. Massage the neck muscles lightly, trying to work out any tension.

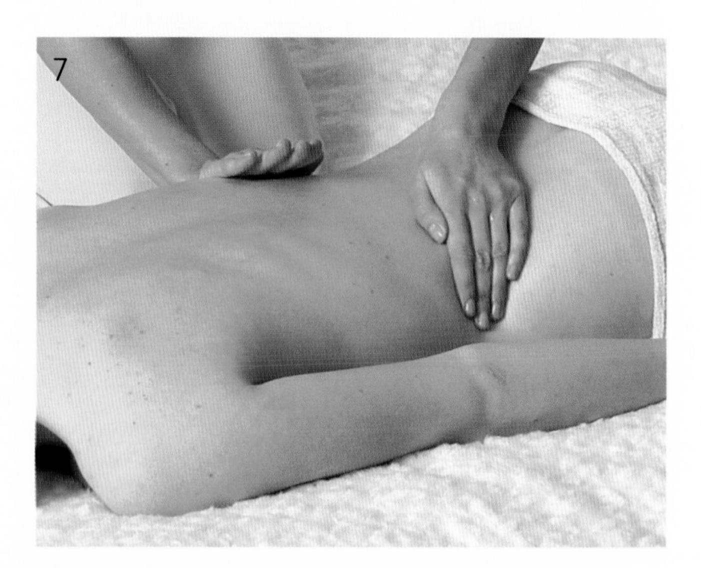

7 Wringing across the back: Kneel facing your partner's side. Place the hands on opposite sides of the torso with your fingertips facing away from you. Think of wringing out a towel as you lift the flesh up on both sides bringing the hands towards each other. Make sure the hands are at least 5 cm apart as they pass, allowing the skin to twist without causing pain. Continue the hands sliding until they reach the opposite side from which they started. Repeat a few more times, thinking of lifting the muscle away from the bone.

8 Friction to the base of the spine: Place the thumbs on either side of the spine at the top of the buttocks. Lock the thumb joint and make small circles, using the whole arm around the base of the spine. The areas where the spine and pelvis meet can hold a lot of tension. Think of massaging the muscle away from the bone with small, circular movements. Remember not to press directly on the spine.

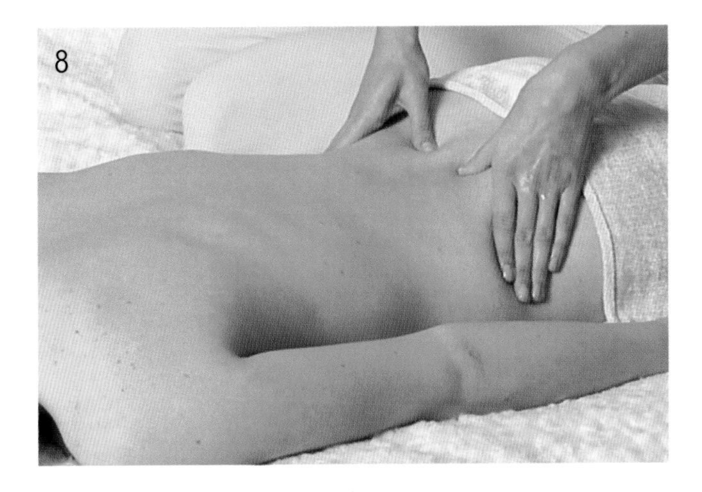
8

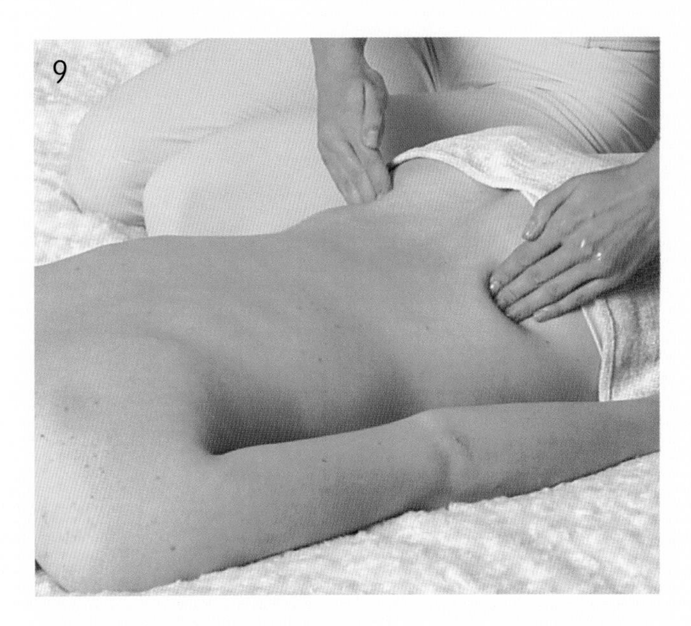
9

9 Friction with the fingers: Place the fingers over the hip and buttock area. Make circles with the tips of the fingers into the fleshy area of the top of the buttocks. Make circles around the hips and top of the buttocks.

10 Alternating effleurage: Place both hands at the base of either side of the spine. Start one hand sliding up the side of the spine and across the shoulder. As the hand glides down the outside of the body, start the opposite hand sliding up the other side of the spine. Think of waves rolling in the ocean as you do this. It is a soothing stroke with a relaxing, calming rhythm.

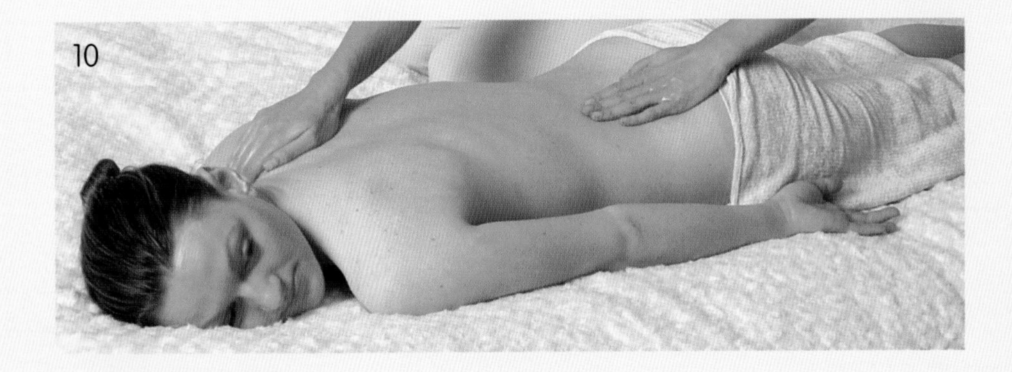
10

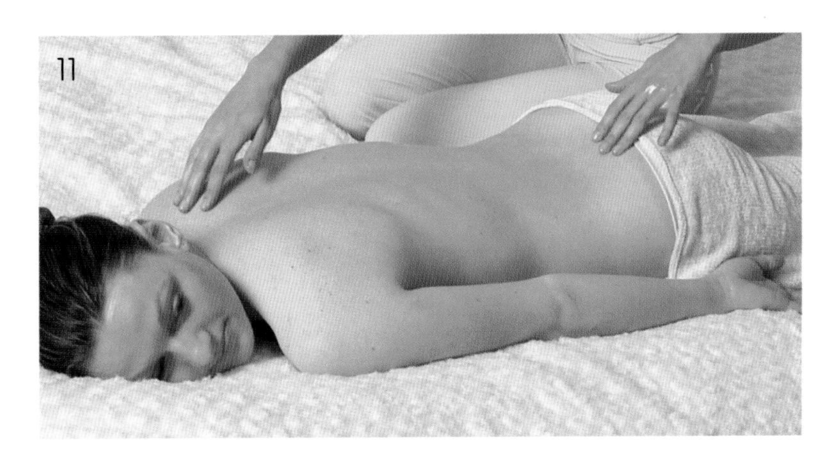
11

11 Feather stroking: Lightly touch the top of the back with the fingertips of one hand. Separate the fingers as you gently brush down the back. When the fingers are almost at the base of the spine, start the other hand brushing down the back. Repeat a few times.

Ending: Cover the back with a towel. If you did not use essential oils, lightly press the towel down across the back. This will absorb any extra oil remaining on the surface of the skin. If using essential oils you want them to remain on the skin as long as possible so that they may be absorbed into the blood stream through the skin.

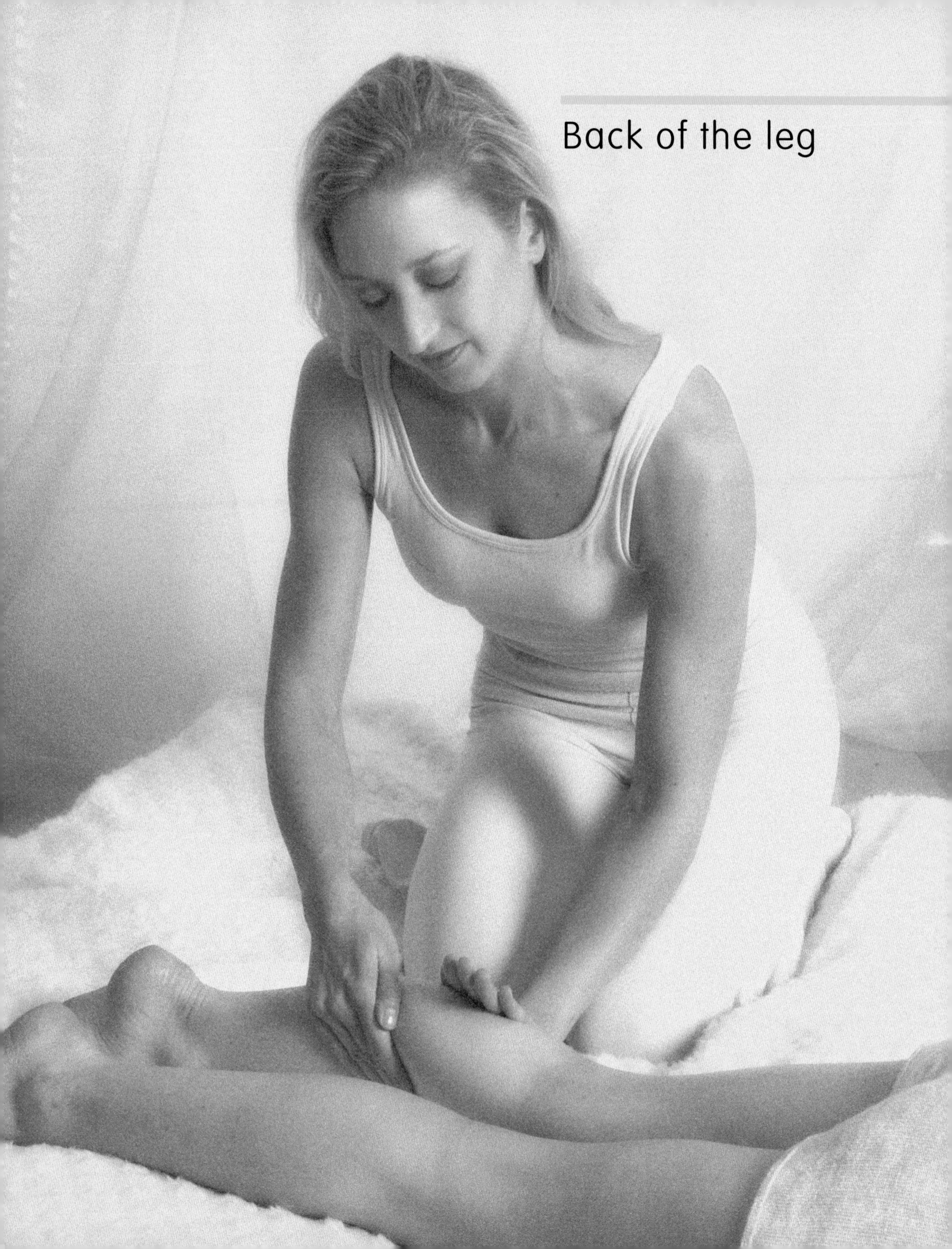

Back of the leg

Spreading the oil: Start by uncovering the leg you are working on. You want to be able to see the hip joint while maintaining your partner's modesty. Place a small amount of oil into your hand. Rub your hands together before spreading the oil from the ankle up towards the hip.

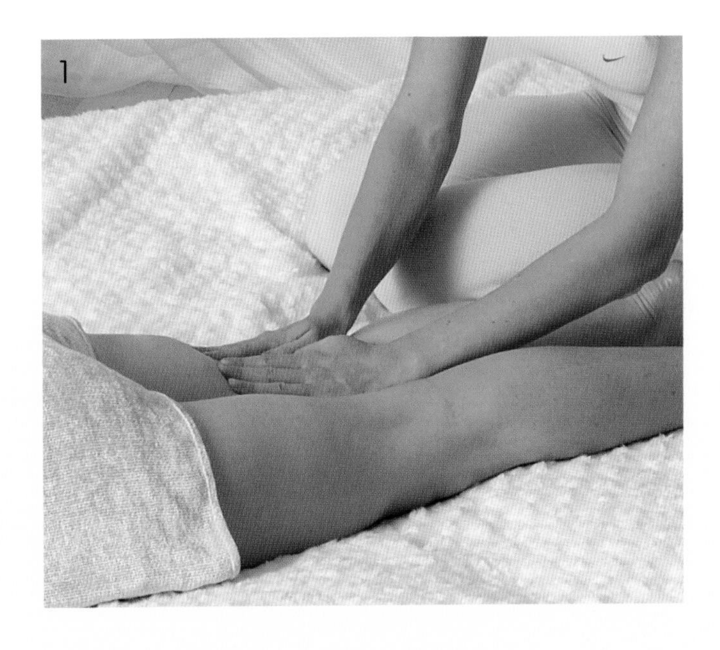
1

1 **Basic effleurage:** Place both hands on the ankle with the fingertips facing the hip. Keeping the hands together, slide the hands along the length of the leg towards the hip. Separate the hands and lightly glide them along the outsides of the legs back to their original position. Press firmly on the way up the leg, avoiding the back of the knee, and press gently on the return. Repeat a few more times. Repeat to the thigh only, preparing the thigh for the next sequence.

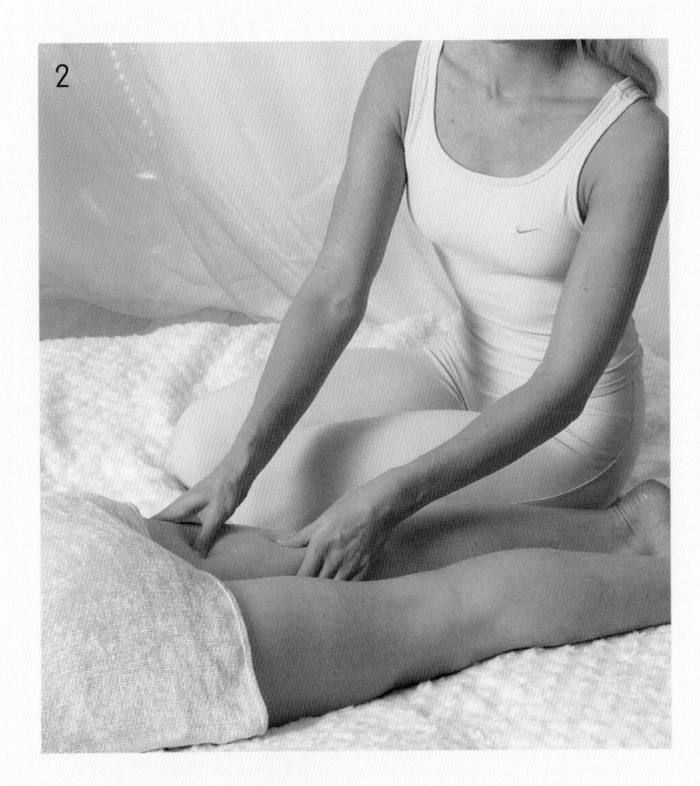
2

2 **Friction to the thigh:** Place the thumbs just above the knee with the fingers to the sides. Make alternating circles with the thumbs and move across the whole thigh area. If you keep the thumb joint still and make small circles with the arm, deeper pressure can be achieved. This stroke works deeply into the belly of the hamstring. Be sure to check with your partner that the pressure is desirable.

3 **Kneading the inner thigh:** Kneel facing the thigh with your hands placed on the inner part of their leg. The fingers should be facing down with the elbows and thumbs out. Knead the inner thigh by picking up the flesh with one hand and sliding it across to the other. Shift your weight from side to side with the rhythm of the movement.

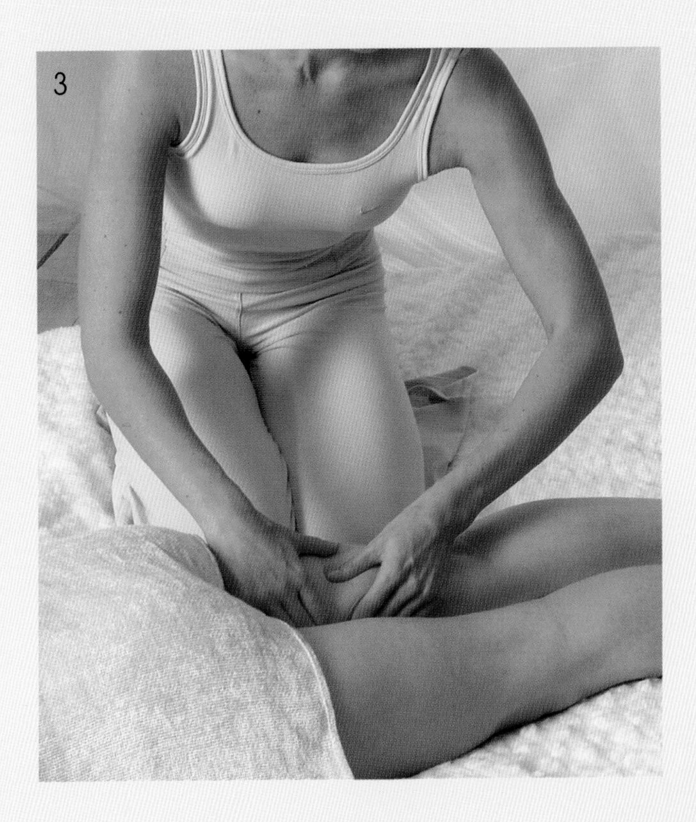
3

4 Wringing the thigh: Place one hand on either side of the thigh with the fingertips away from you just above the knee. Lift the muscle up as you slide the hands towards each other. Cross the hands with 5 cm in between them as they relax down to the opposite side. You should see the flesh slightly twist between the hands. Repeat, going back in the opposite direction as you work your way up the thigh towards the hip.

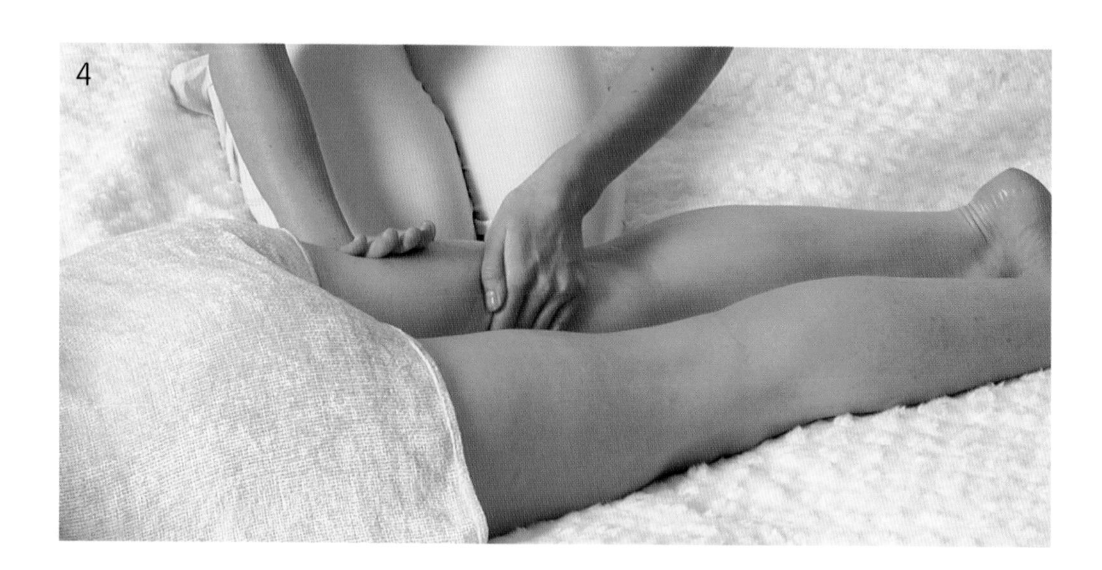

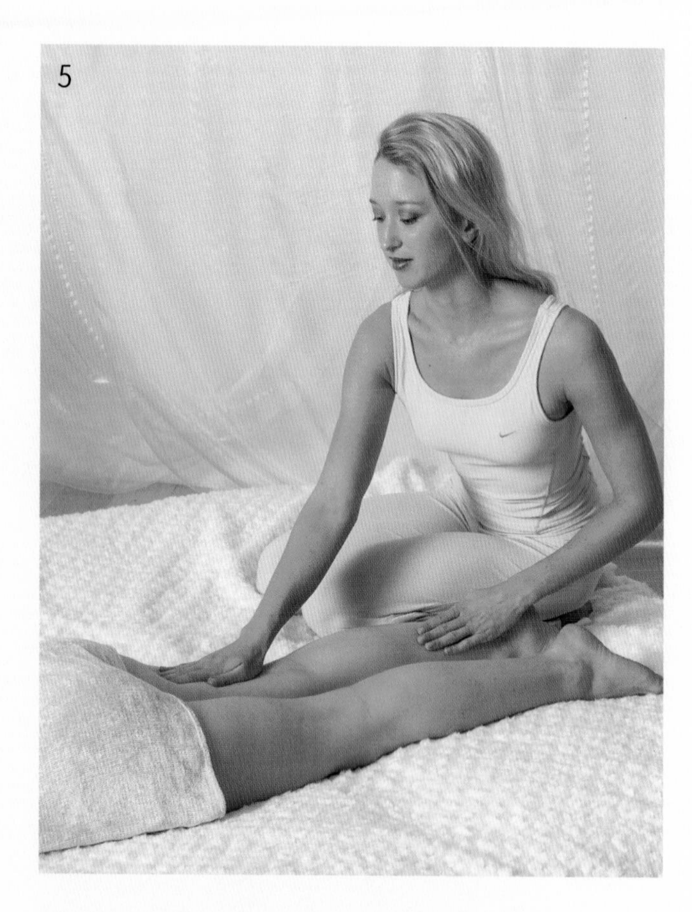

5 Basic effleurage: Stroke the thigh from the top of the knee towards the hip to help flush the toxins towards the lymph nodes. Repeat the effleurage movement, starting from the ankle and working all the way up to the hip. Avoid the back of the knee. Repeat one more time just focusing on the calf. Work from the ankle up to the beginning of the knee.

6 Friction to the calf: Start with the thumbs at the ankle and the fingers to the sides. Work the thumbs in continuous circles up the calf, making sure to cover the whole area. This can be tender so make sure to check with your partner that the pressure is accurate.

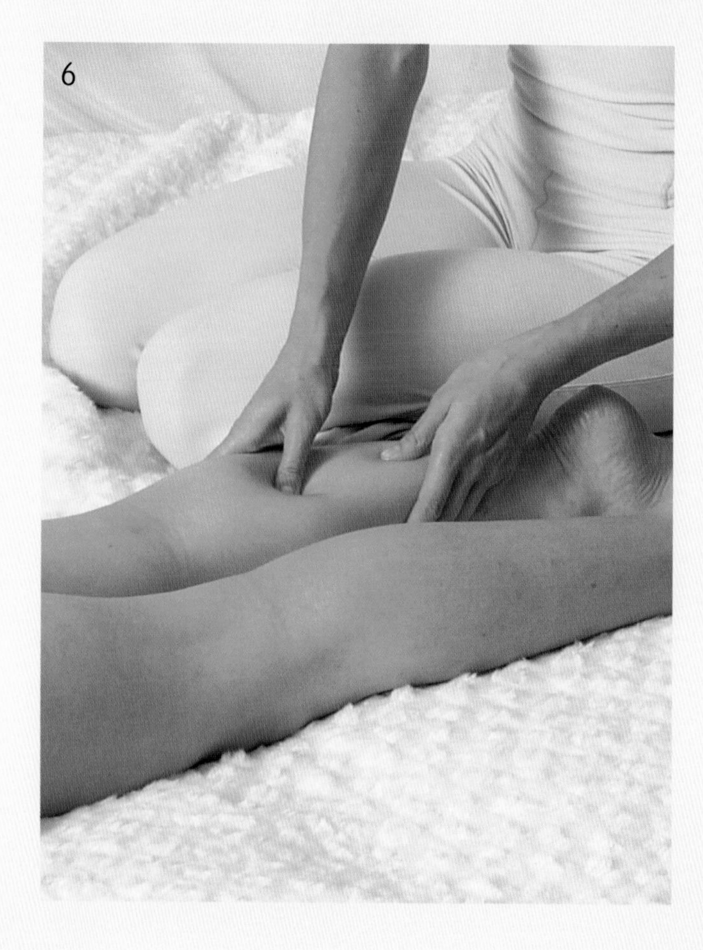

7 Wringing the calf: Move to the side of your partner. Start with the hands on either side of the ankle. The fingertips should be facing away from you. Think of lifting the muscle off the bone as you bring the hands towards each other. Allow space between the hands as you slide them across and down to the opposite sides from which they started. Repeat, working your way up to the knee and continuously alternating the hands.

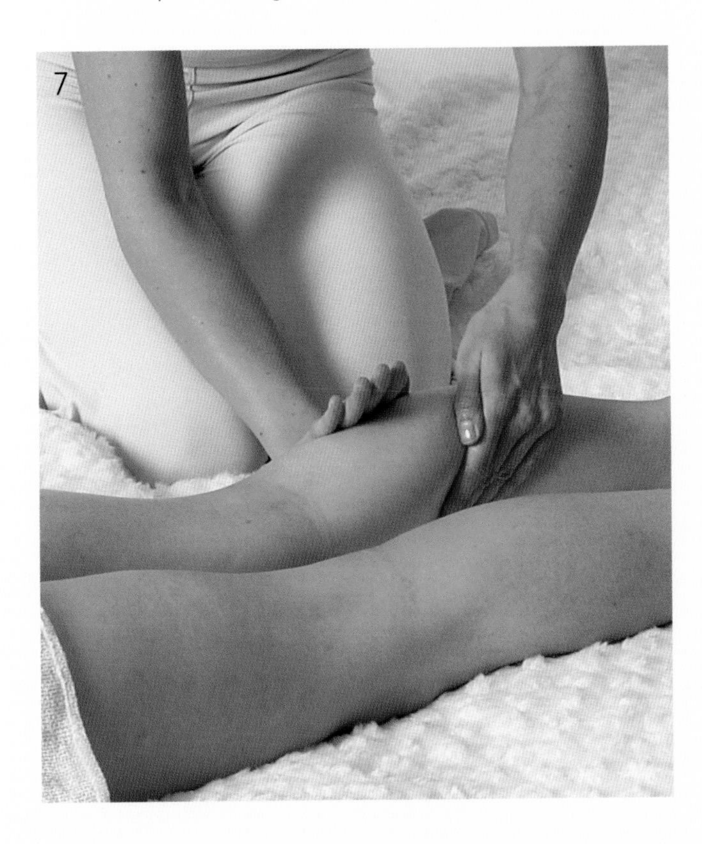
7

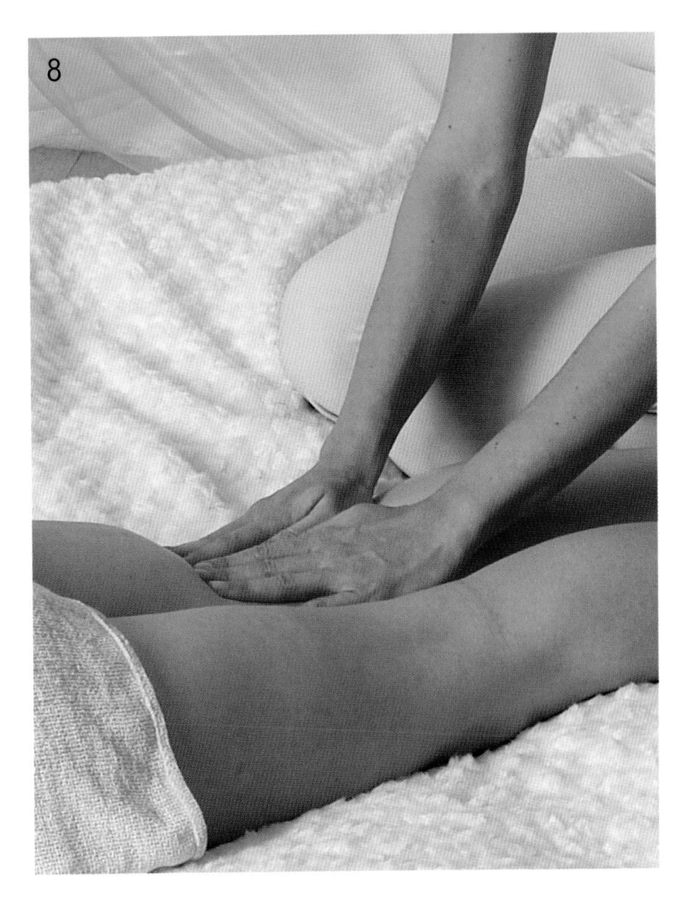
8

8 Alternating effleurage: Place the hands on the ankle with the fingertips facing the hip. Glide one hand up towards the hip and then back down along the outside of the leg, avoiding the back of the knee. As the hand is reaching the ankle, glide the other hand up to the hip. Repeat a few times in slow, fluid movements.

9 Feather stroking: Place the fingertips of one hand lightly at the top of the thigh. Gently stroke down the leg. As the hand gets to the ankle, start your other hand at the top of the thigh. repeat several times.

Ending: Cover the leg and repeat the whole sequence to the other leg. Then lift the towel slightly, at a diagonal away from you, so that your partner can turn over onto their back.

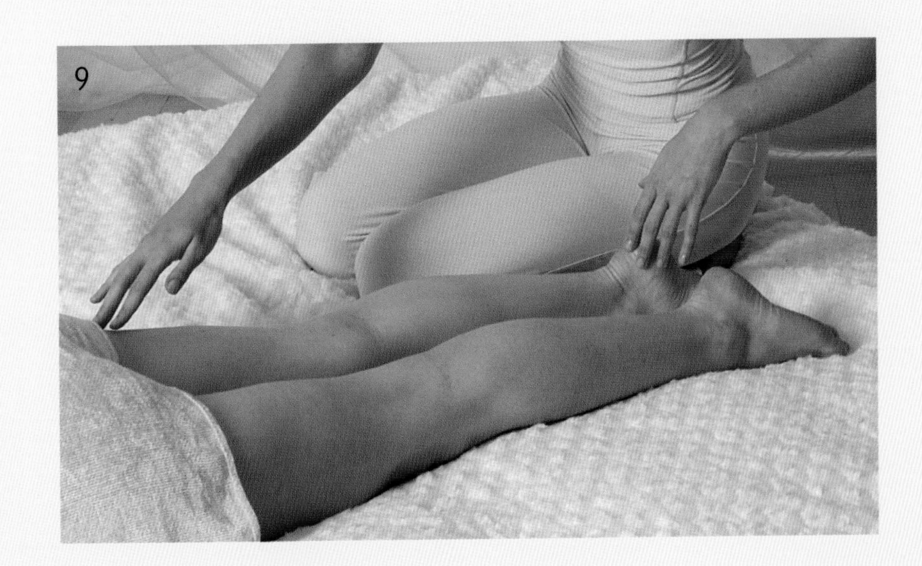
9

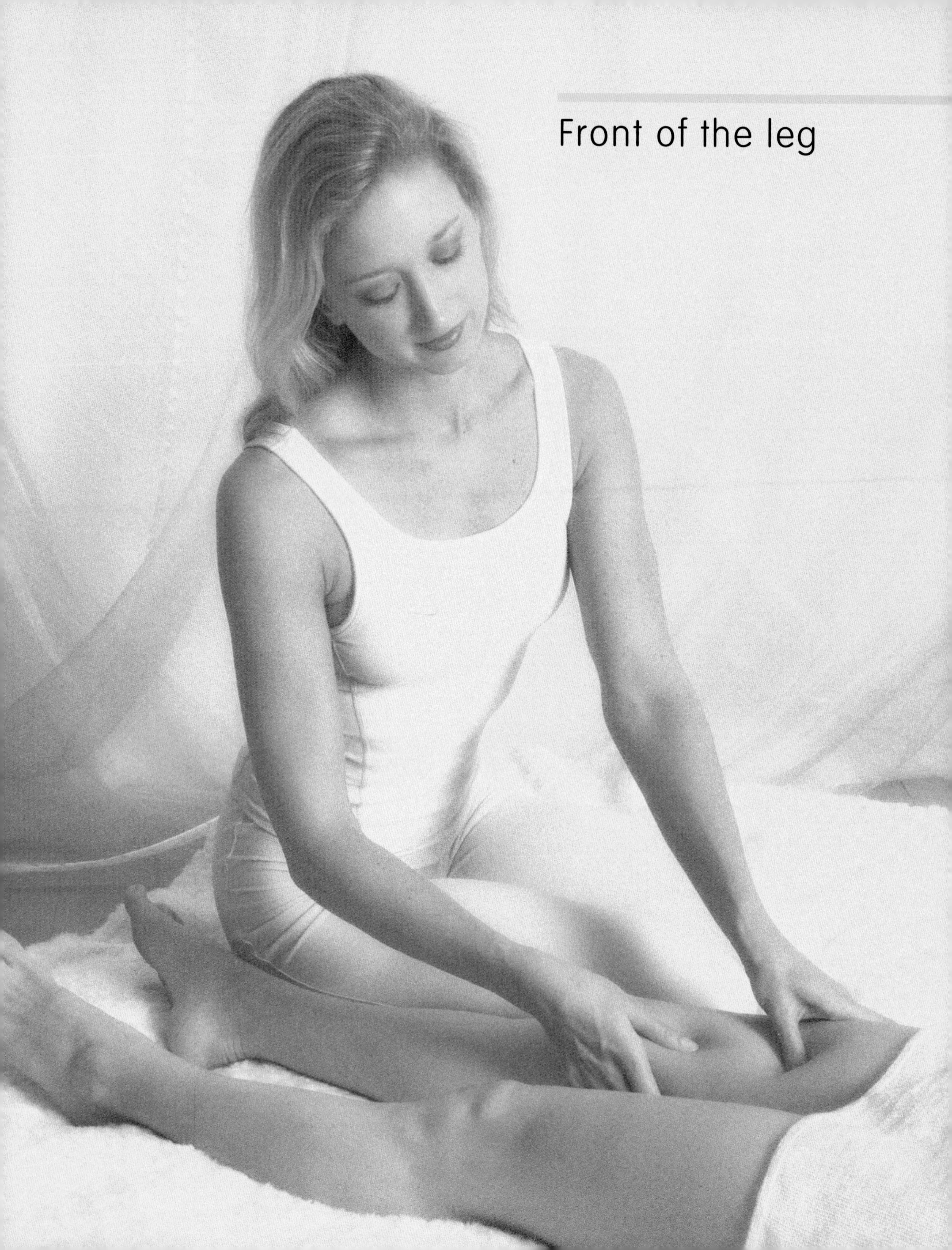

Front of the leg

Spreading the oil: Uncover the leg so that you can see your partner's hip but you are still keeping their modesty. Pour some oil into your hands. Rub your hands together and spread the oil onto the leg, starting at the ankle and working your way up to the hip.

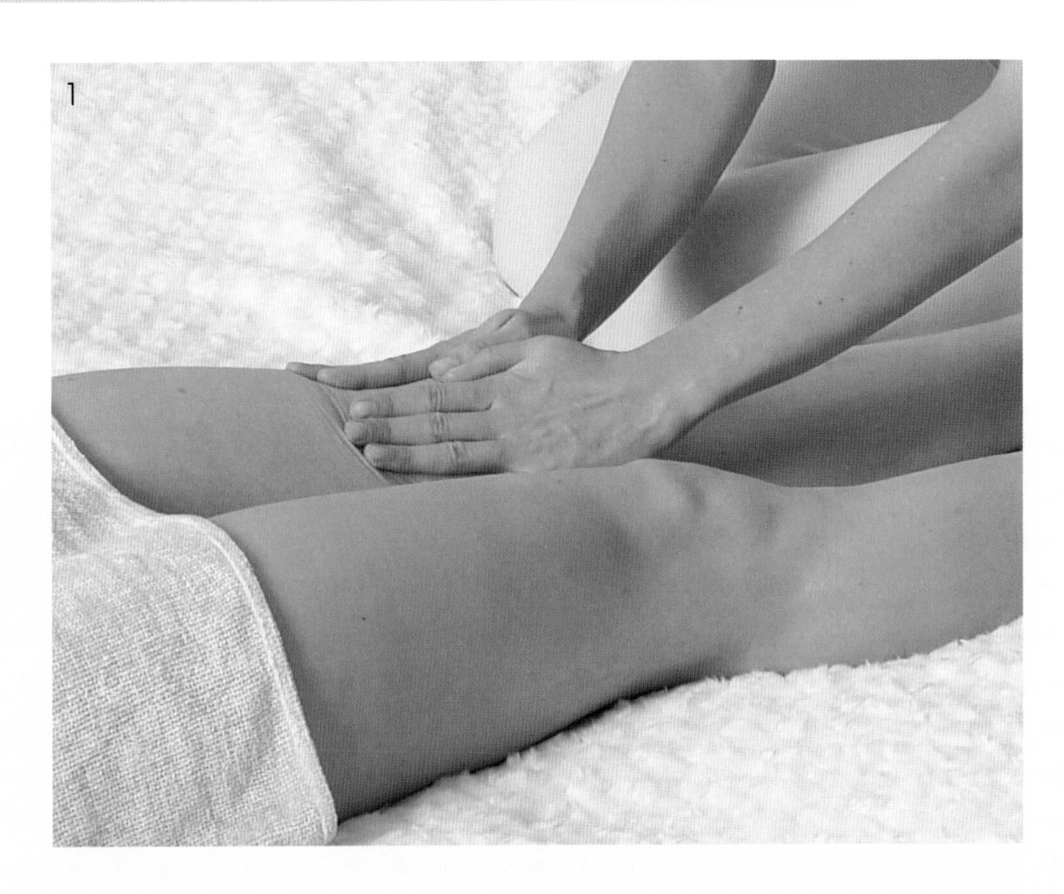

1 **Basic effleurage:** Starting at the ankle, place both hands on the leg with your thumbs together and your fingers facing the hip. Slide the hands up the leg to the hip, avoiding the top of the kneecap. Separate the hands and glide the hands back down the outside of the leg. Repeat a few times. Then place the hands above the knee and repeat only on the front of the thigh.

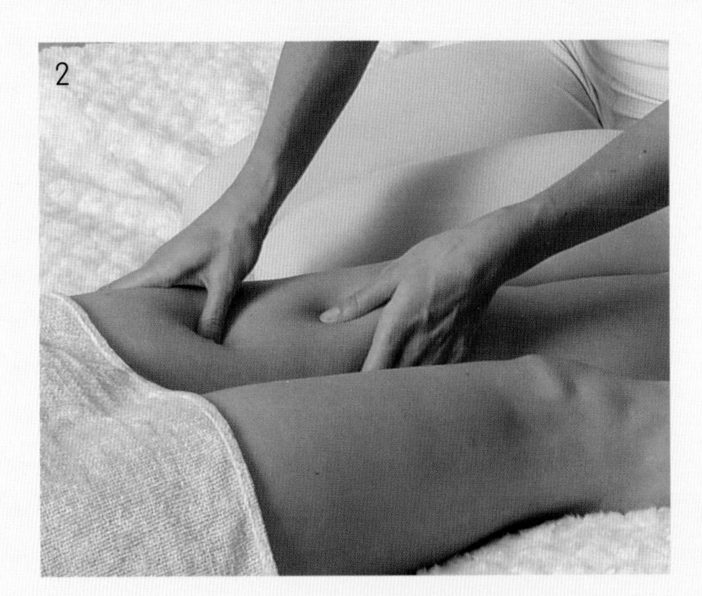

2 **Friction to the thigh:** Place the thumbs just above the knee. With circular motions, sweep the thumbs over the entire thigh area. This can be a deep movement, working out any toxins or tightness you might find. Be sure to check with your partner that the pressure feels right.

3 **Kneading the inner thigh:** Kneel facing your partner's thigh. Place your hands on the opposite side of the thigh with your fingers facing away and your thumbs and elbows out to the sides. Pick up some flesh with one hand and gently squeeze it as you slide it over to your opposite hand. As you release it, pick it up with your opposite hand. Move the flesh back and forth as you shift your body weight from side to side.

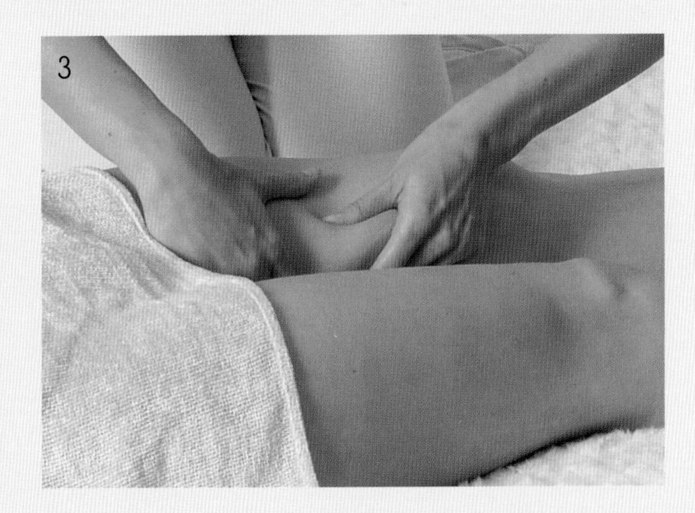

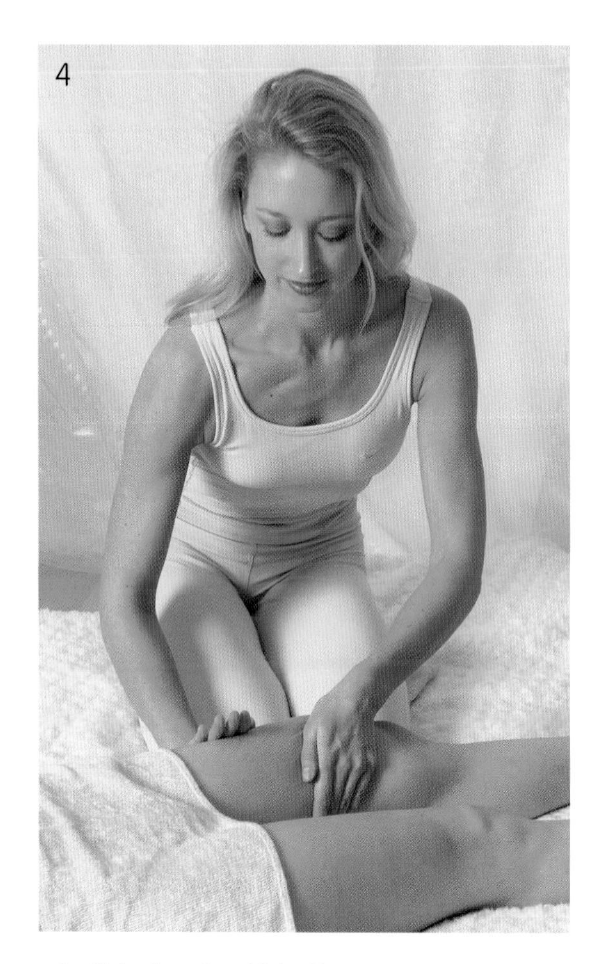

4 Wringing the thigh: Place one hand on either side of the thigh with your fingers facing away from you. Think of gently lifting the muscle off the bone as you slide the hands in opposite directions across the muscle to the other side. Make sure the hands are at least 5 cm apart so that the muscle twists without causing pain.

5 Friction to the outside of the leg: The outside of the legs are often tight. Face your partner's leg and hold the ankle with your nearest hand. With your other hand start with the thumb above the knee on the outside of the leg and make small circles, travelling up to the hip. Slide the hand down to the starting position and repeat twice.

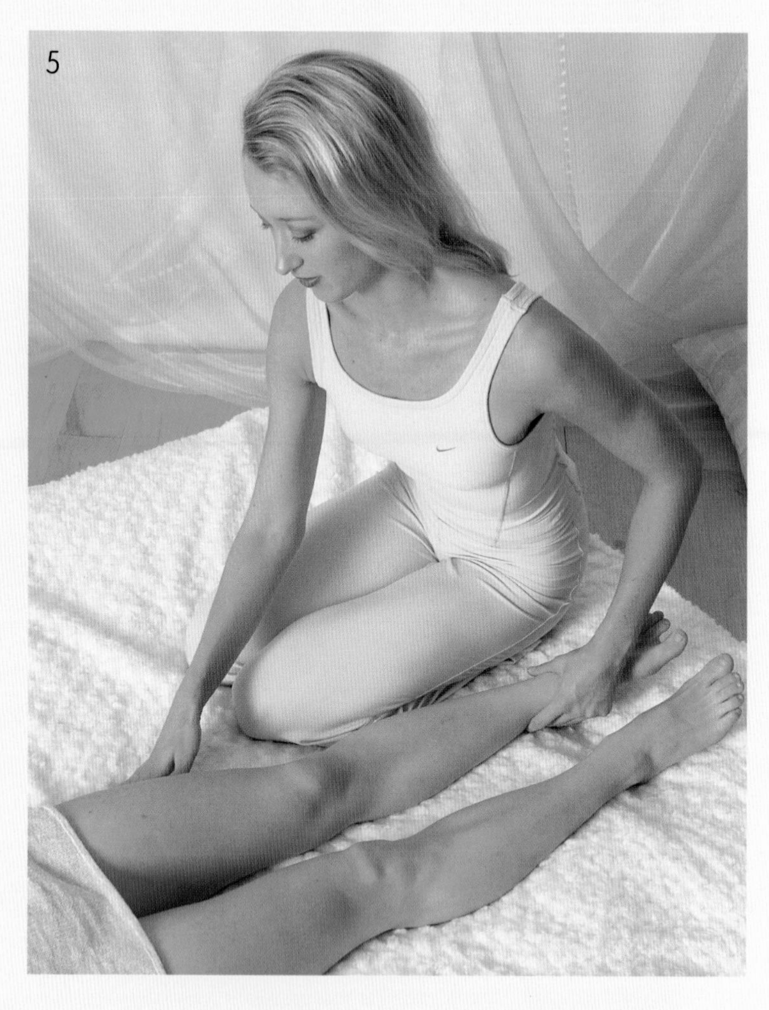

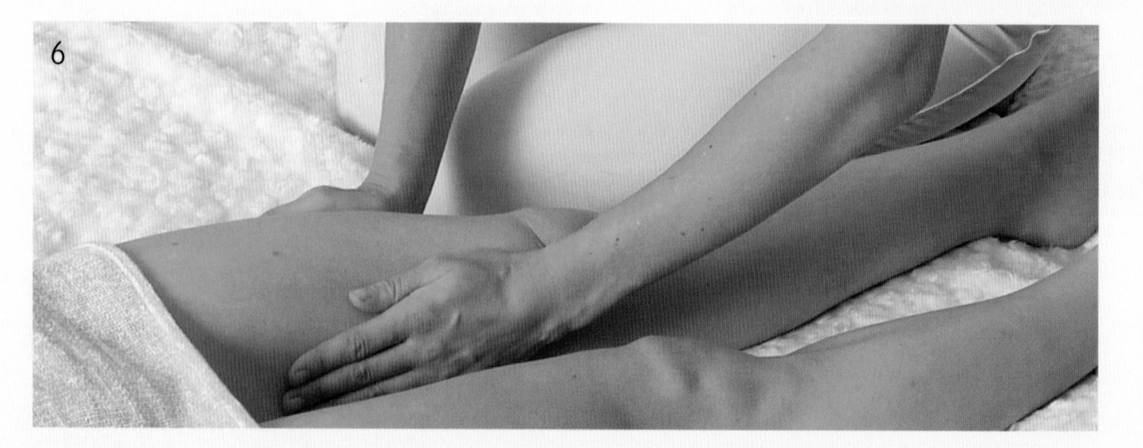

6 Basic effleurage: Place the hands above the knee with the fingertips facing the hip. Sweep the hands up to the hip, open and slide them back down the outside of the leg. Repeat a few times to help any toxins that you might have dislodged go towards the lymph nodes.

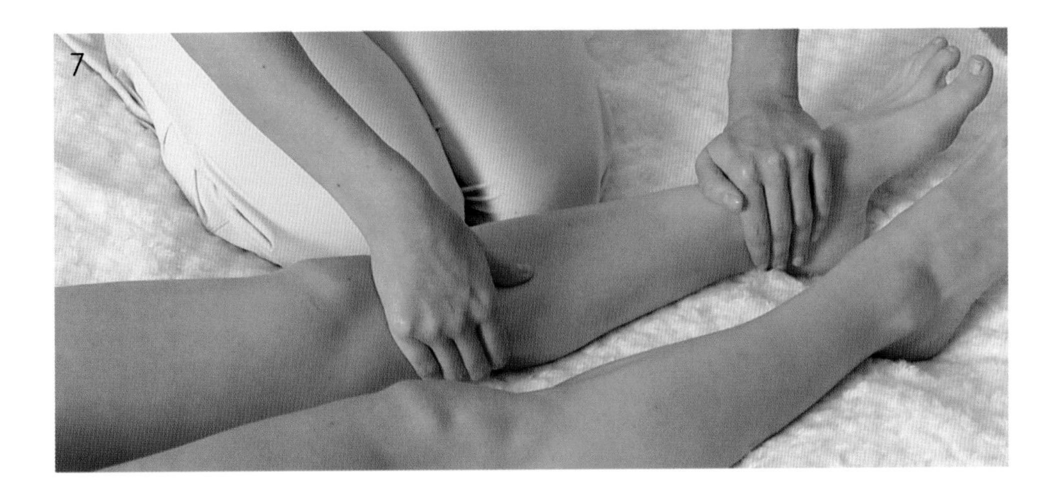

7 Friction down the shin: Place one hand on the ankle and the other hand on the inside of the leg just below the knee. Your fingers should be slightly under the calf with the thumb on top, touching the shin. Circle the thumb down towards the ankle as you squeeze the calf with the fingers underneath. Think of pushing the muscles away from the shin. When you reach the ankle, circle the anklebone with your thumb 3 times. Repeat the whole sequence 3 times.

8 Alternating effleurage: Place both hands on the ankle with the fingertips facing the hip. Slide one hand up the leg towards the hip, avoiding the top of the knee. Glide the hand down the outside of the leg. Repeat immediately with the other hand. This should feel like waves coming rhythmically over the leg.

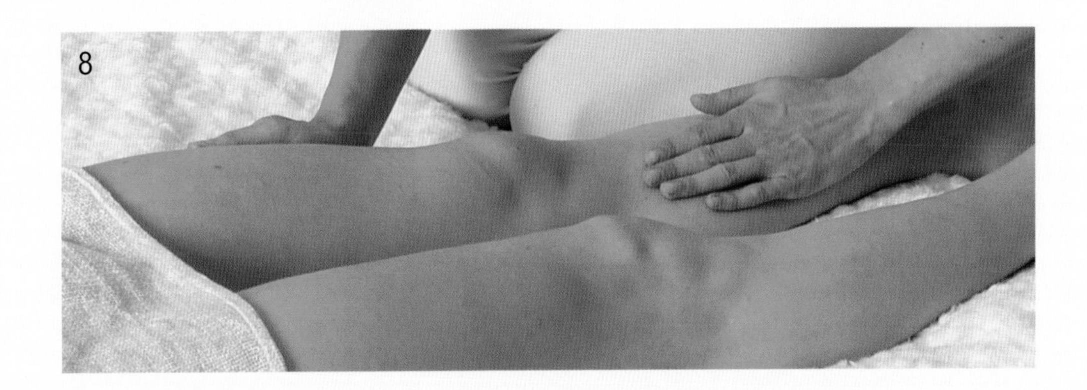

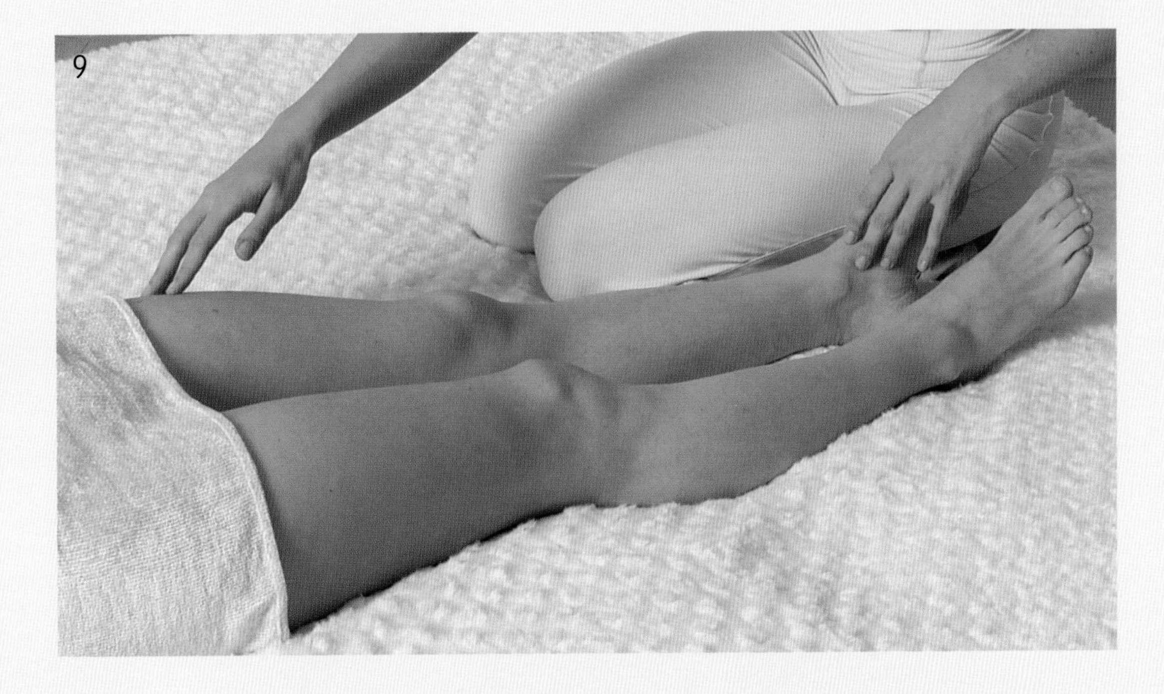

9 Feather stroking: Start with the fingertips of one hand at the top of the leg. Lightly stroke the fingers down the leg towards the ankle. Before that hand finishes the stroke, start the other hand at the top of the hip.

Ending: Cover the leg and move to the other side of the table. Uncover the other leg and repeat the whole sequence.

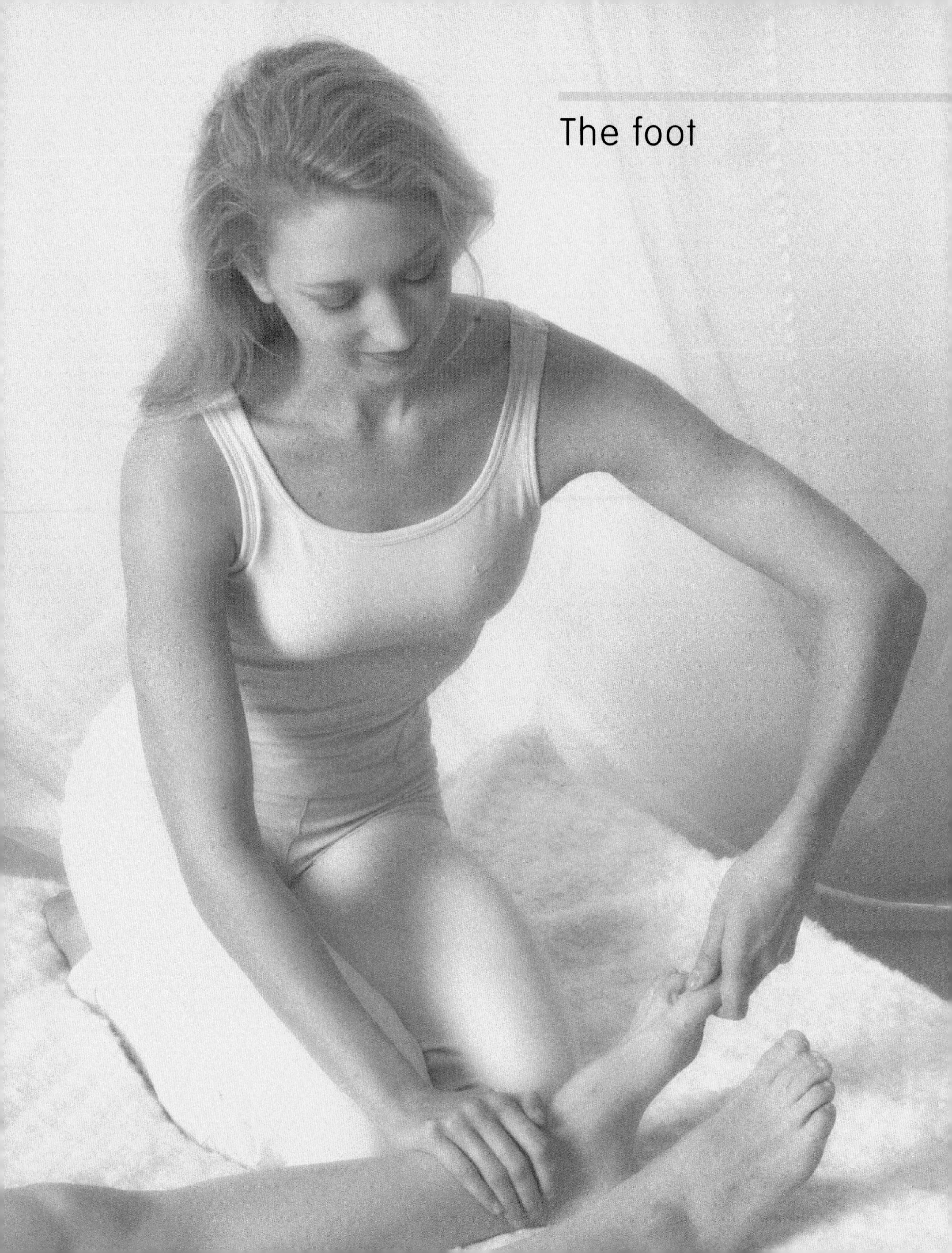

The foot

Spreading the oil: Place a small amount of oil onto the palm of your hand. Rub your hands together and then spread the oil over the foot.

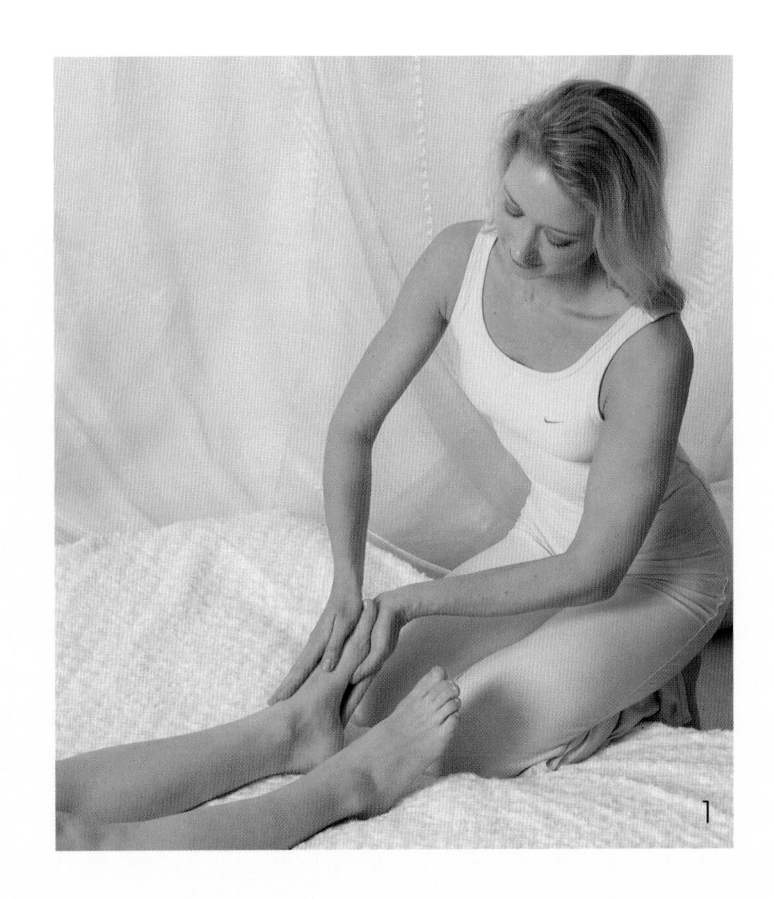

1

1 **Sandwiching:** Place both hands on either side of the foot. The palms should be flat against the foot with the fingertips facing the ankle. Press your hands into the foot as you slide them together and away. Change the hands so that the hand that was on the bottom of the foot is now on the top of the foot. Repeat the movement, alternating the hands as you do this.

2 **Friction:** Place the thumbs on the top of the foot. Make small circles with the thumbs as you move them around the whole area. Repeat this action to the sole of the foot.

3 **Toe massaging:** Place the thumb and forefinger at the base of one of the toes. Squeeze the toe gently as you circle your fingers. Work your way up the entire length of the toe and gently pinch the toe as you pull and release. Start at the base of the next toe and repeat until all the toes have been released.

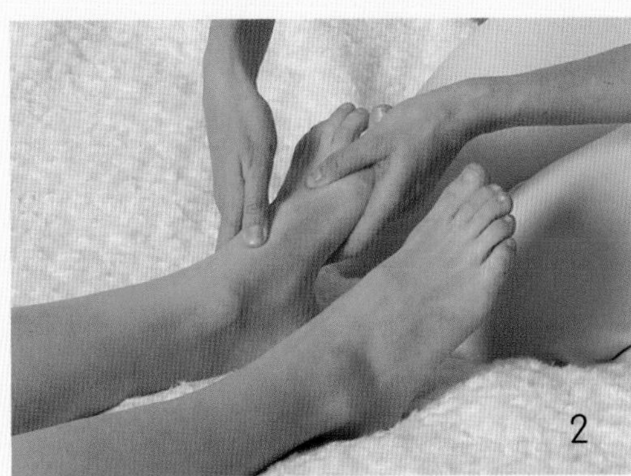

2

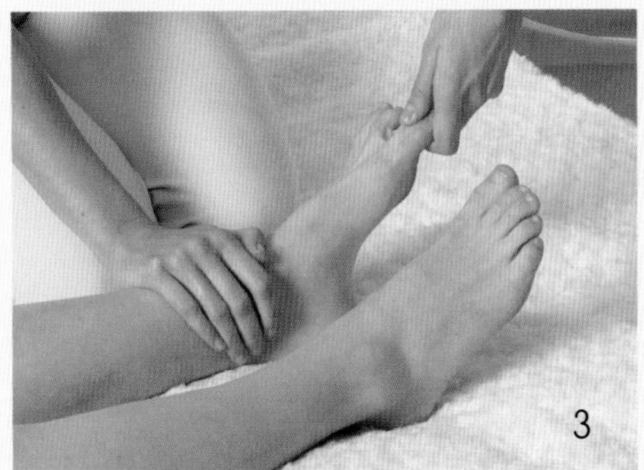

3

4

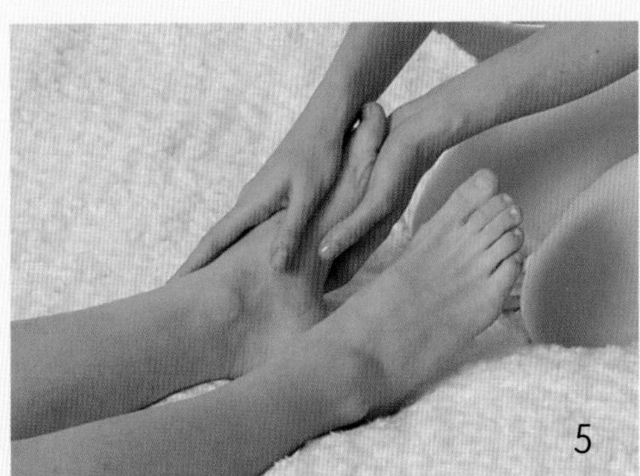

5

4 **Squeezing the foot:** Wrap your hands around the foot and squeeze it. Change the placement of your hands and repeat a few times.

5 **Holding the foot:** Place your hands lightly on the foot and hold for a few moments.

Ending: Cover the foot with a towel and repeat to the other side.

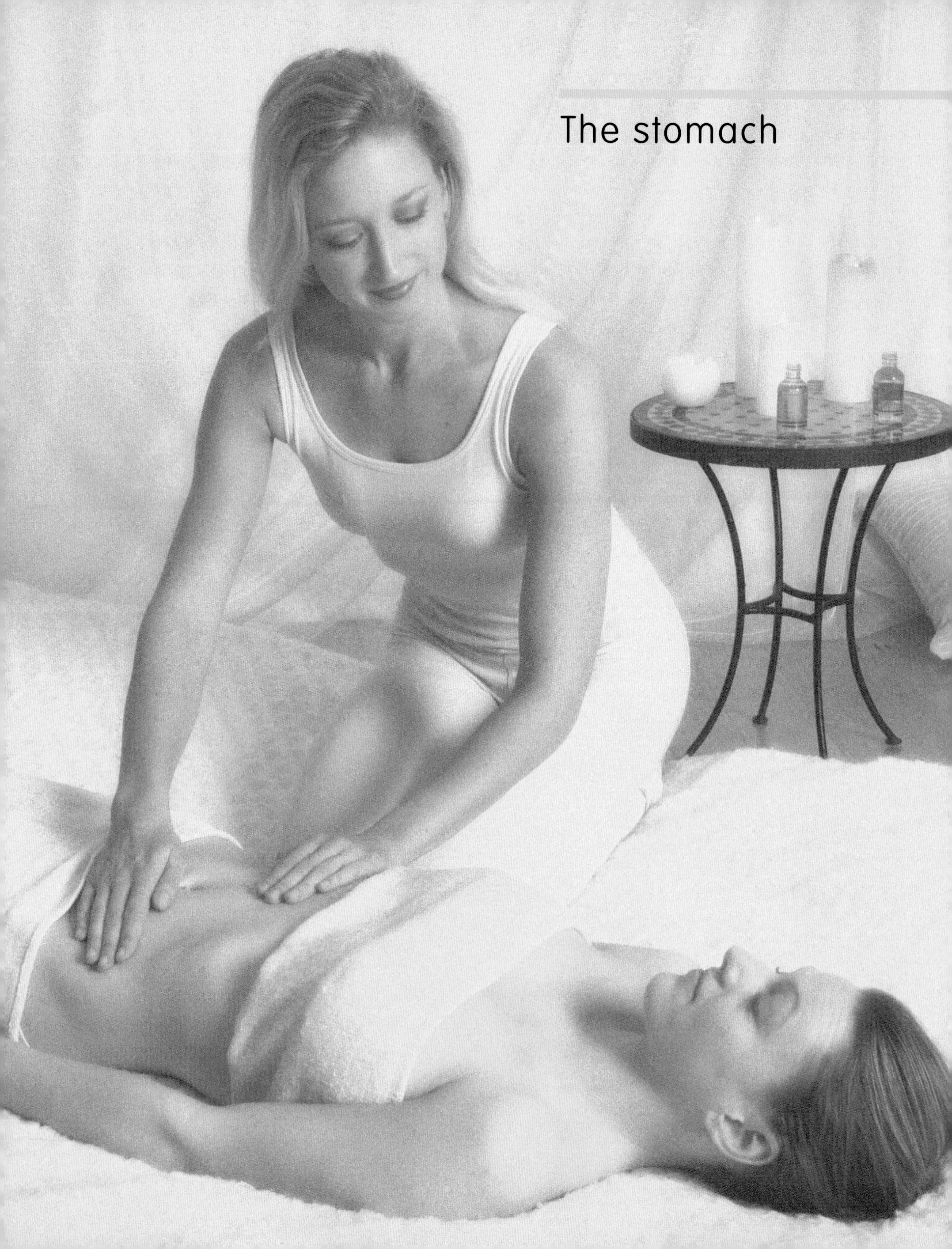

The stomach

The stomach is a very delicate area of the body, so work gently without invasion. The comfort of your partner is extremely important, so take extra care when removing the towels to expose the stomach only. If you are working on a woman, place another towel across the chest on top of the one already in place. Move the bottom towel down to expose the stomach.

Spreading the oil: Place a small amount of oil into your hand. Rub your palms together to warm the oil before placing it on the stomach.

1 **Circling:** The best image to think of is stirring a pudding. Place the hands flat on top of the stomach. Circle the hands in a clockwise direction, picking them up and placing them back down as necessary. Work slowly and rhythmically. This is the transition movement between strokes and you will come back to it often.

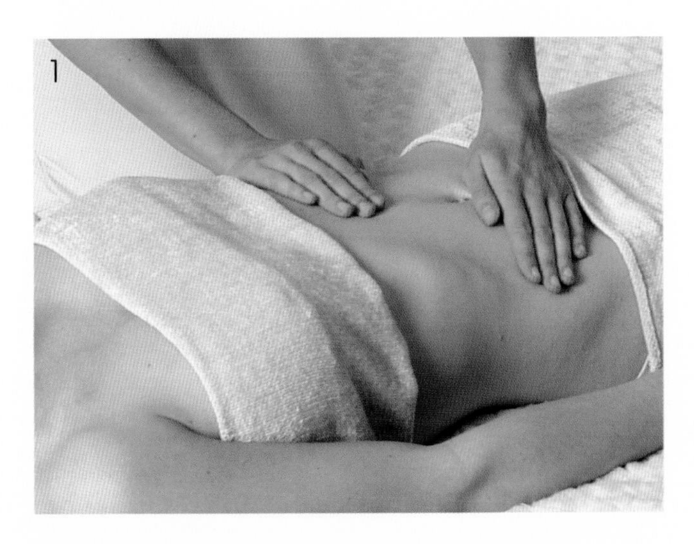
1

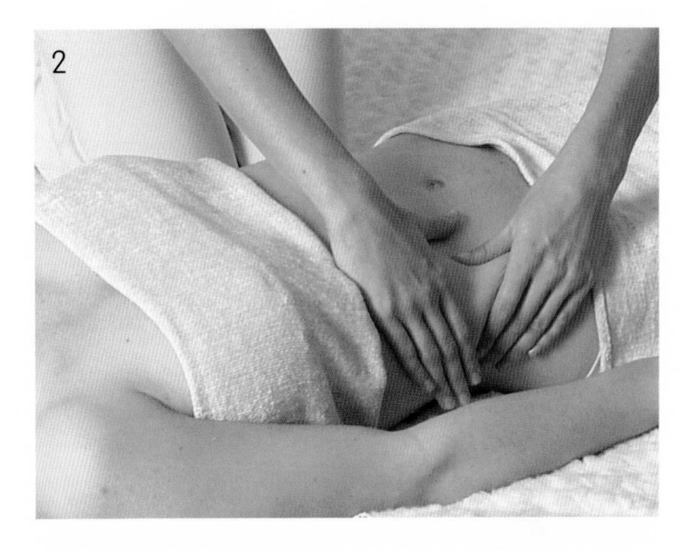
2

2 **Kneading the waistline:** Place both hands on the opposite side of your partner's waist with the fingers facing down and the thumbs out. Working lightly, pick up the flesh in one hand and pinch it as you slide it towards your opposite hand. As you release the flesh, pick it up with your other hand and repeat. Do not forget to shift your weight with the movement. Repeat to the other side.

3 Circling: Repeat step 1.

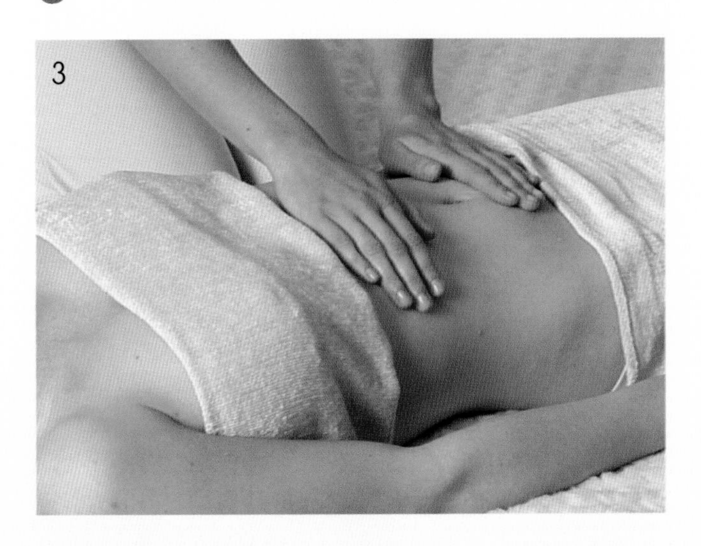
3

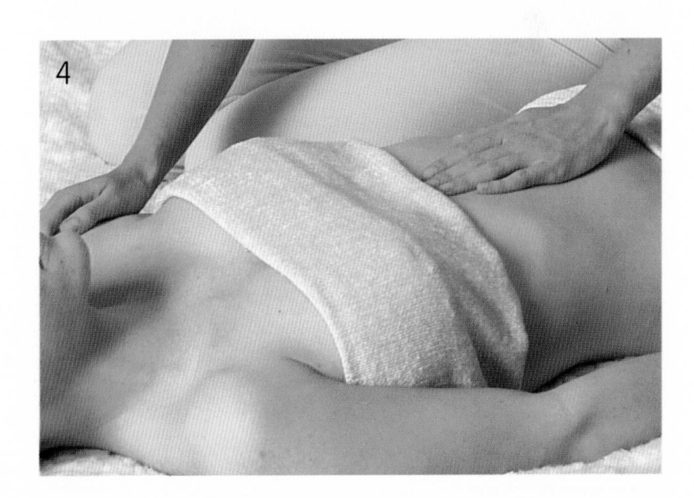
4

4 **Rub solar plexus:** Place one hand on your partner with the fingertips just below the point where the ribs end and the palm towards the belly button. Make small, gentle circles with the fingers in a clockwise direction.

Ending: Cover the stomach with a towel.

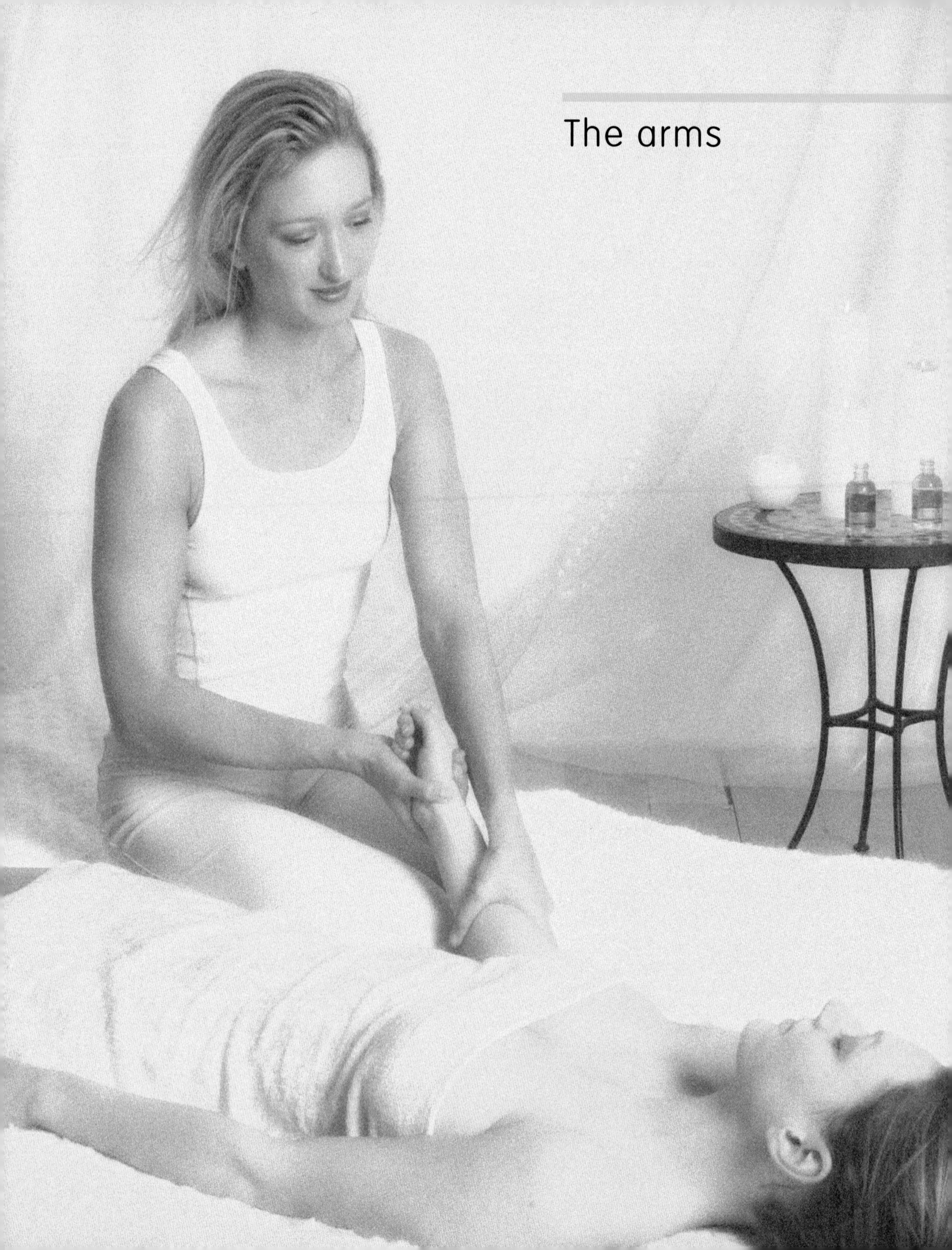

The arms

Spreading the oil: Take the arm out from underneath the towel and place it on top. Pour a small amount of oil onto the palm of your hand. Rub your hands together and spread the oil up the arm, starting at the wrist. Make sure you cover the whole arm because you will be working on the underneath as well as on top.

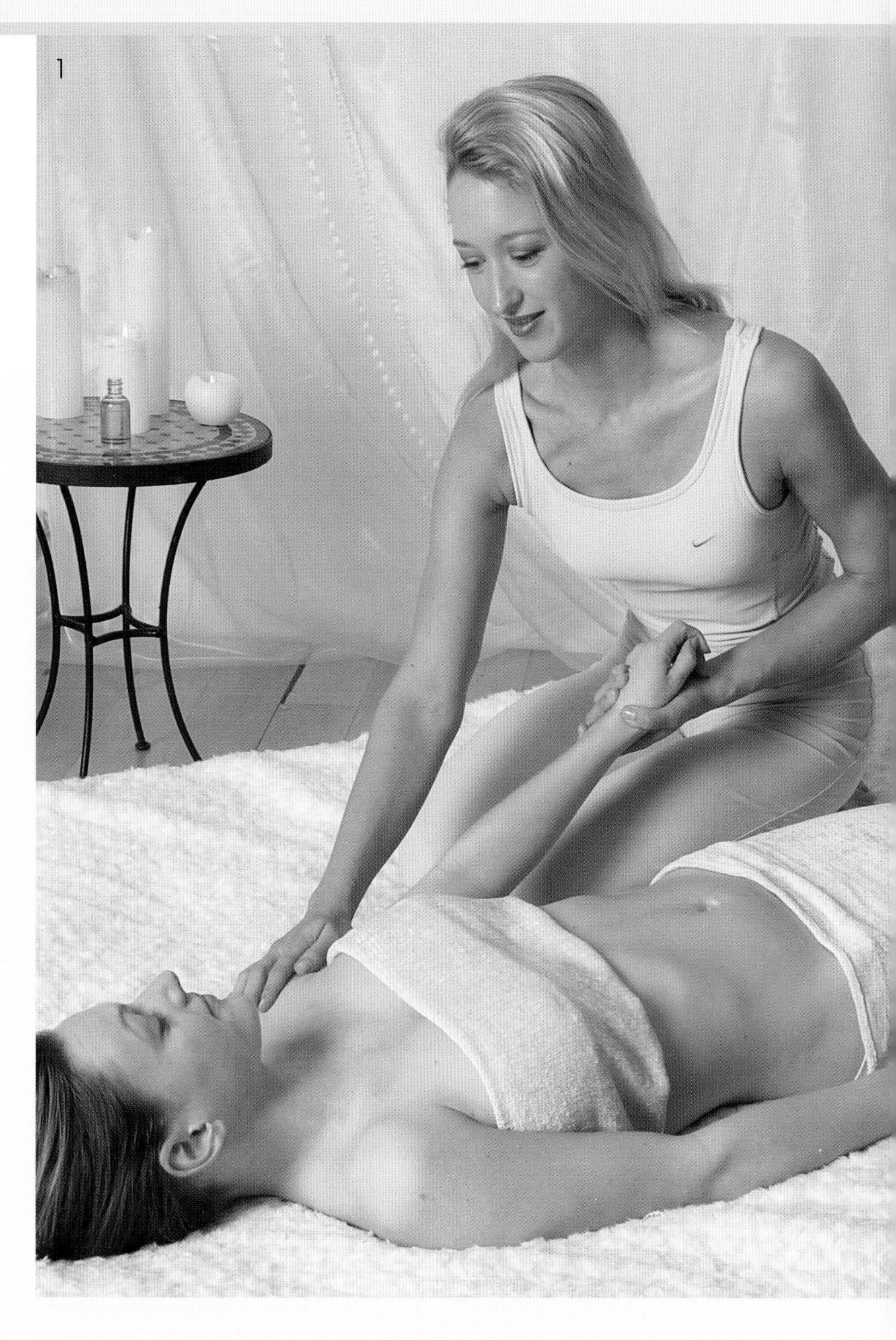

1

1 **Alternating effleurage:** Hold the wrist with one hand and place the other flat above the wrist with the fingers pointing towards the shoulder. Moulding your hand to the contours of the arm, slide the hand up towards the shoulder. Circle the shoulder with your whole hand and slide the hand back down the outside of the arm. Change hands and repeat the movement. Put light pressure on the way up and less pressure on the way back to the wrist.

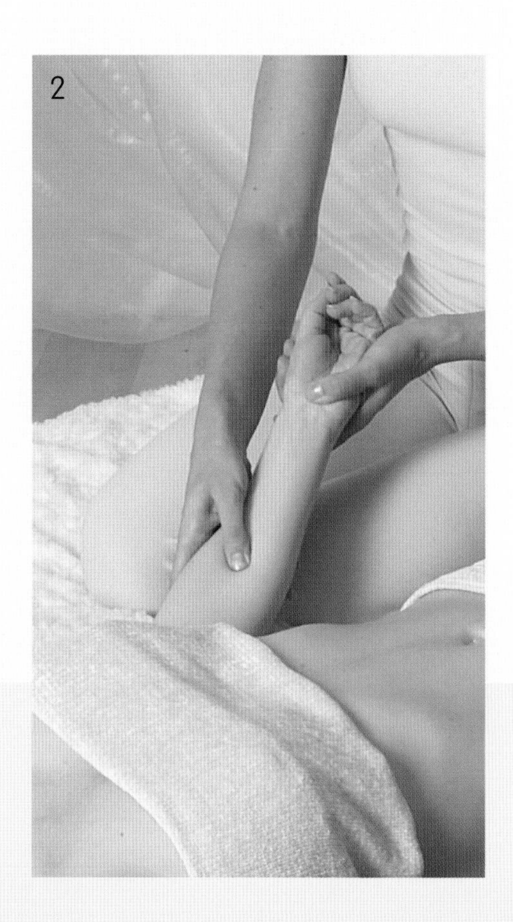

2

2 **Friction to the forearm:** Continue holding the wrist and turn the palm over so it is facing you. Place the thumb of one hand on the wrist. Make small circles with the thumb, going up towards the elbow. Stop before you get to the elbow and repeat twice. Turn the palm over and repeat to the top of the lower arm.

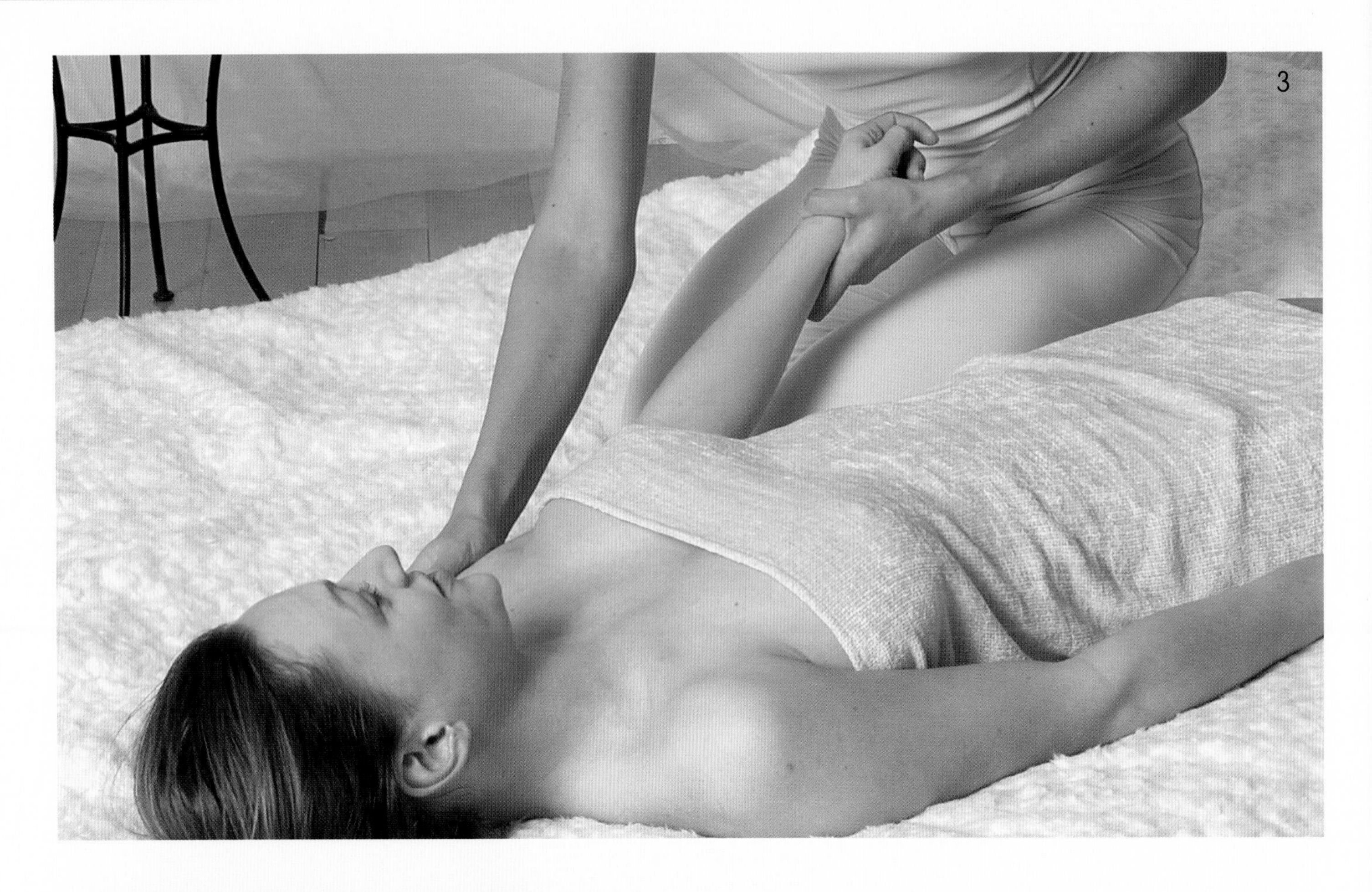

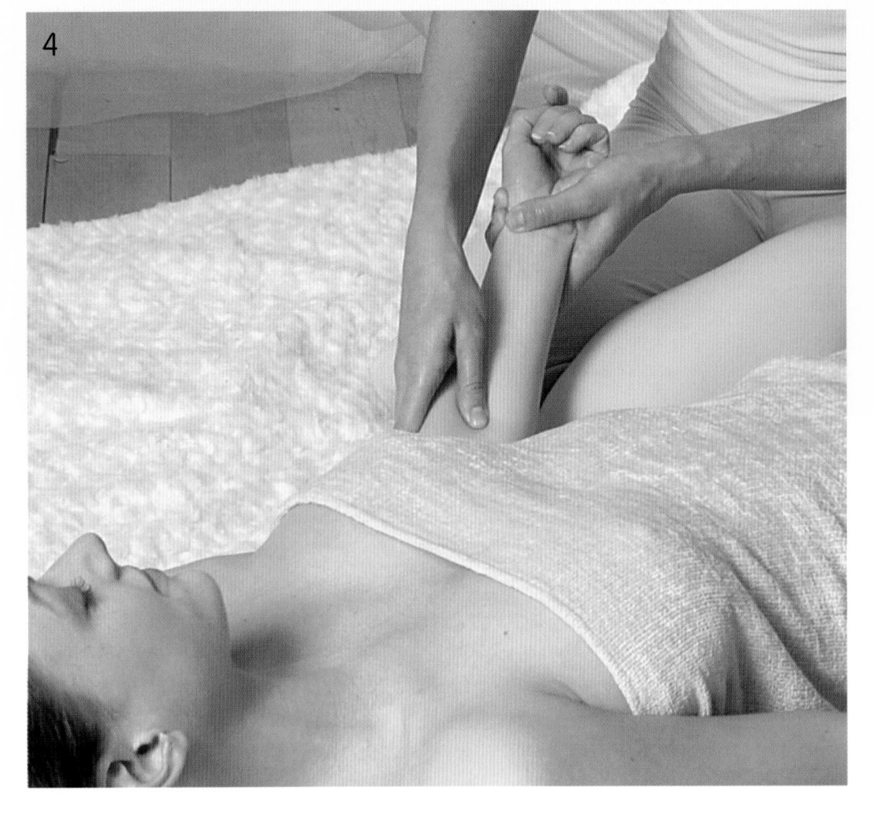

3 **Alternating effleurage:** Hold the wrist with one hand and place the other flat above the wrist with the fingers pointing towards the shoulder. Moulding your hand to the contours of the arm, slide the hand up towards the shoulder. Circle the shoulder with your whole hand and slide the hand back down the outside of the arm. Change hands and repeat the movement. Put light pressure on the way up and less pressure on the way back to the wrist.

4 **Friction to the forearm:** Continue holding the wrist and turn the palm over so it is facing you. Place the thumb of one hand on the wrist. Make small circles with the thumb, going up towards the elbow. Stop before you get to the elbow and repeat twice. Turn the palm over and repeat to the top of the lower arm.

5 Friction to the hand: Hold the hand in both of yours. Place the thumbs on top of the hand and make circles covering the whole hand and wrist area. Turn the palm up to face you and continue making circles with your thumbs across the palm.

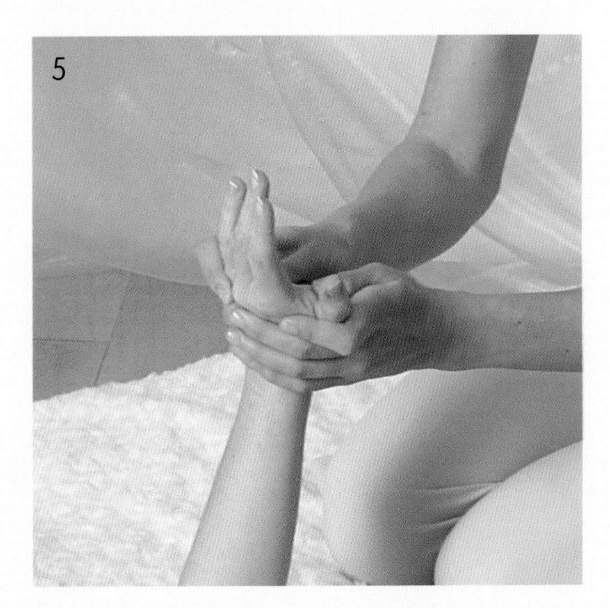
5

6 Finger massage: Hold the wrist with one hand. Place your thumb and forefinger at the base of one of your partner's fingers. Massage the finger with small circles as you work your way up to the tip. Repeat with the next finger until all the fingers have been massaged.

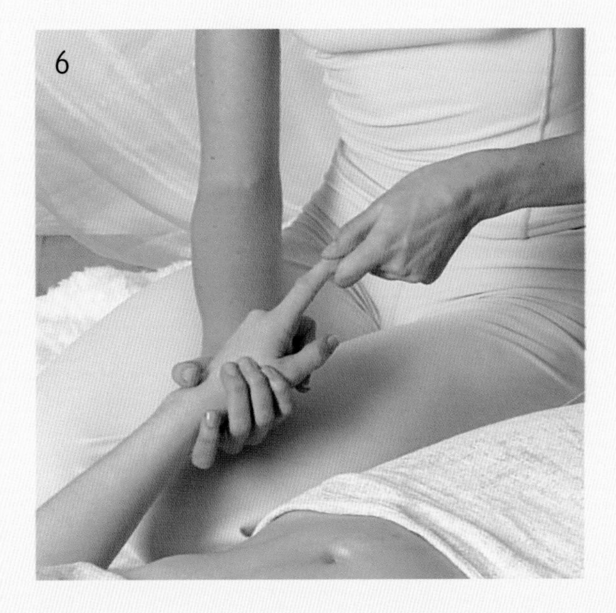
6

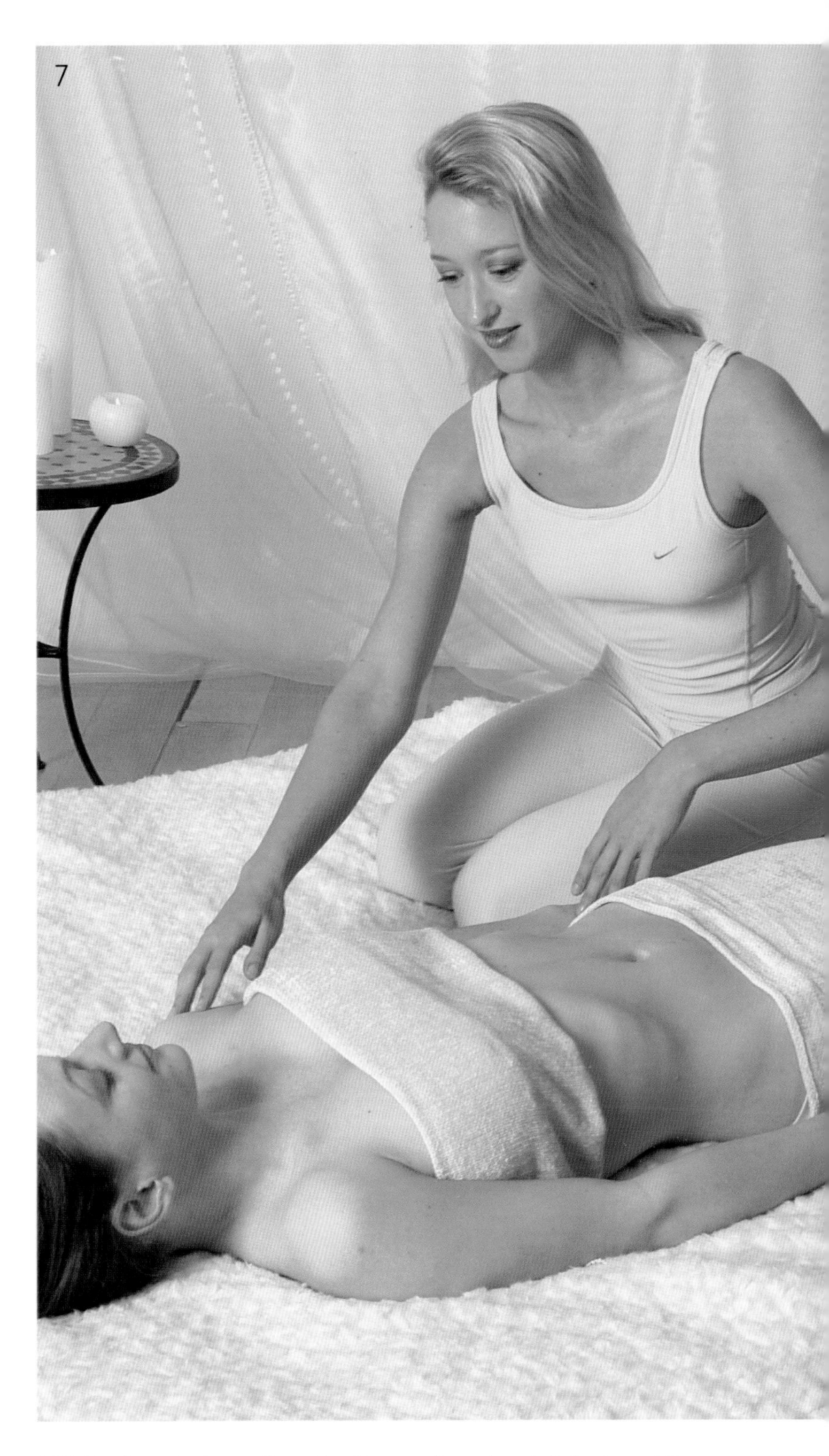
7

7 Feather stroking: Place the fingers of one hand at the top of the arm. Gently let them caress the arm slowly down to the wrist. Repeat with the other hand.

Ending: Place the arm underneath the towel and move to the other side to repeat the sequence.

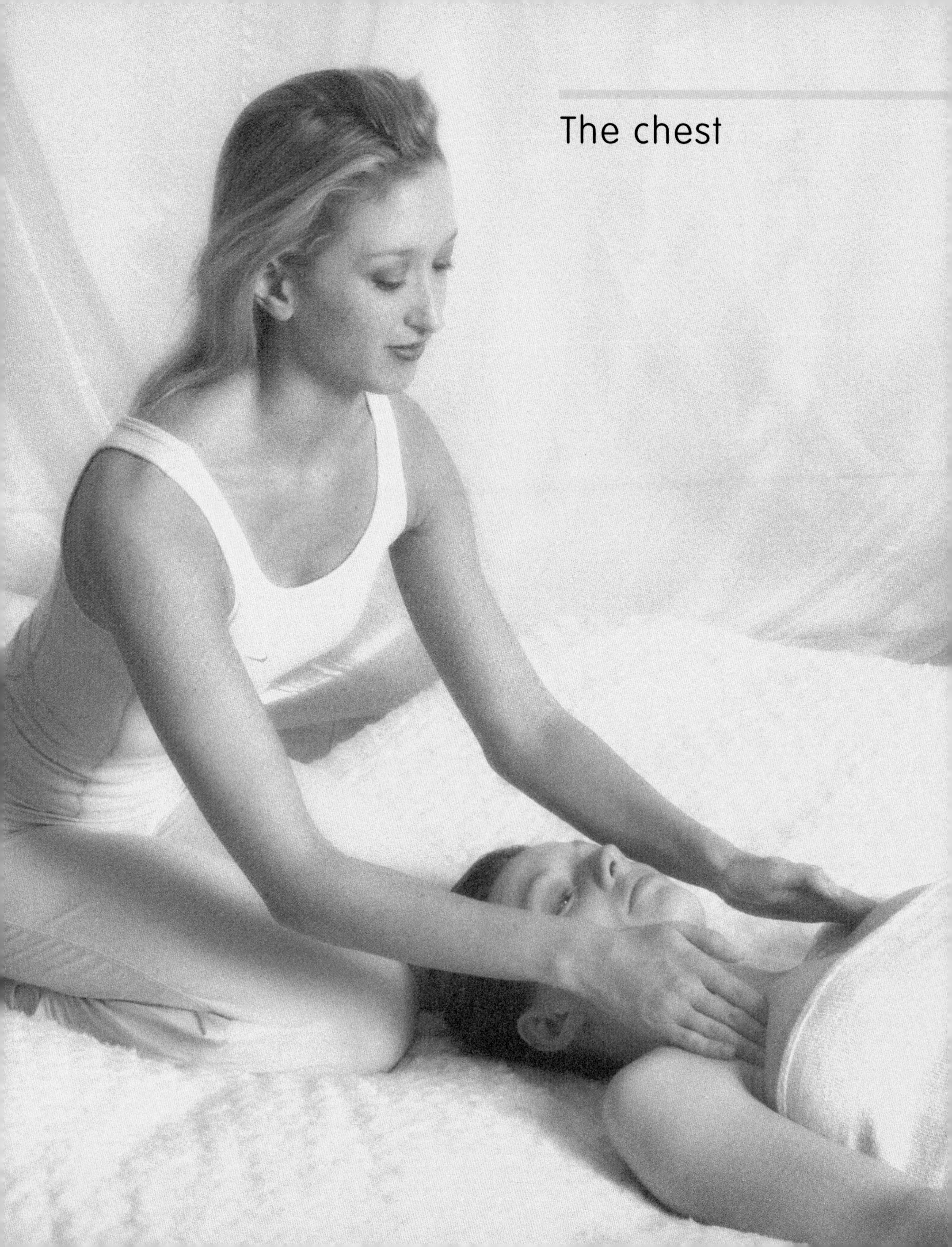

The chest

The chest is a very delicate area. Fold the towel back so that you can work on the chest without exposing your partner. Work lightly, avoiding the front of the neck. If you get too close to the front of the neck area, your partner may feel as if you are choking them.

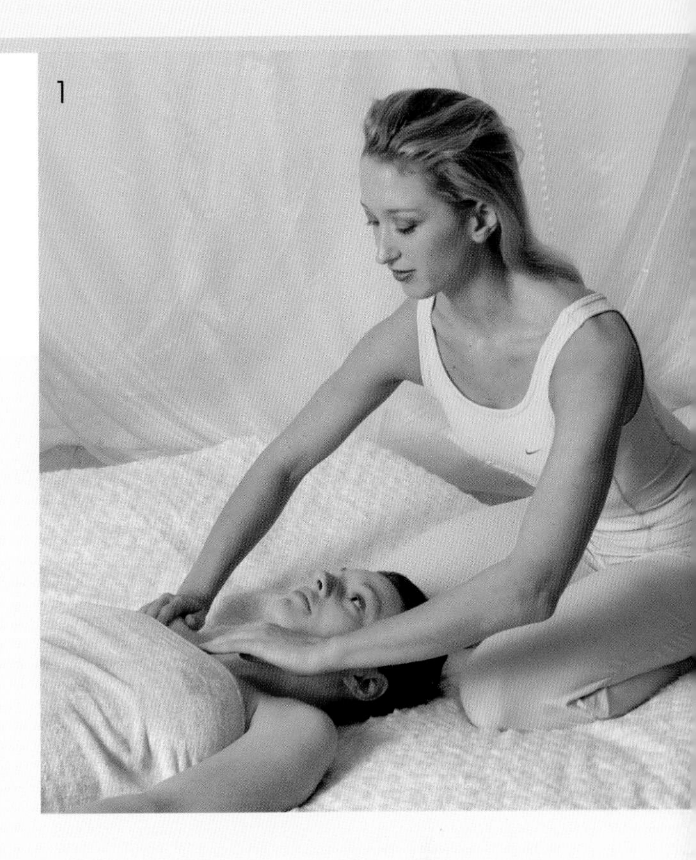

Spreading the oil: Place a small amount of oil in one hand. Rub the oil between your hands. Place the hands on the chest with the fingers facing each other and your elbows out to the sides. Gently press the hands out to the sides towards the shoulders, spreading the oil. Then, place the hands underneath the neck. Slide them out along the neck towards the shoulders. Repeat this action above and below the shoulders until the oil is evenly spread.

1 **Alternating effleurage:** Place the right hand on the chest below the neck with the fingers facing the left shoulder. Press and slide the hand towards the right shoulder. Then repeat the action with the left hand towards the left shoulder. Repeat the action with slow, rhythmic movements.

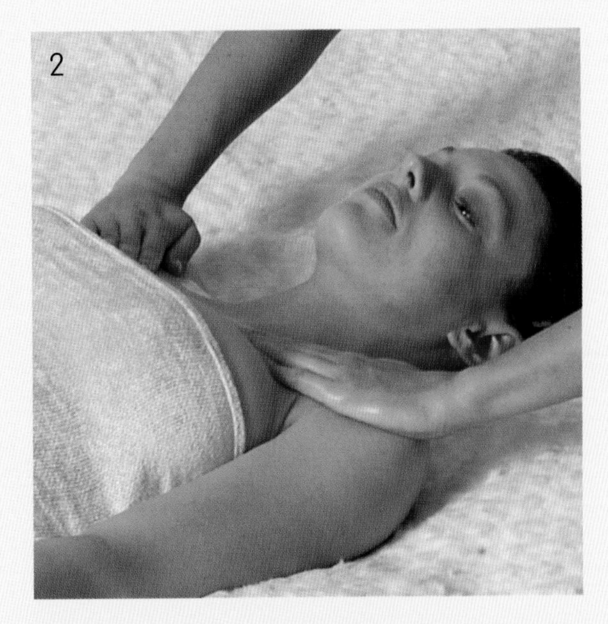

2 **Circling chest, neck and shoulders:** Place both hands on the chest with the fingertips together and the elbows out to the sides. Slide the hands in opposite directions towards the shoulders. Circle the shoulders with your hands. Slide the hands along the back of the shoulders until they are at the base of the neck. Bring the hands together and slide them up the neck to the base of the head. Repeat this a few times.

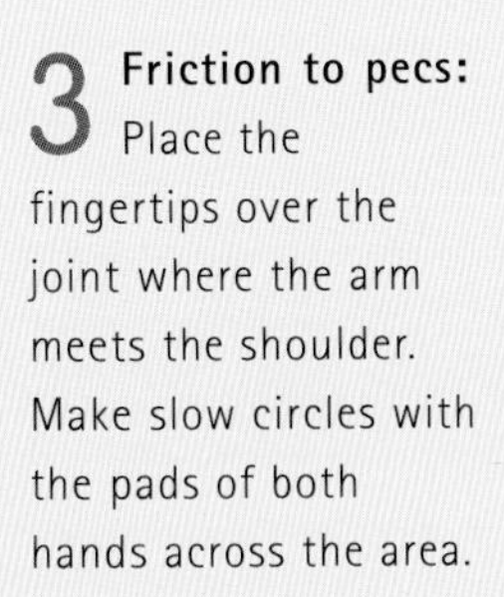

3 **Friction to pecs:** Place the fingertips over the joint where the arm meets the shoulder. Make slow circles with the pads of both hands across the area.

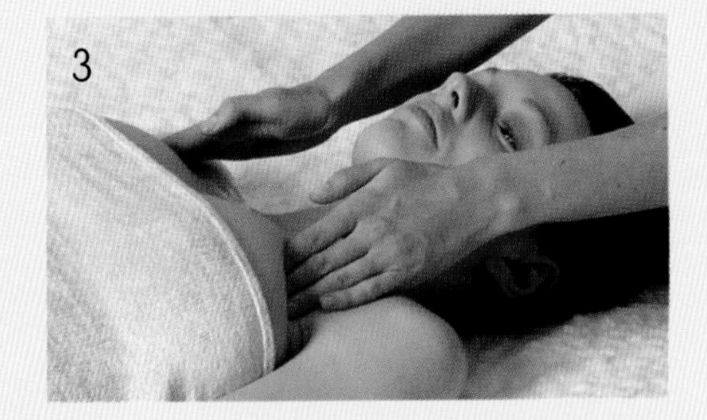

4 **Circling chest, neck and shoulders:** Repeat step 2.

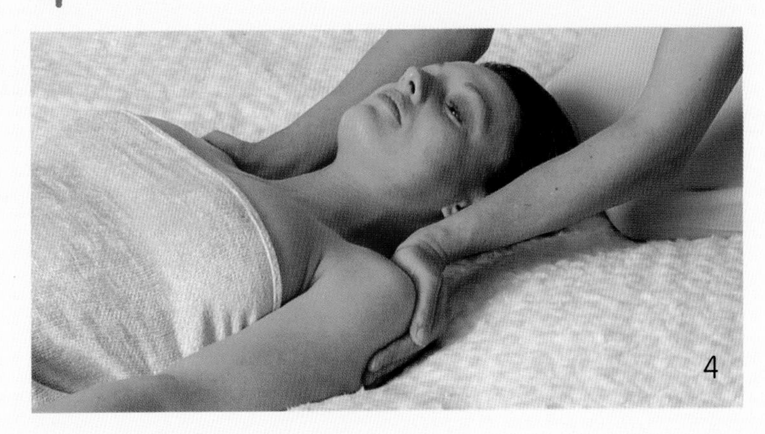

The neck and head

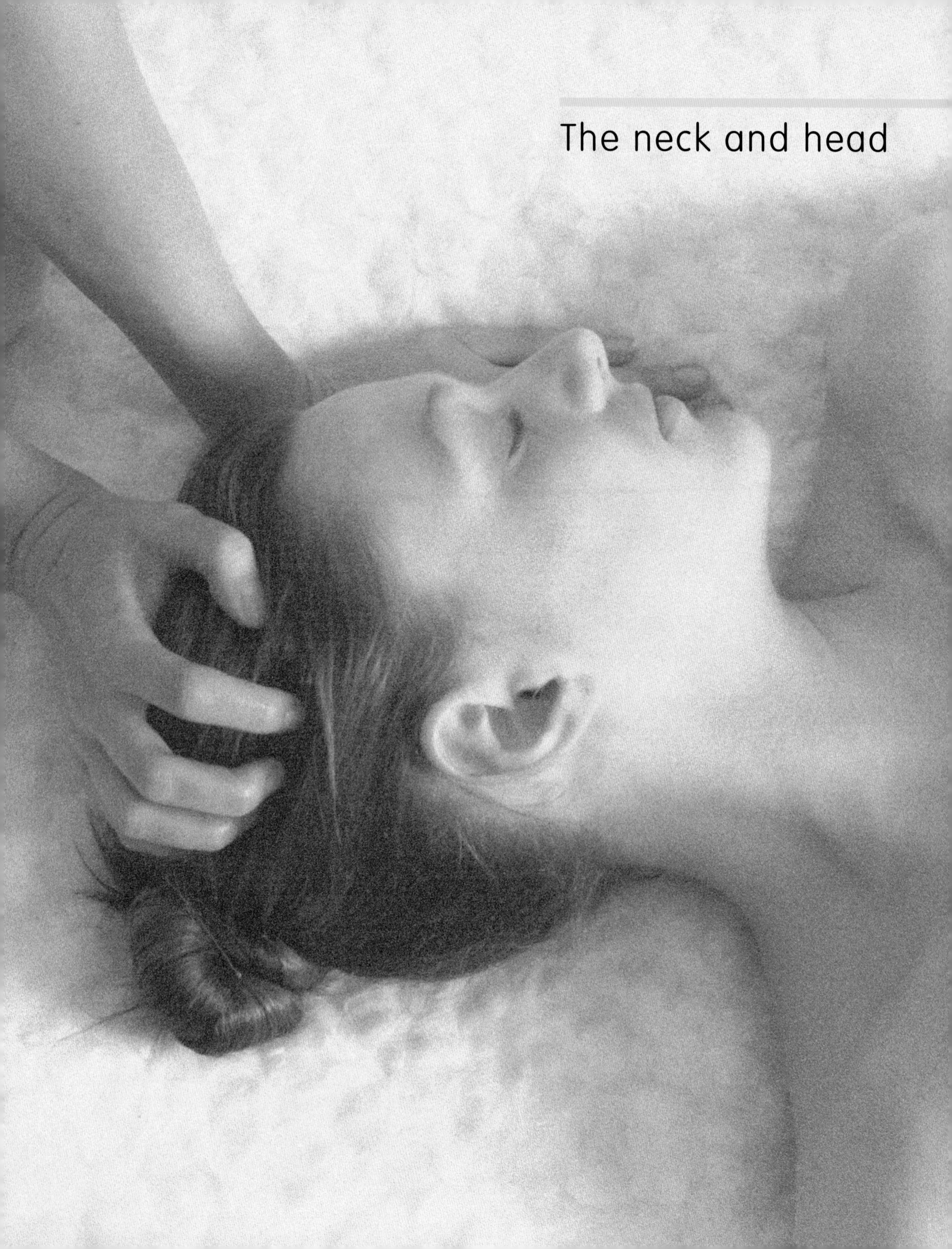

1 Gently roll the head to the right side. Place the right hand in front of the head so that it does not move around. Make sure the head is not tilting out of alignment.

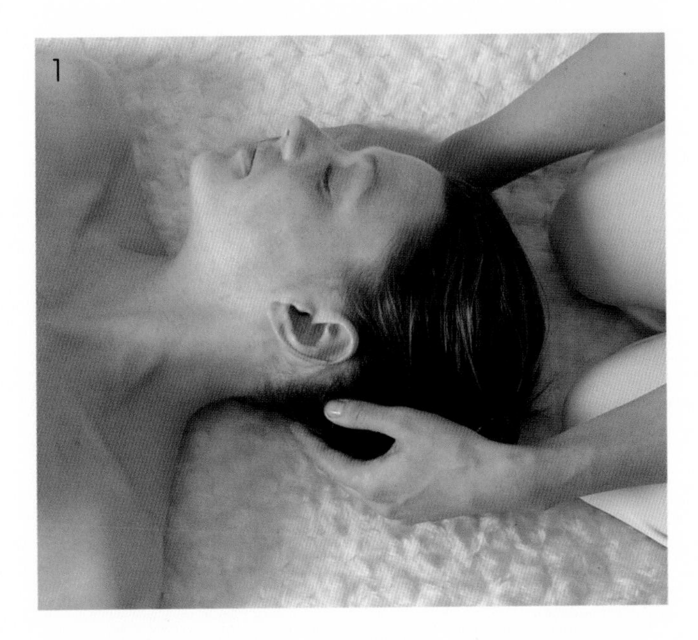

2 **One hand effleurage:** Place the fingertips down towards the floor with the thumb out. Place the hand at the base of the skull. Slide the hand along the neck towards the shoulders with the thumb following the contour of the neck. Wrap the hand around the shoulder and slide the hand back along the neck exactly as it went before. The fingers should remain down and the thumb up the whole time. Keep your hand flat and use the inside of the forefinger to massage the neck.

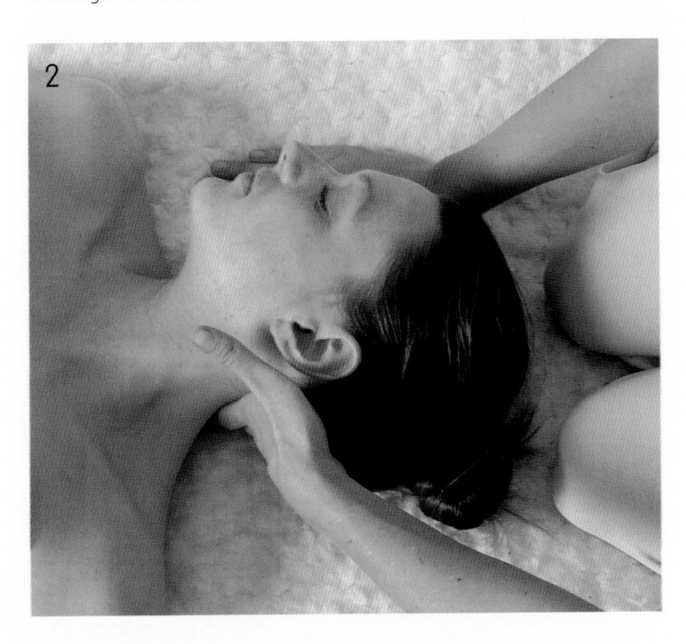

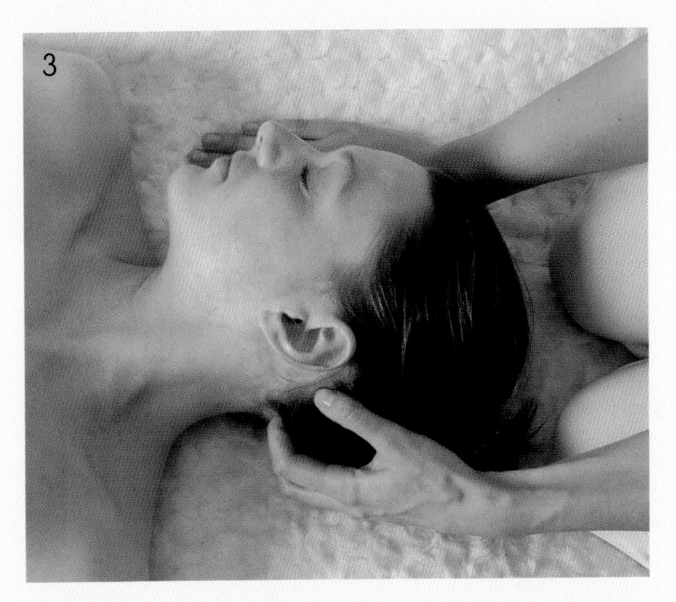

3 **Friction to base of head:** Place the fingertips of the left hand in the groove at the base of the head. Spread your fingers out and form a loose claw with your hand. Make small, slow circles with the pads of the fingers. Wipe the oil off your hands.

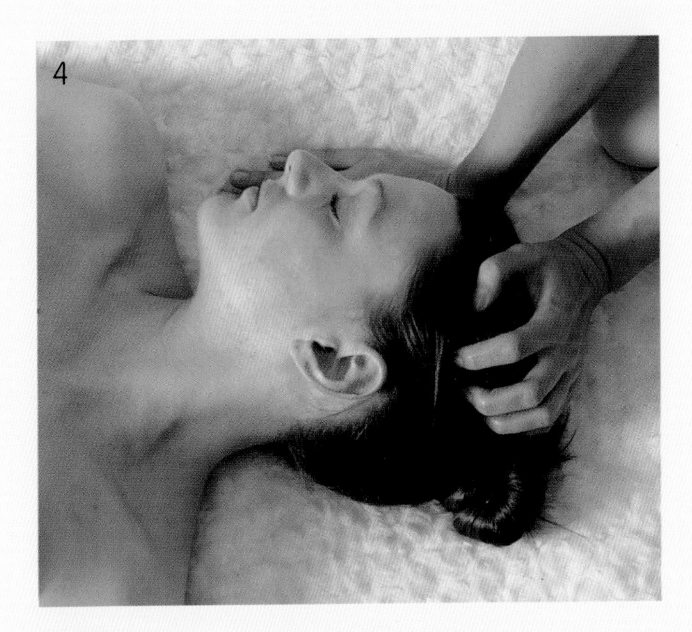

4 **Head massage:** Form a claw with your left hand. Start at the base of the skull and make slow, small circles with your fingertips. Make sure the scalp moves. Do not think of washing hair! The point is to move the skin over the bone. Slowly work your way up to the top of the head. Repeat, this time starting closer to the ear.

Ending: Slowly roll the head over to the other side. Repeat the whole sequence.

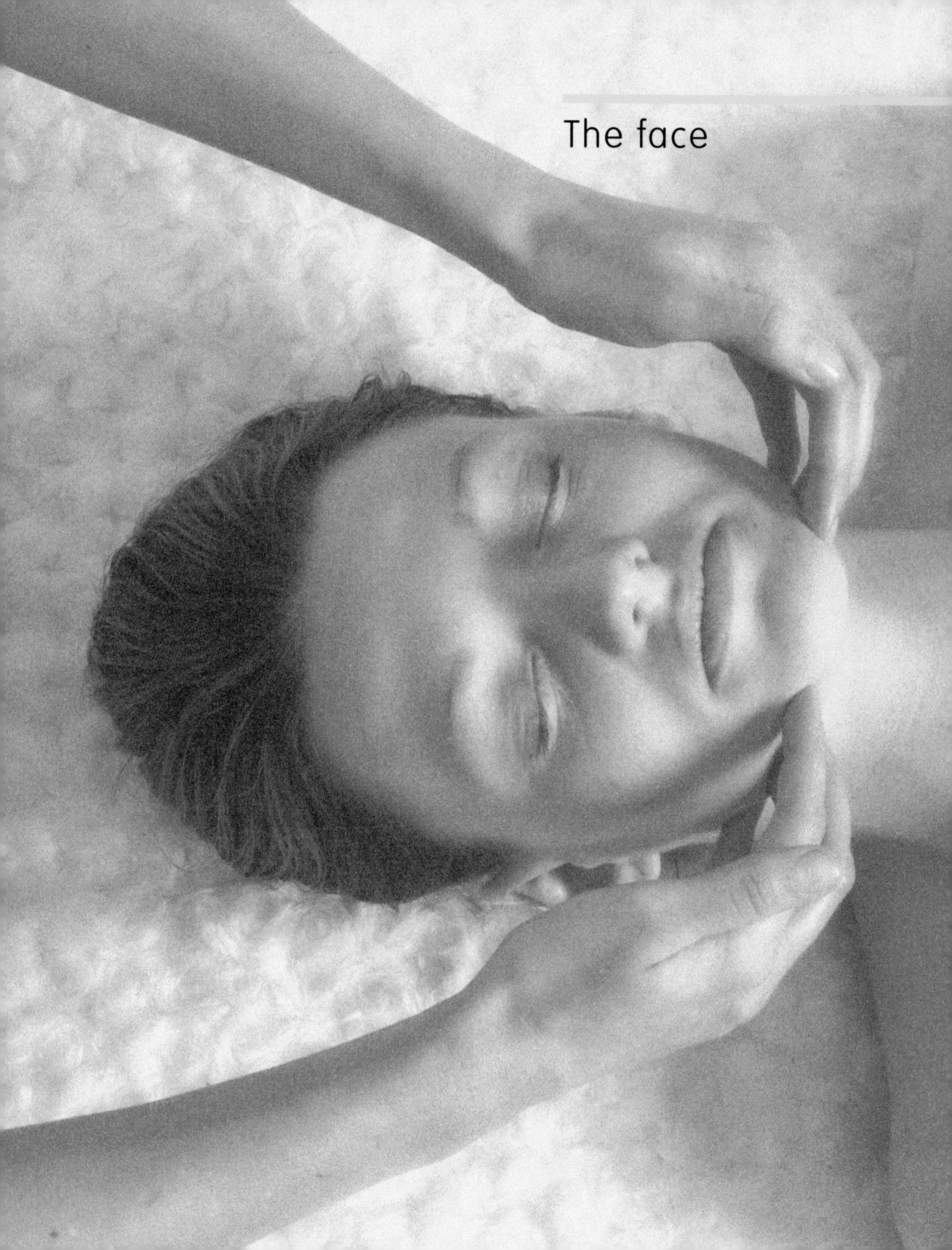

The face

The face is a very delicate area of the body. Work extremely gently and carefully.

Spreading the oil: Only put one or two drops of oil onto your fingertips. This is so that your fingers can slide along the skin without clogging the pores of your partner.

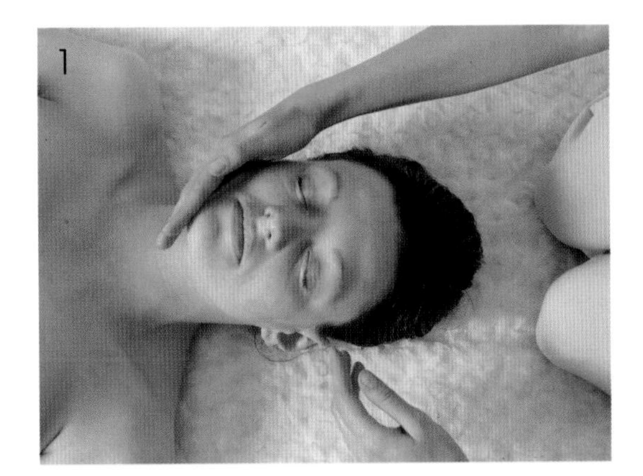

1 **Effleurage to the chin:** Place the fingertips lightly underneath the chin with your elbows out to the sides. Caress the chin with one hand up towards the ear. Then caress the chin with the other hand up to the ear. Repeat, with soft, sweeping movements. Then repeat with both hands on the same side, alternating as they move from the chin to the ear. Repeat to the other side.

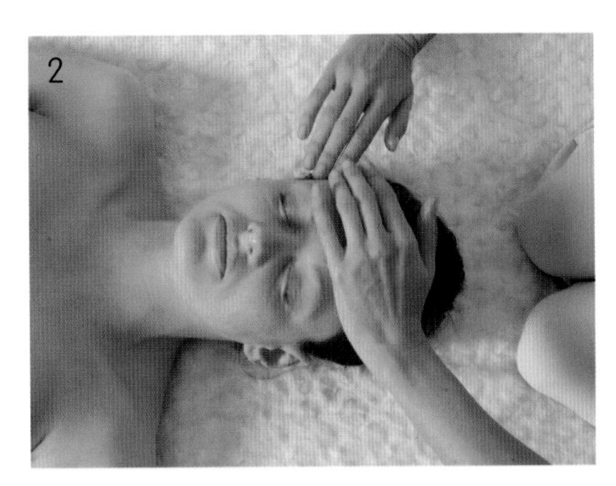

2 **Effleurage to the forehead:** Place one hand gently on the forehead with the palm of the hand sideways and the fingers facing the opposite ear. Slide the hand gently across the forehead, replacing it with the other hand.

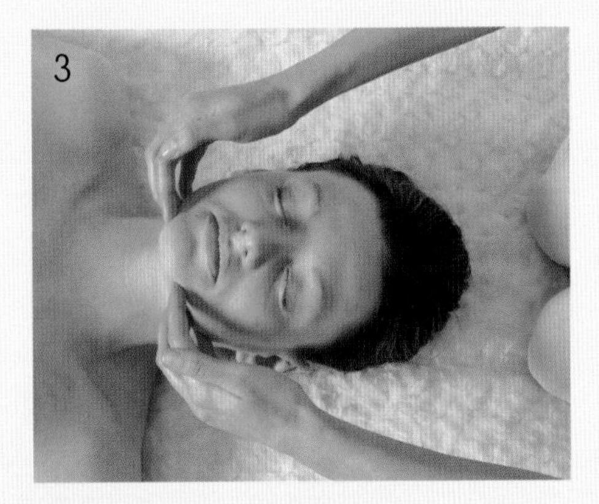

3 **Friction:** Place the fingertips underneath the chin. Spread them out and make small circles, staying in one place. Move the fingers towards the jaw and repeat. Move the hands to the space between the upper lip and chin. Then move them below the lower lip.

4 **Massaging the ears:** Place the thumb and fingers on one ear. Rub the ear between the fingers. Gently pull the ear away as you continue rubbing. Repeat with the other ear.

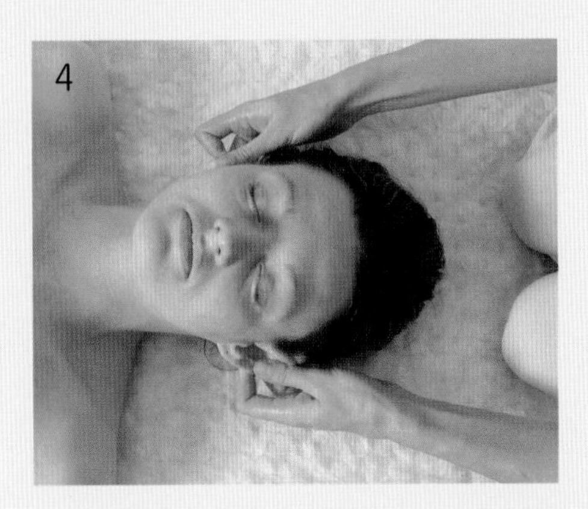

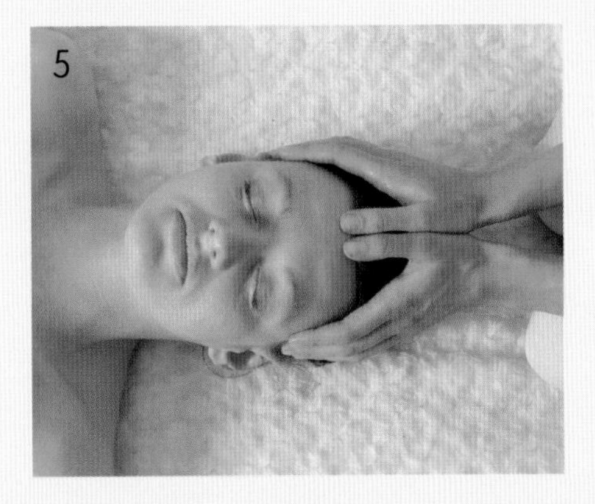

5 **Ending:** Place the thumbs on the forehead with the fingers around the head towards the ears. Hold the head for a few moments.

Ending the massage

Move to the side of your partner. Place your hands on both of their shoulders and gently squeeze. Move your hands down to their hips and gently squeeze. Continue moving your hands down their body to their knees. Gently squeeze the knees. Slide your hands down towards their feet. Hold their feet for a few moments. Release and shake out your hands.

Quick guide – back

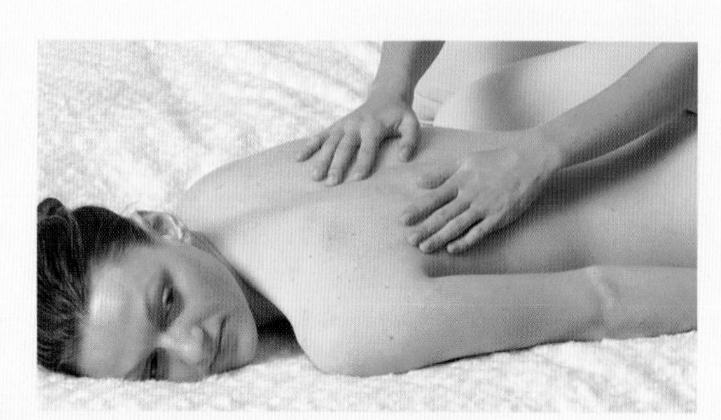
1. Spreading the oil

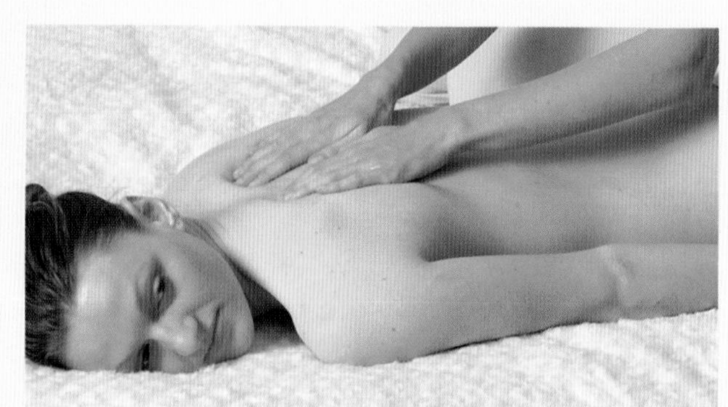
2. Basic effleurage

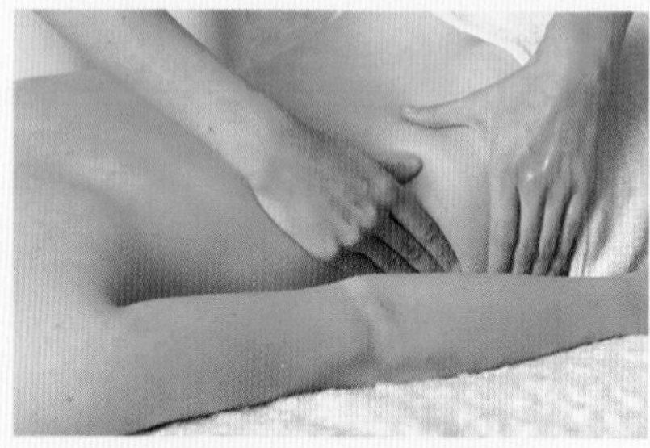
3. Kneading to the sides

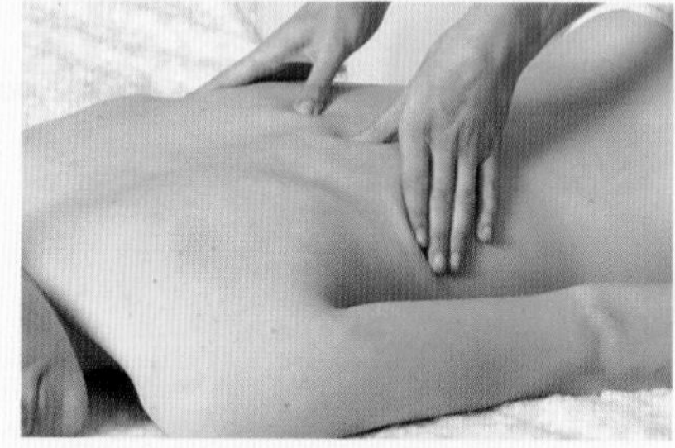
4. Friction up the spine

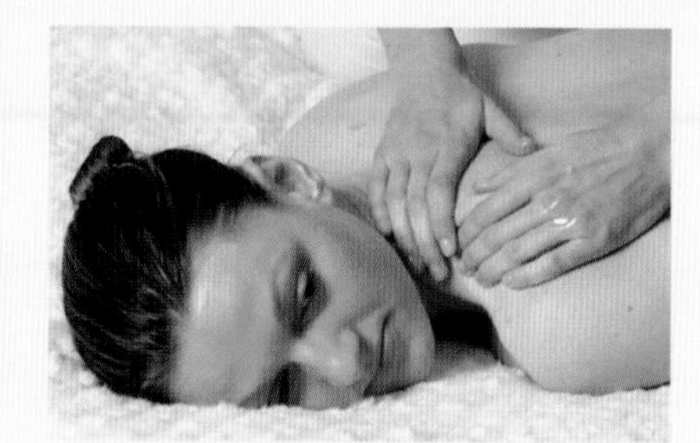
5. Kneading to the shoulders and neck

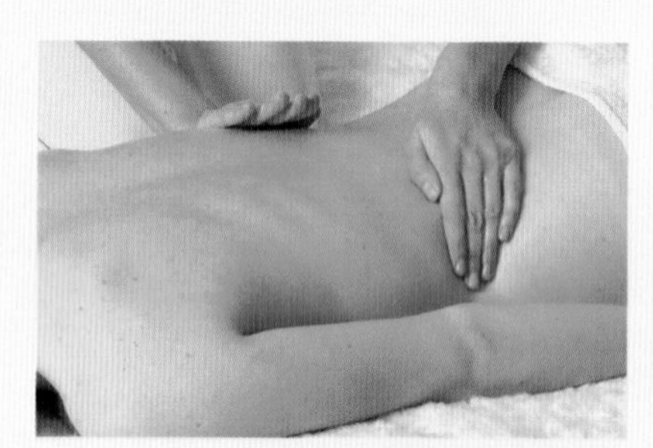
6. Wringing across the back

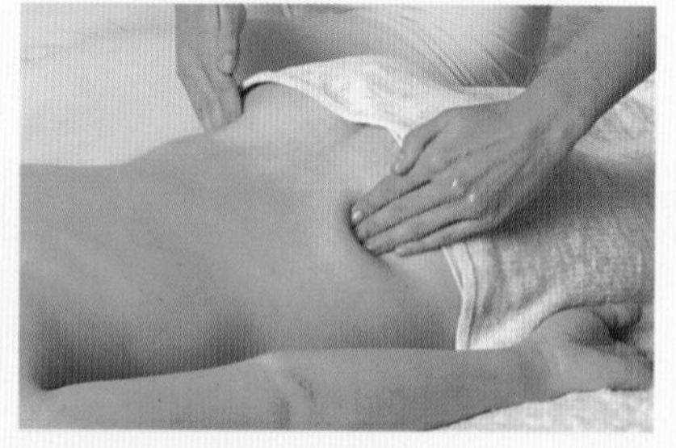
7. Friction to the base of the spine

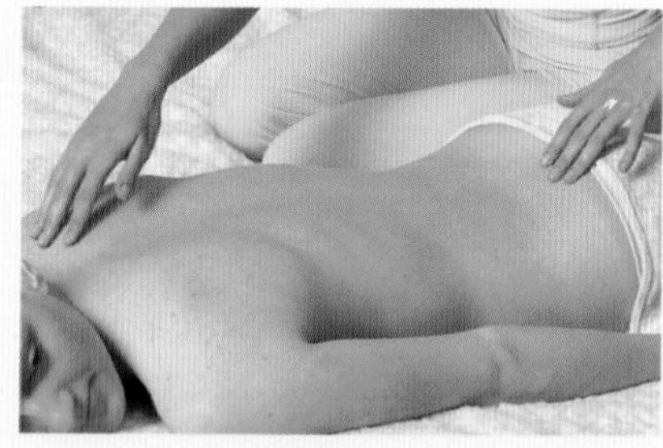
8. Feather stroking

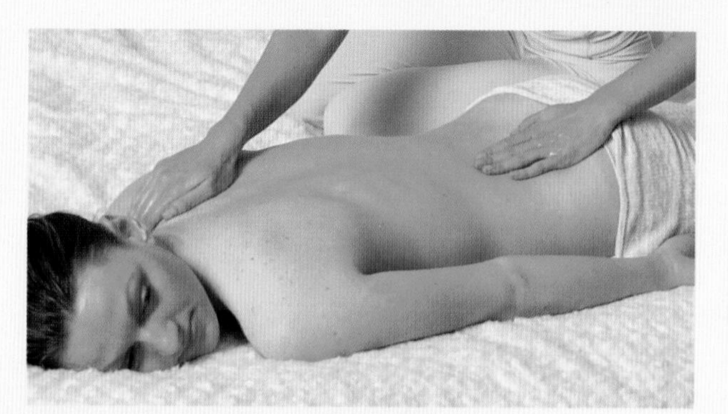
9. Alternating effleurage

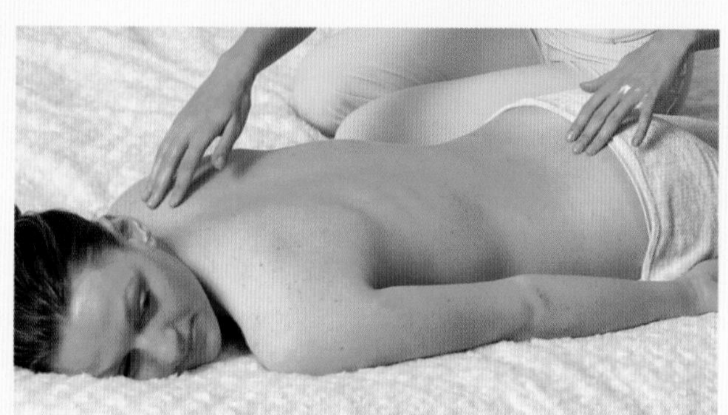
10. Feather stroking

Quick guide – back of the leg

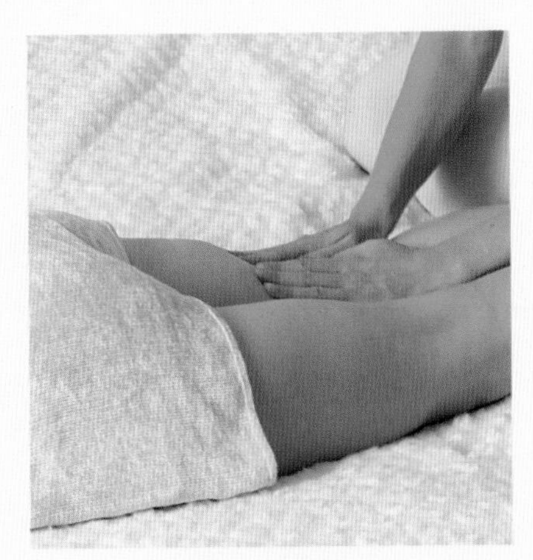
1. Basic effleurage

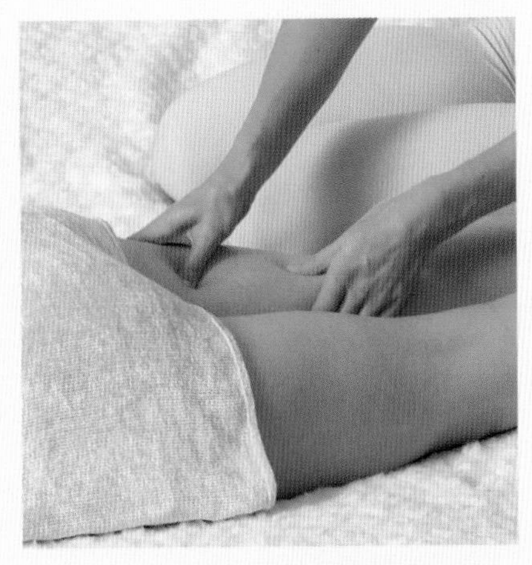
2. Friction to the thigh

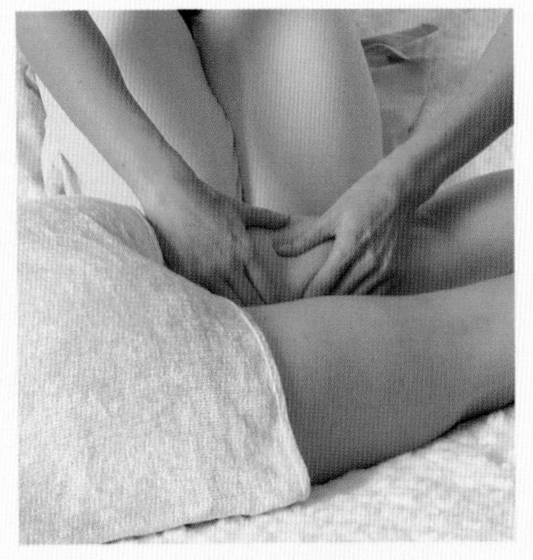
3. Kneading the inner thigh

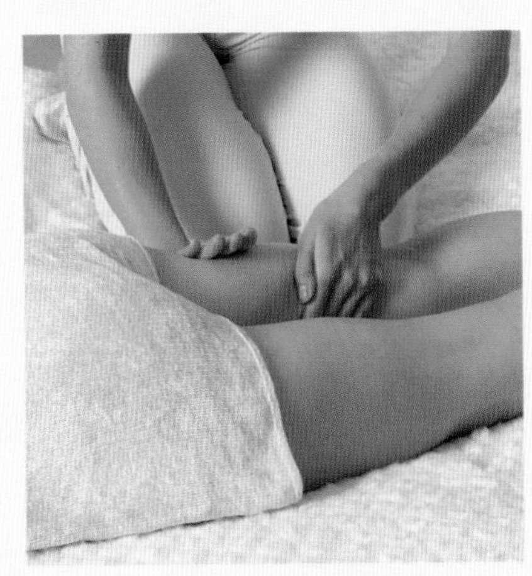
4. Wringing the thigh

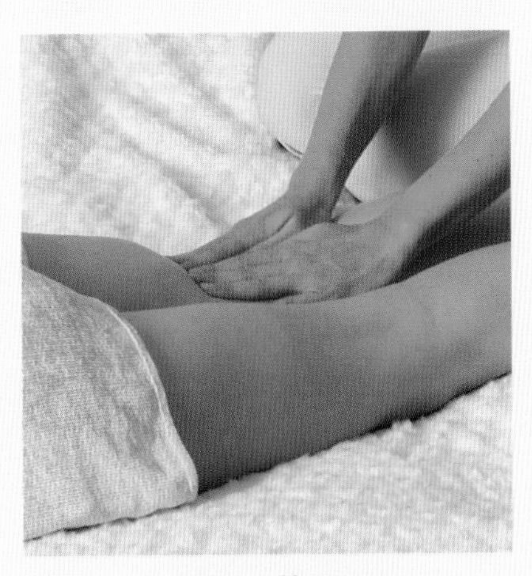
5. Basic effleurage

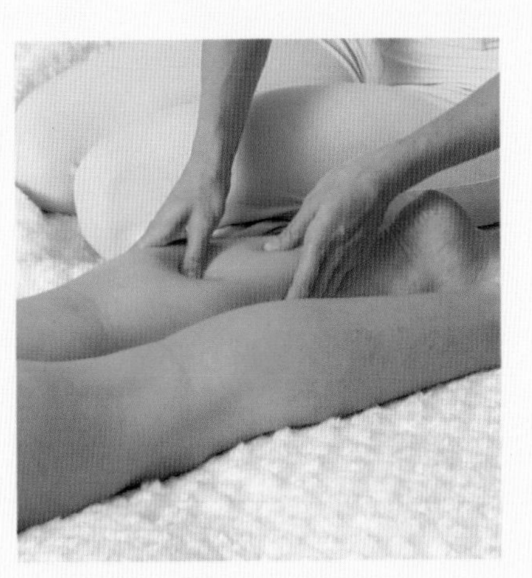
6. Friction to the calf

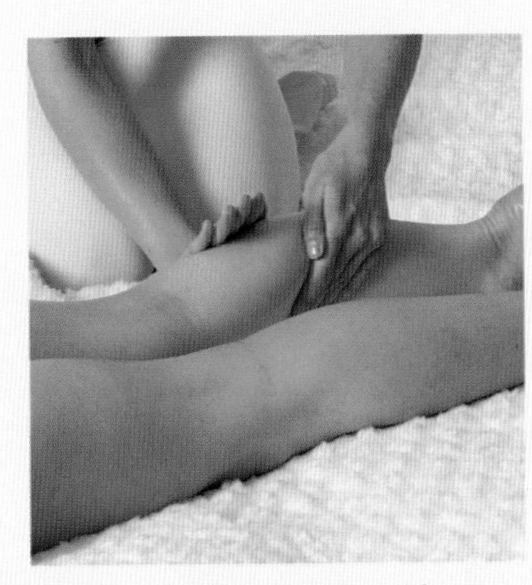
7. Wringing the calf

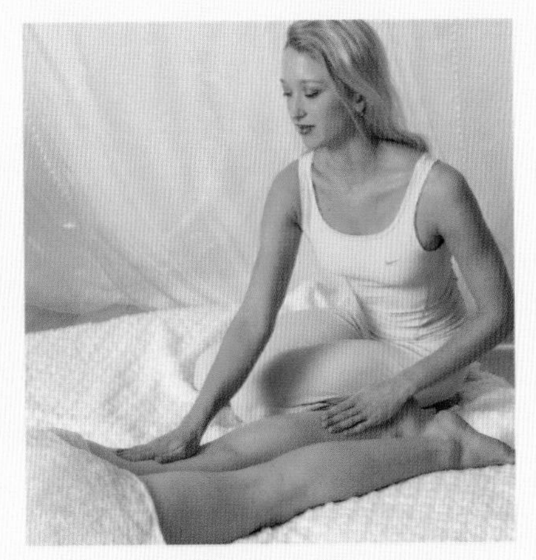
8. Alternating effleurage

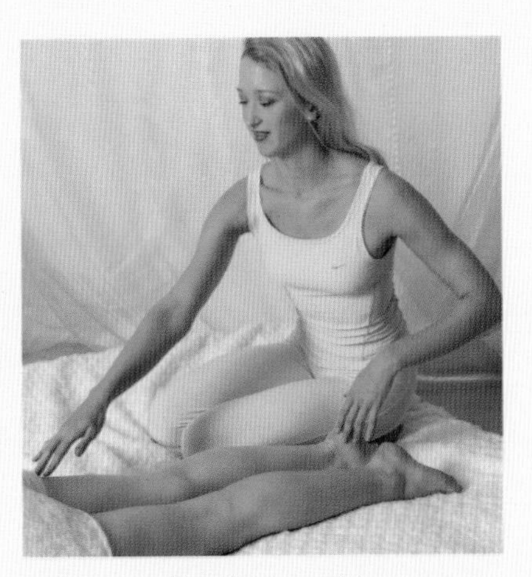
9. Feather stroking

Quick guide – front of the leg

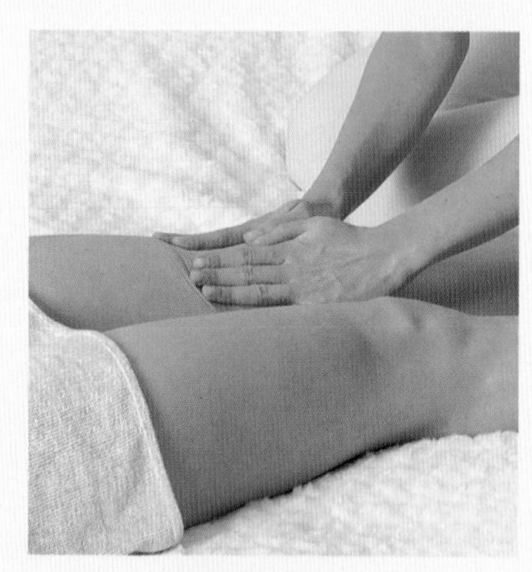

1. Basic effleurage

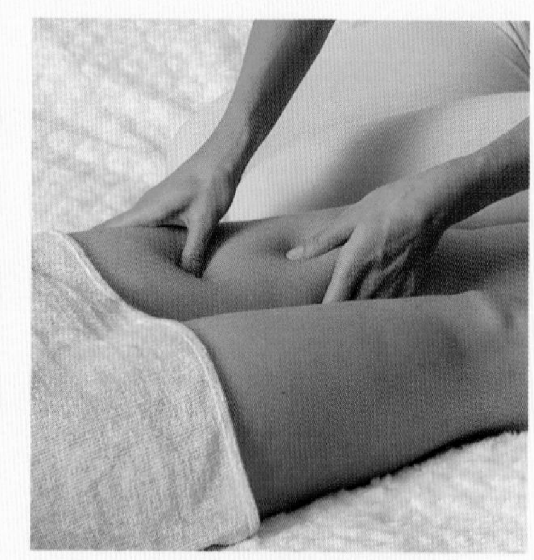

2. Friction to the thigh

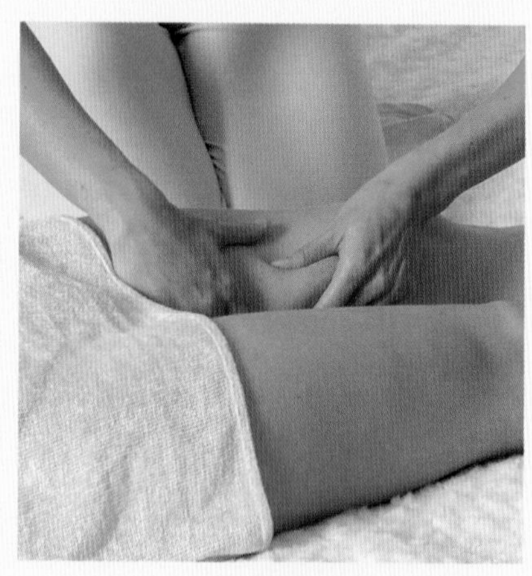

3. Kneading the inner thigh

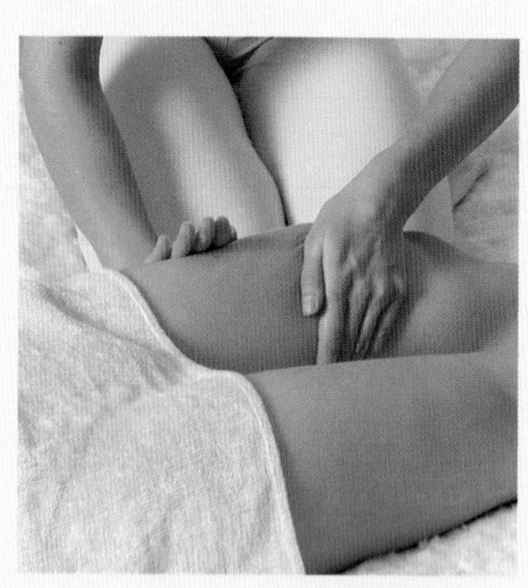

4. Wringing the thigh

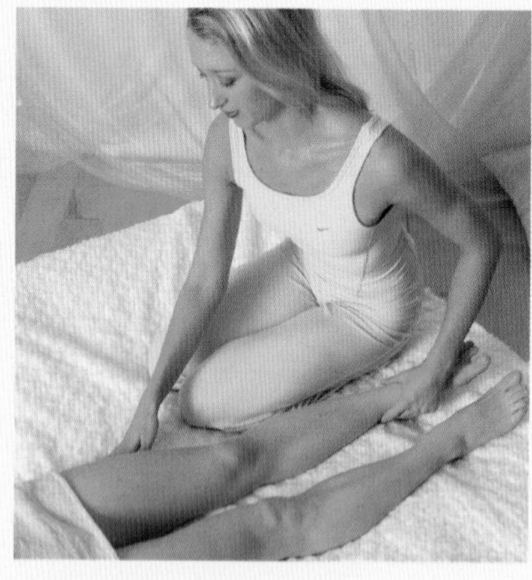

5. Friction to the outside of the leg

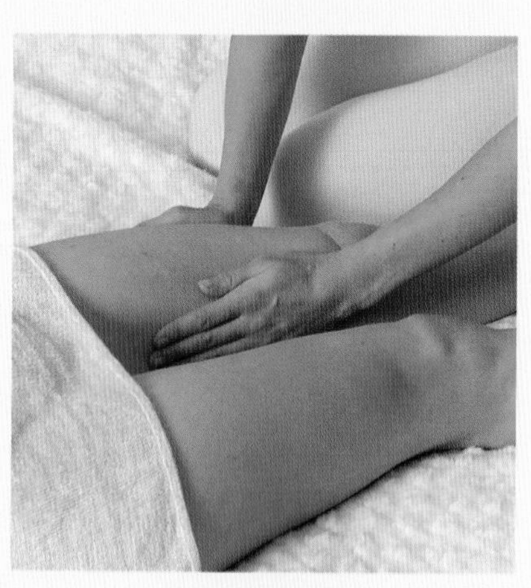

6. Basic effleurage

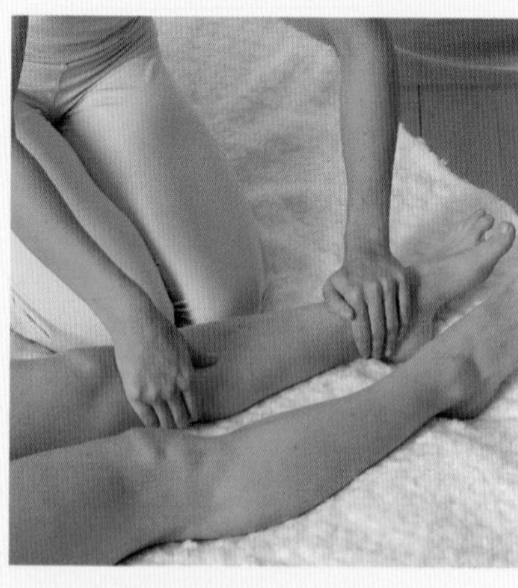

7. Friction down the shin

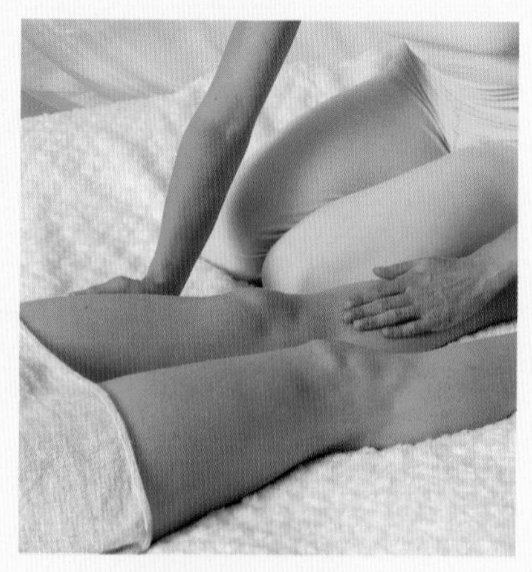

8. Alternating effleurage

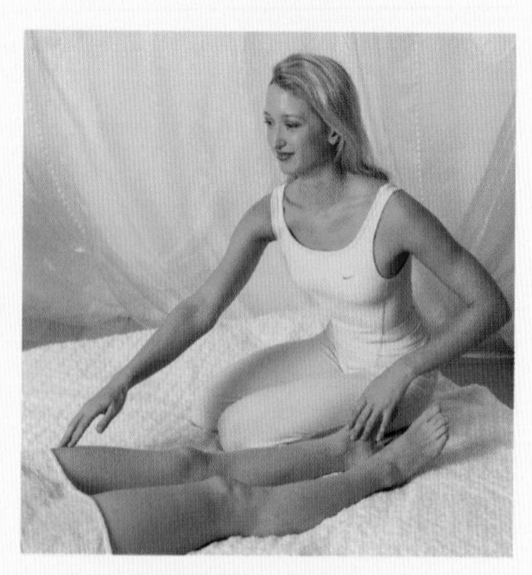

9. Feather stroking

Quick guide – foot

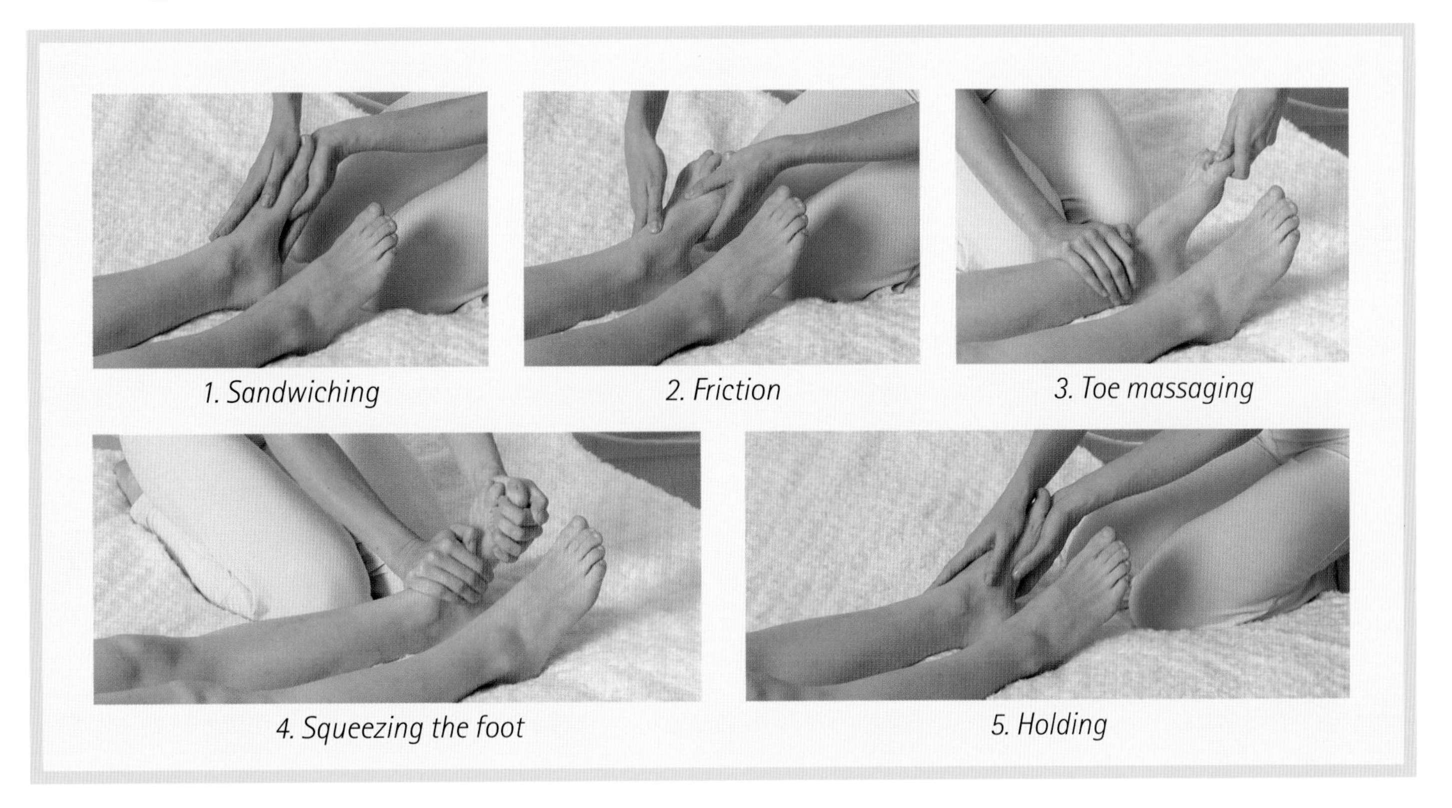

1. Sandwiching
2. Friction
3. Toe massaging
4. Squeezing the foot
5. Holding

Quick guide – stomach

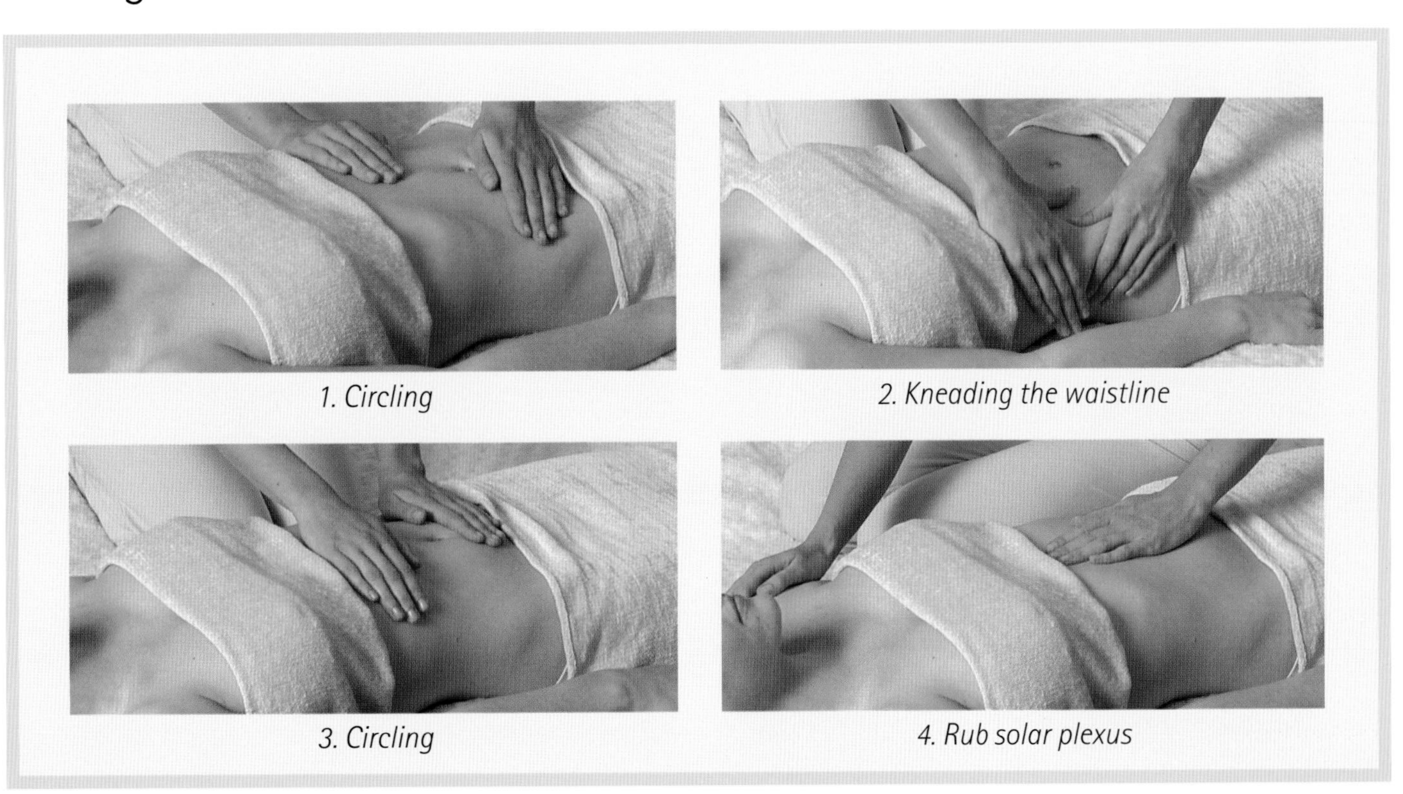

1. Circling
2. Kneading the waistline
3. Circling
4. Rub solar plexus

Quick guide – arm

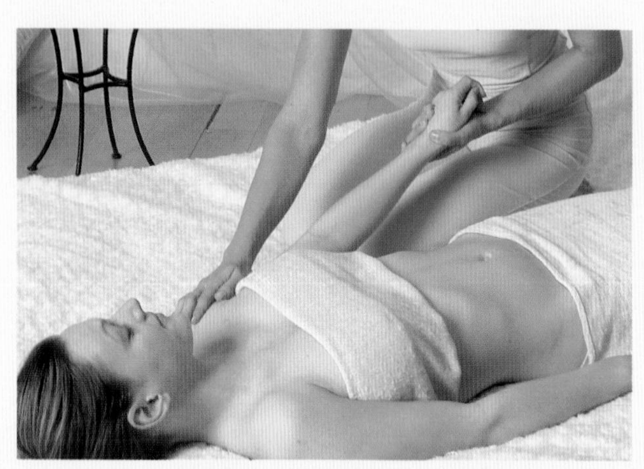

1. Alternating effleurage

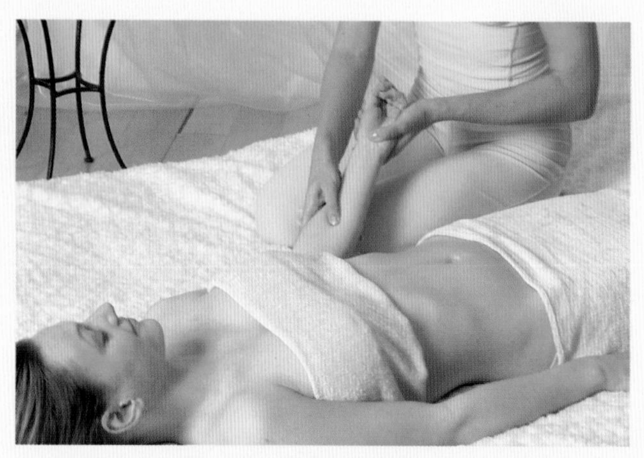

2. Friction to the forearm

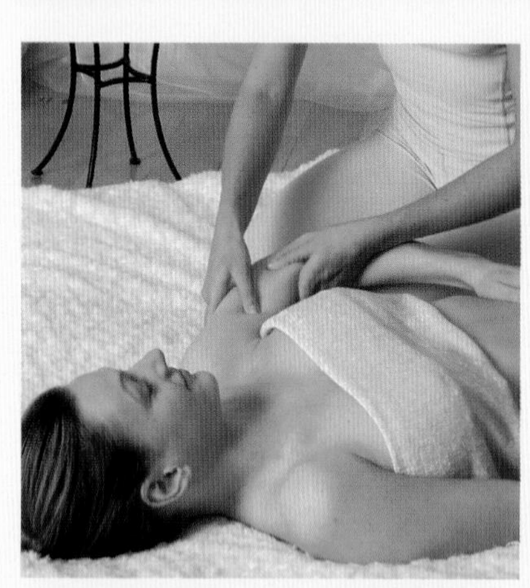

3. Friction to the upper arm

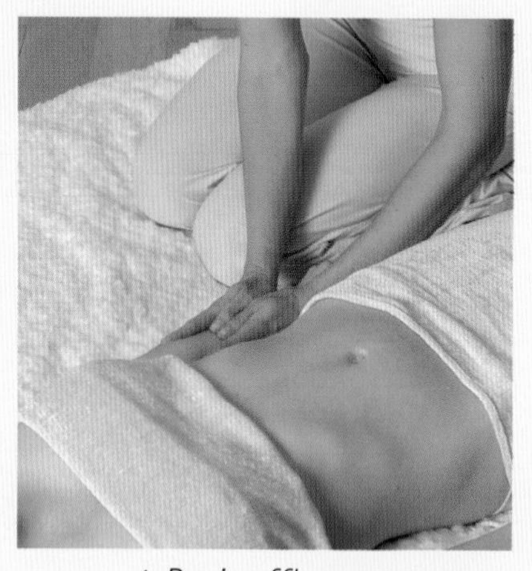

4. Basic effleurage

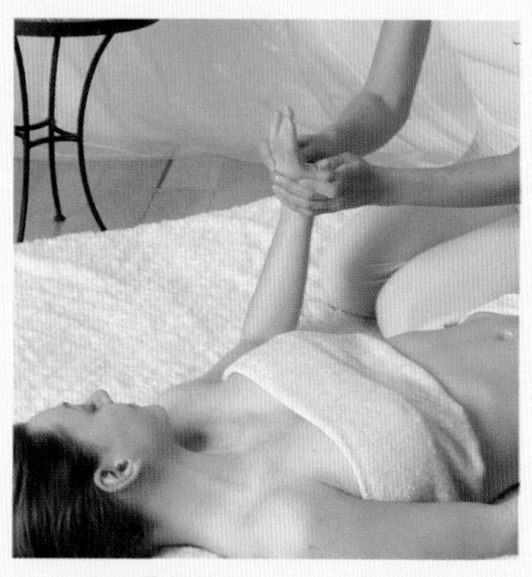

5. Friction to the hand

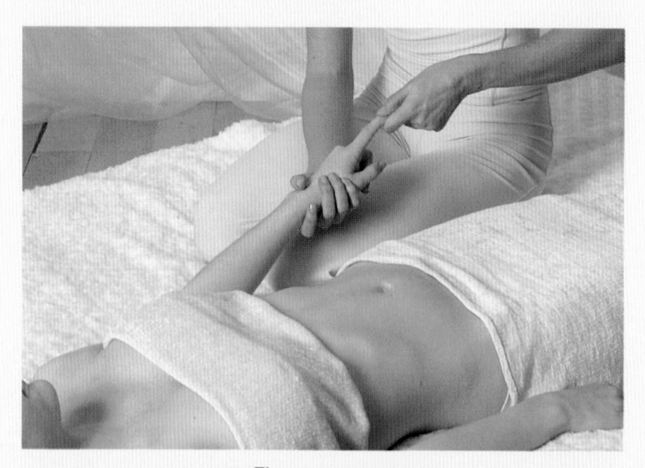

6. Finger massage

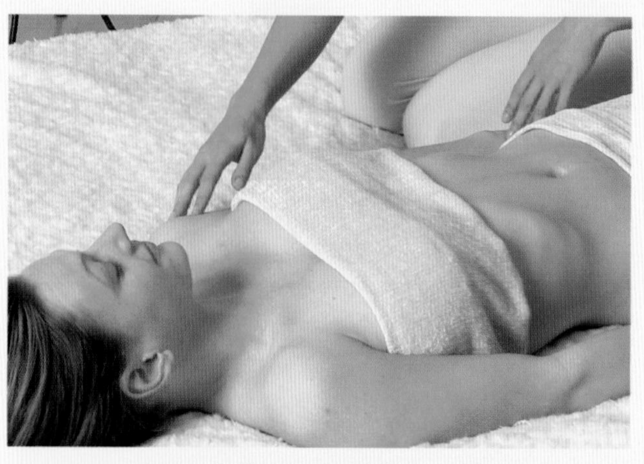

7. Feather stroking

Quick guide – chest

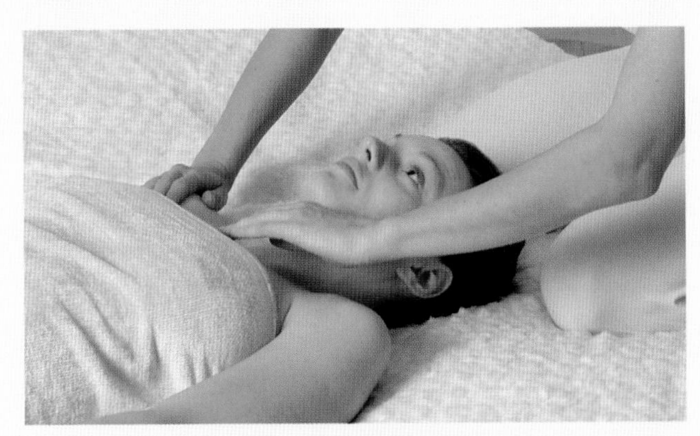

1. Alternating effleurage

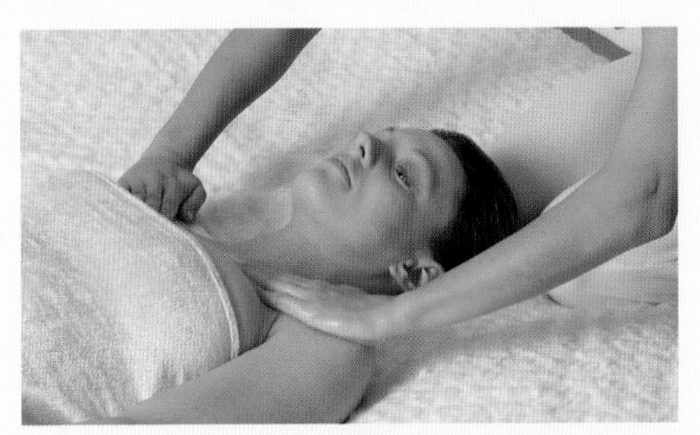

2. Circling chest, neck and shoulders

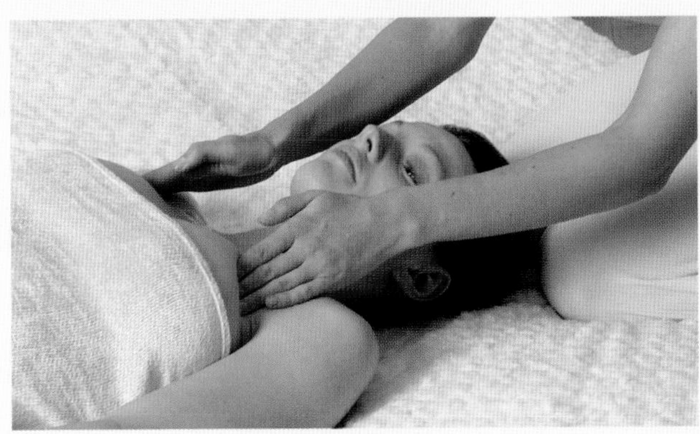

3. Friction to pecs

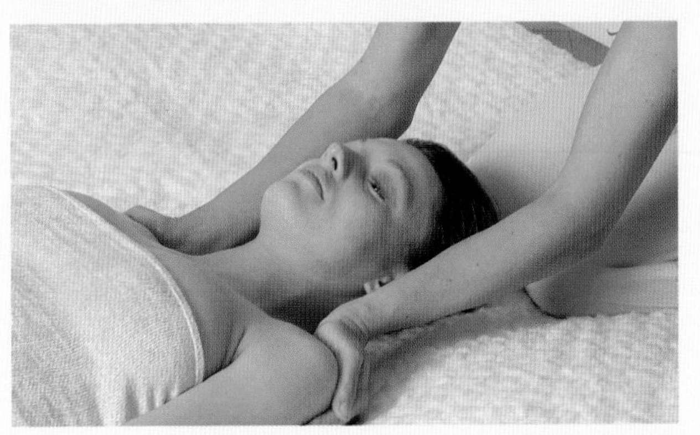

4. Circling chest, neck and shoulders

Quick guide – neck and head

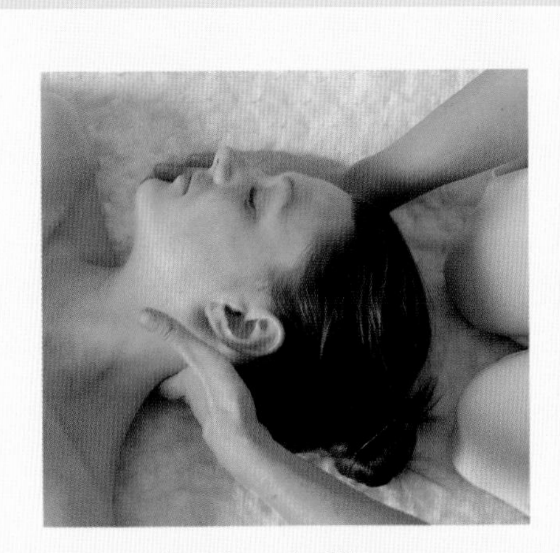

1. One hand effleurage

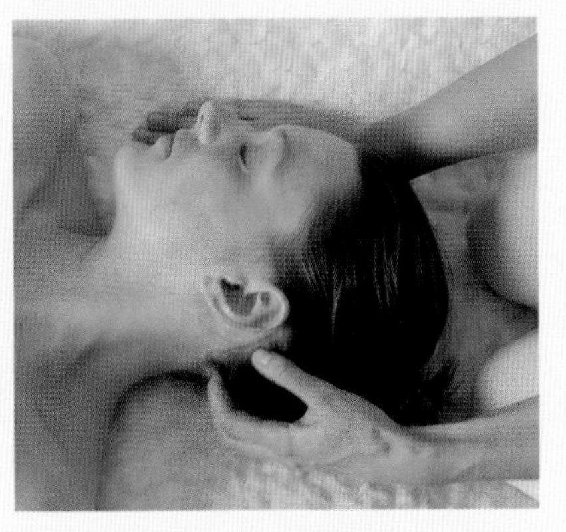

2. Friction to base of head

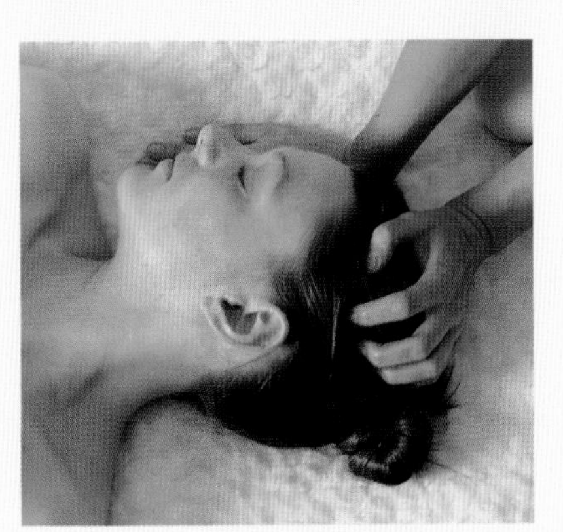

3. Head massage

Quick guide – face

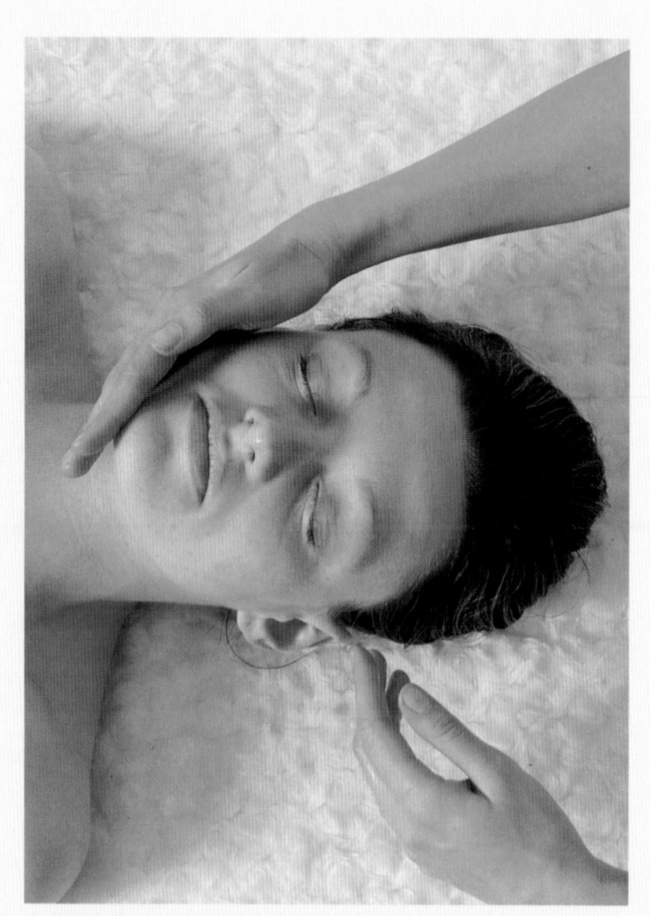

1. Effleurage to the chin

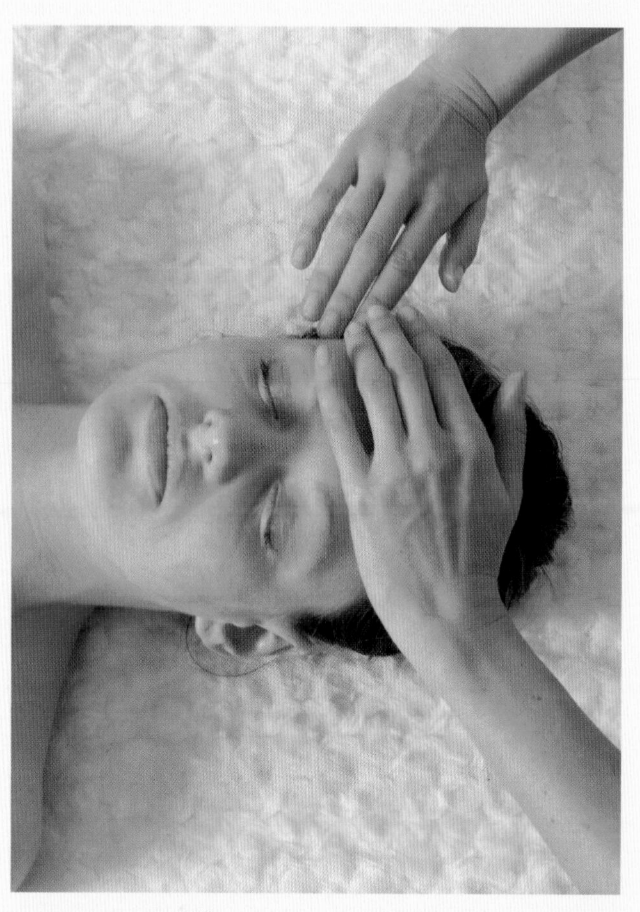

2.Effleurage to the forehead

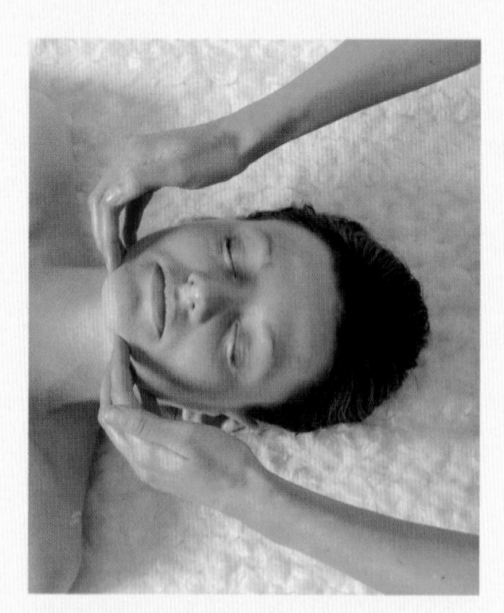

3. Friction

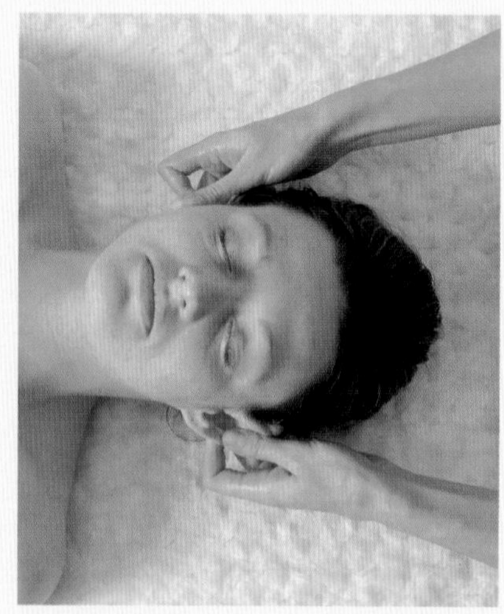

4. Massaging the ears

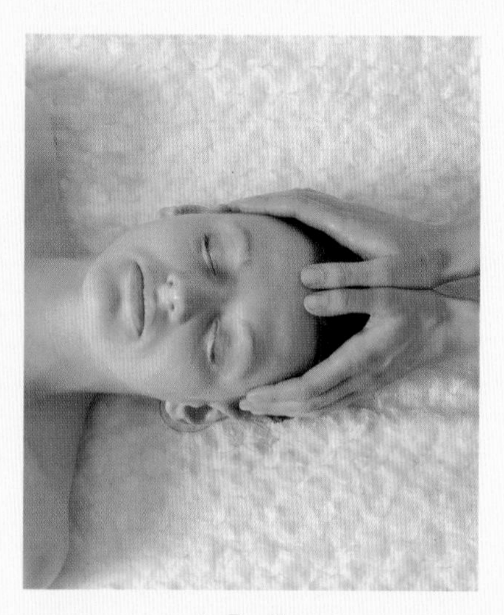

5. Ending

Further techniques

Once you have mastered the basic massage strokes, it is time to move on to further techniques. The massage strokes in this section are more advanced than the previous ones. While the basic techniques relax and soothe, some of the strokes in this section are performed more quickly. Some of the new strokes will invigorate the muscles by drawing blood to the surface of the skin.

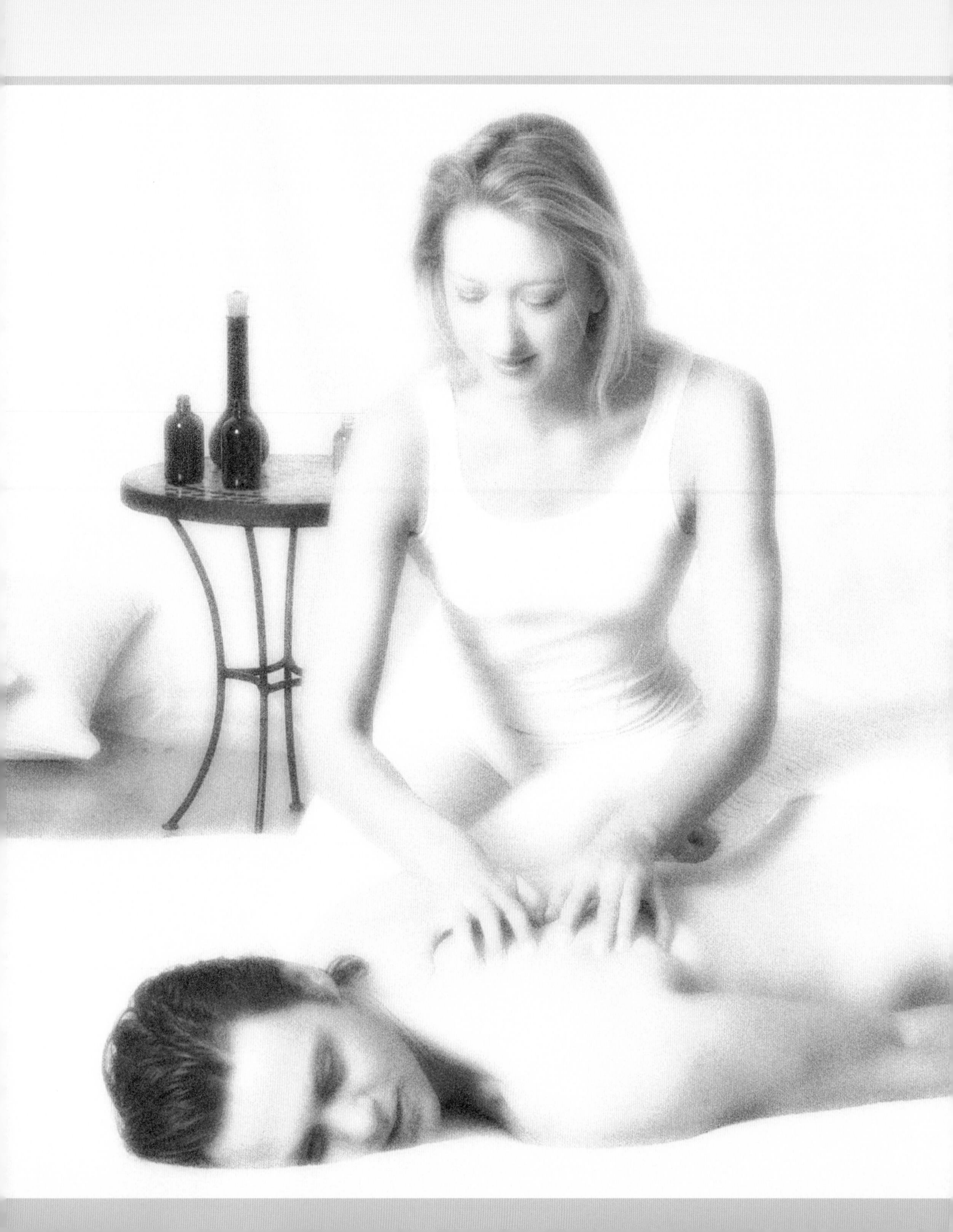

Strokes

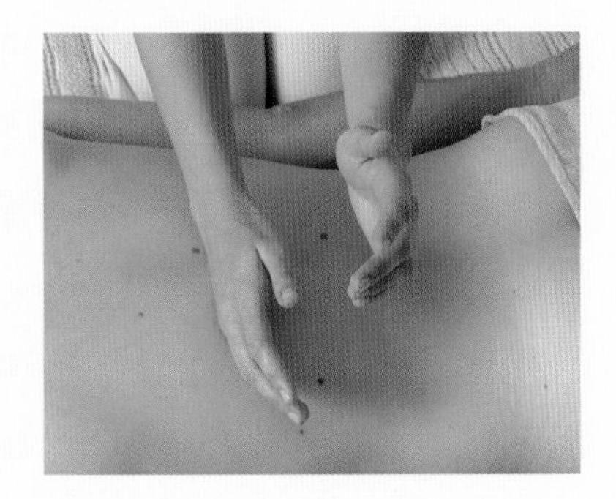

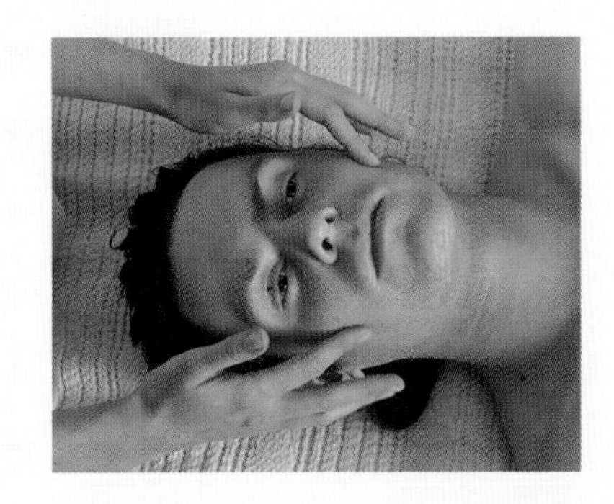

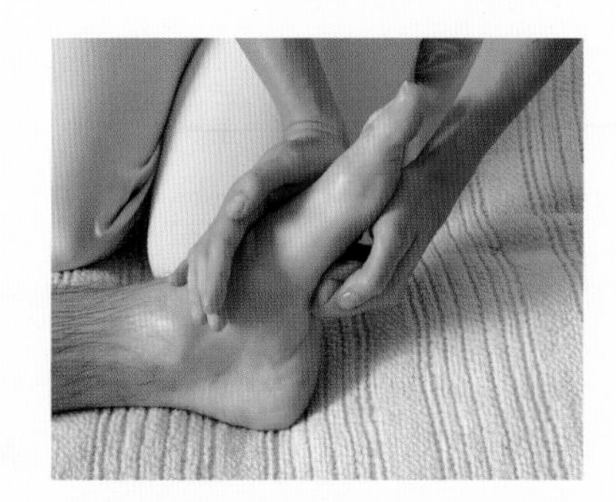

These strokes are more challenging than earlier ones, but offer a greater depth to the massage. As in the previous section, practise the strokes individually and then incorporate them into a massage routine. Again, the massage routines outlined after the description of the strokes are intended simply as a guideline rather than a strict workout. By this stage you probably know which strokes you prefer, but be creative and use the massage routines as a reference point to get you started.

Softening

This technique is performed above the towel before you expose the part of the body you are going to work on. It prepares the area by relaxing your partner and getting them used to your touch.

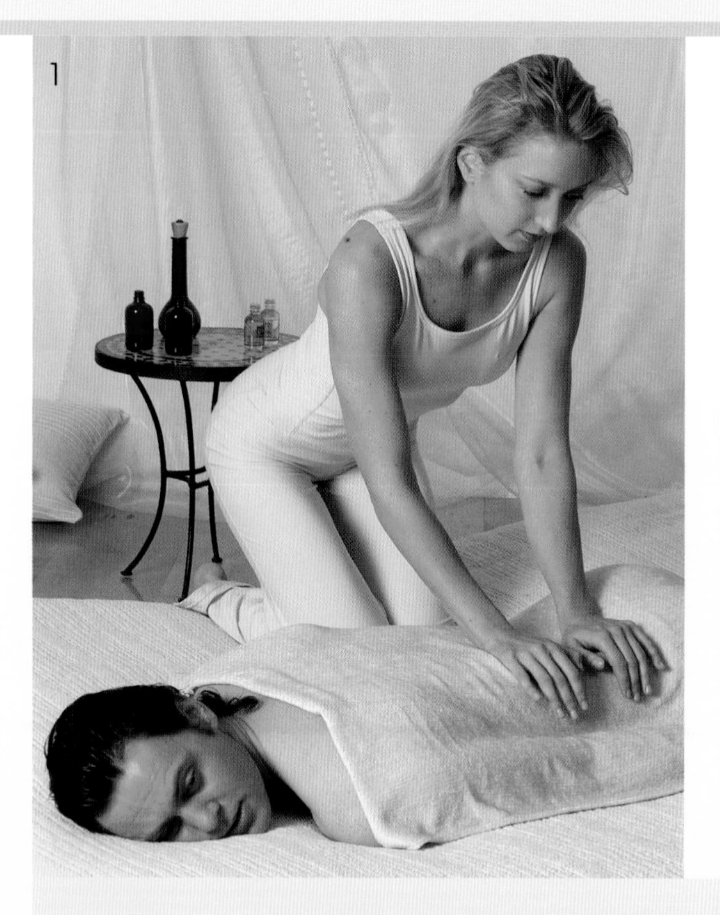

To the back

1 Kneel facing the spine. Place the palms of the hands on one side of the base of the spine. Gently press the palms into the fleshy area next to the spine and release.

2 Slowly work your way up to the base of the neck. Repeat to the other side.

3 Place the hands flat on the towel. Vigorously rub all over the back.

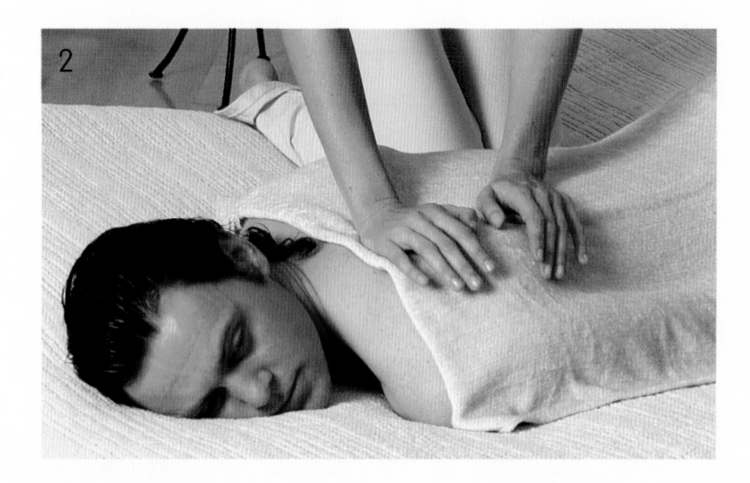

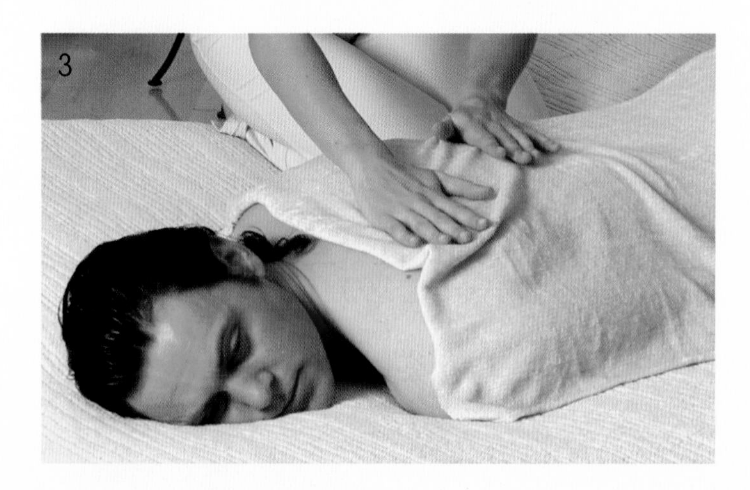

To the arms and legs

Place the hands over the towel. Squeeze the flesh underneath the towel and release. Do this up and down the limb you are working on. Vigorously rub up and down the limb with the hands above the towel.

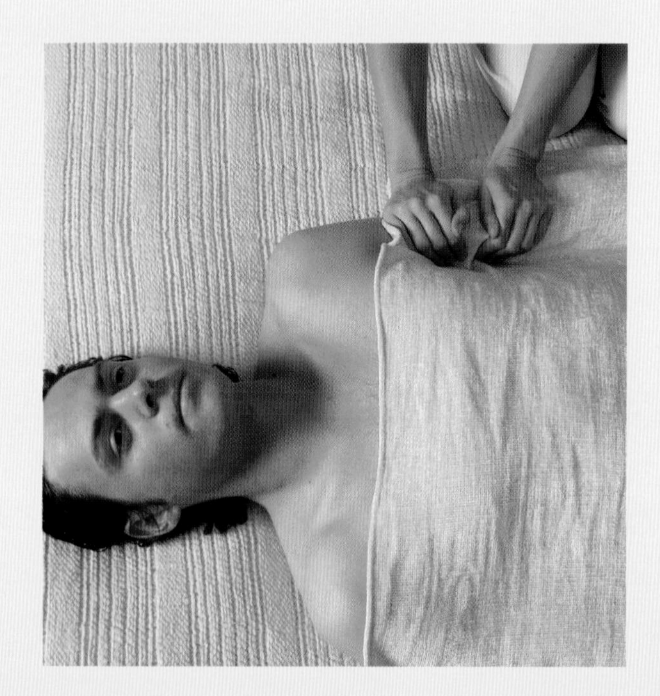

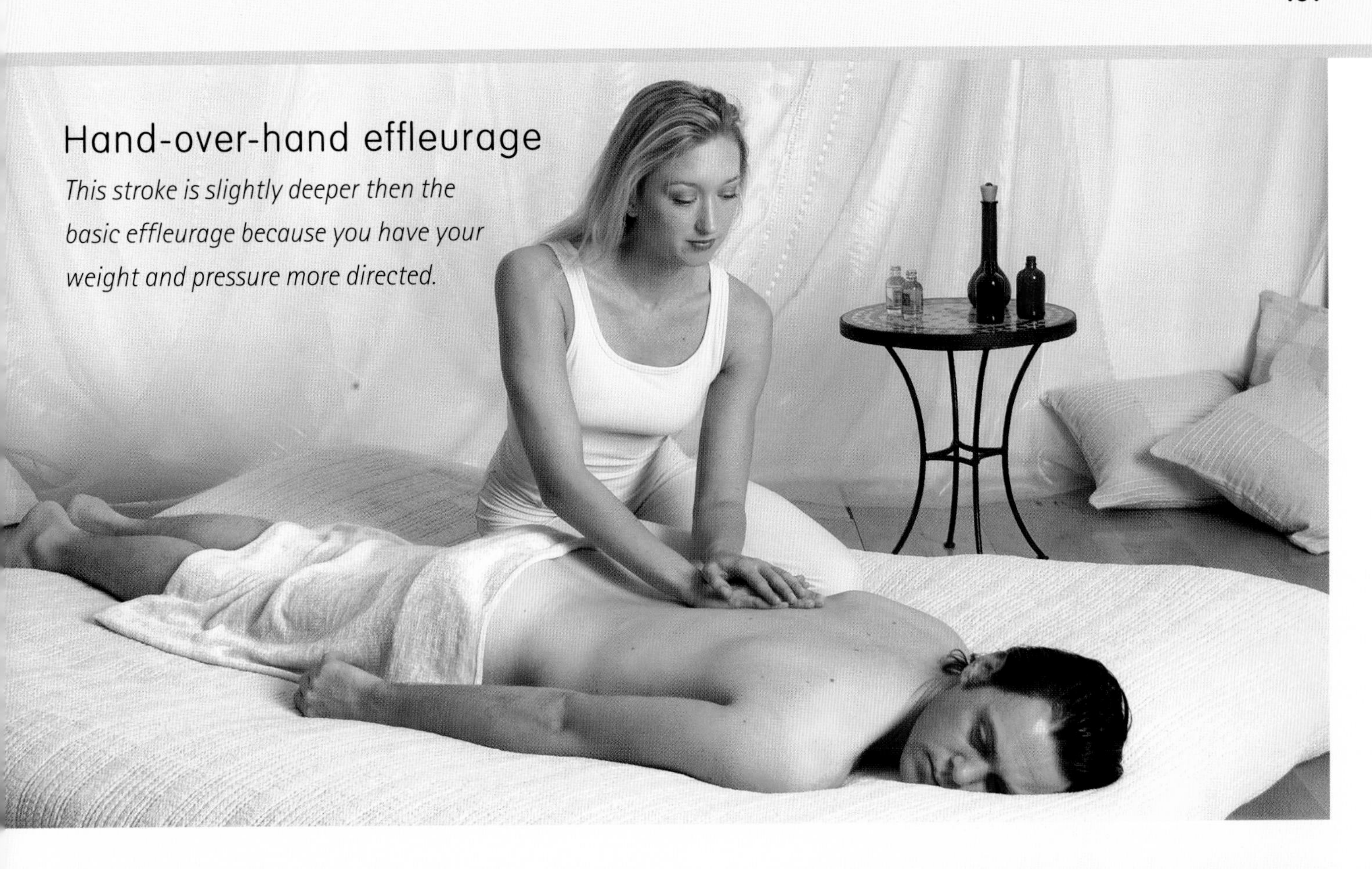

Hand-over-hand effleurage

This stroke is slightly deeper then the basic effleurage because you have your weight and pressure more directed.

To the back

1 Place one hand on top of the other. Start with the palm of your bottom hand at the fleshy area next to the base of the spine.

2 Press with the palms of your hands up the side of the spine.

3 Slide the hands across the shoulder (on the same side of the body) and then lightly back down. The fingertips should mould to the contour of the body.

Repeat 3 times on this side, and then move to the other side of the body and repeat. Make the stroke one continuous sweeping circle, pressing firmly on the way up, and more lightly on the way back up.

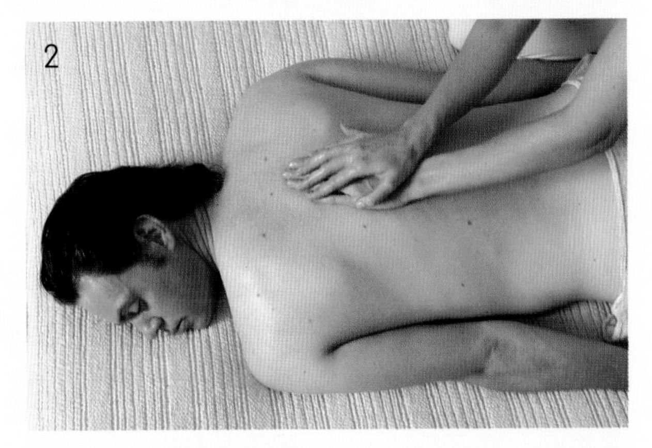

2

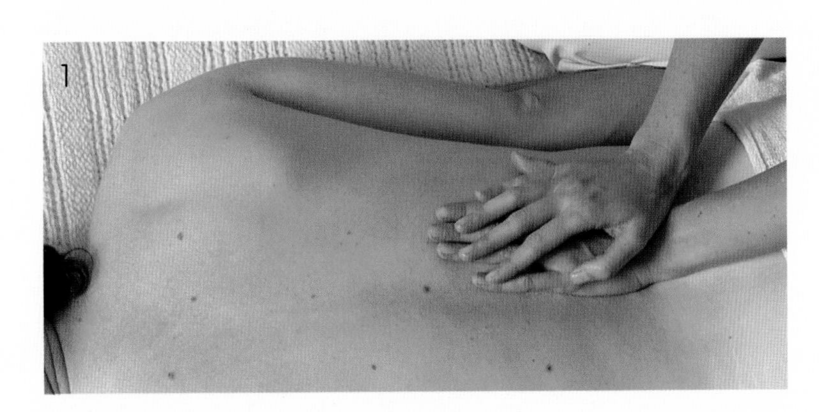

1

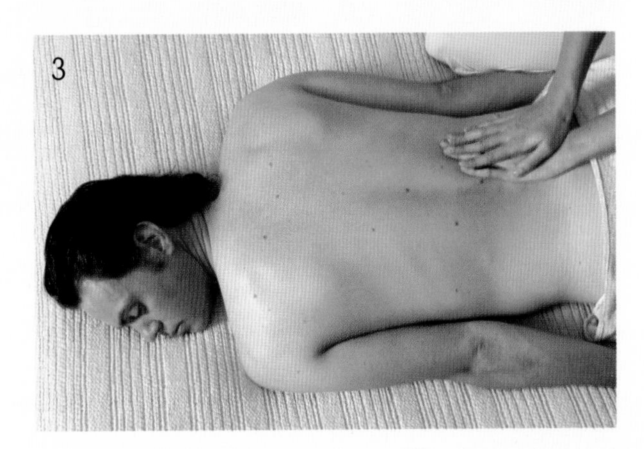

3

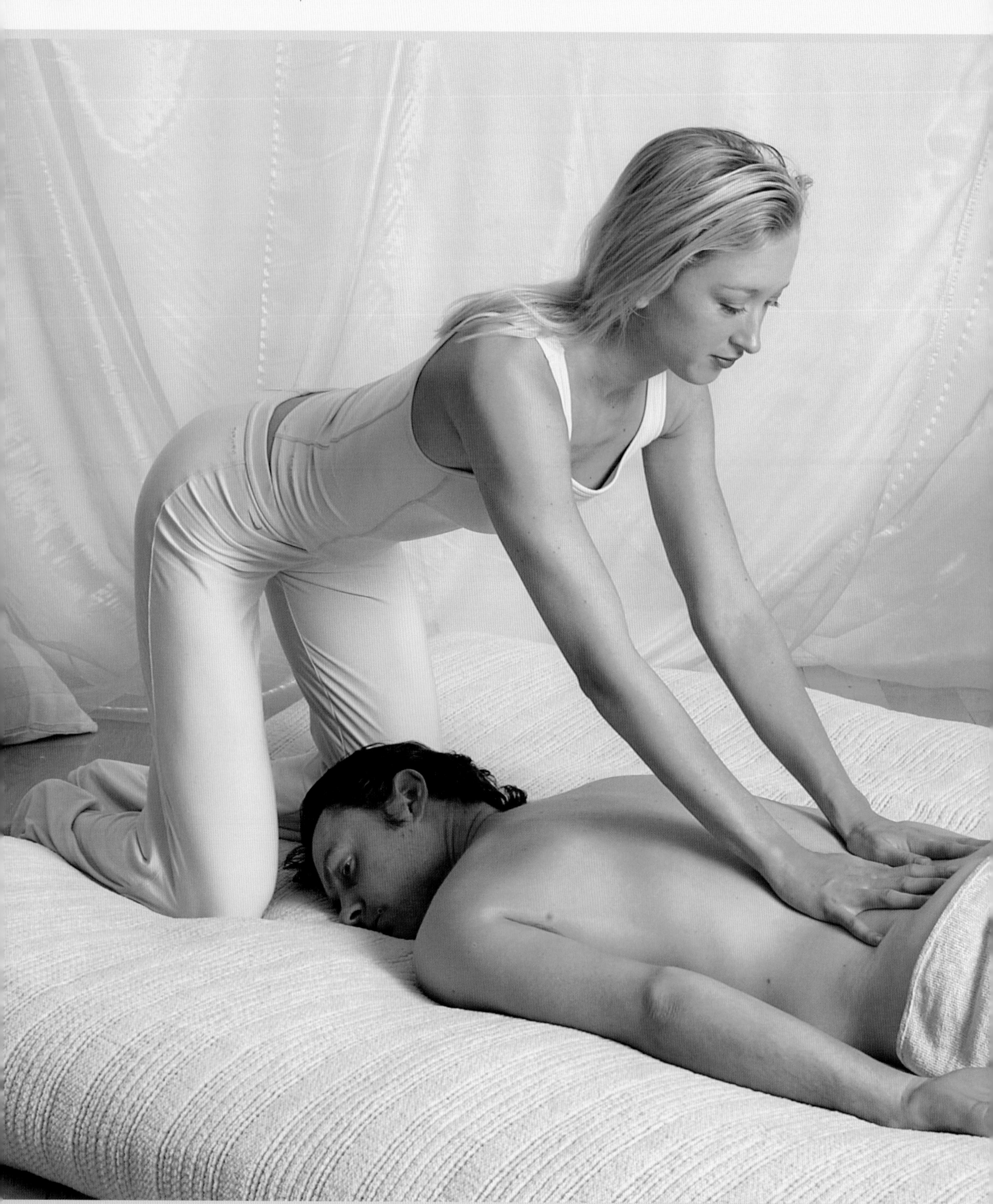

Pull-ups

This is a very soothing stroke that can be performed in several ways.

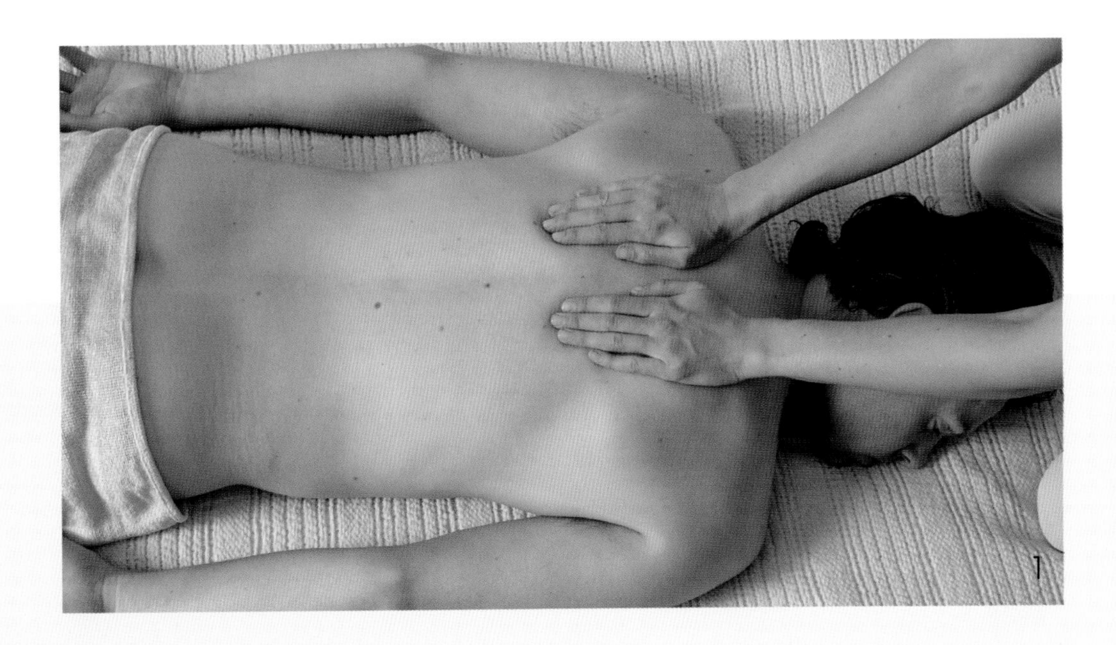

Across whole back

1 Kneel at the head of your partner facing their feet. Place your hands flat on either side of the spine towards the neck.

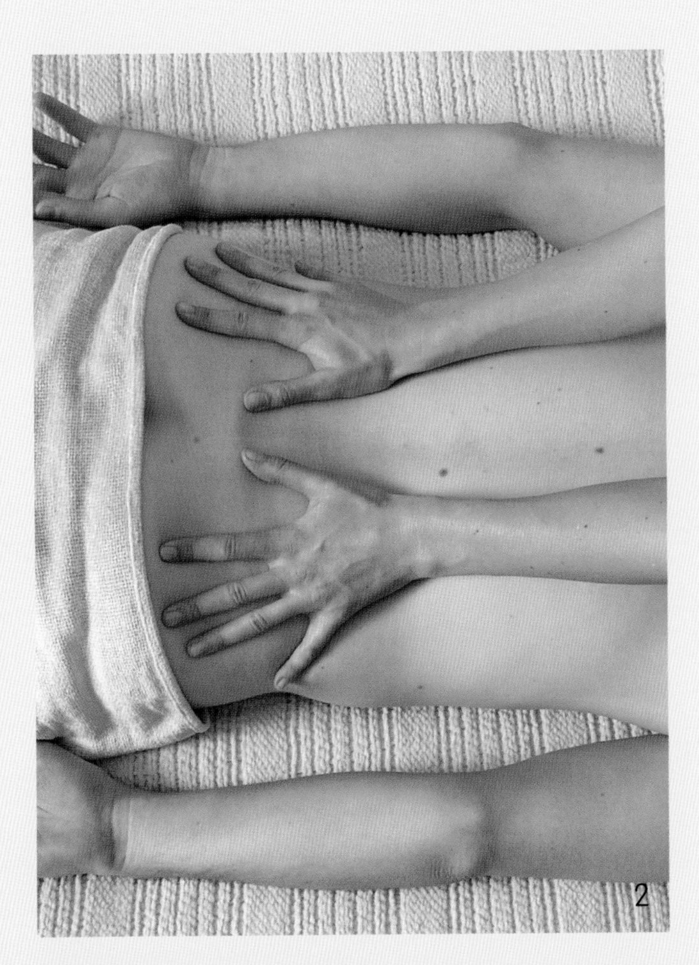

2 Very lightly, slide the hands down towards the buttocks and across the hips.

3 Change the hands so that they are holding the hips with the thumb on top and the fingers underneath. Firmly pull the hands all the way up the sides to the shoulders.

Repeat three times.

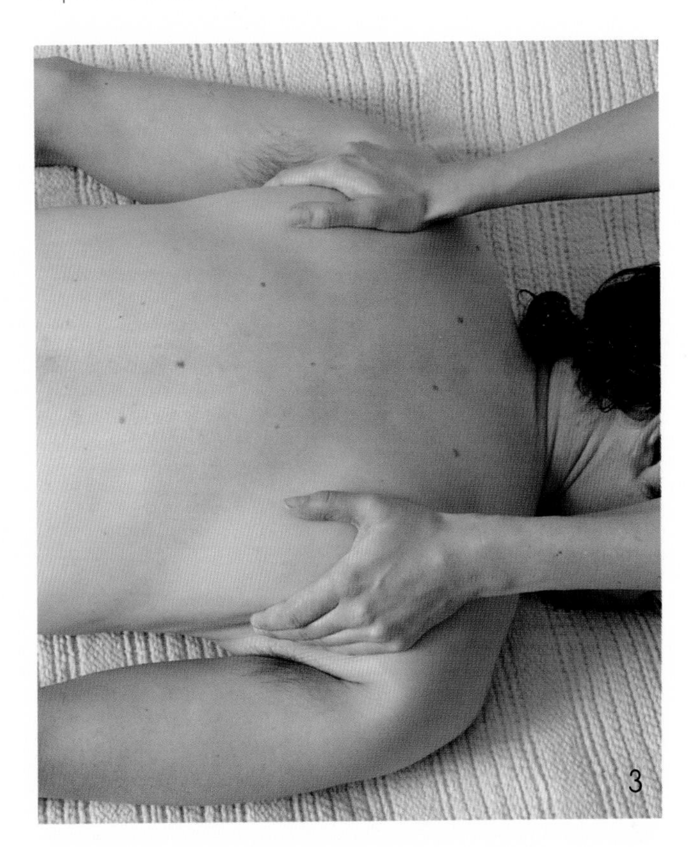

To the waistline

This stroke is performed on the back or stomach, depending on how your partner is lying.

Kneel to the side of your partner. Reach to the opposite side and think of lifting up the flesh from underneath, alternating hands. Keep the pressure smooth and relaxed.

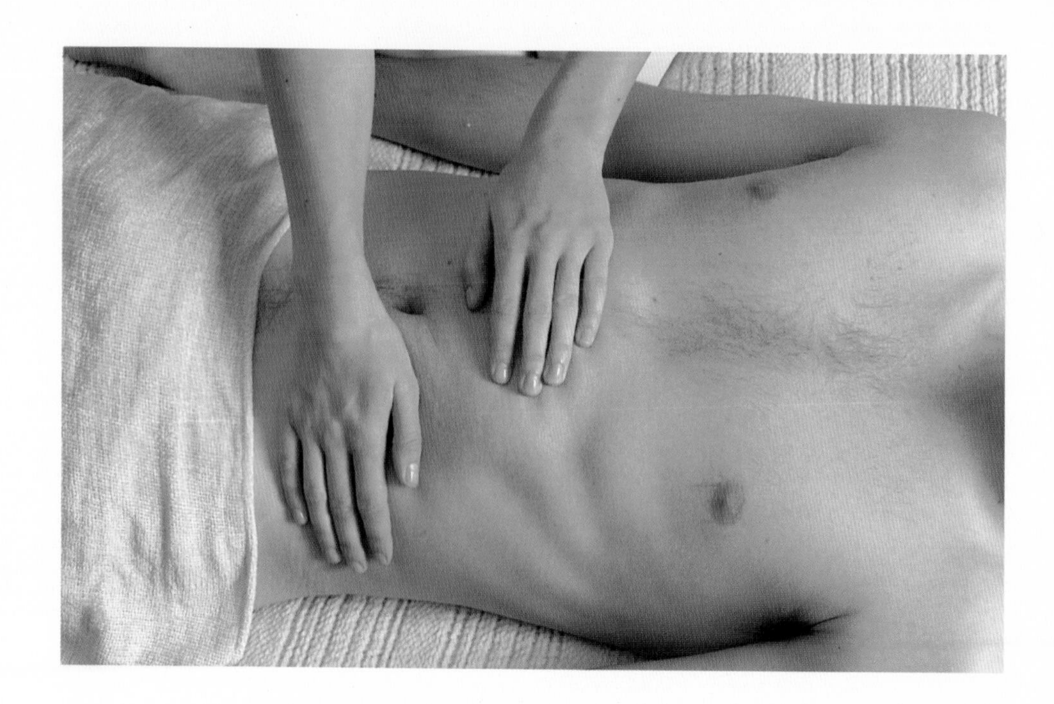

To the shoulders

Kneel to the side of your partner, facing their head. Place one hand on the underneath side of the shoulder with the fingers facing down. Pull gently on the shoulder as you slide the hand towards their pelvis. As soon as the hand moves from the shoulder, replace it with your other hand. Keep alternating hands on one shoulder. Repeat to the other shoulder.

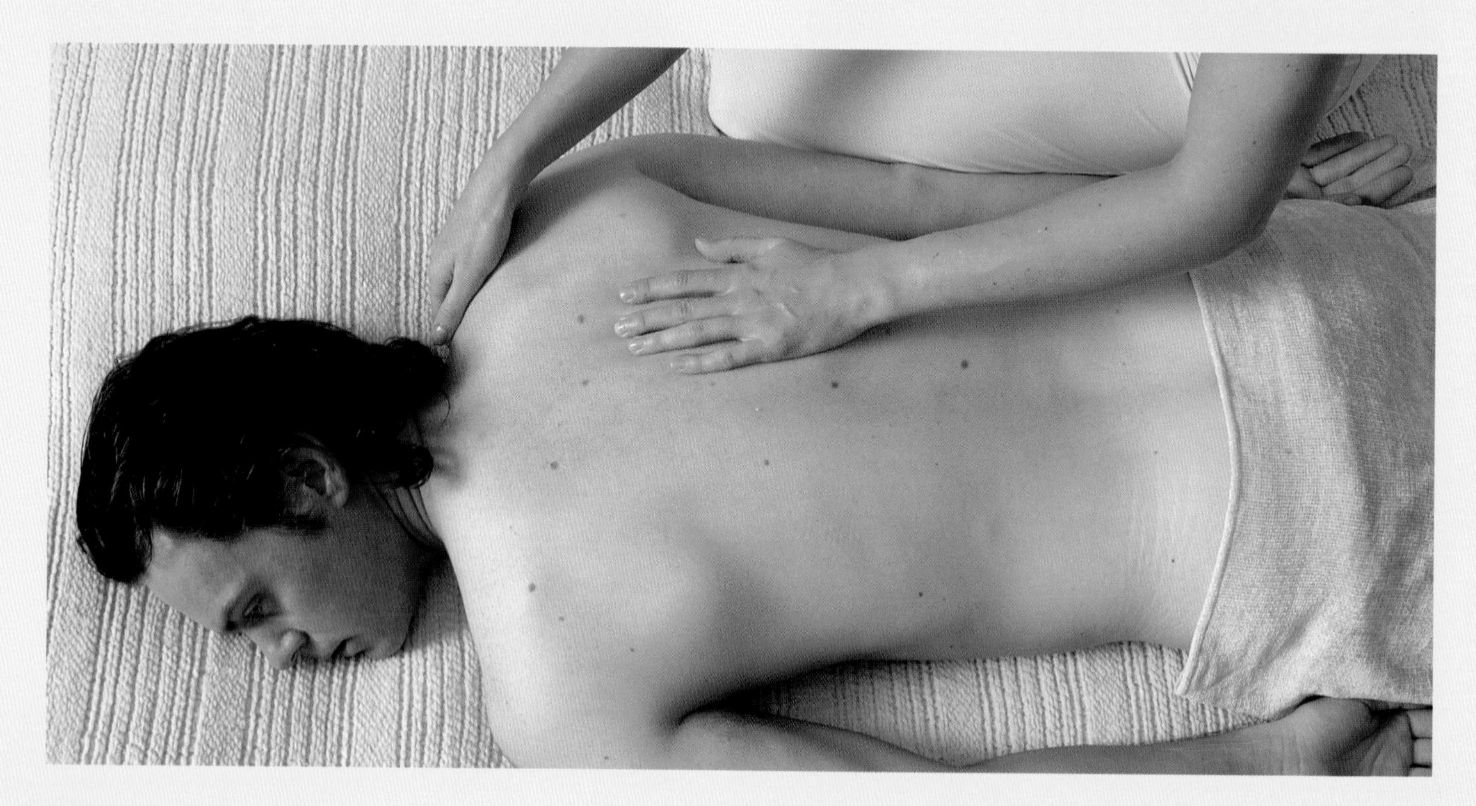

Fanning

This stroke is performed on the back.

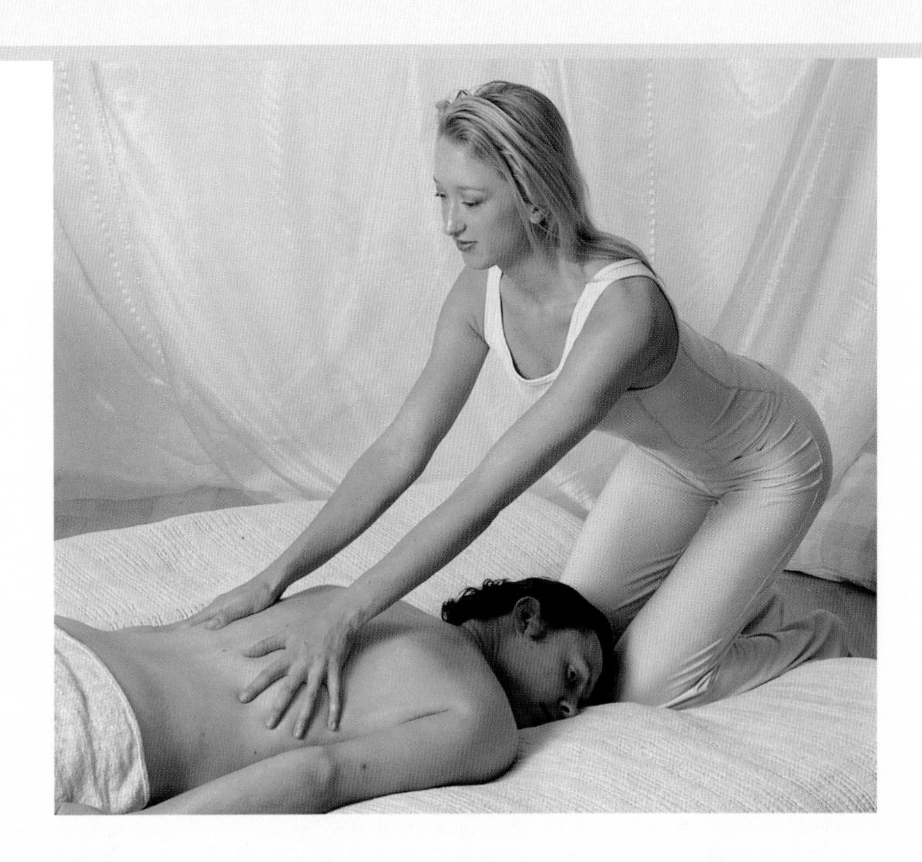

1 Kneel at the head of your partner. Place the hands flat on either side of the spine towards the neck.

2 Lightly slide the hands down towards the hips and spread your fingertips out at the base of the spine. Make slow, small circular motions with the fingertips 3 times. Move the hands up and across the ribs and circle 3 times. Move the hands up to the point where the arm meets the back and repeat.

Repeat the whole movement 3 times.

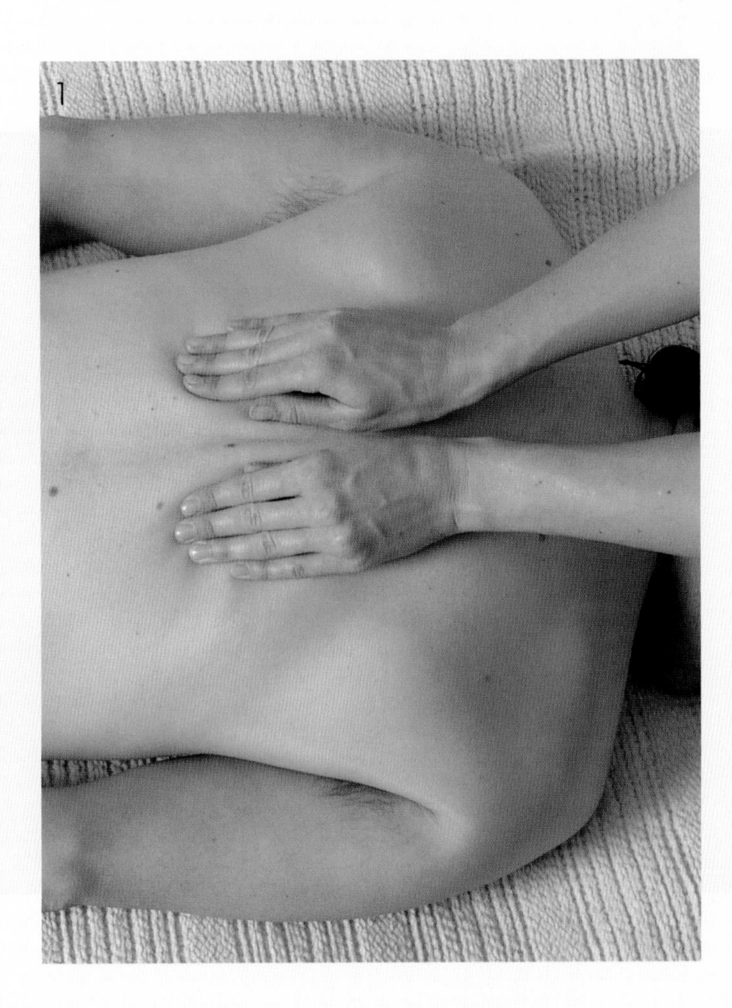

1

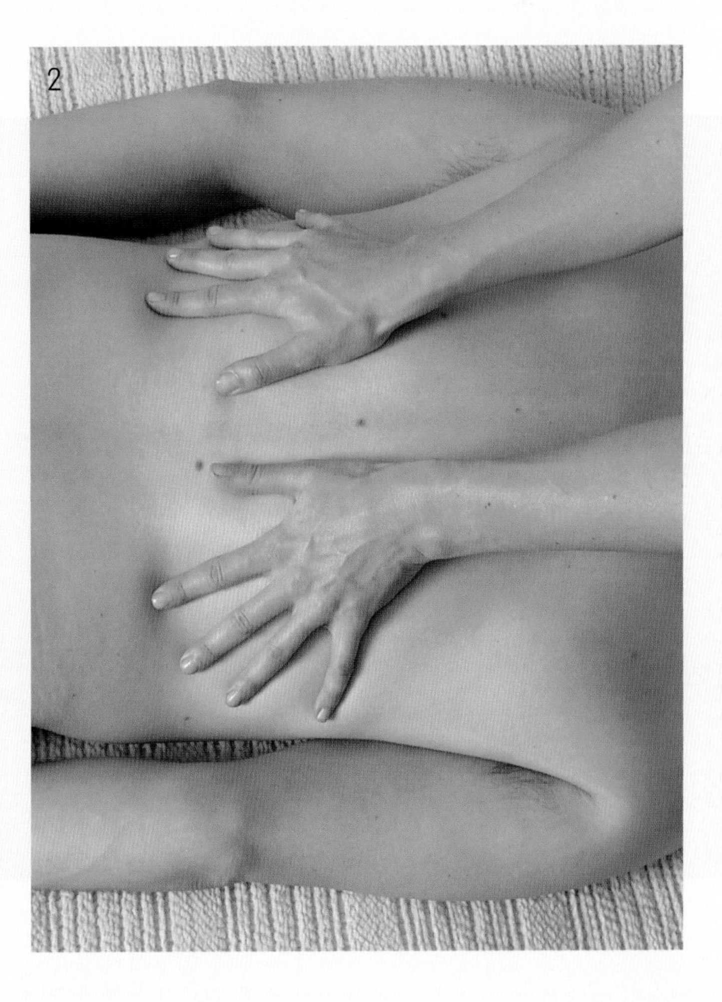

2

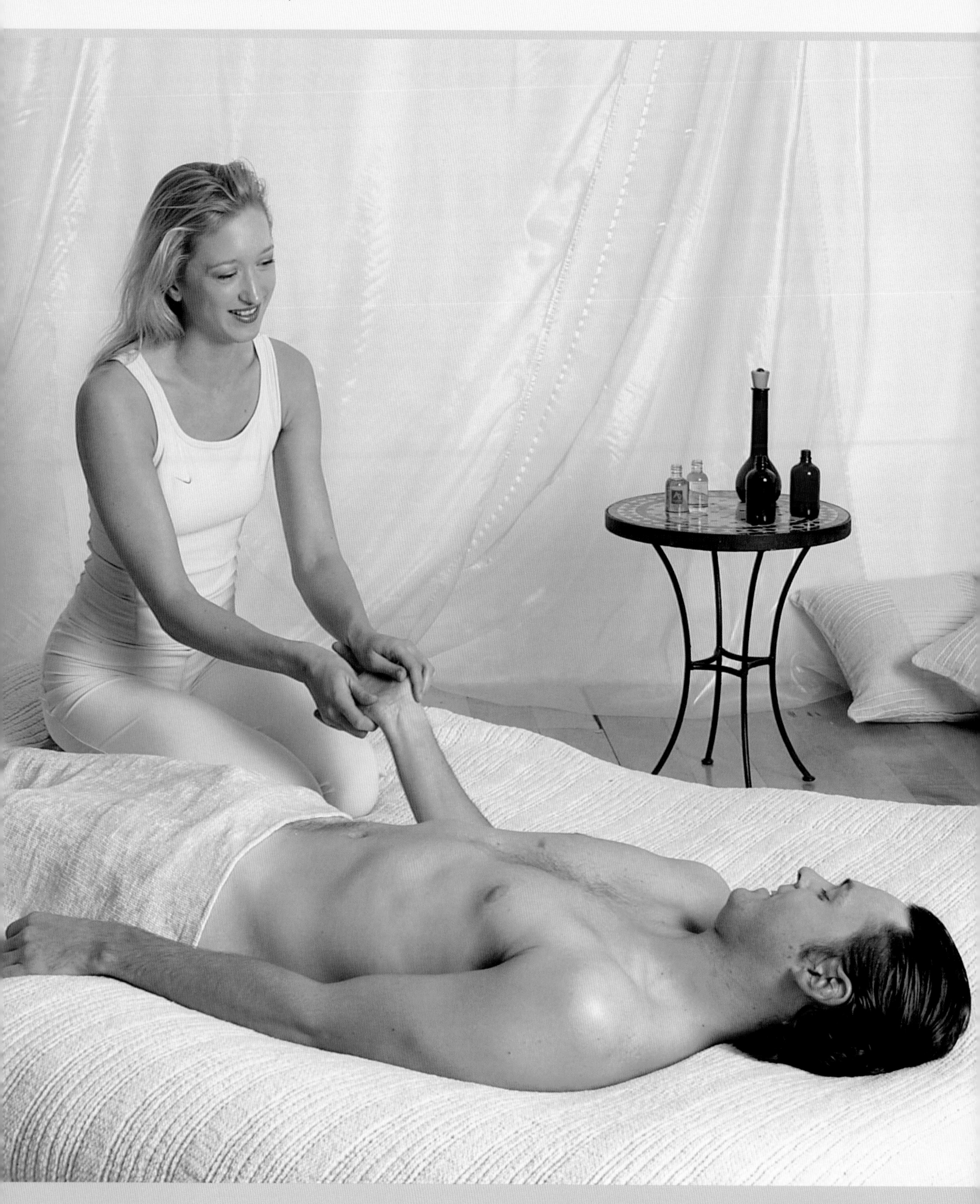

Opening

This stroke has a wonderfully soothing effect and should be performed on the smaller areas of the body like the hands, feet and knees.

On the tops of the knees

1 Place the lengths of the thumbs together with the thumbs facing towards your partner's head.

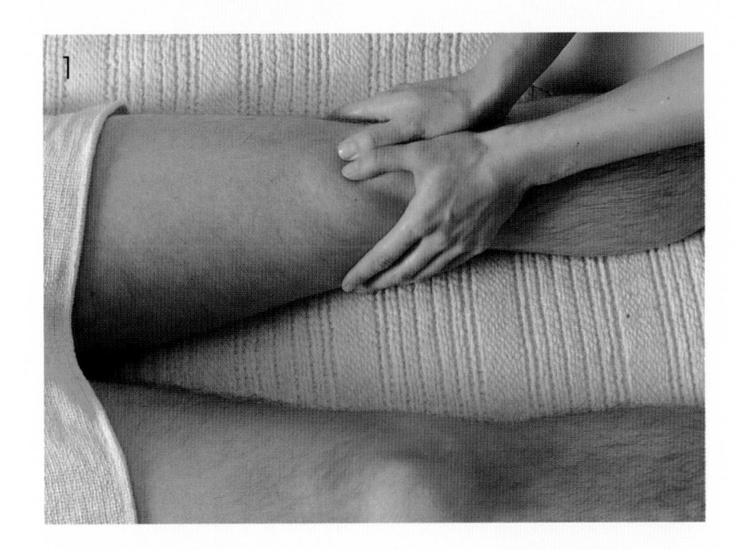
1

2 Gently press the thumbs out to the sides of the knee while circling the knee with the pads of the thumbs.

Repeat three times.

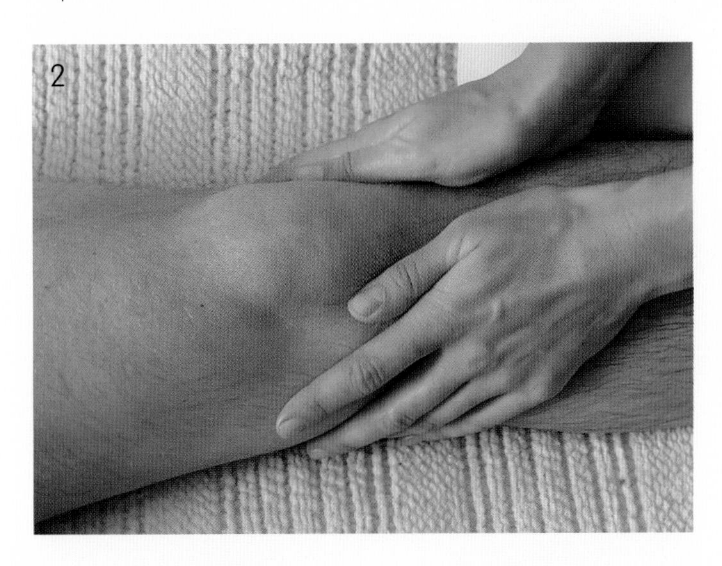
2

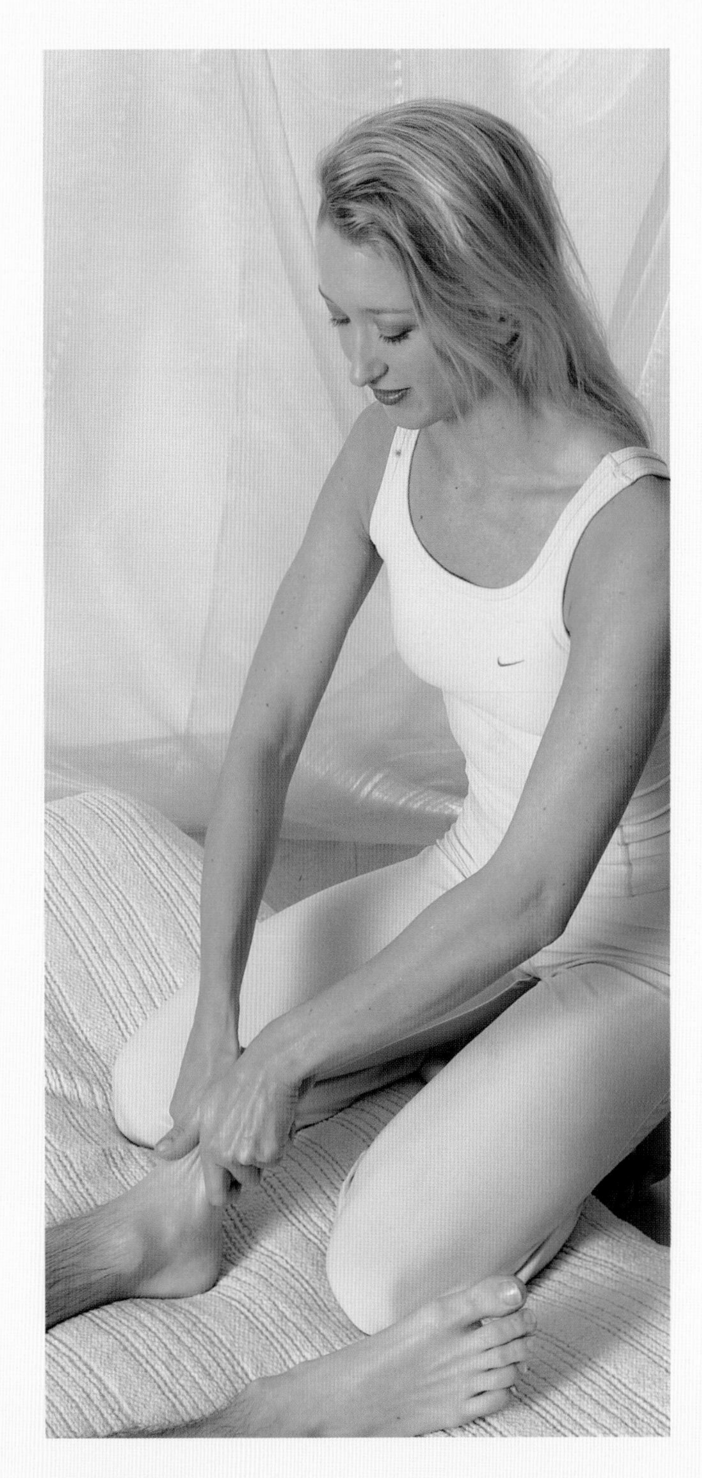

On the feet

Place the palms of the hands on the top of the foot with the fingers wrapped around to the sole of the foot. Press the hands against the foot while rolling the fingers to the outside of the foot. Think of opening up the foot as you would open a book.

On the hands

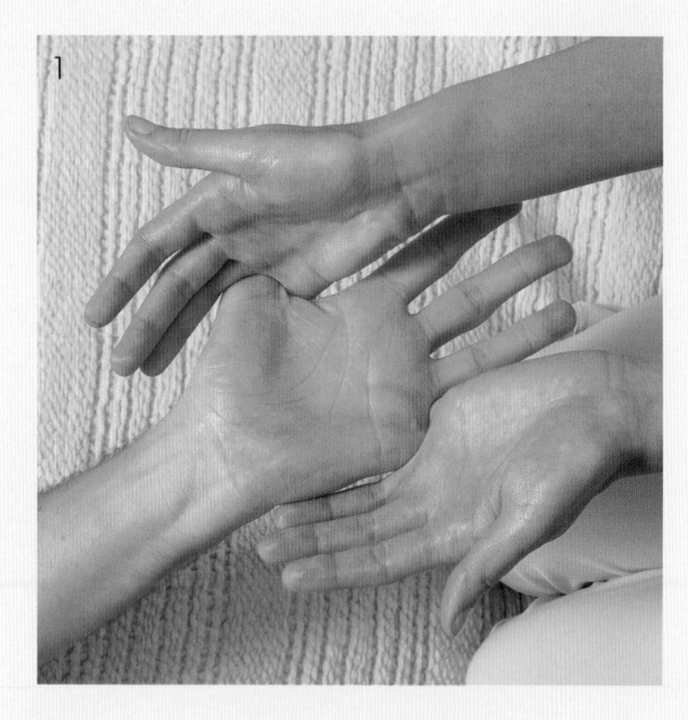

1 Turn your partner's palm up and lace your pinkies between their thumb and pinkie.

2 Place the length of your thumbs together on the centre of their palm.

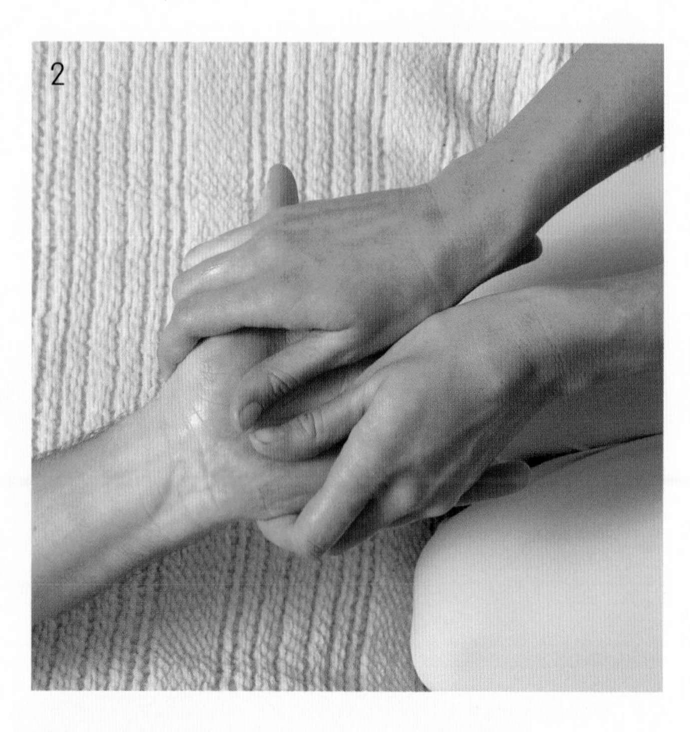

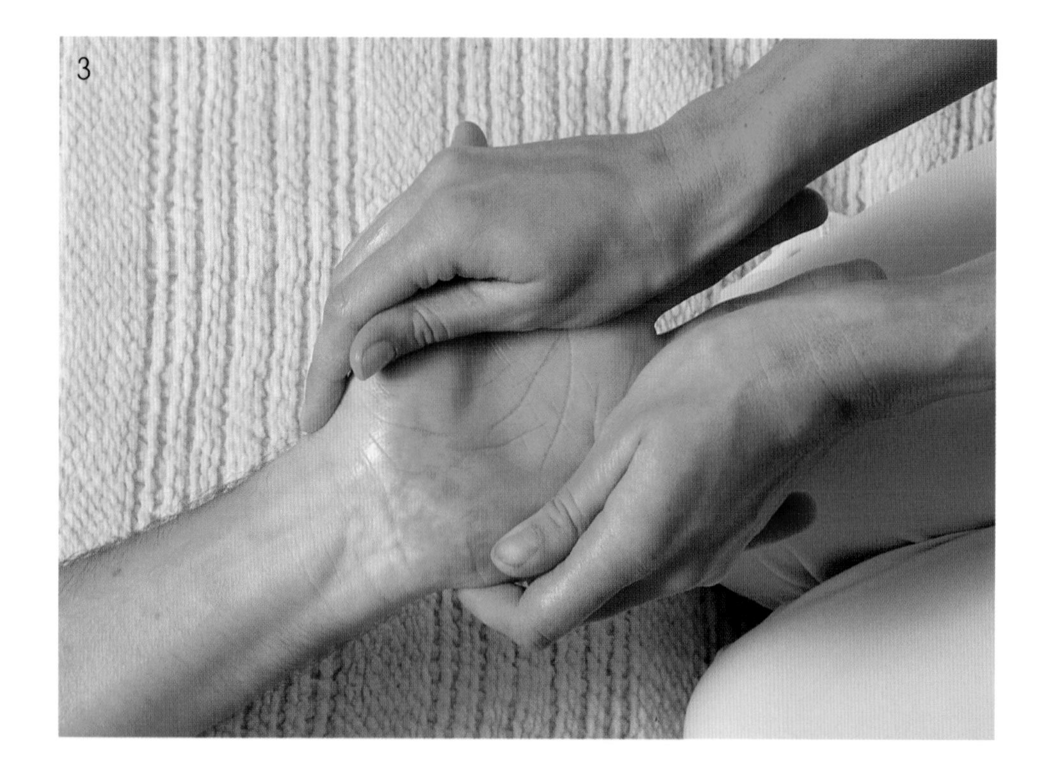

3 Gently press your thumbs into their palm and open, stretching the hand back.

Note: leave the hand in this position and massage the palm with circular strokes using your thumbs. Wonderful!

Vibration

Vibration strokes help to release tension and relax the body. They allow the blood to come to the surface of the skin and help people to let go.

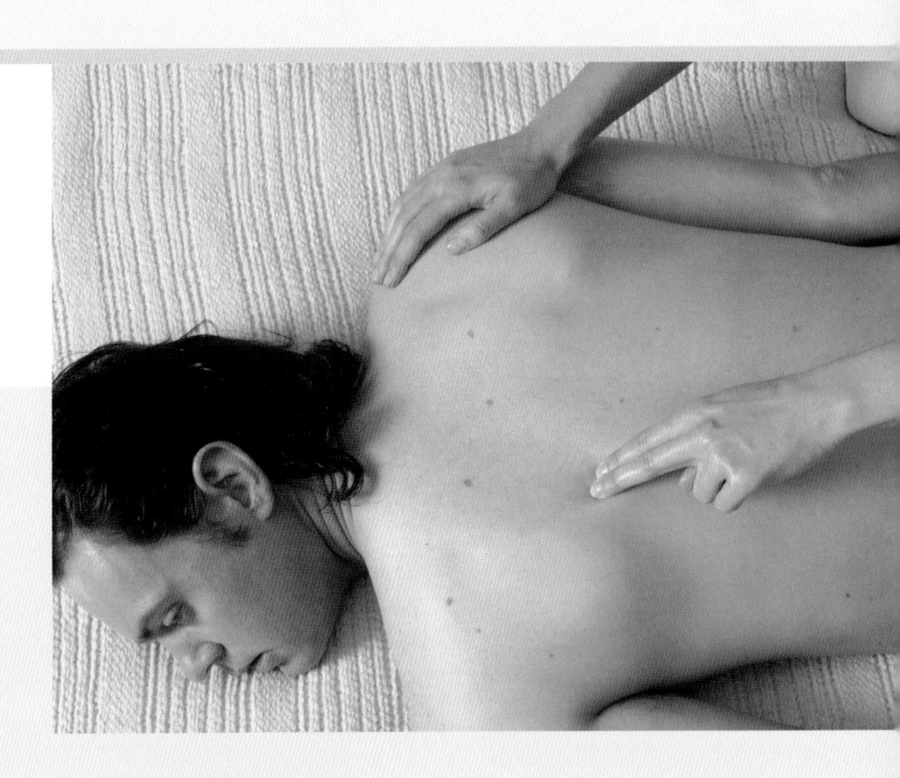

On the back

Kneel at your partner's side. Straighten your first two fingers and curl the rest under. Place the fingers of one hand on the side of the spine. Quickly zigzag down the back, allowing the fingers to shake the flesh as they go. When you reach the base of the spine, lift the hand off and bring it back to the top to start again. Change the starting position each time to cover the whole back.

For extra vibration:

1. Hand on back
2. Hand under shoulder
3. Vibration in shoulder

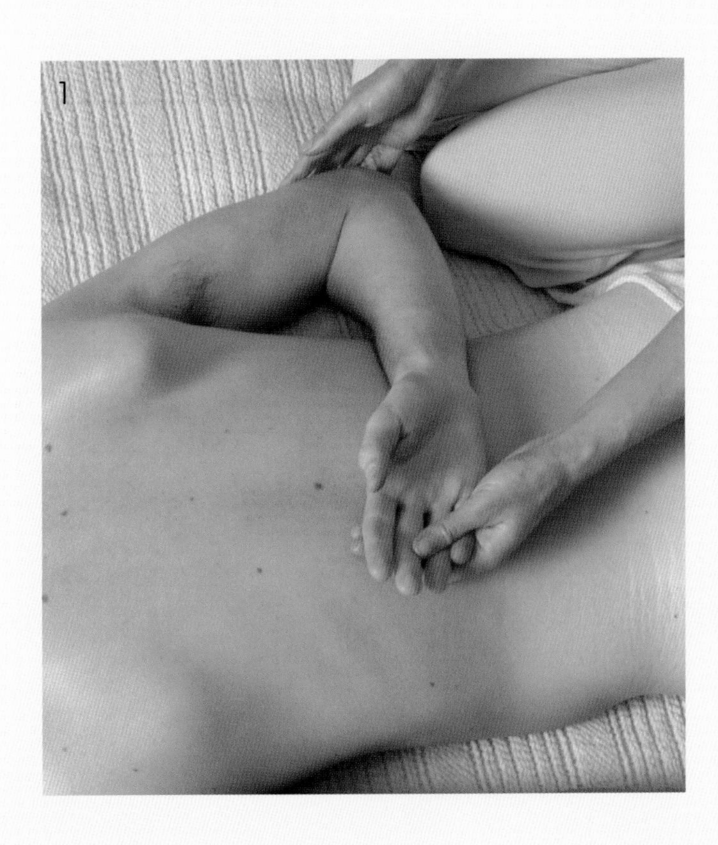
1

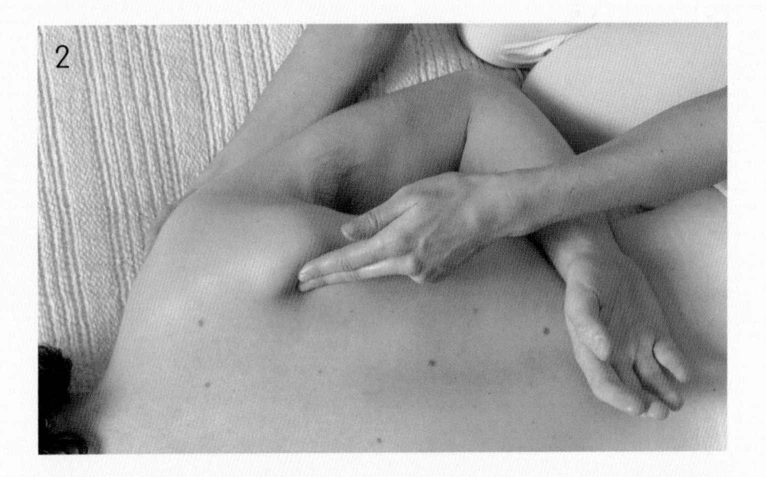
2

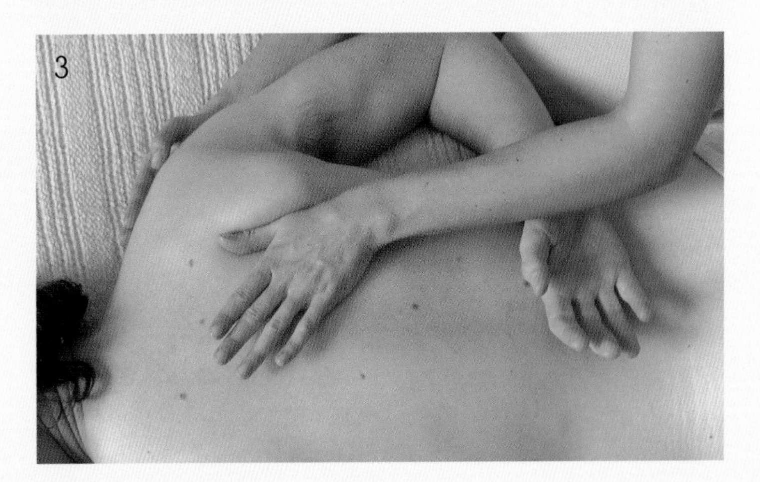
3

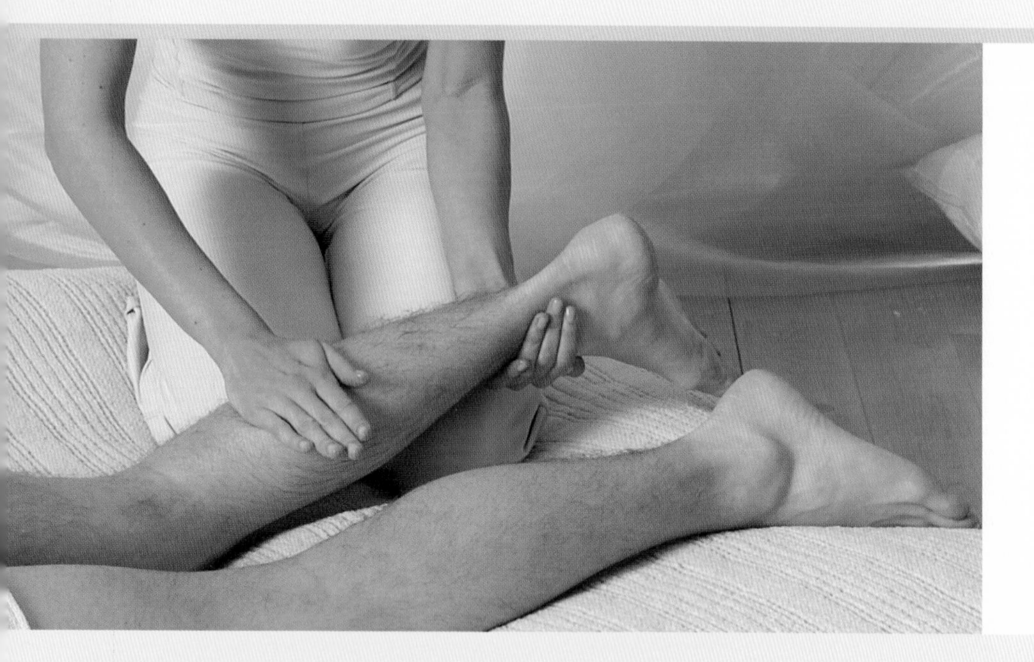

On the calf

Lift up the ankle with one hand. Place the other hand flat across the bulk of the calf muscle with your fingers facing away from you. Vigorously shake the calf, moving your hand back and forth across the muscle.

On the foot

1 Kneel facing the sole of your partner's foot. Extend both hands along either side of their foot with the palms flat and facing inward.

2 Shake the foot vigorously back and forth between your hands.

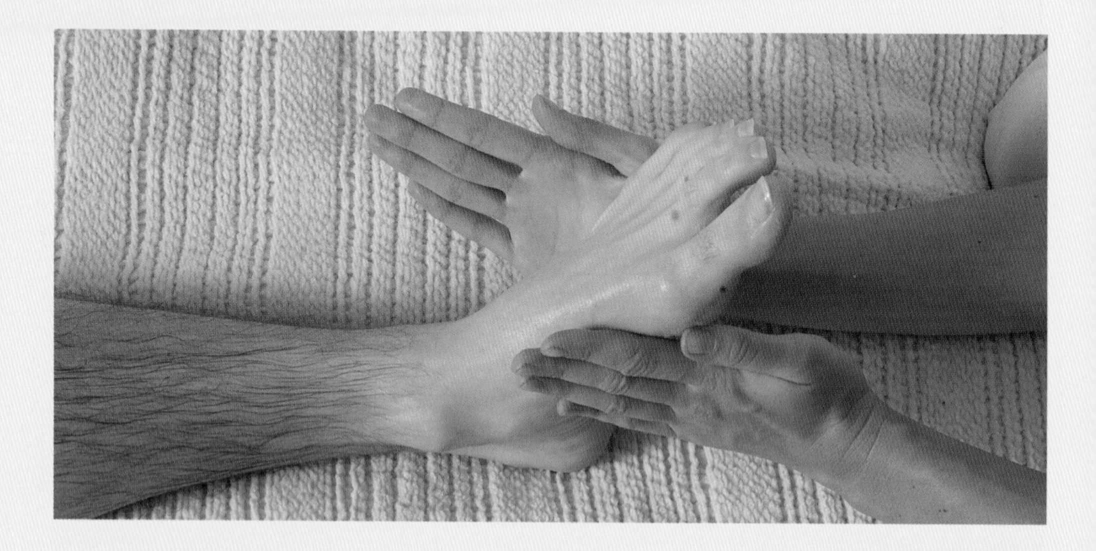

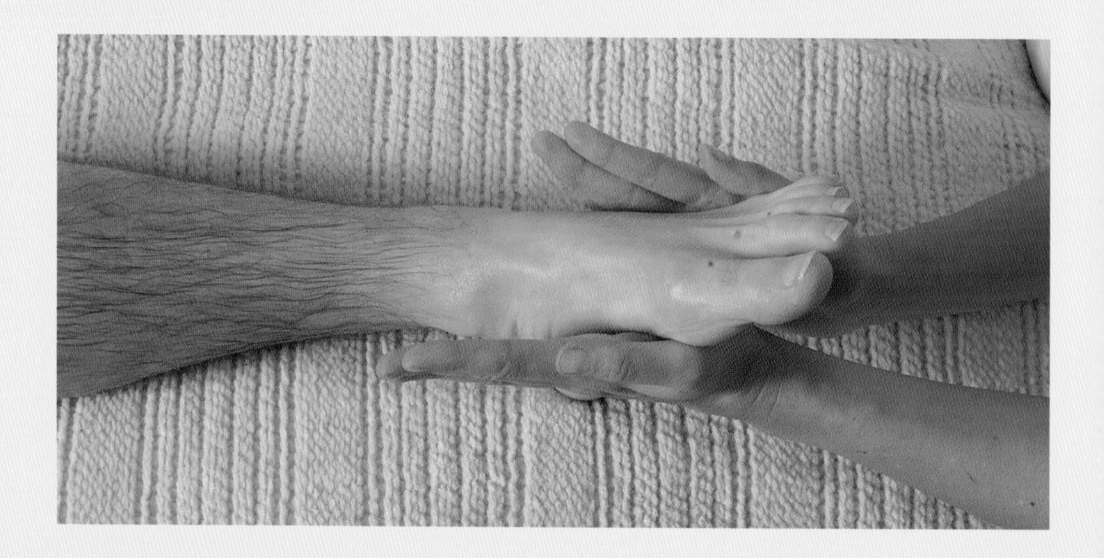

Percussion

Percussion strokes are quick, rhythmic strokes used to awaken and enliven the muscles. The hands quickly and gently strike the skin to stimulate circulation, bringing the blood to the surface and breaking up toxins in the body. It is important to have the correct posture while doing this stroke. Kneel facing your partner. Keep your upper back and head lengthening towards the ceiling. The tendency is to round the back, creating stiffness and causing the back to suffer undue pressure.

Hacking

For this stroke, bring your palms to face each other about 8 cm apart. The outside of your pinkie fingers gently comes in contact with the body. The action of the wrists flicks up and down, alternating quickly along the body.

On the back

Kneel to the side of your partner facing their back. Place the palms facing each other with the pinkies about 5 cm away from the skin. Lightly flick the wrists up and down, quickly moving the hands along the back. This should create a soothing percussive sound as you do it.

Note: avoid the kidney area.

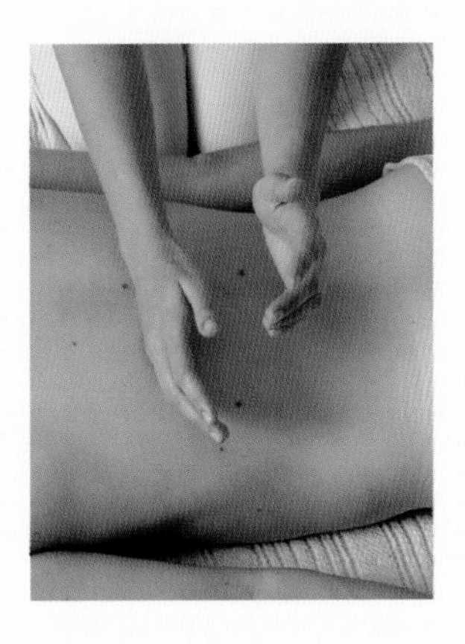

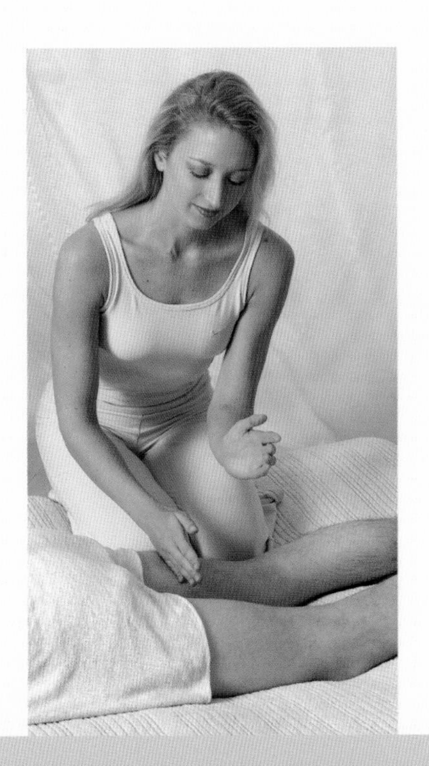

On the legs

Kneel facing the thigh. Your hands should be facing each other with the pinkies just above the skin. Quickly flick the hands against the skin along the whole length of the thigh.

Repeat the motion to the calf.

Tapoment

This is a percussive stroke used across the chest and on the face. It is a very light movement involving just the fingertips. Place the hands above the area to be worked on. Very quickly and lightly let the fingertips fall separately onto the body. This should feel like light raindrops falling on the surface of the skin.

To the chest

Sit or kneel at your partner's head, facing their feet. Place your fingertips lightly above their chest. Let your fingertips fall separately along their chest and shoulders like raindrops falling on their skin.

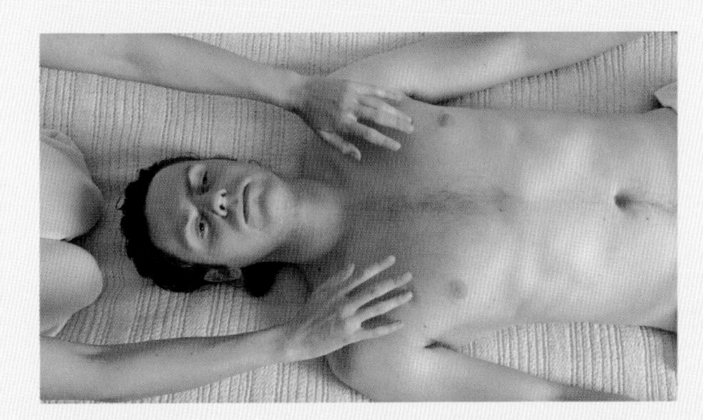

To the face

Place your hands above your partner's face. On this stroke, avoid the eyes, nose and mouth. Lightly tap the forehead, cheeks and chin, letting each of the fingers fall separately onto the surface of the skin.

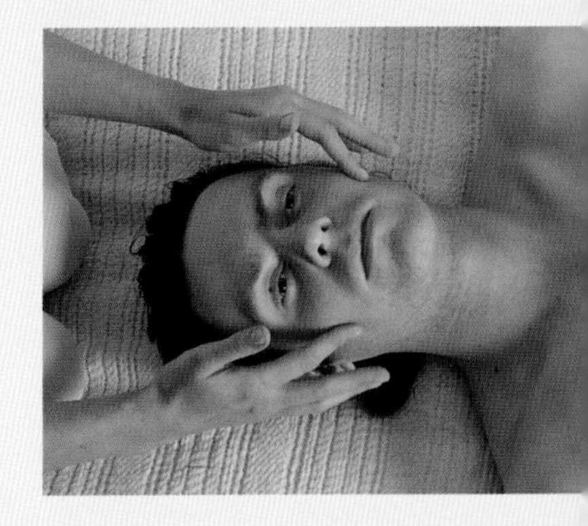

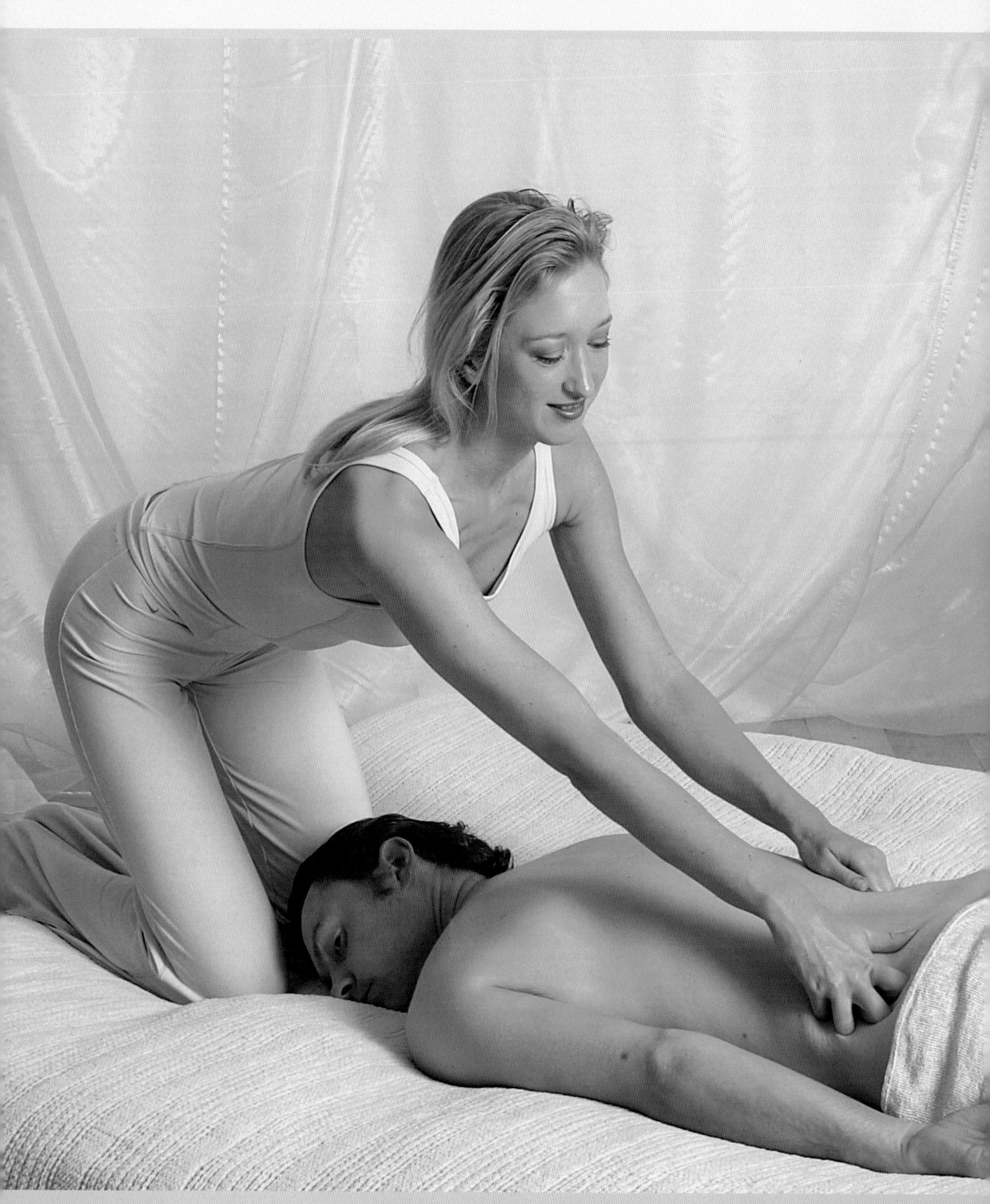

Knuckle roll

This stroke breaks up tension and releases toxins. It is a great stroke to add if your fingers are getting tired and need a short rest.

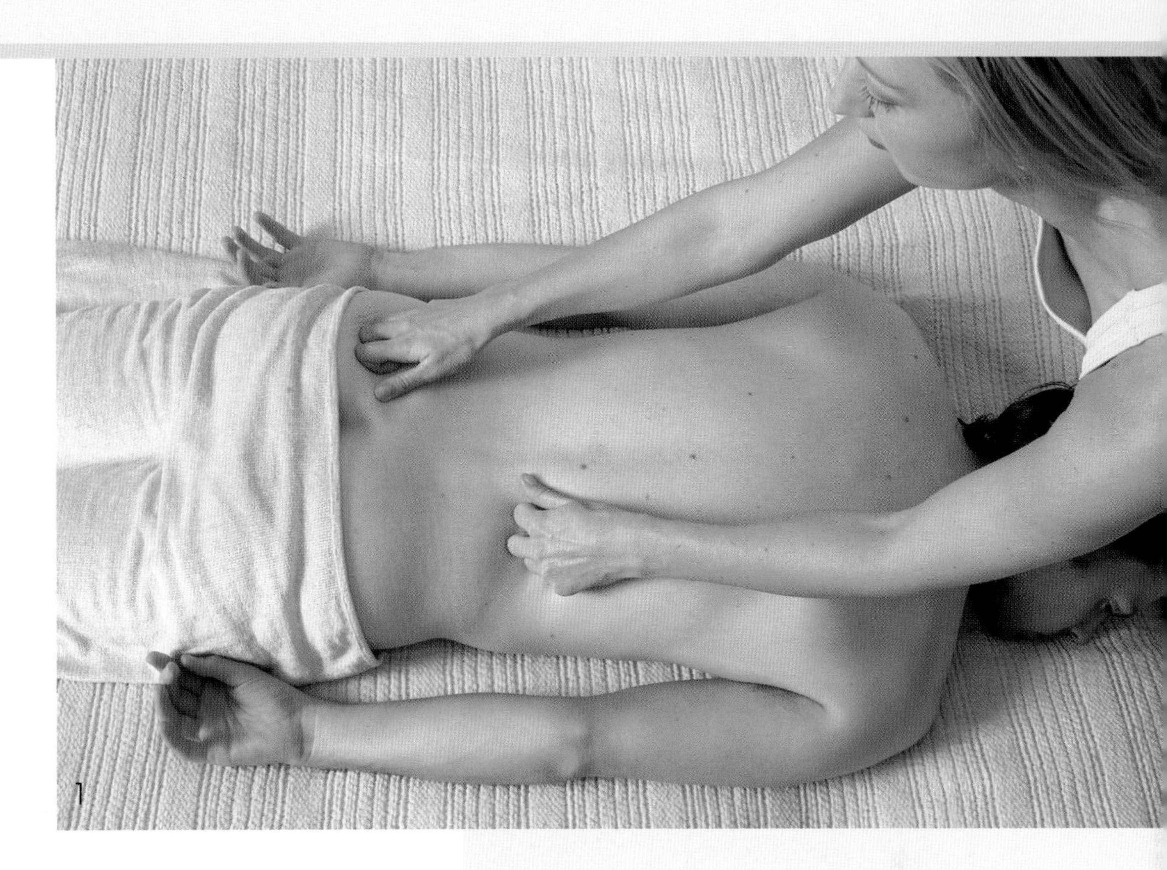

On the back

1 Kneel at the head of your partner facing their feet. Curl your fingertips in so that the knuckles are touching the surface of the skin. One hand should be placed above each of the buttocks.

2 Roll the knuckles gently but firmly across the base of the spine and hips. Roll one hand and then the other, alternating as you go.

Note: the pressure depends on your partner. Ask them how it feels and adjust accordingly.

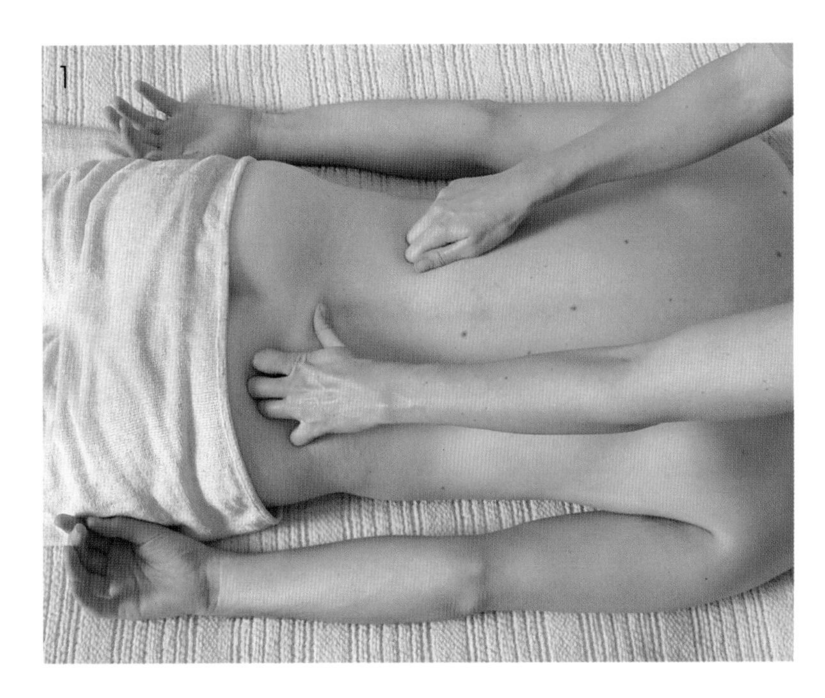

To the foot

Curl one hand so that the pads of the fingers are touching the palm of your hand. Place the knuckles on the base of the foot. Roll the knuckles massaging the underneath side of the foot. Make sure you do not stay in one place but cover the entire sole of the foot.

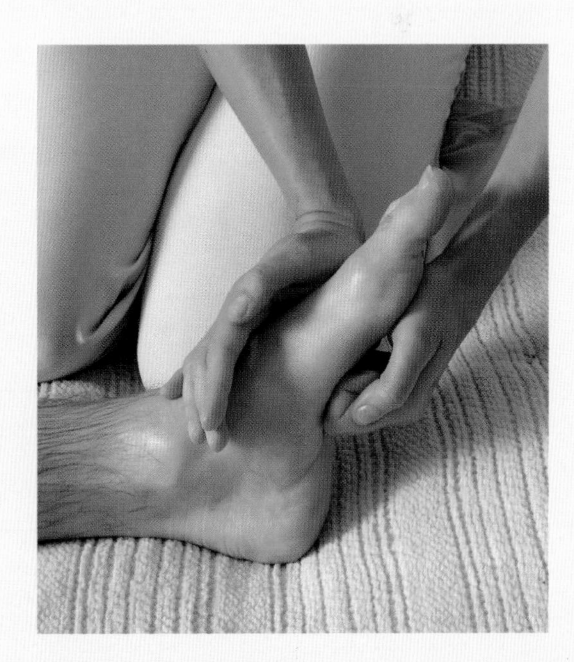

Knuckle slide

This stroke is great for large, fleshy areas of the body. It can be used in place of effleurage strokes or incorporated whenever your fingers are in need of a rest.

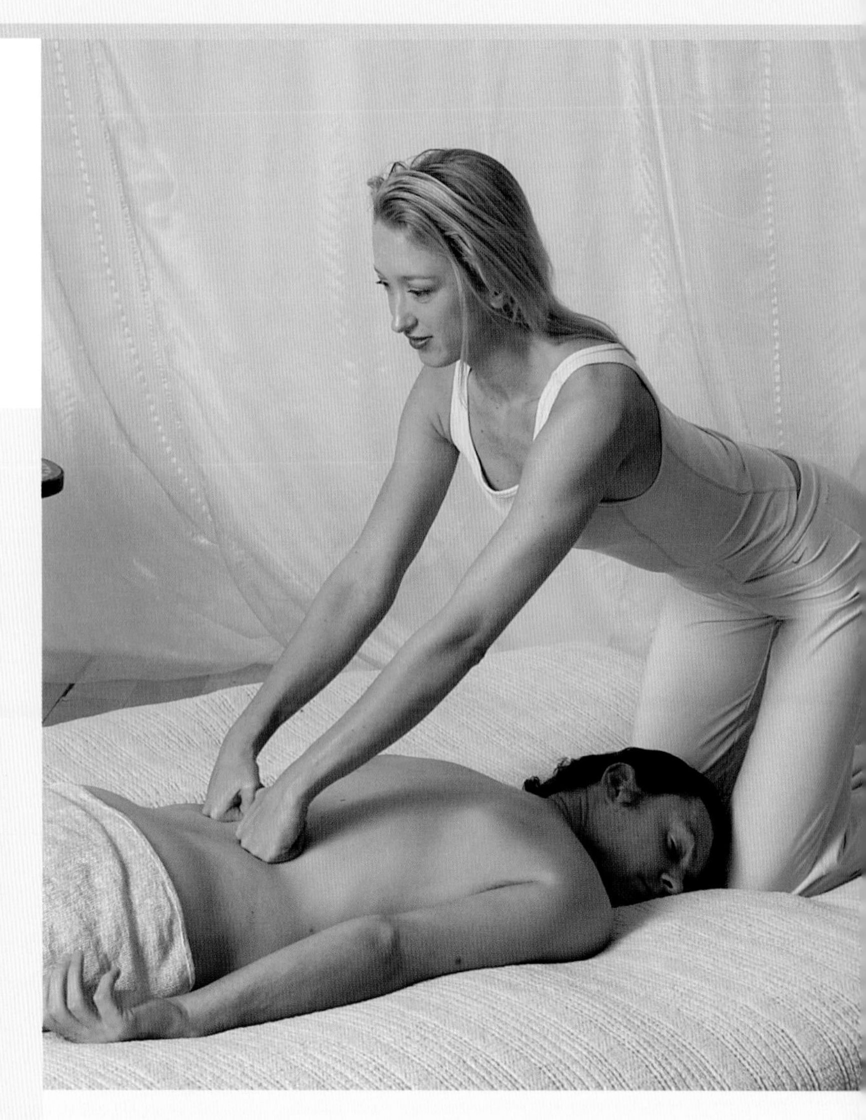

To the back

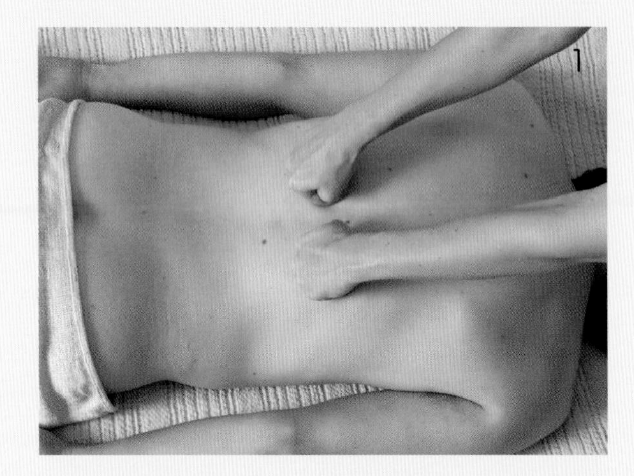

1 Kneel at your partner's head facing their feet. Touch the pads of the fingers of both hands to the palms, forming fists. Place the flat part of your hands just below the knuckles on your partner's back, either side of the spine, near their neck. Slide the knuckles down the sides of the spine towards the pelvis.

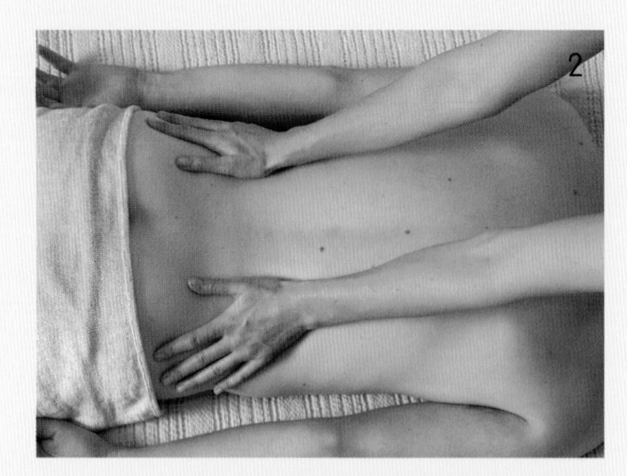

2 Uncurl the hands and place the palms flat at the base of the spine. Slide the hands across the pelvis to the hips and glide them back up to the starting point.

To the leg

Form fists with both hands. Place one fist above the knee, or at the base of the calf (whichever area you are working on). Slide the hand up the leg to the hip (or the knee if working on the calf). When one hand reaches the top, start the other hand at the base. Make sure at least one hand has contact with the body the whole time.

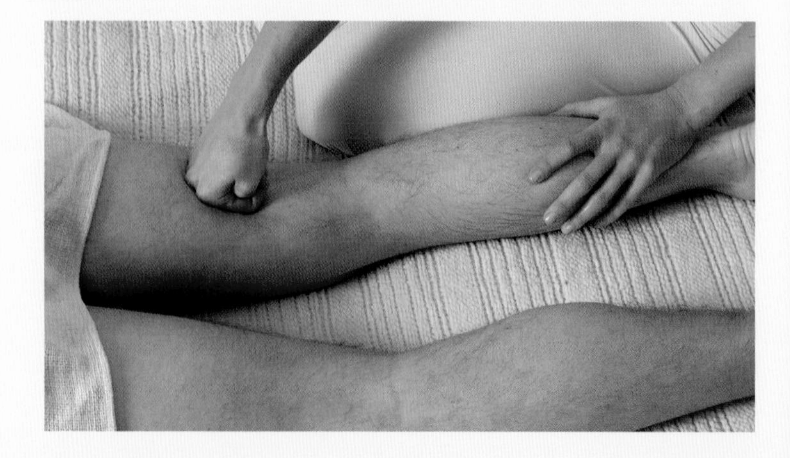

Lion claw

To the shoulders

1 Kneel on the opposite side of the shoulder you are working on. Make a claw shape with both of your hands. Place both hands slightly under the shoulder.

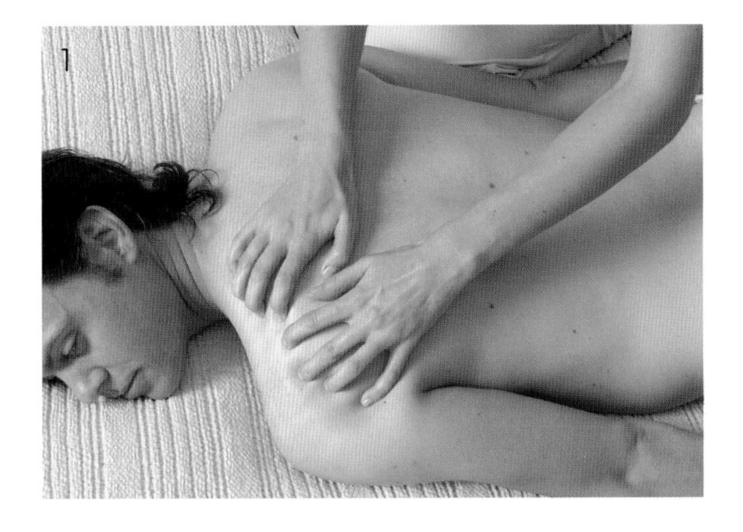

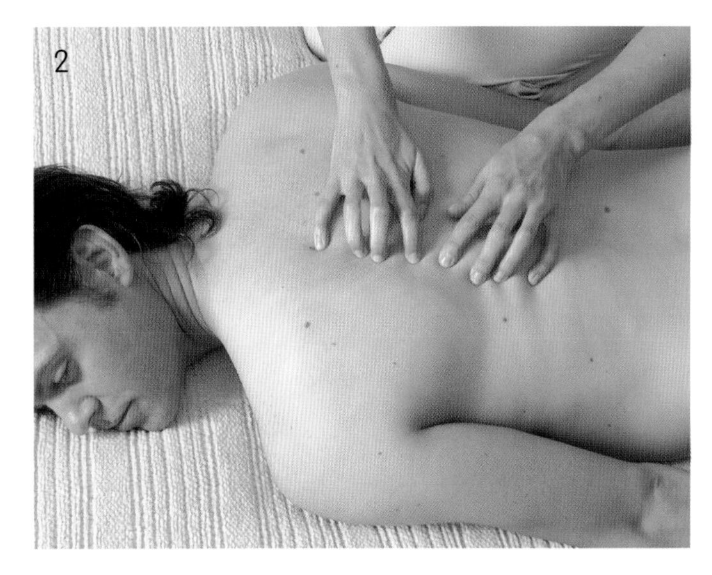

2 Keeping your hands in a claw position, drag them along the back diagonally towards the spine.

Repeat 3 times. Repeat to the other shoulder.

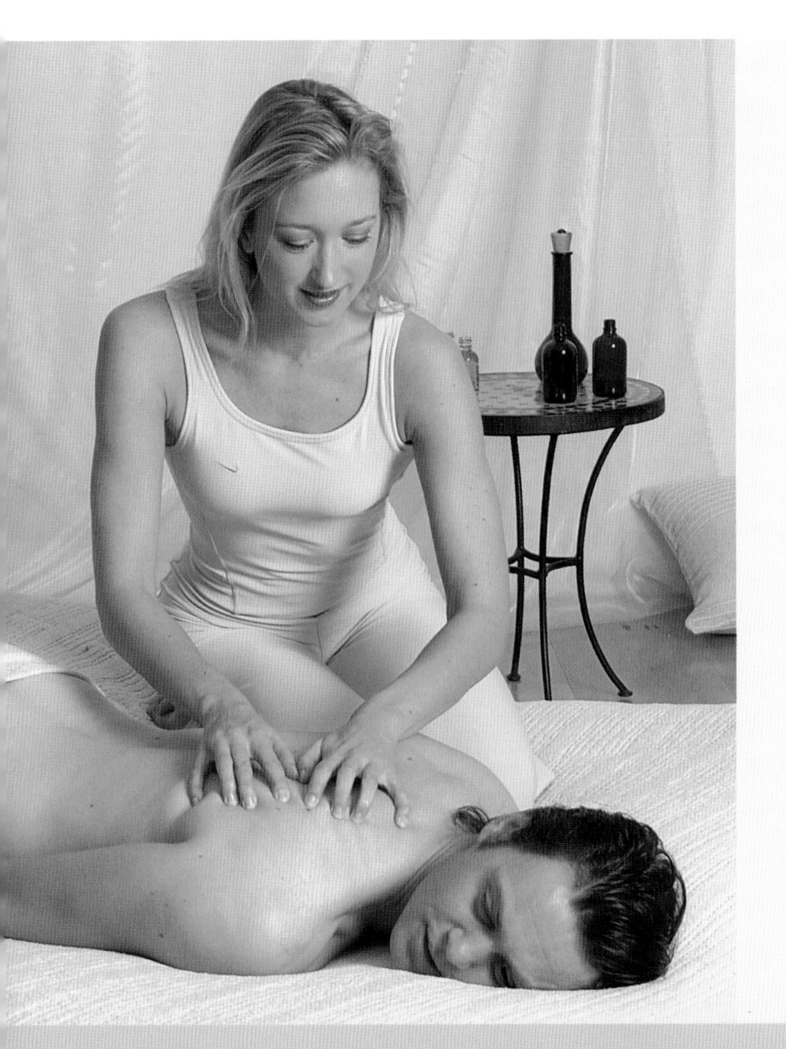

Circling

1 Place your hands on either side of your partner's foot. The palms of the hands should cover the toes, just above the ball of the foot.

2 Slowly circle the palms of your hands around each other. Your partner's foot should make a slight rolling motion.

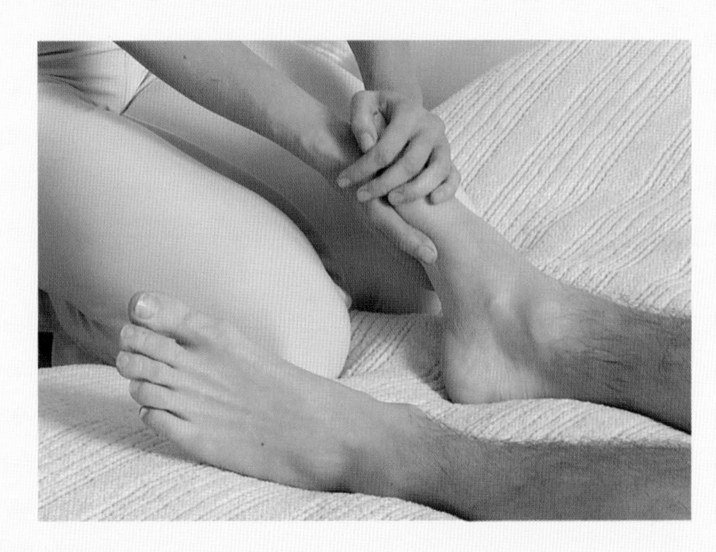

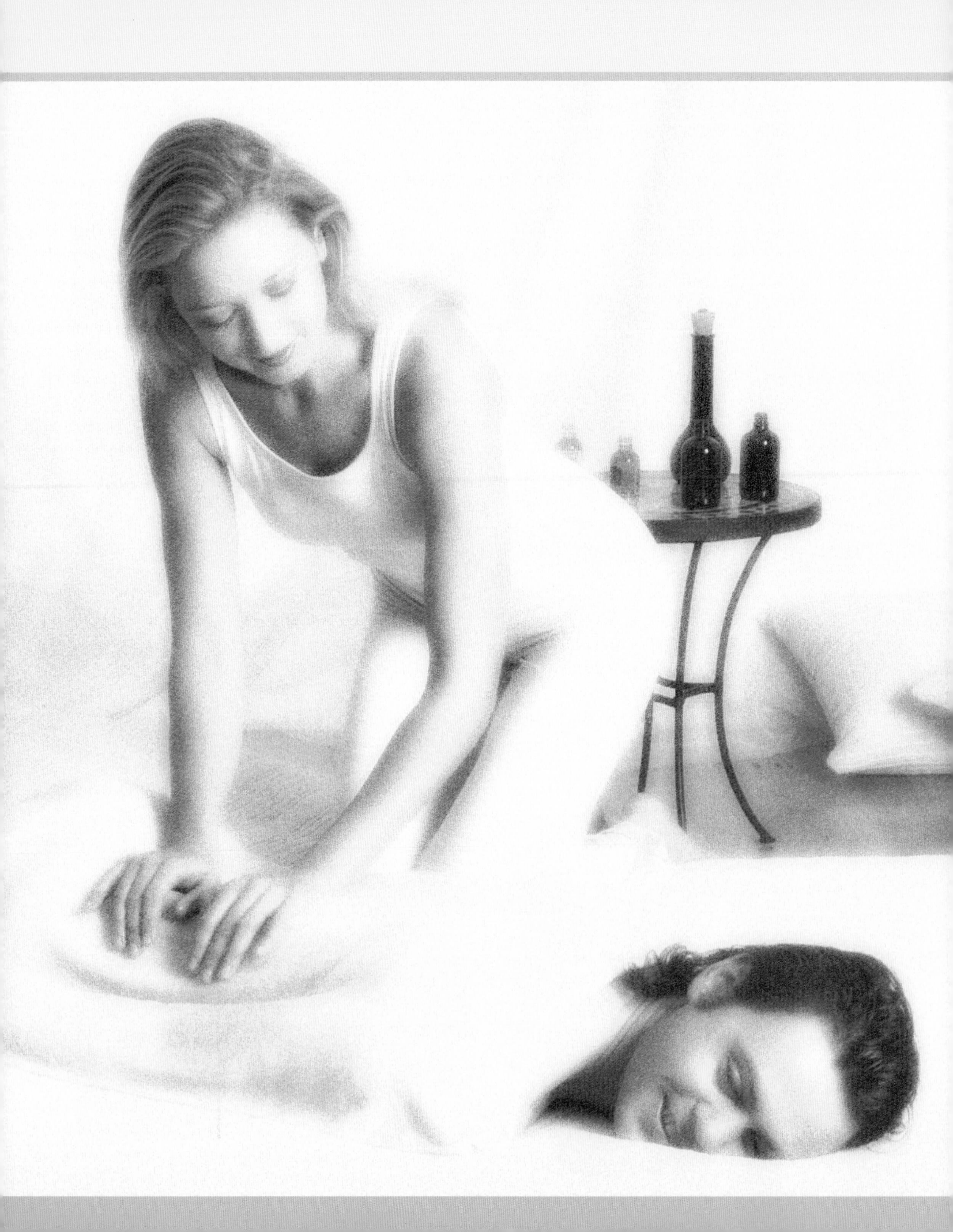

Stimulating massage

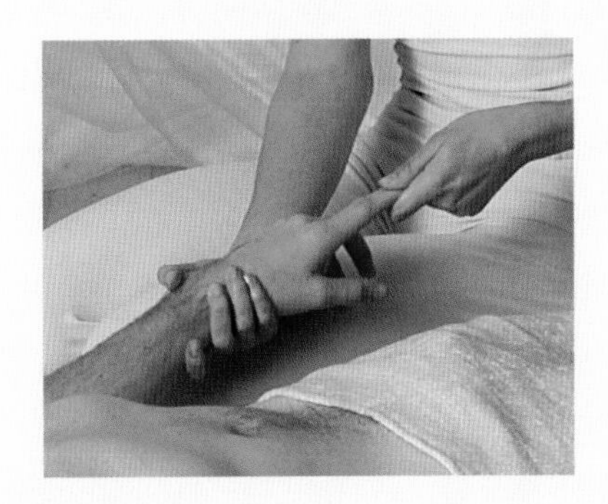

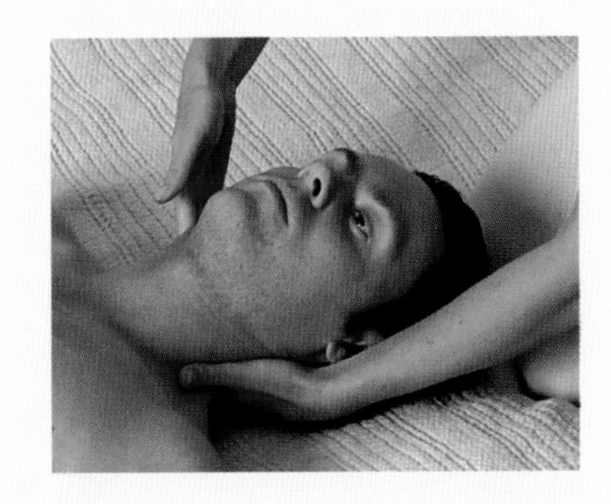

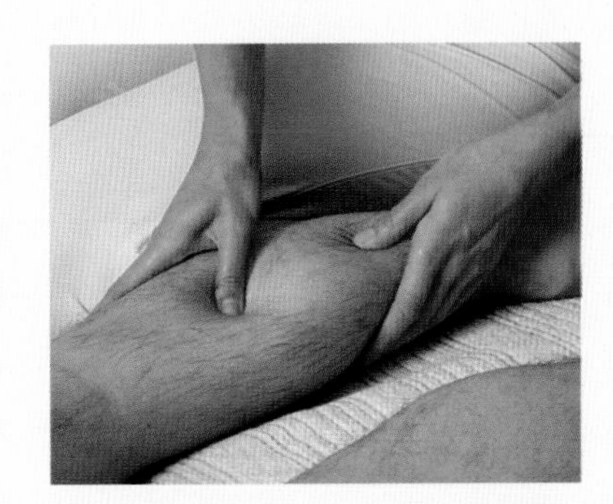

This massage incorporates all the strokes and techniques you have learned while offering slight variations that you can experiment with. Develop your own style and rhythm using the techniques that work for you. Check with your partner occasionally to make sure the pressure is not too strong or too light.

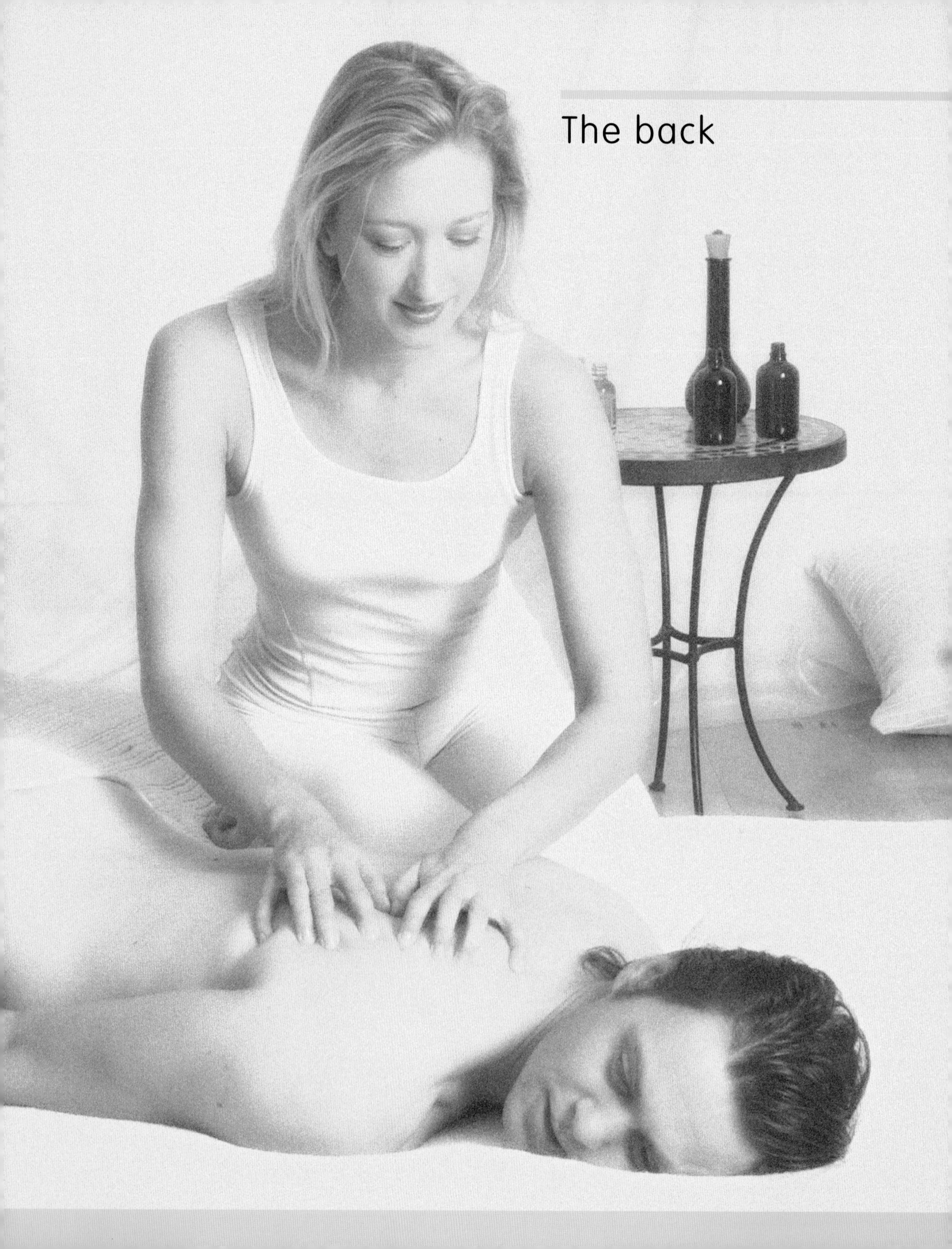

The back

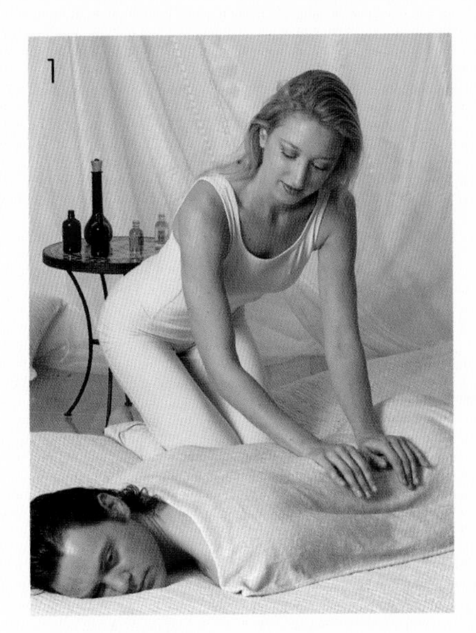

1 Softening: kneel to the side of your partner facing their spine. Place your hands above the towel with your palms on the fleshy area on one side of the base of the spine. Press the palms into the flesh and release. Work your way up to the neck and then repeat on the other side of the spine. Now place your hands flat on the back and rub vigorously all over the back above the towel. Slide the towel down to uncover the back to the top of the buttocks.

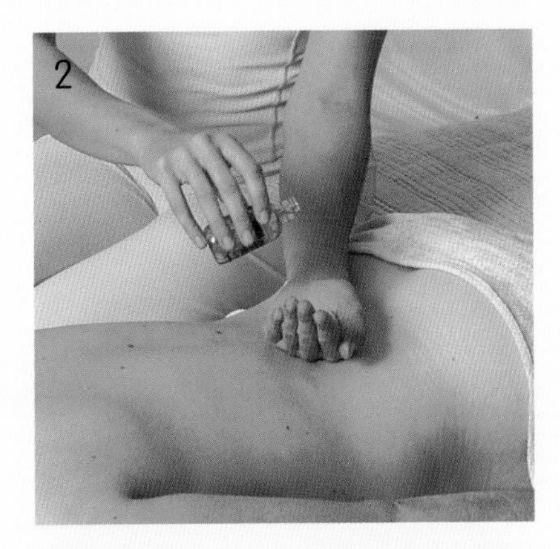

2 Spreading the oil: Kneel at the head of your partner, facing their head. Pour a small amount of oil into your hand and rub your hands together. Spread the oil, starting at the base of their back and working your way up to their shoulders.

3 Effleurage: Place your hands on the base of your partner's spine, with the thumbs together and your fingertips facing their head. Slide your hands up the back to their neck. Separate your hands and glide them across to the shoulders and lightly down the outside of the back of the hips. Circle back to the base of the spine and repeat three times.

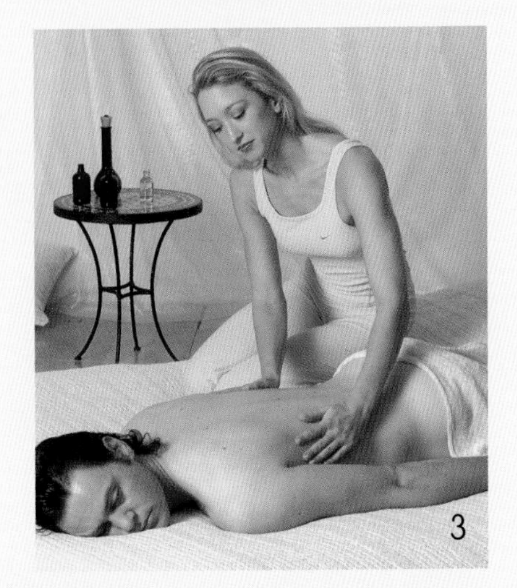

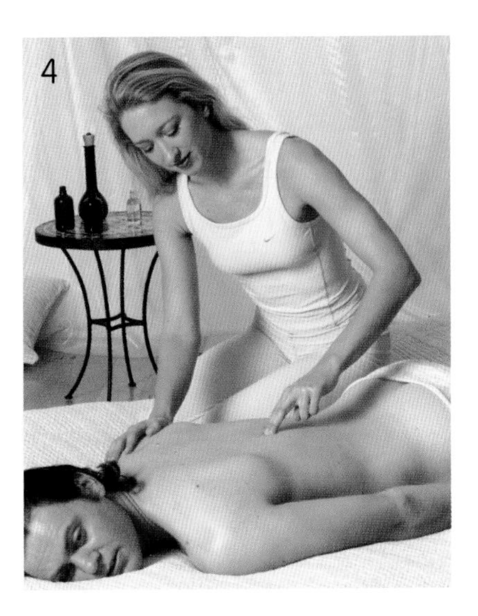

4 Vibration: Place two fingers of one hand together at the top of your partner's back on one side of the spine. Vigorously rub a tight zigzag down the back towards the hips. Start again at the top a little farther away from the spine. Repeat a third time even further away, and then repeat to the other side of the spine.

5 Wringing across the back: Place your hands on either side of the waistline with fingertips facing away from you. Wring across the back, remembering to keep your hands a few centimetres apart. Repeat a few times.

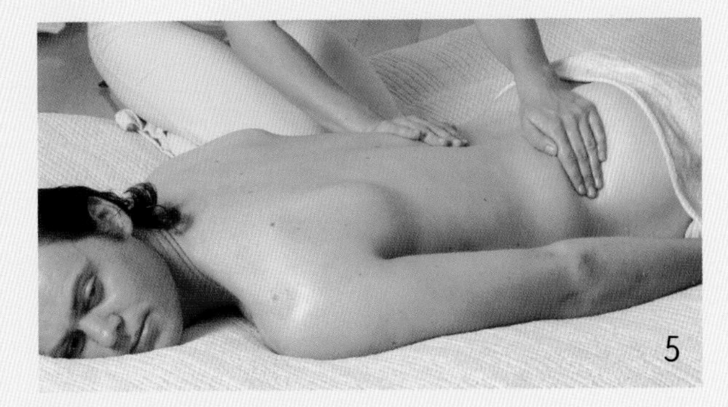

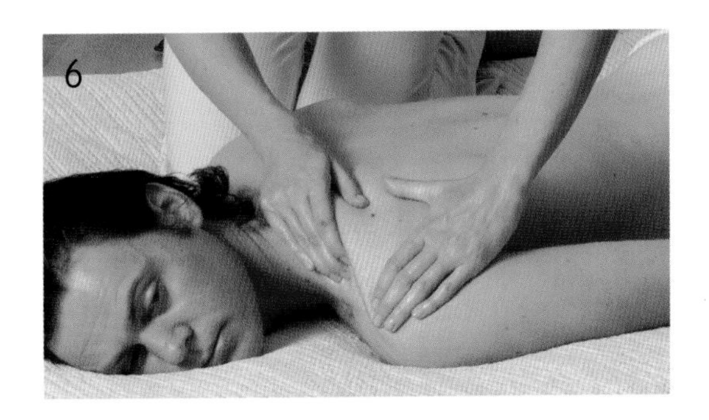

6 Kneading to the shoulders and neck: Place both hands on one shoulder and glide the flesh back and forth between them, releasing the tension. Remain for about 30 seconds on each shoulder. Remember to use only one hand when massaging the back of the neck.

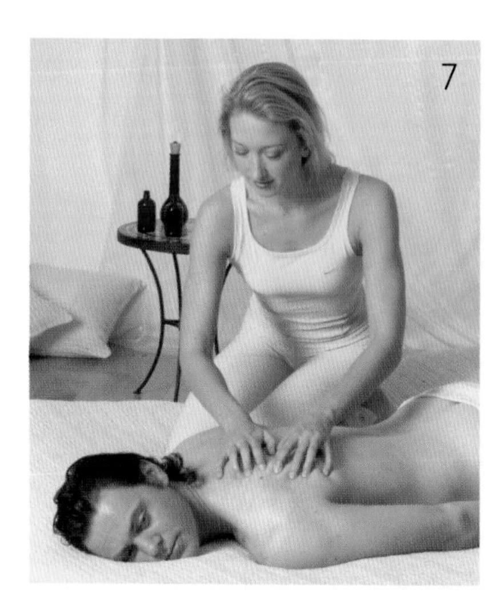

7 Lion claw: Form a claw with both hands and place them on the opposite shoulder to the side you are kneeling on. Pull the flesh back on a diagonal towards the spine. Repeat a few times and then do the opposite side.

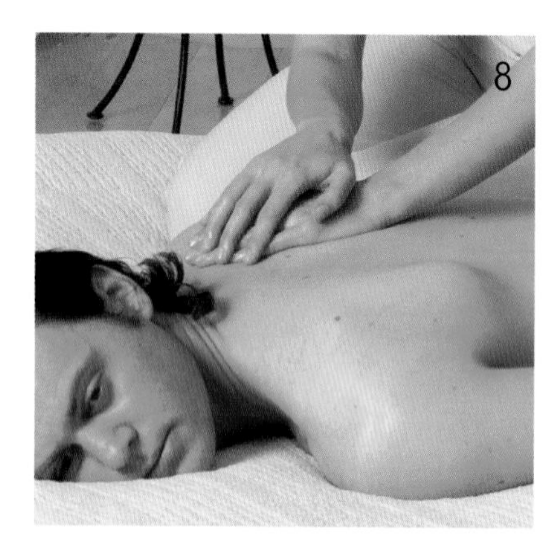

8 Hand-over-hand effleurage to the shoulder: Kneel to the right side of your partner to work on the right shoulder. Place your right hand on top of your left and both of your hands on the inside of their left shoulder blade. Press the hands up towards the neck and across the shoulder. Sweep the hands down around the shoulder blade and back to your starting position. Press firmly as your hands slide up and across the shoulders and lighter as they circle back to your starting position. Repeat to the other side.

9 Friction to the shoulder blade: Kneel on the right side of your partner. Pick up their right hand and place it on their back. Take your right hand and place it underneath their right shoulder. Press the shoulder up slightly so that the shoulder blade wings out. Place two fingers in between the shoulder blade and the spine. Make small circles up the inside of the shoulder blade, thinking of releasing the muscle from the bone. Repeat 2 more times.

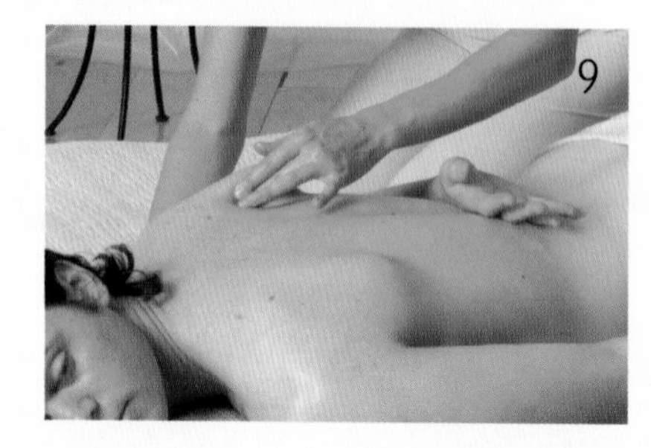

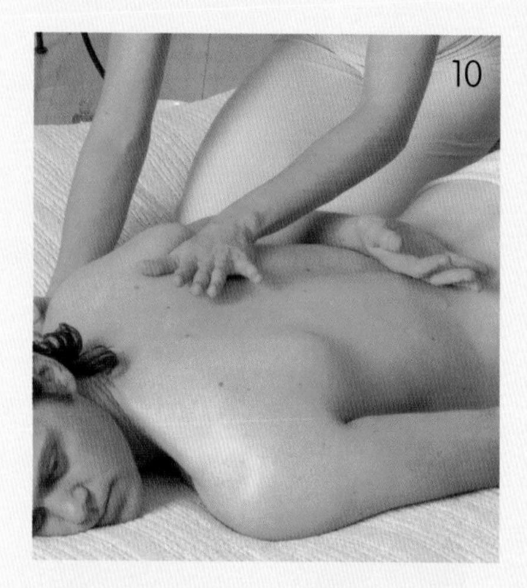

10 Vibration to the shoulder blade: Continue holding the shoulder with the right hand. Change your hand position so that the length of the thumb is along the ridge of the shoulder blade. Quickly and gently vibrate the hand against the shoulder blade.

11 Repeat steps 8 through 10 to the other side.

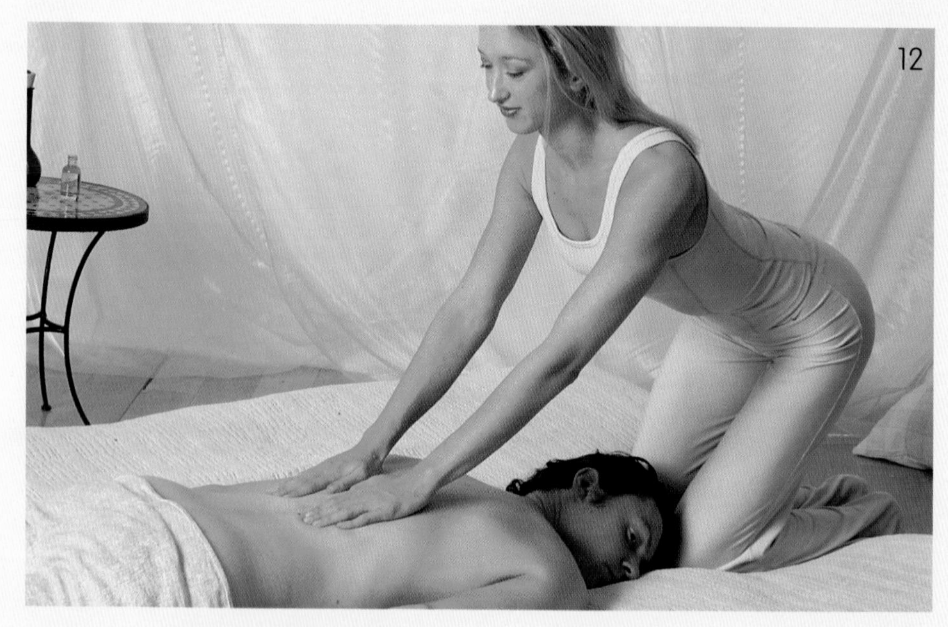

12 Pull-ups: Kneel at the head of your partner facing their feet. Slide the hands down the back and out along the hips. Hold the hips as you pull the flesh towards you. Repeat three times.

13 Knuckle rolls: Staying at your partner's head and facing their feet, slide the hands down the spine one more time. When the fingers reach the base, roll them over so that the knuckles are touching the skin. Roll the knuckles in a circular motion around the hips, lower back and buttocks.

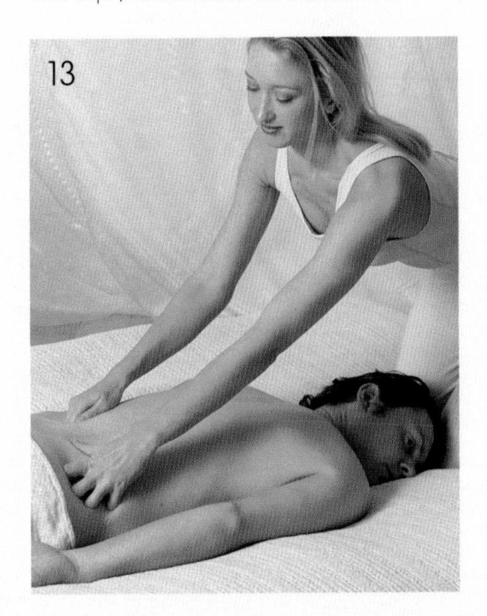

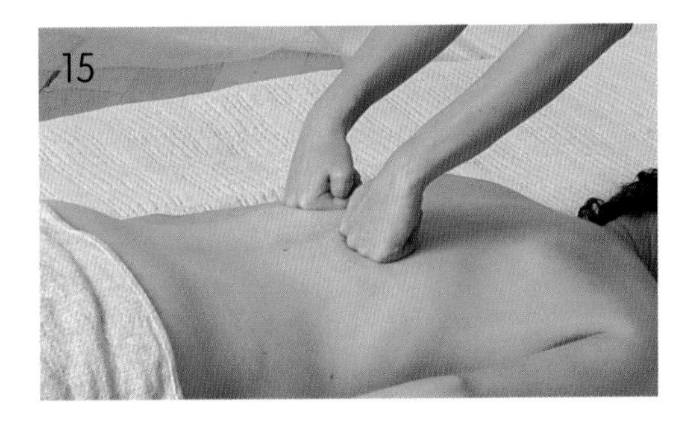

15 Knuckle slide: Remain kneeling at your partner's head. Make fists and place the flat part of the hands on your partner's back either side of the spine near the neck Slide the knuckles down to the pelvis. Uncurl the hands, then slide them across the pelvis to the hips and glide them back up to the starting point.

16 Hacking: Move to the side of your partner so that you are kneeling facing their back. Hold your hands 5 cm above your partner with your palms facing each other. Lightly flick the skin alternating with your pinkies. This is a quick wrist action moving along the spine. Be sure not to hit the kidney area as you do this.

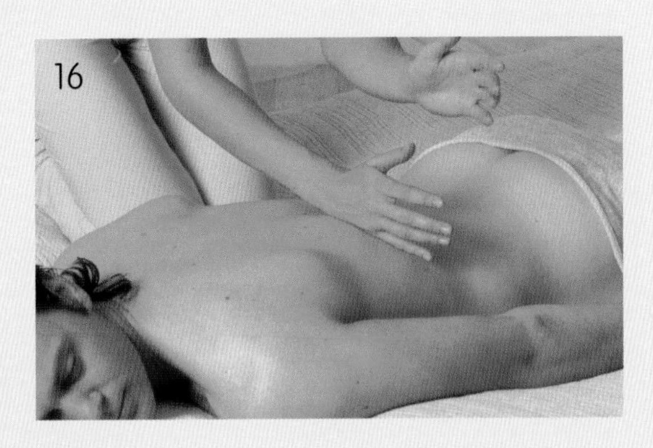

14 Fanning: Continue kneeling at your partner's head. Slide the hands down the back and spread the fingers out along the base of the spine. Circle the fingers 3 times. Move the hands up to the ribs and repeat. Move the hands up to the shoulders and repeat. Repeat the whole sequence 3 times.

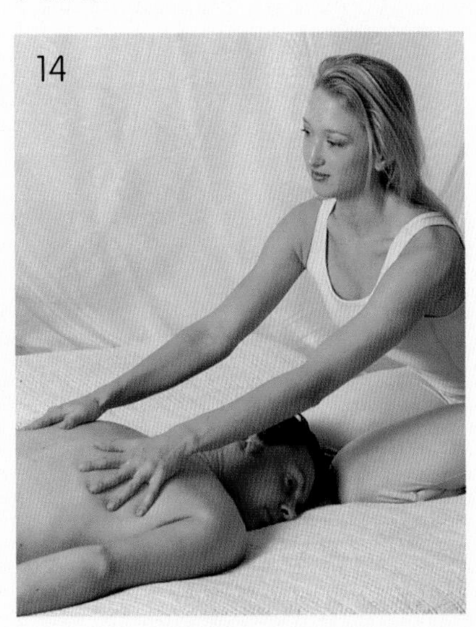

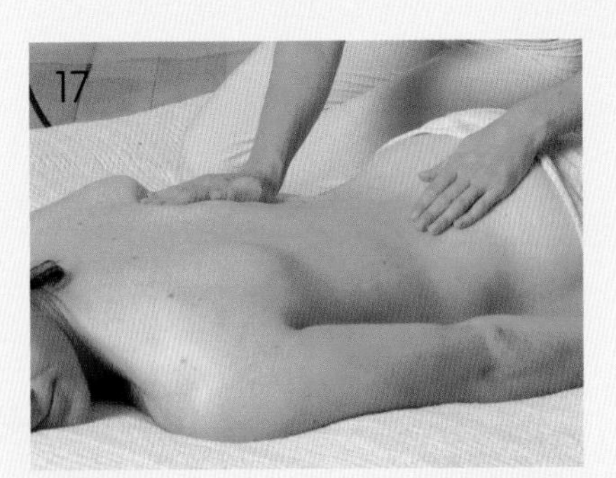

17 Alternating effleurage: Start with the hands on either side of the base of the spine with the fingertips facing the head. Slide one hand up, across the shoulder and down the outside of the back. Repeat with the other hand in smooth, rhythmic motions.

18 Feather stroking: Lightly stroke down the back with your fingertips. Alternate the hands as you gently caress the back.

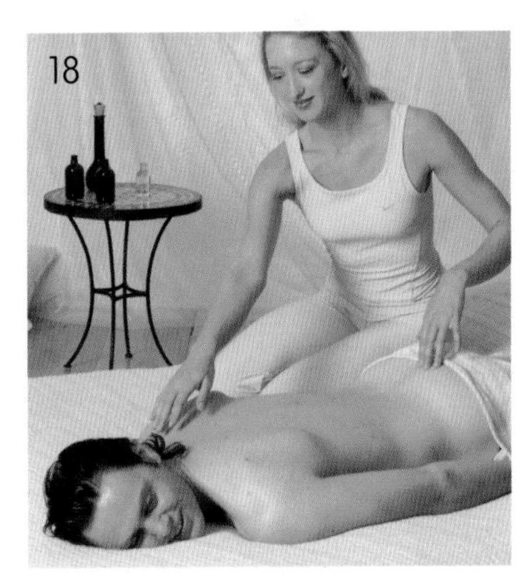

Ending: Pull the towel back up across the back. Place one hand between the shoulder blades and one hand on the base of the spine. Press the hands out and down, gently trying to stretch the spine.

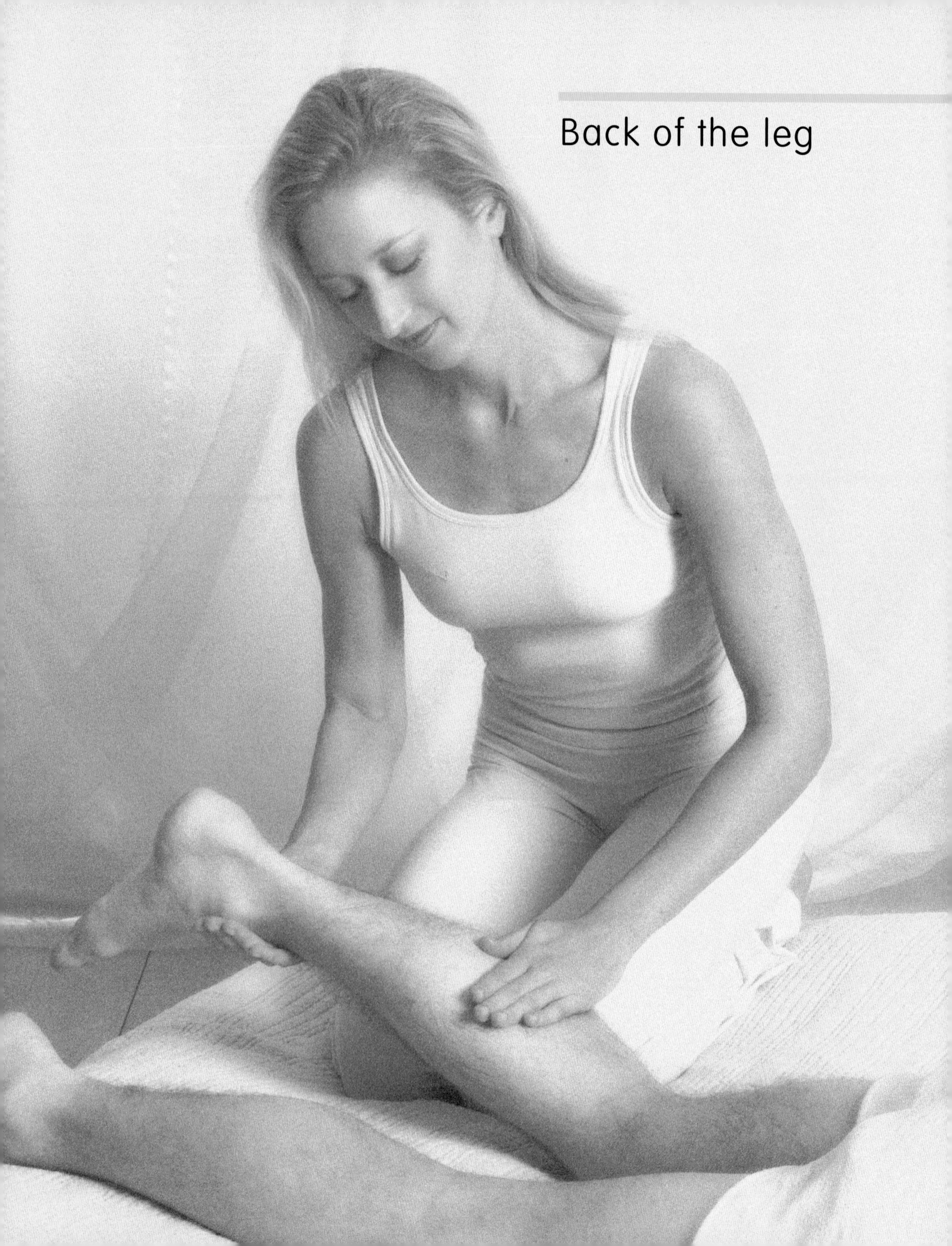

Back of the leg

Softening: Place your hands above the towel with the palms on one side of the leg and the fingers on the other. Pinch the flesh underneath the towel and release. Move to a different area of the leg and repeat until you have covered the whole leg. Place the hands flat above the towel and rub the leg vigorously.

Spreading the oil: Uncover the leg so you can see the hip while retaining your partner's modesty. Pour a small amount of oil into your hand and rub your hands together. Start at the ankle and spread the oil up the leg towards the hip.

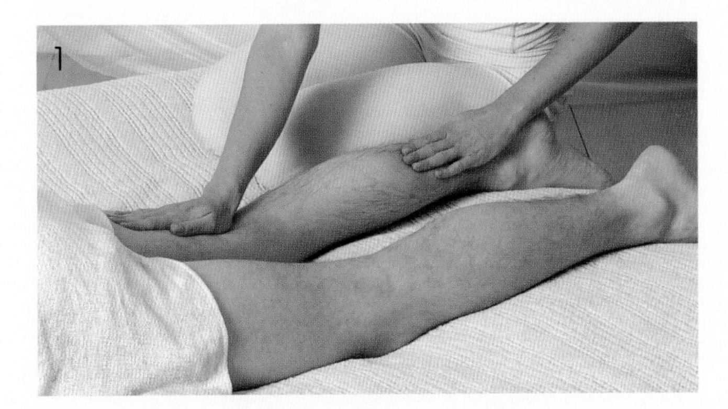

1 **Alternating effleurage:** Place both hands on the ankle with the fingers facing the hip. Slide one hand up the leg to the hip, avoiding the back of the knee. Glide the hand to the outside of the leg and back down to the ankle. As the hand reaches the ankle, slide the other hand up the leg. Remember to press firmly on the way up and gently on the way down.

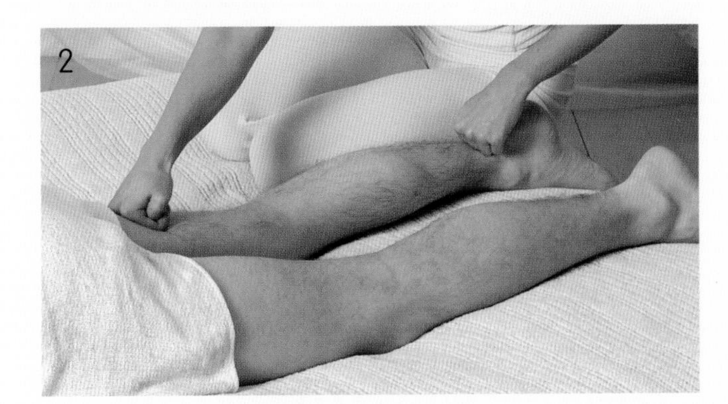

2 **Knuckle slide:** Form a fist with both hands. Place the flat part of the fist near the knuckles of one hand at the ankle. Slide the hand up to the hip, avoiding the back of the knee. As the hand reaches the top, start the other hand sliding up. Repeat a few times, and imagine waves rolling up the leg.

3 **Kneading the inner thigh:** Kneel to the side of your partner facing their thigh. Place your hands on their inner thigh with the fingers facing down. Pick up the flesh with one hand and slide it across to the other hand. Release the flesh as you pick it up with the opposite hand. Shift your weight as you think of kneading dough.

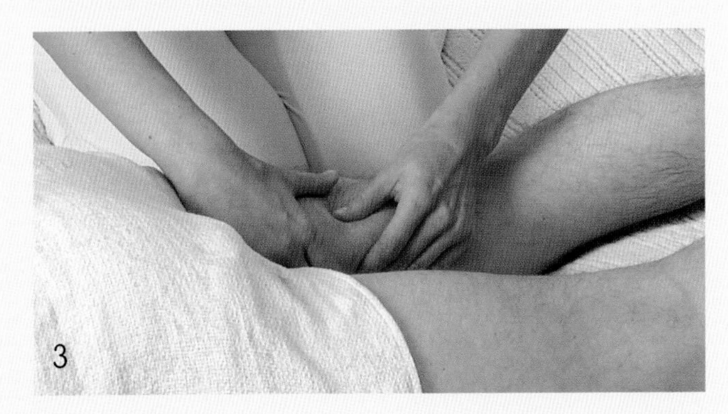

4 **Wringing the thigh:** Place your hands on either side of the thigh with your fingers facing away from you. Think of lifting the flesh off the bone as you slide the hands past each other in opposite directions. Remember to keep the hands a few centimetres apart so that the flesh twists without causing a burning sensation.

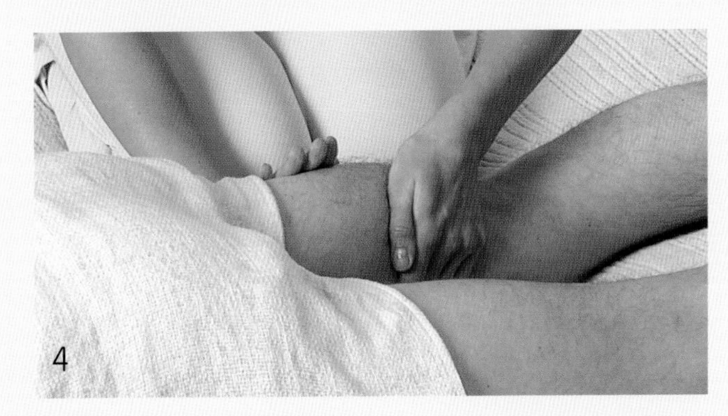

5 **Friction to the thigh:** Place the thumbs just above the knee with the fingers to the sides. Circle the thumbs, covering the whole thigh area.

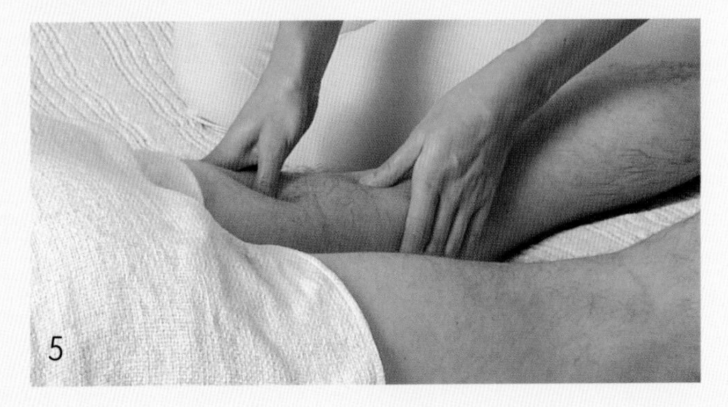

6 Hacking: Kneel facing the thigh with the hands a couple of centimetres above the thigh and the palms facing each other. Quickly strike the thigh with alternating hands, allowing the pinkies only to touch the thigh.

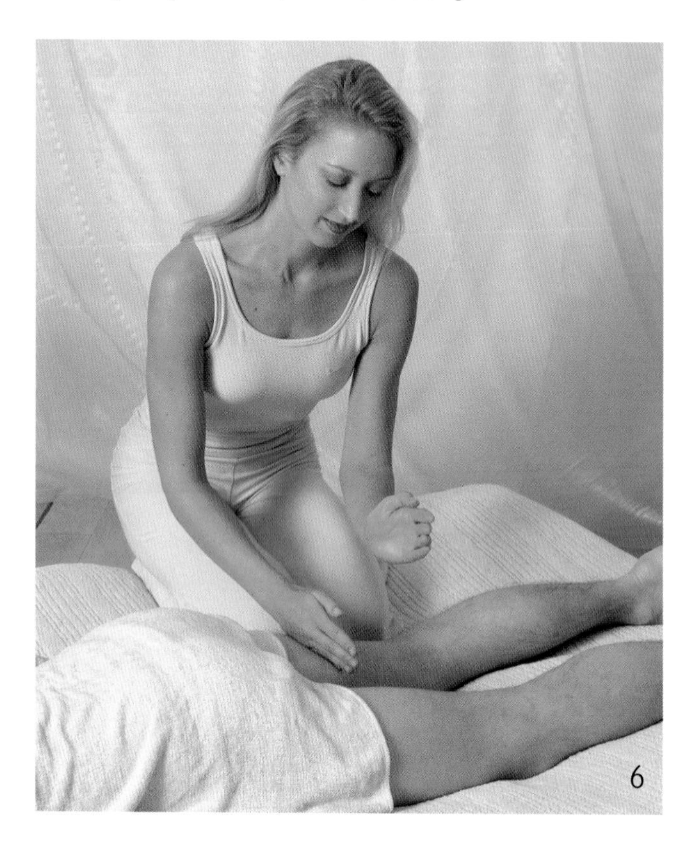

6

7 Basic effleurage: Place both hands just above the knee with the fingers facing the hip. Slide the hands towards the hip, open to the sides, and glide the hands back down to the original position. Repeat 3 times. Now repeat to the whole leg 3 times, starting at the ankle. Then again just to the calf.

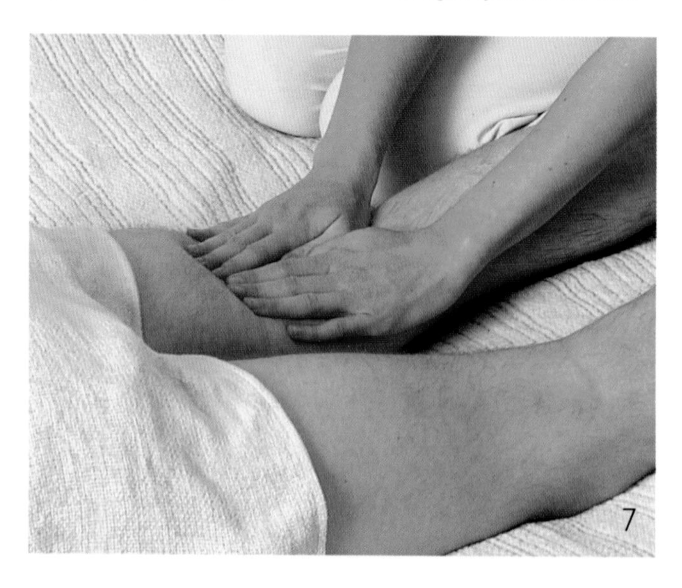

7

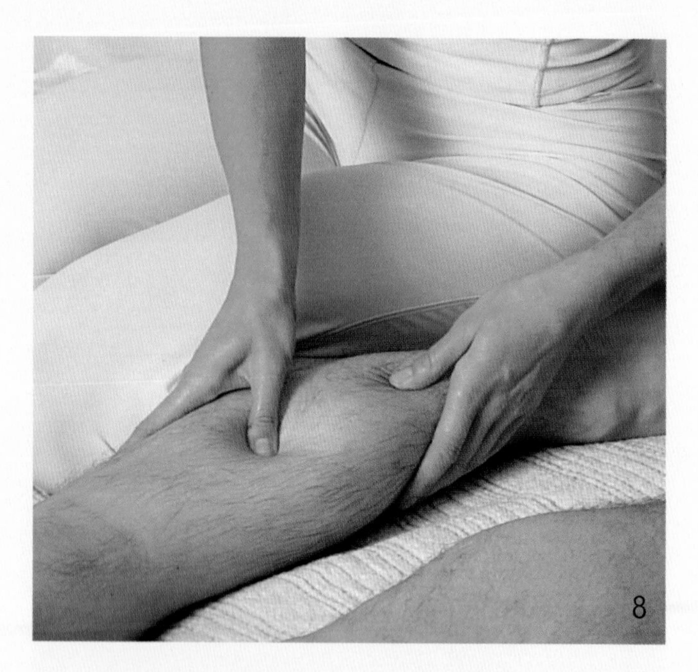

8

8 Friction to the calf: Start with the thumbs at the ankle with the fingers out to the sides. Using the whole arm, make circles with the thumbs across the whole calf muscle. This area might be tender, so work lightly!

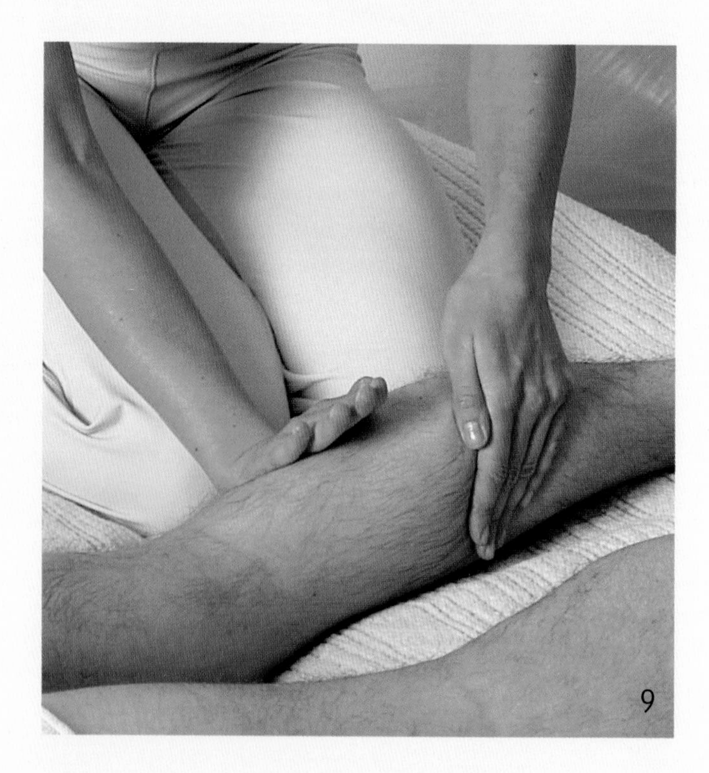

9

9 Wringing the calf: Sit or kneel to the side of your partner, facing the calf. Place the hands on either side of the calf with the fingers facing away from you. Wring the calf with the hands a few centimetres apart causing the flesh to twist in opposite directions.

10 Vibration: Pick up the ankle with the opposite hand to the leg you are working on. As you do this, place the other hand flat against the belly of the calf. Vigorously move the hand back and forth across the belly of the calf causing it to shake. Continue for about 10 seconds, and then release the leg back onto the table.

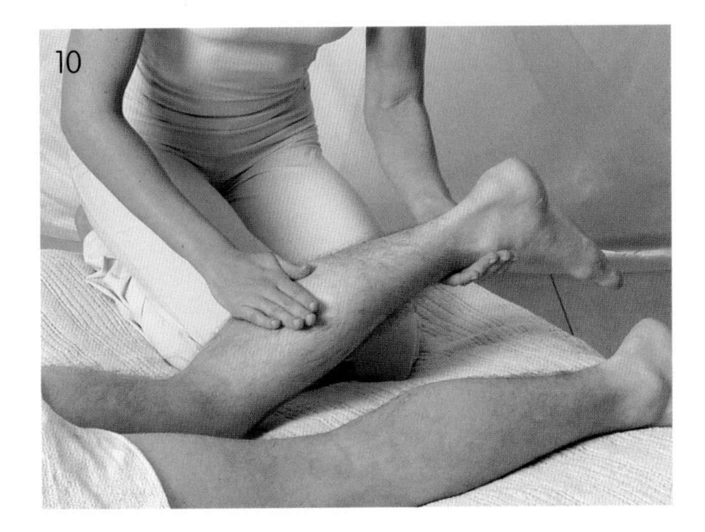

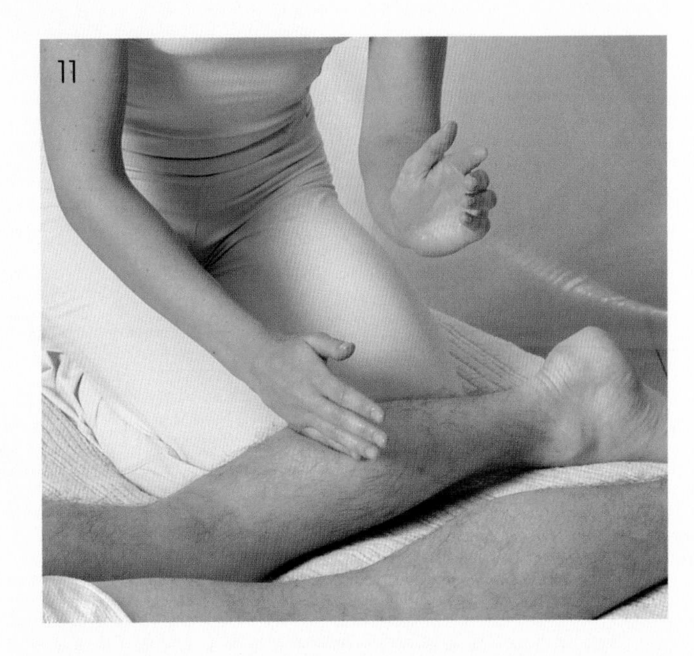

11 Hacking: Lightly strike the fleshy part of the calf with the palms facing each other. Perform quick, alternating rhythmic movements awakening the muscle.

12 Alternating effleurage: Place both hands on the ankle with the fingers facing the hip. Slide one hand up the leg to the hip, avoiding the back of the knee. Glide the hand to the outside of the leg and back down to the ankle. As the hand reaches the ankle, slide the other hand up the leg. Remember to press firmly on the way up and gently on the way down.

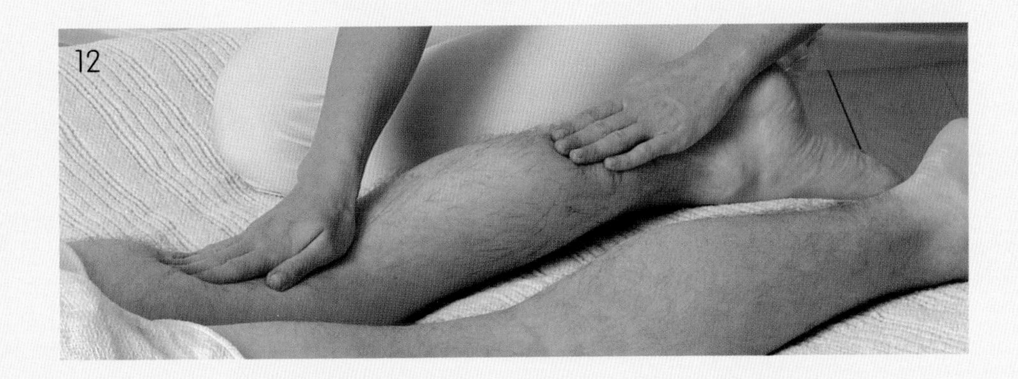

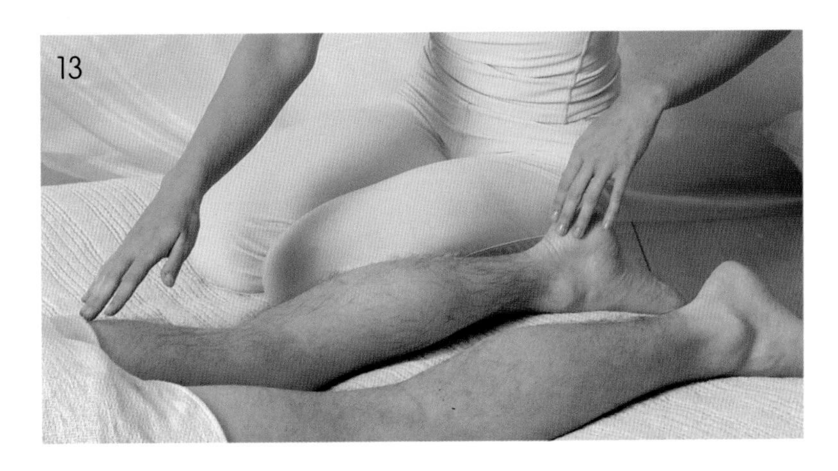

13 Feather stroking: Place the fingertips lightly at the top of the leg. Stroke the fingers down the leg just barely caressing the leg as you do this. When the hand gets to the ankle, start the fingertips of your opposite hand stroking down the leg.

Ending: Cover the leg. Move to the other side of your partner. Uncover the leg so that you can see the hip joint. Repeat the whole sequence to the other side.

Help your partner to turn over. Hold the towel slightly above them, at a diagonal away from you, so that they can turn easily without getting tangled in the towels.

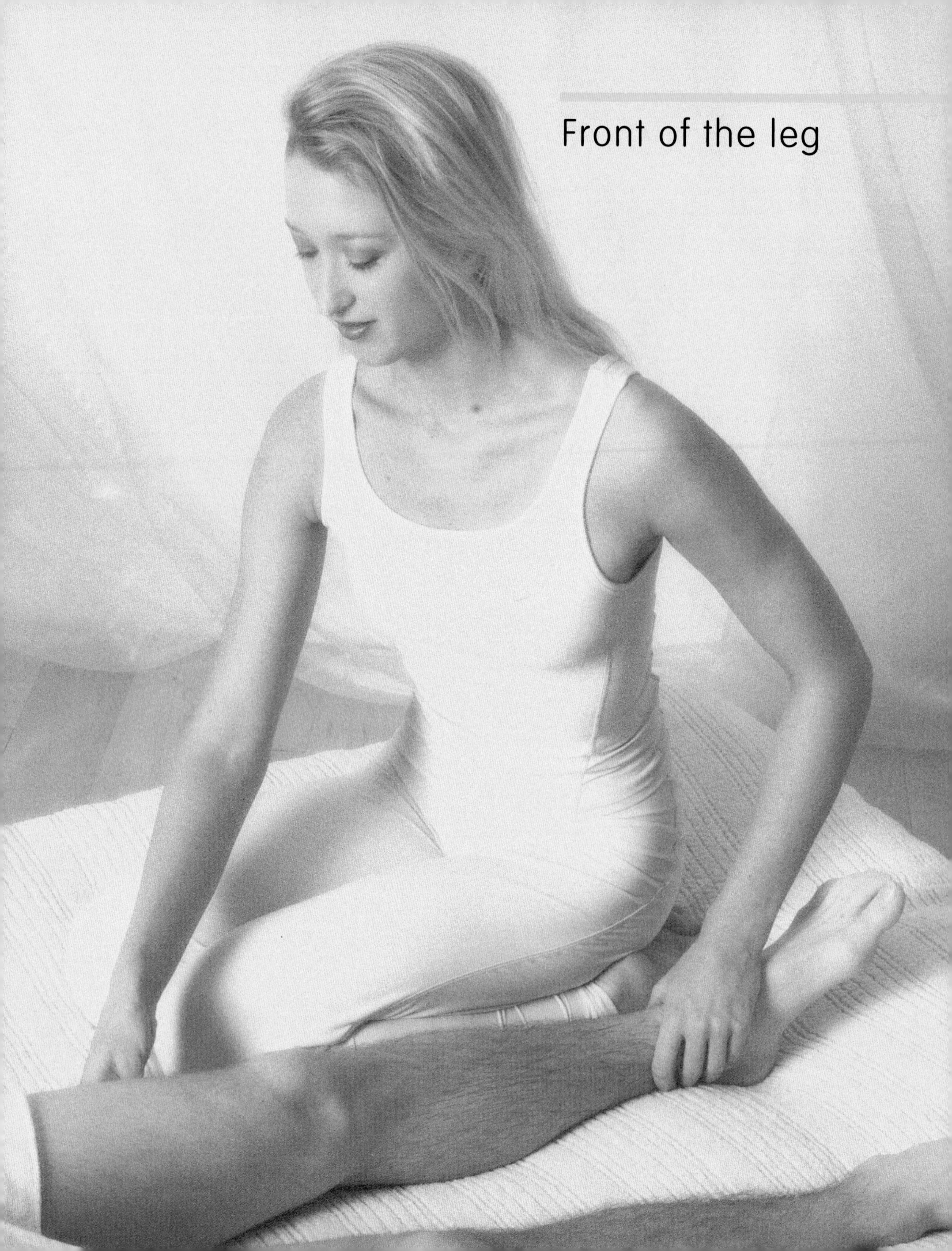

Front of the leg

Softening: Kneel or sit to the side of your partner facing their leg. Place the hands above the towel with the palms on one side of the leg and the fingers on the other. Pick up the flesh and release. Cover the whole area of the leg. Place the hands flat and rub the leg vigorously.

Spreading the oil: Uncover one leg to the hip joint. Pour a small amount of oil into your hand. Rub your hands together and spread the oil, starting at the ankle and working your way up to the hip.

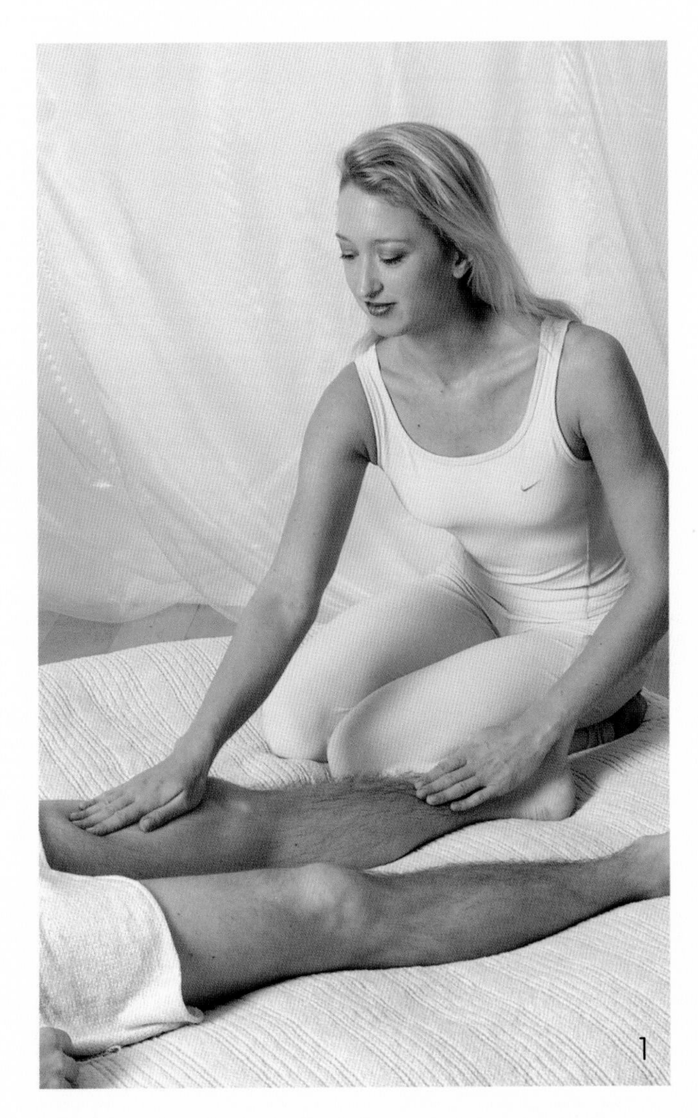
1

1 **Alternating effleurage:** Place the hands on the ankle. Slide one hand up the ankle to the hip, avoiding the knee. Slide the hand to the outside of the leg and glide it back down to the ankle. Repeat with the other hand. Repeat a few more times.

2 **Knuckles up thigh:** Place the flat part of one fist just above the knee. Slide the hand up to the hip. Place your other hand in a fist just above the knee. Slide that hand up to the hip while the first hand is lifting off to start again.

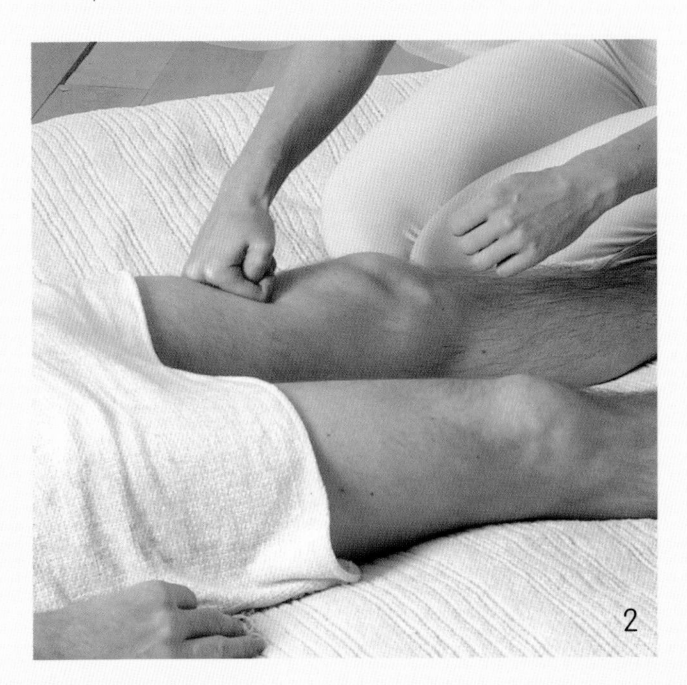
2

3 **Wringing the thigh:** Continue kneeling, facing the thigh. Place one hand on either side of the thigh with the fingers facing away from you. Slide the hands across the thigh in opposite directions as you twist the flesh when the hands cross. Repeat this action, thinking of lifting the flesh off the bone.

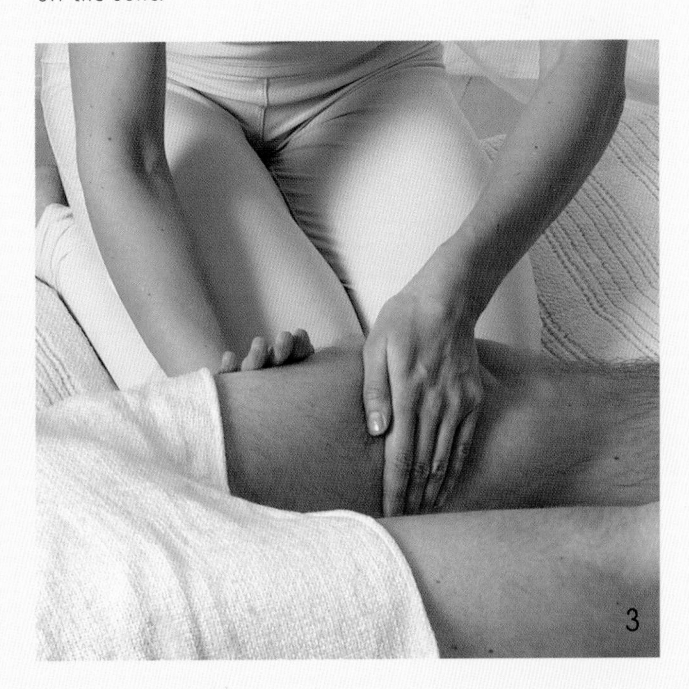
3

4 Hacking: Kneel facing your partner's leg. Hold your hands a couple of centimetres above your partner's thigh with your palms facing each other. Quickly strike the thigh with alternating hands, moving along the entire length of the thigh.

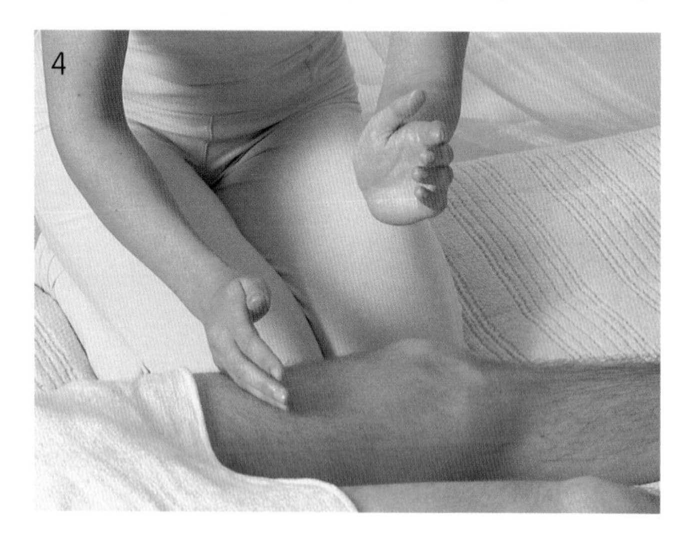
4

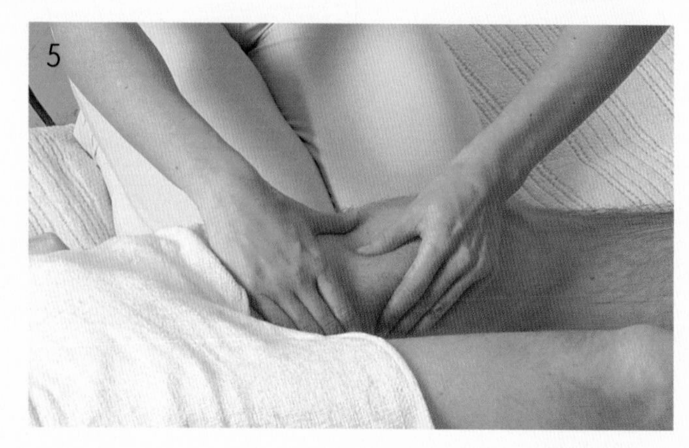
5

5 Kneading the inner thigh: Kneel facing the thigh. Place your hands on the inner thigh with your fingers facing down and your thumbs out to the sides. Pick up the flesh with one hand. Gently squeeze it as you slide the hand across to the other one. As you release the flesh, pick it up with the other hand. Continue sliding the flesh back and forth as you switch your weight from side to side with the movement.

6 Friction to the thigh: Place the thumbs just above the knee. Lock the thumb joint and make small circles with the whole arm, using the pads of the thumbs to cover the whole thigh.

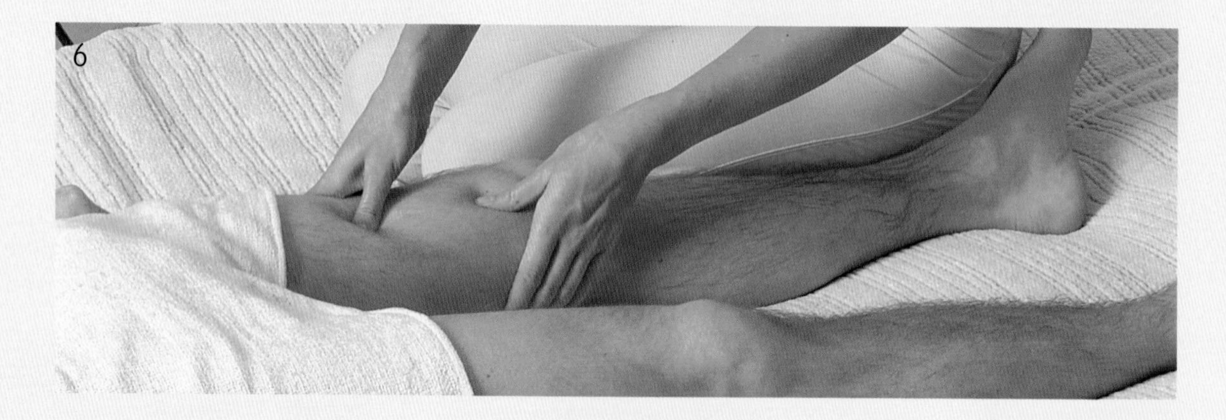
6

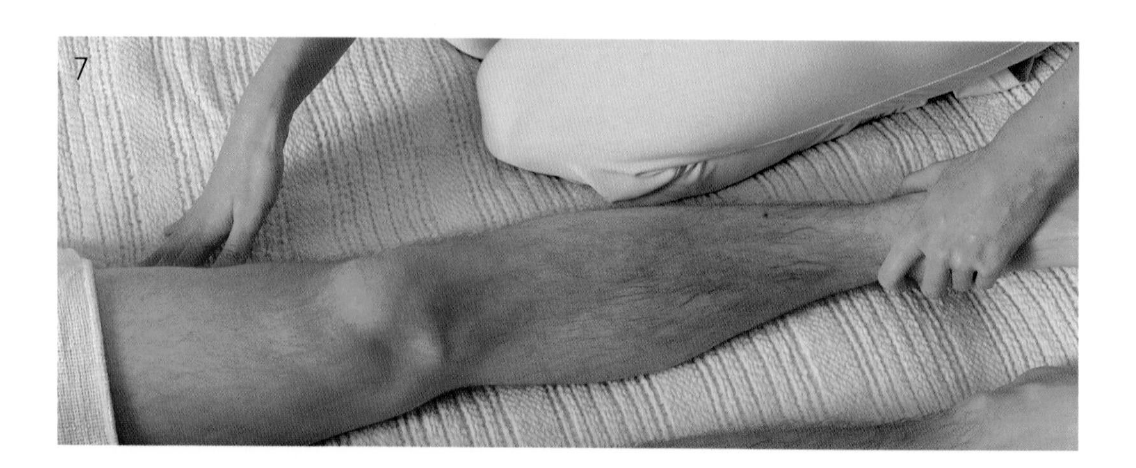
7

7 Friction to the outside of the leg: Place one hand on the ankle and slightly rotate the leg inwards. Take the thumb of your opposite hand and place it on the outside of the leg just above the knee. Make small circles with the thumb, going up towards the hip. Circle the hip a few times and repeat twice.

8 Opening the knee: Place the thumbs lengthwise on the knee with the thumbs towards the hip and the fingers to the sides. Slide the thumbs away from each other while circling the knee with the pads of the thumbs. Repeat this 3 times.

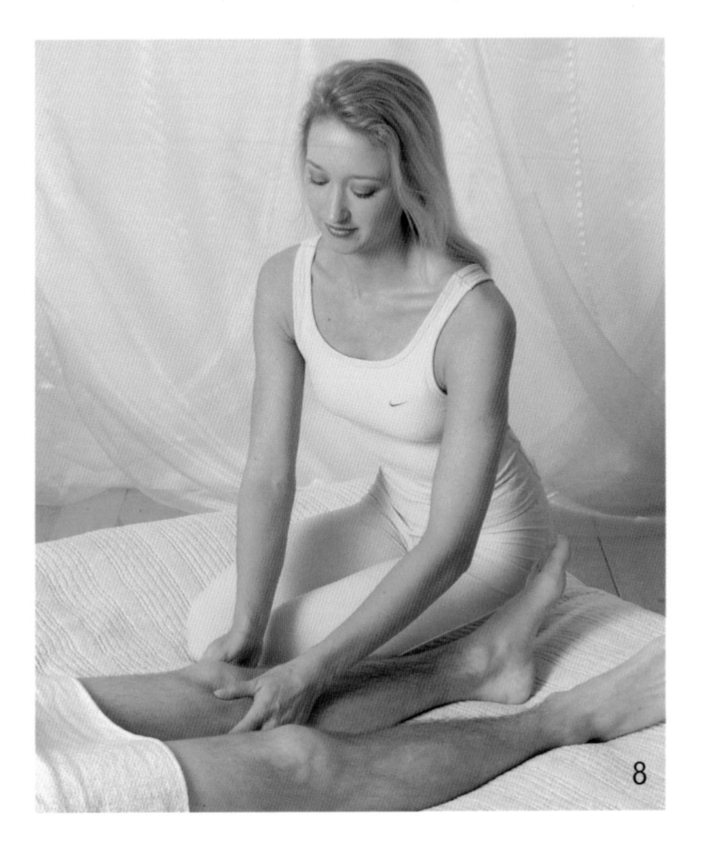

8

9 Kneading the calf: Kneel facing your partner's leg. Place the hands on the inside of the shin and pick up the fleshy part of the calf. Slide one hand across to the other taking the flesh with it. As you release the muscle, pick it up with your other hand. Slide the flesh back and forth between your hands.

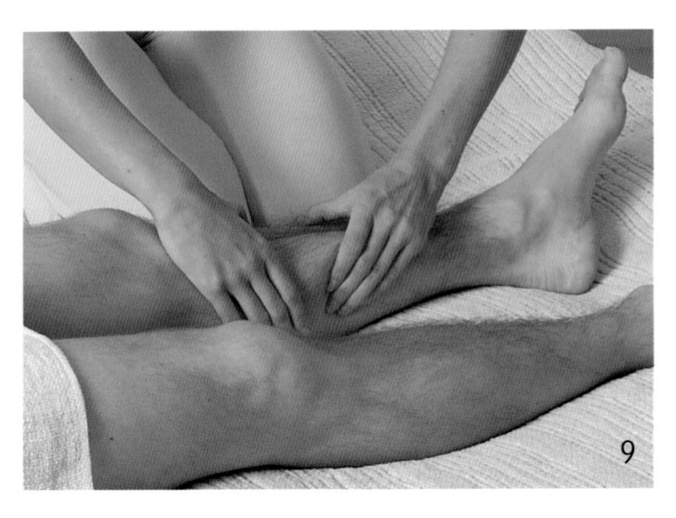

9

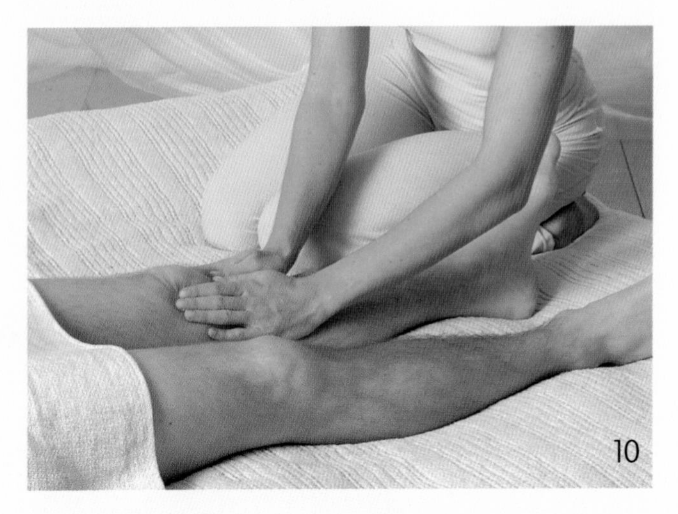

10

10 Basic effleurage: Place both hands on the ankles with the fingers facing the hip. Slide the hands up the leg to the hip, avoiding the knee. Open the hands to the sides of the leg and glide them back down. Repeat the movement 3 times. Place the hands just above the knee. Repeat the sequence to the thigh.

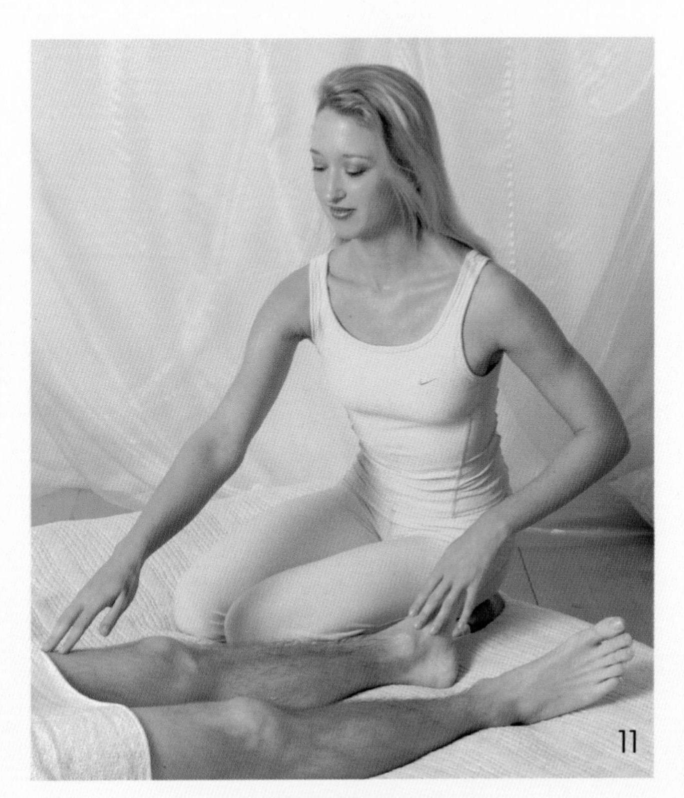

11

11 Feather stroking: Start with the fingertips of one hand at the top of the leg. Gently stroke down the leg, letting the fingers mould to the contour of the leg. As the hand gets to the ankle, repeat with the opposite hand.

Ending: Cover the leg and repeat to the other side.

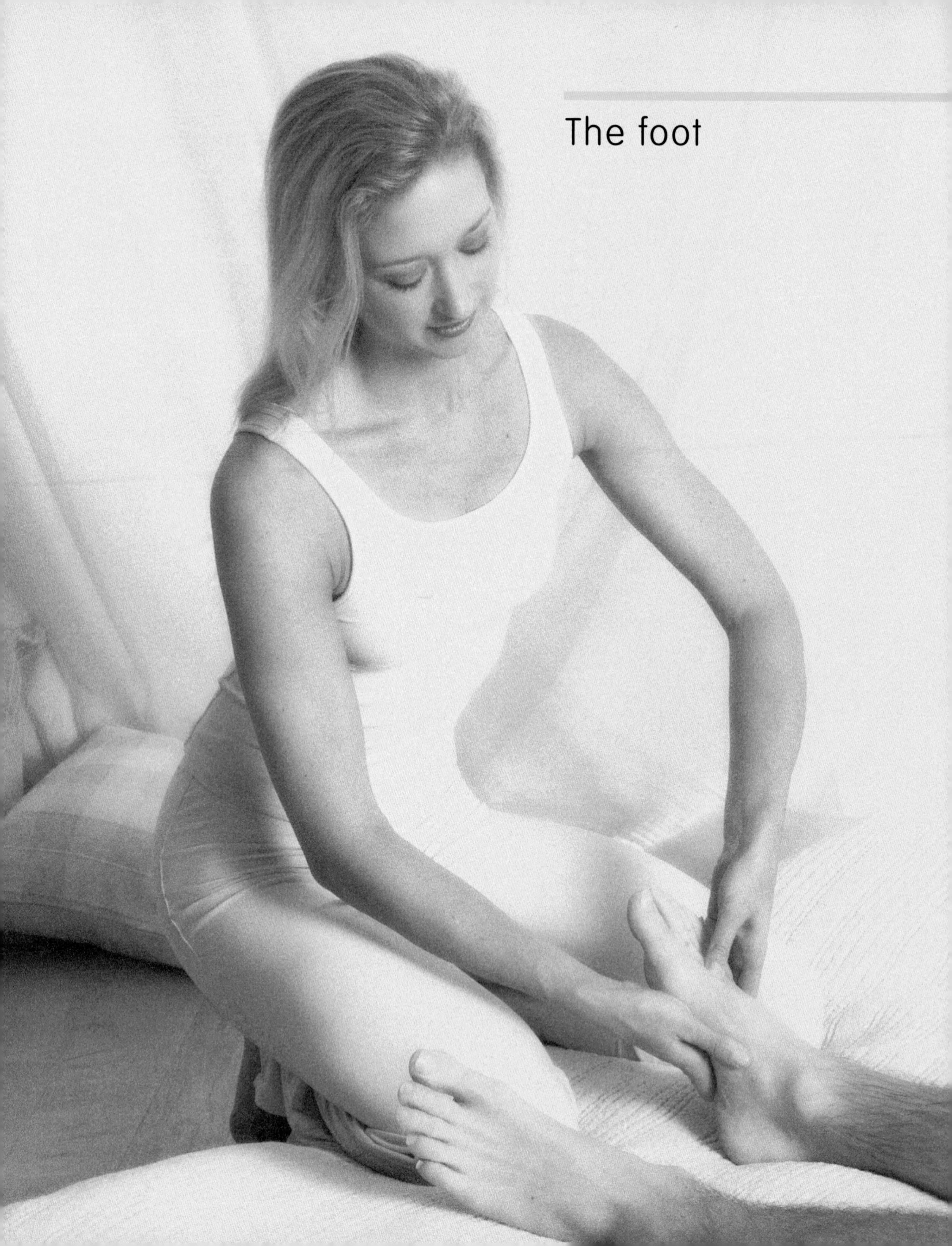

The foot

Spreading the oil: Pour a pea-size amount of oil into one palm. Rub your hands together and spread the oil to cover the entire foot.

1 **Sandwiching:** Place the palms of both hands on either side of the foot with the fingers facing the ankle. Press the foot as you slide the hands away, bringing the palms of your hands together. Repeat, changing the side of the foot that the hands were on.

2 **Circling the anklebones:** Place the fingertips of both hands on either side of the ankle. Slowly circle the anklebones. This is incredibly relaxing.

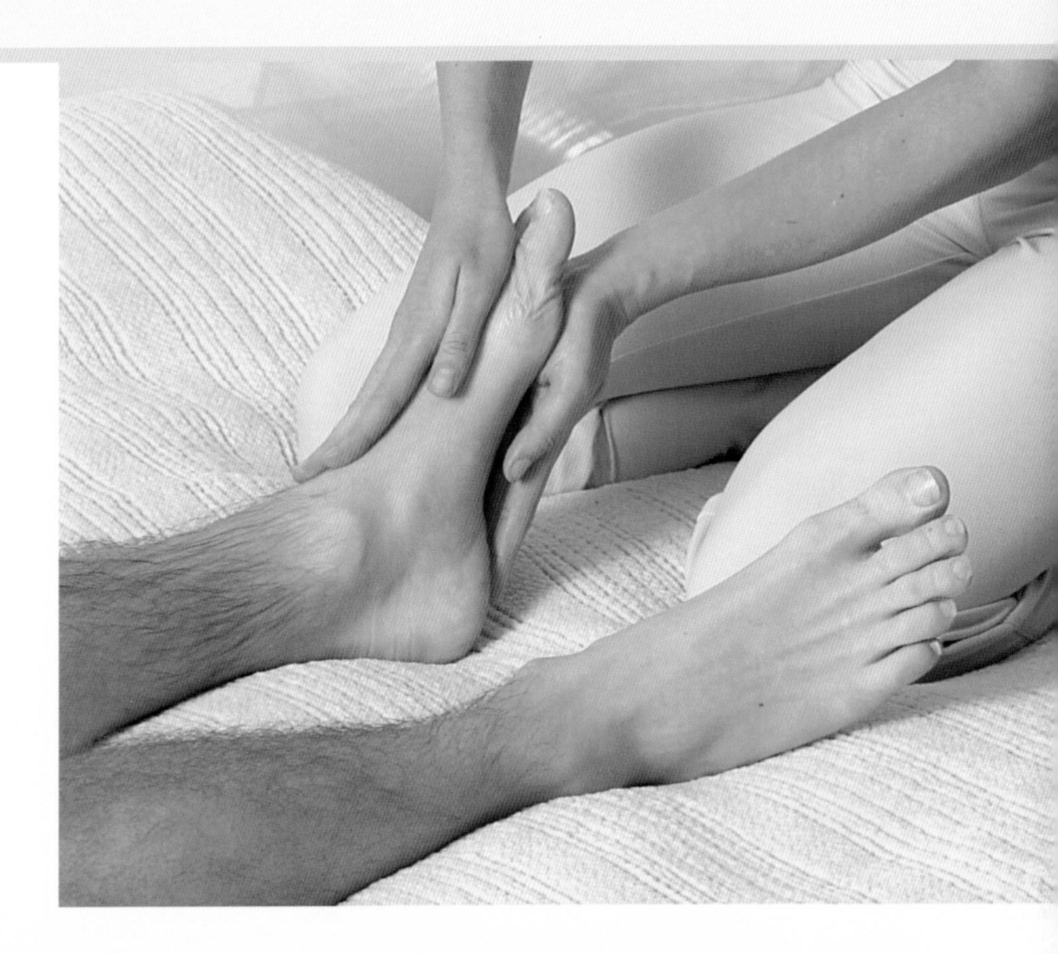

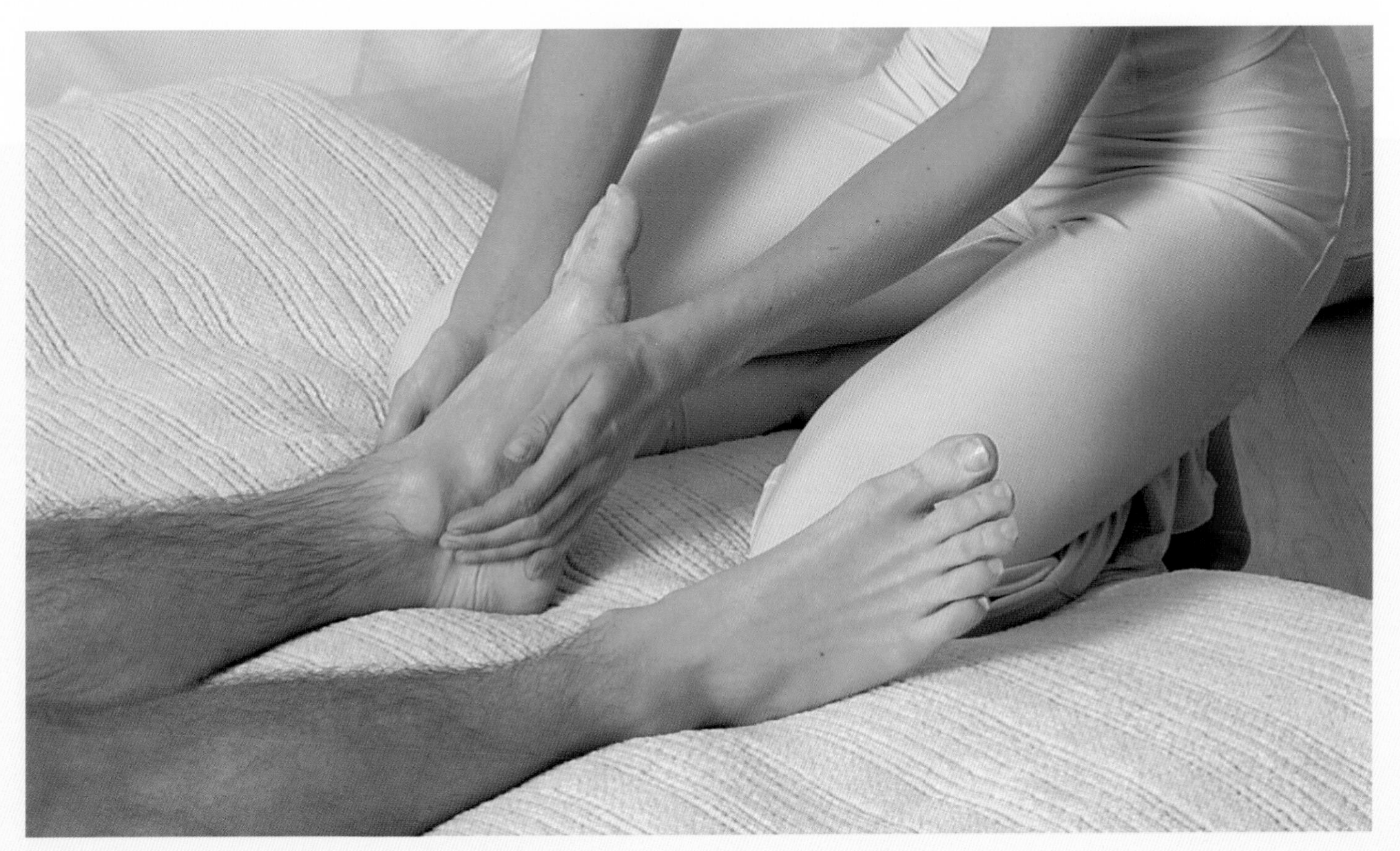

3 Friction: Place the thumbs on the top of the foot. Circle the thumbs across the entire area. Then switch the thumbs to the bottom of the foot. Cover the bottom of the foot with circles, trying to work out any knots.

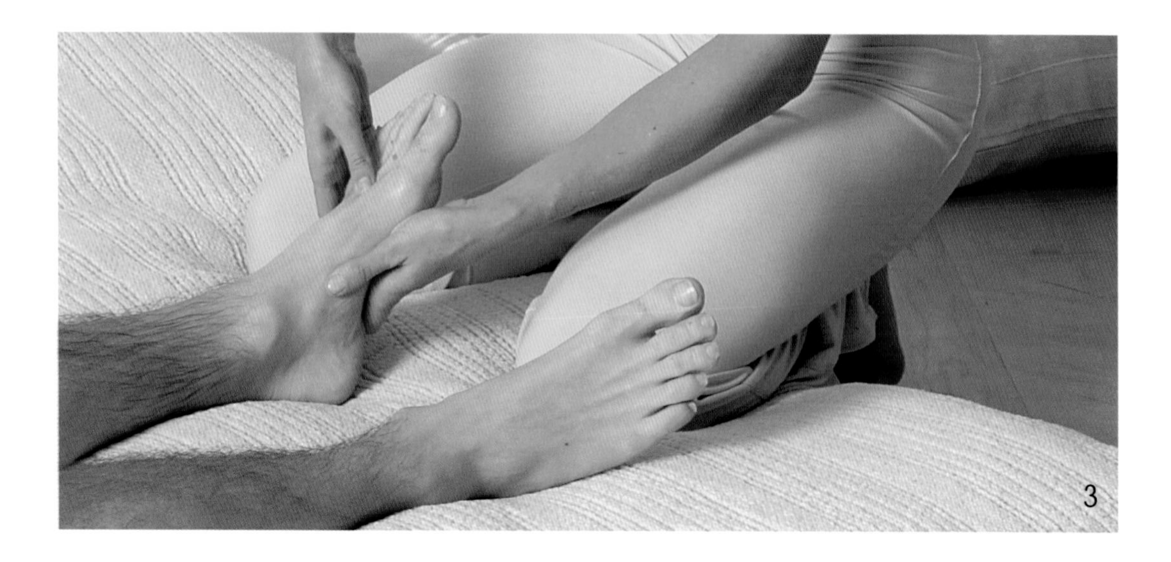

3

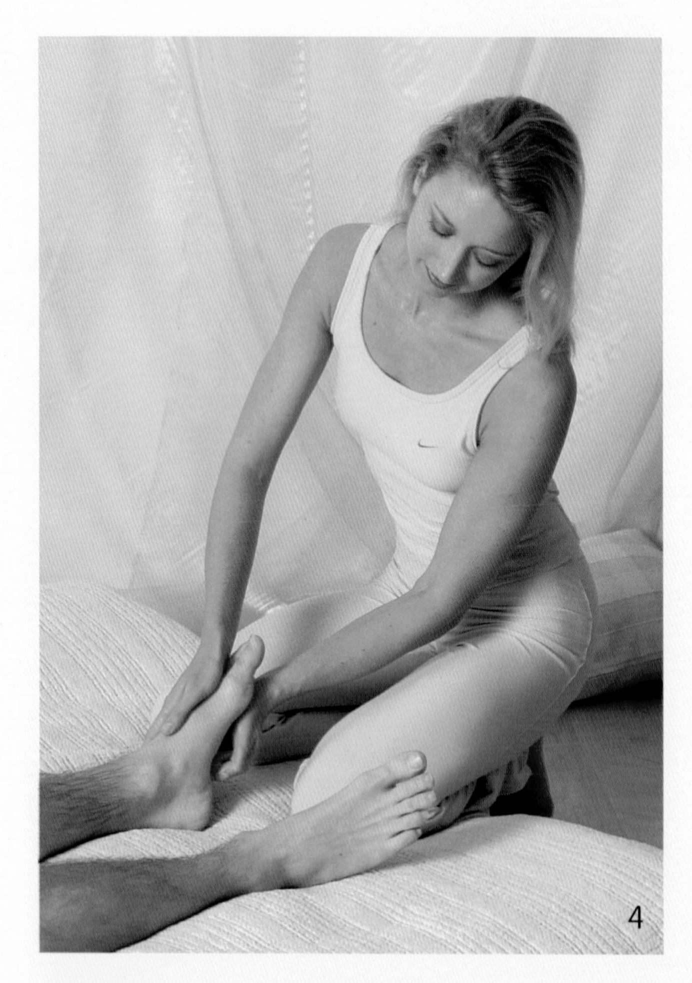

4

4 Knuckle rolls to sole of foot: Touch the fingers to the palm on one of your hands. Place the knuckles facing downwards onto the foot. Roll the knuckles over the entire length, massaging the sole of the foot.

5 Toe massage: Place the thumb and forefinger on either side of the base of the toe. Make small circles as you gently pull the toe, working your way out to the tip. Pinch the toe as you release it and move on to the next toe. Keep repeating until all the toes have been massaged.

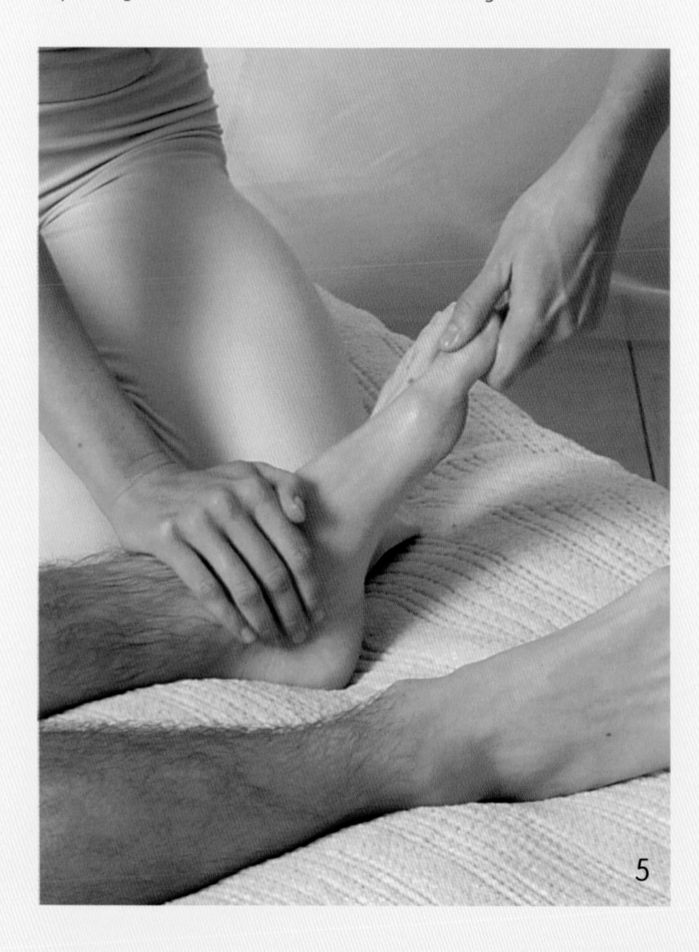

5

6 Vibration: Place the hands on either side of the foot. Your palms should be flat with the centres touching the edges of the foot. Move the foot quickly back and forth between the hands causing the foot to shake.

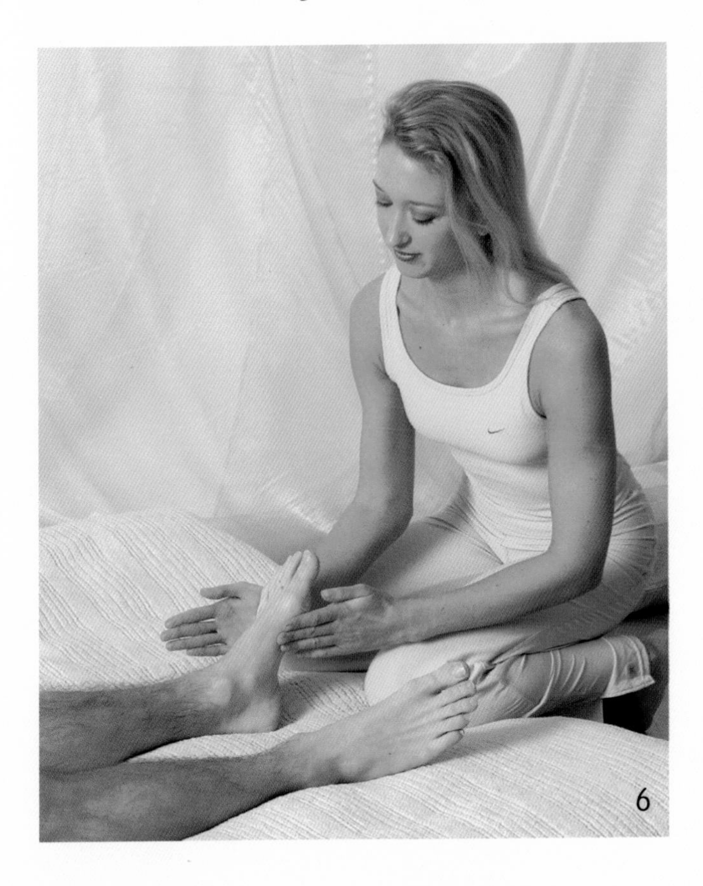
6

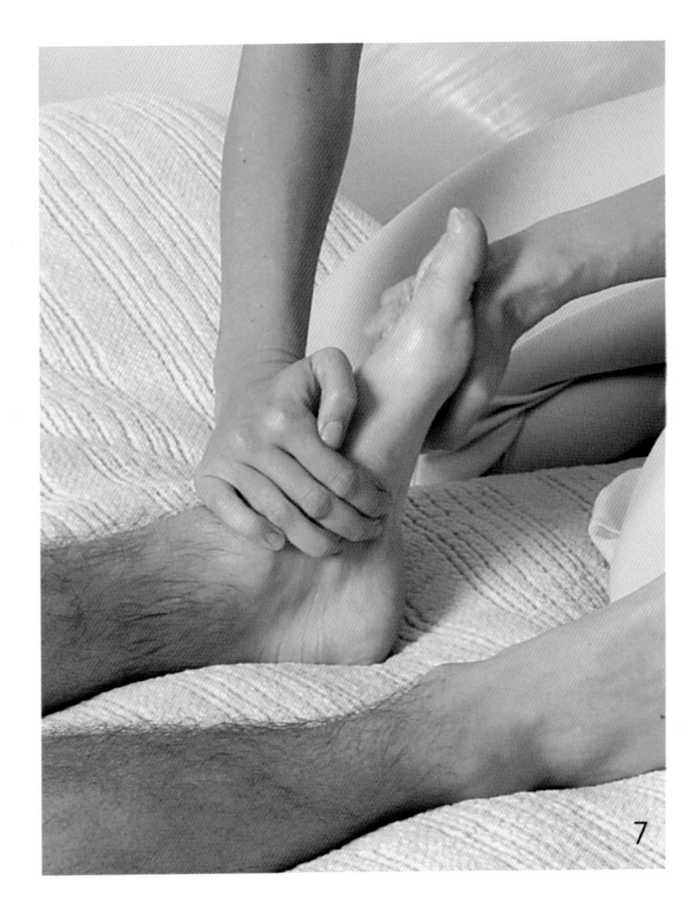
7

7 Squeeze foot: Place both hands around the whole foot. Gently squeeze the foot and then change hand positions. Repeat this a few times.

8 Holding: Wrap the hands around the foot. Hold the foot for a few seconds. This has a very nurturing and reassuring feeling for your partner.

Ending: Wrap the foot in a towel and repeat the sequence to the other foot.

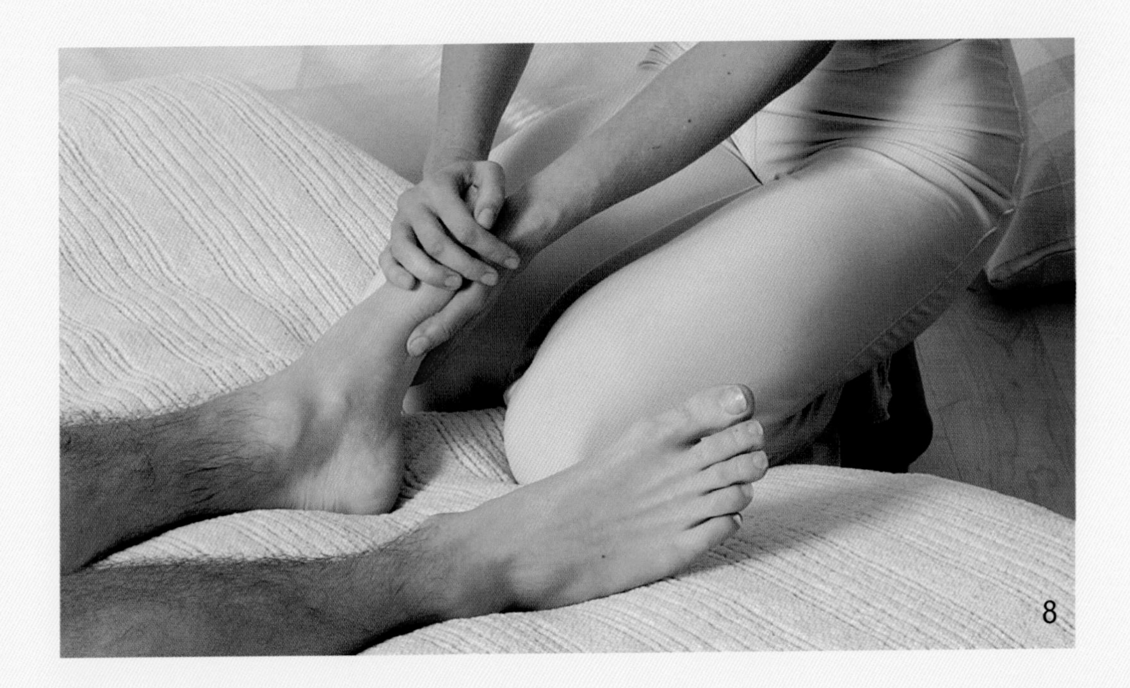
8

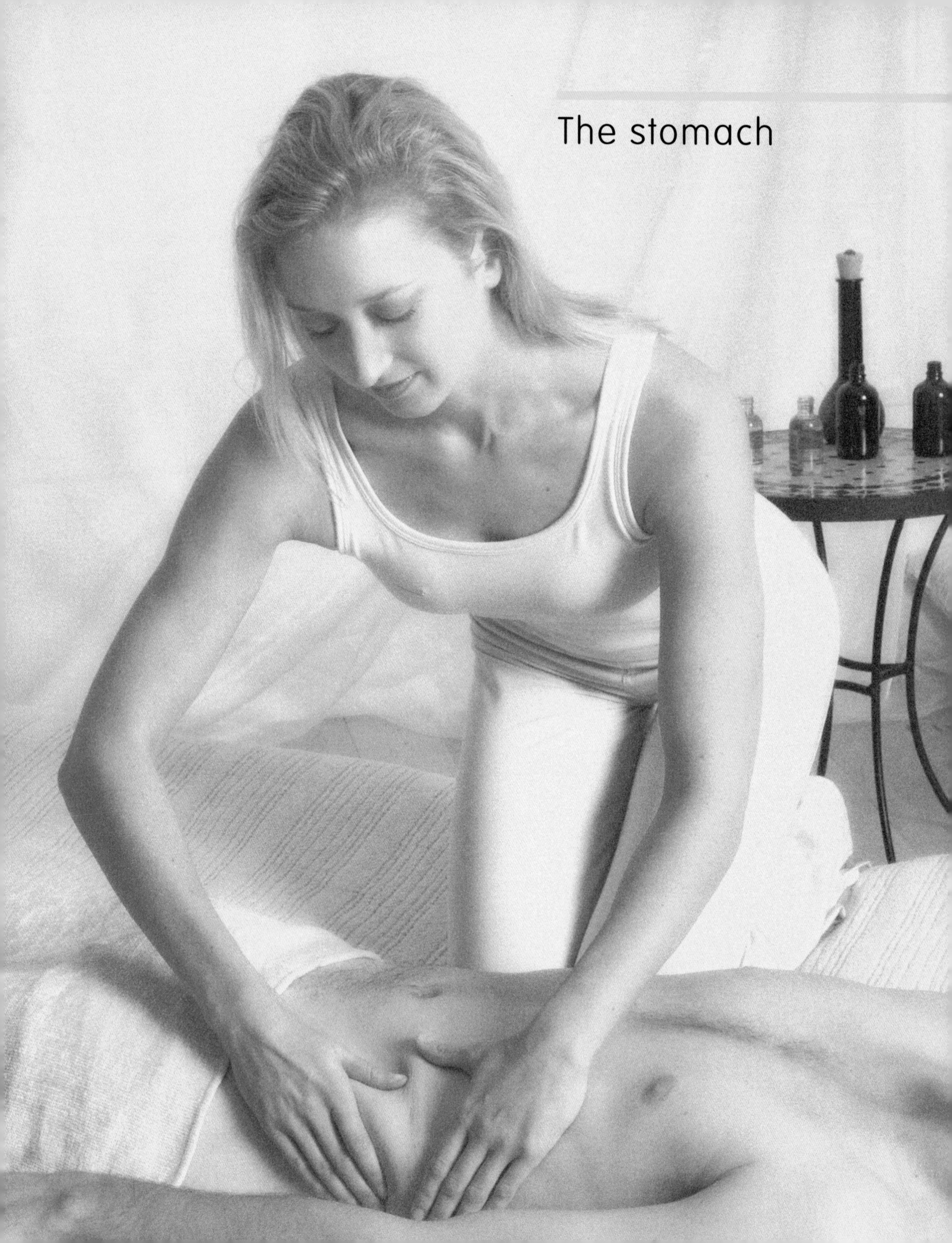

The stomach

Spreading the oil: If you are working with a woman, place a towel across your partner's chest on top of the one already in place. Slide the bottom towel down without moving the top towel. Uncover the stomach, folding the towel down to the hips. Pour a pea-size amount of oil into your hand. Rub your hands together.

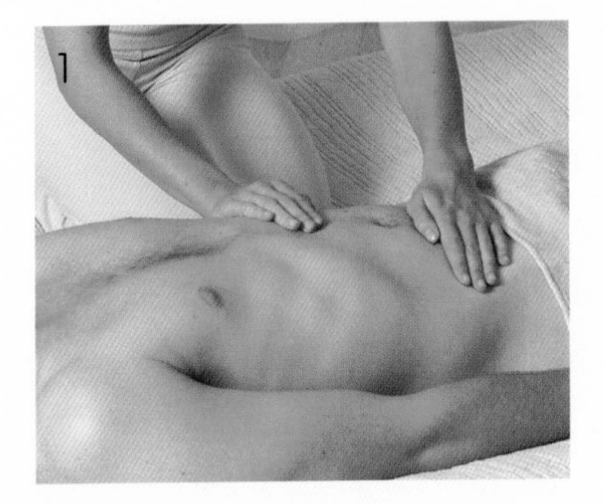

1 Circling: Place the hands flat on your partner's tummy on either side of their belly button. Circle the hands in a clockwise direction, picking them up and placing them back down as necessary.

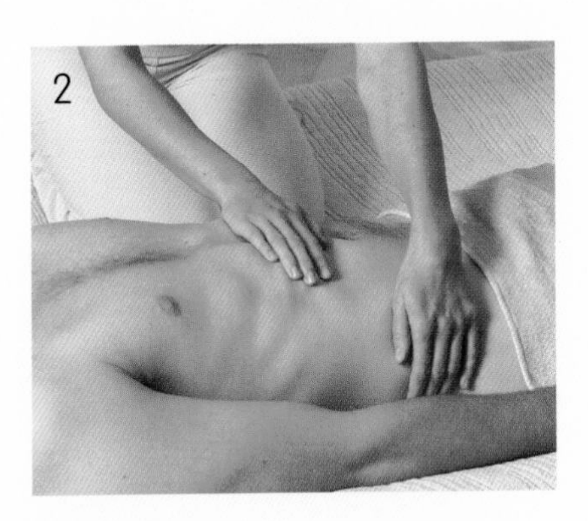

2 Pull-ups: Reach your hands across to the opposite side of your partner and place your hands underneath the waistline with your fingers facing down. Pull up on the flesh and across to the stomach. Return that hand to the starting position as you slide the opposite hand across towards the belly button. Keep repeating with smooth, rhythmic motions.

3 Kneading the waistline: Reach to the opposite side of your partner and place the hands on their waist with the fingertips facing down and the thumbs out to the sides. Gently pick up the flesh with one hand. Squeeze it as you slide the hand towards the other one. Release the flesh as you pick it up with your other hand. Slide the flesh back and forth shifting your weight as you do so.

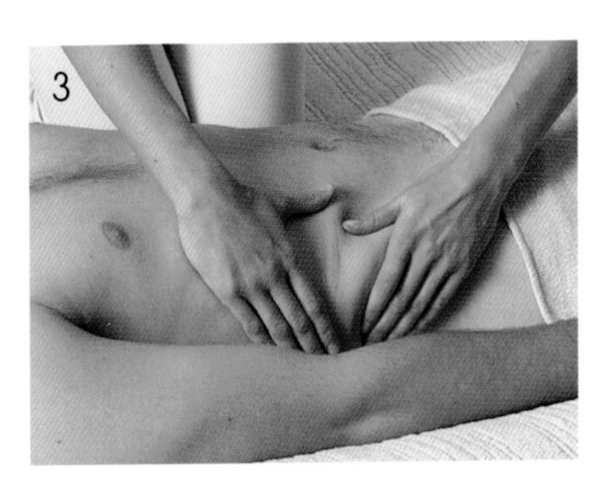

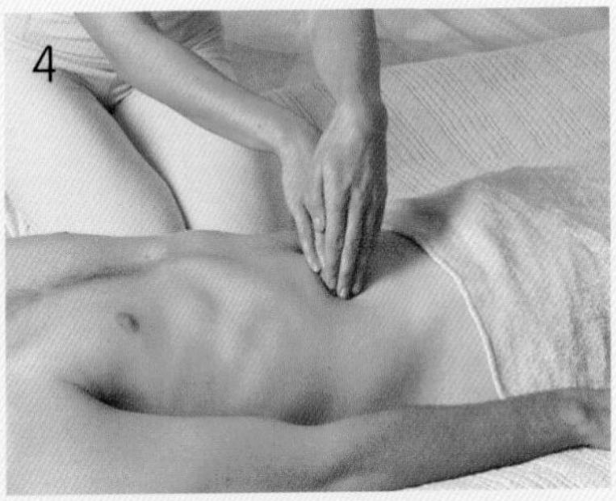

4 Double-handed circles: Kneel on the right side of your partner. Place one hand on top of the other with the fingertips just below the belly button on the right side. Imagine a square around the belly button. You are going to make tiny circles on 3 sides of the square. Circle up towards the ribs, across towards the other side and down the other side only. Repeat the action 3 times. This stroke massages the digestive tract.

5 Circling: Repeat step 1.

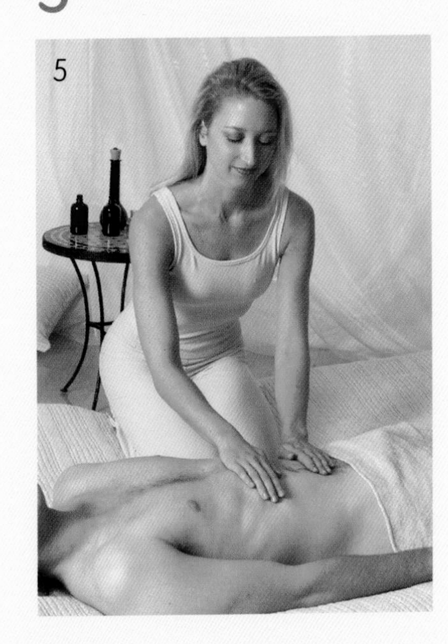

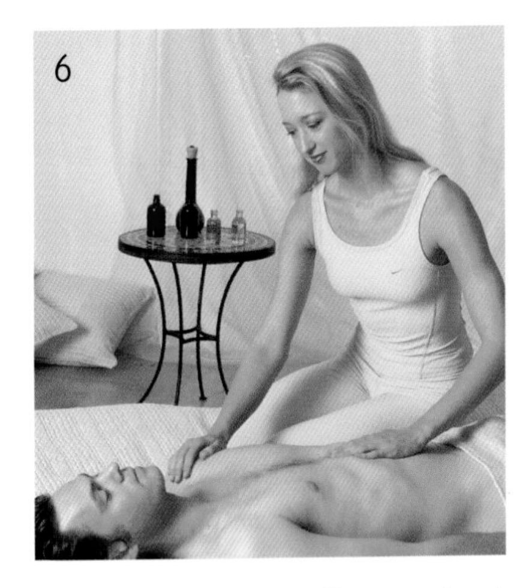

6 Rub solar plexus: Place one hand just beneath the breastbone with the fingertips facing the head. Slowly make barely perceptible small circles with the whole hand. This has a really nurturing effect.

Ending: Pull the towel up over the chest and if you are working with a woman, remove the chest towel by sliding it out carefully from underneath.

The arm

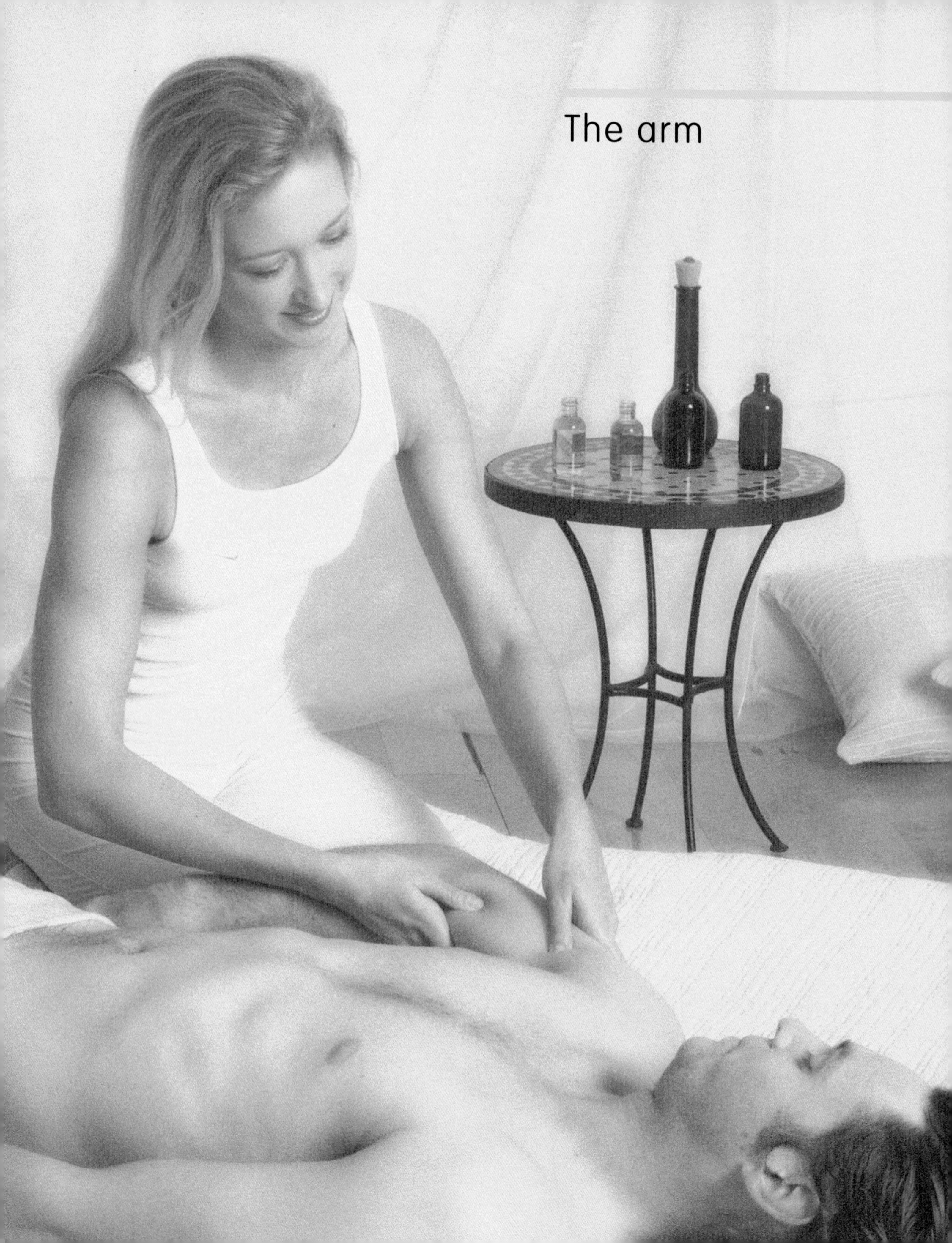

Softening: Place the hands above the towel with the palms on one side and the fingers on the other. Pinch the flesh underneath the towel with the whole hand and release. Work your way along the entire length of the arm. Then rub the arm vigorously.

Spreading the oil: Place one hand on the shoulder and one hand on the wrist above the towel. Press down with both hands gently but firmly. Take the arm out from under the towel. Pour a small amount of oil into one hand and rub your hands together. Starting from the wrist, spread the oil up the arm to the shoulder. Be sure to cover both sides of the arm.

1 **Alternating effleurage:** Hold the wrist with one hand. Slide the other hand up the arm to the shoulder. Circle the shoulder with the whole hand and glide the hand back down to the wrist. Switch hands and repeat the movement with the opposite hand. Press firmly on the way up and gently on the way down.

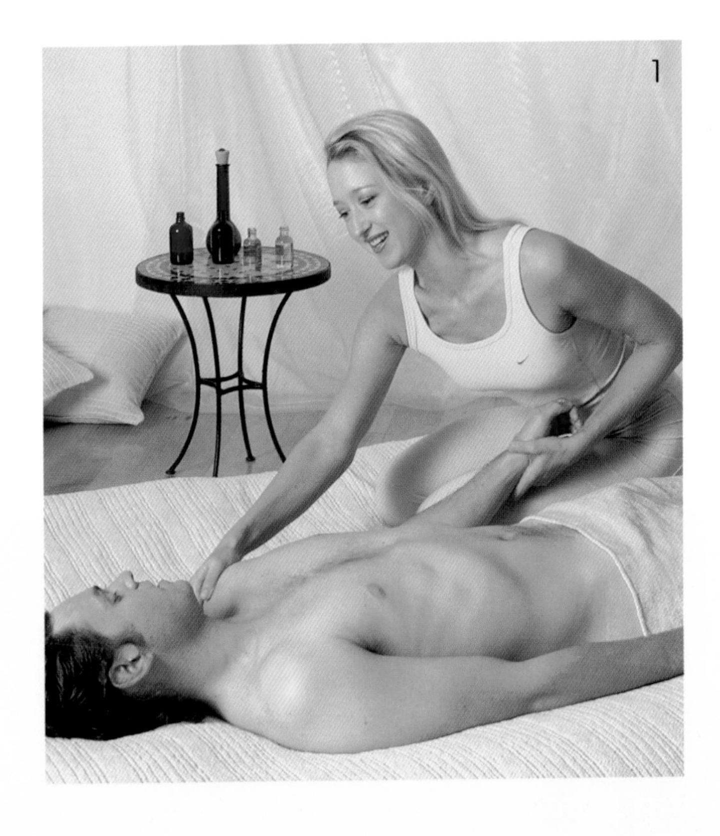

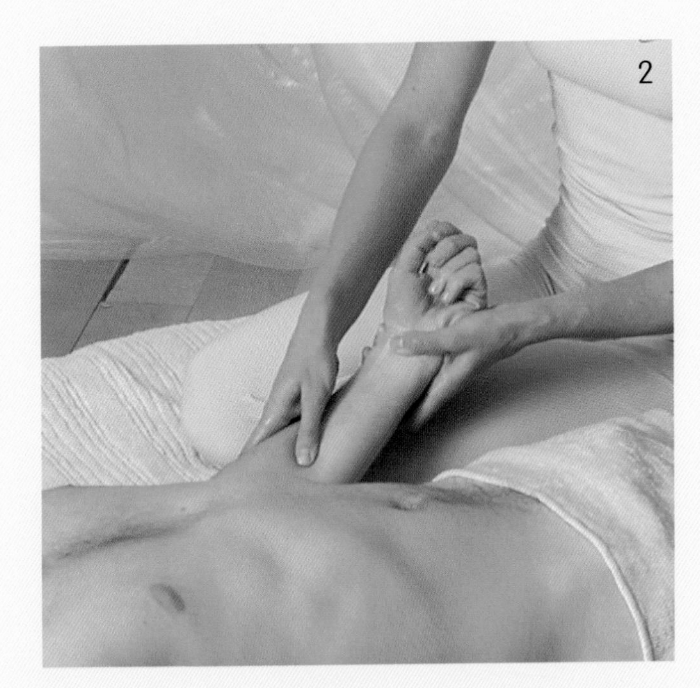

2 **Friction to the forearm:** Turn the palm over so that it is facing up. Place your thumb on the inside of the wrist and slowly circle up towards the elbow. Repeat the action twice, covering the whole inside of the forearm. Turn the wrist over and repeat to the top of the forearm.

3 **Friction to the upper arm:** Hold the upper arm just above the elbow in both hands, placing the thumbs on top of the arm with the fingers underneath. Circle the thumbs up to the shoulder while squeezing the flesh with the fingers underneath.

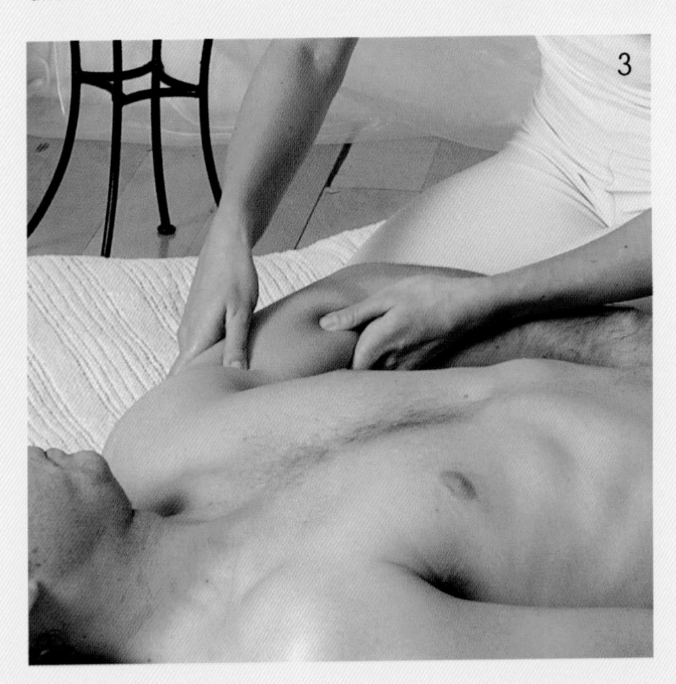

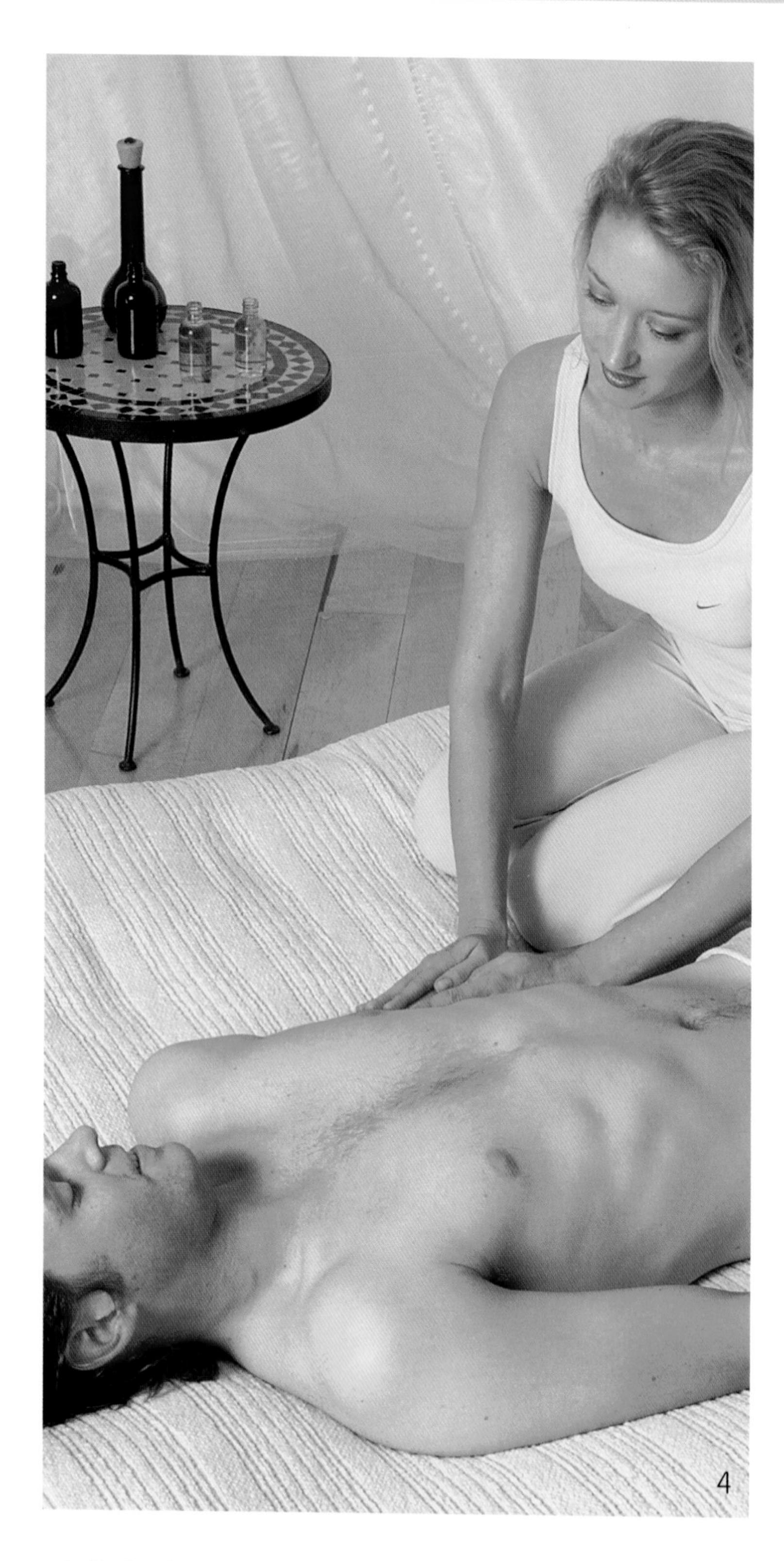

4 **Basic effleurage:** Place the arm on the table with the palms at the wrist and your fingers facing the shoulder. Slide the hands up the arm, separating them as you glide back down to the wrist. Repeat a few times.

5 **Friction to the hand:** Hold your partner's hand in both hands with the thumbs on top and the fingers around the sides. Circle the thumbs, massaging the entire top of the hand as well as the wrist. Turn the hand over and massage the palm with your thumbs.

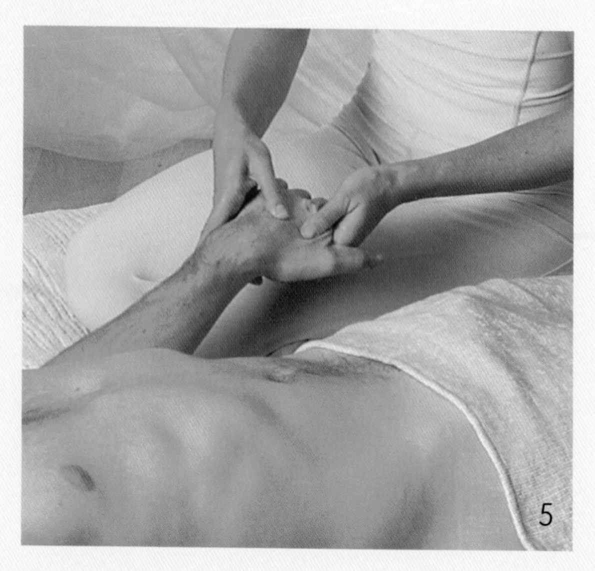

6 **Opening:** Lace your pinkies in your partner's thumb and pinkie with their palm facing you. Place your thumbs together at the base of their palm. As you spread your thumbs apart, open their hand wide with your pinkies. Repeat a few more times. Stay in this position and circle the thumbs throughout the whole palm.

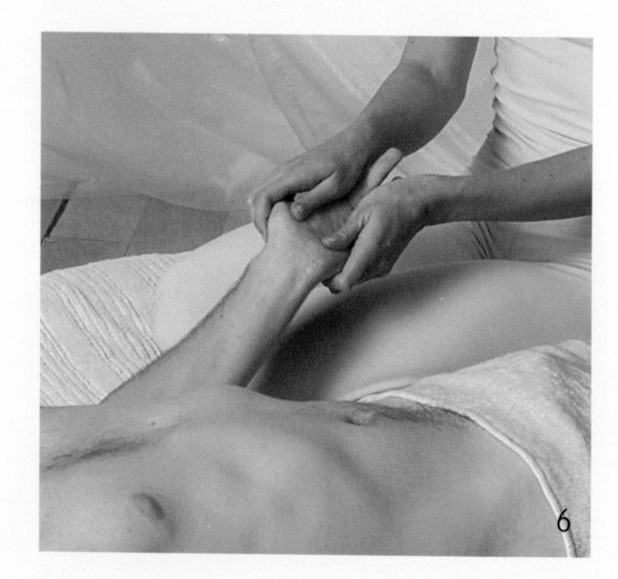

7 **Finger massage:** Hold one finger at the base between your thumb and forefinger. Make small circles as you work your way down to the tip of the finger. Pinch the end as you release. Move to the next finger. Repeat until you have completed all the fingers.

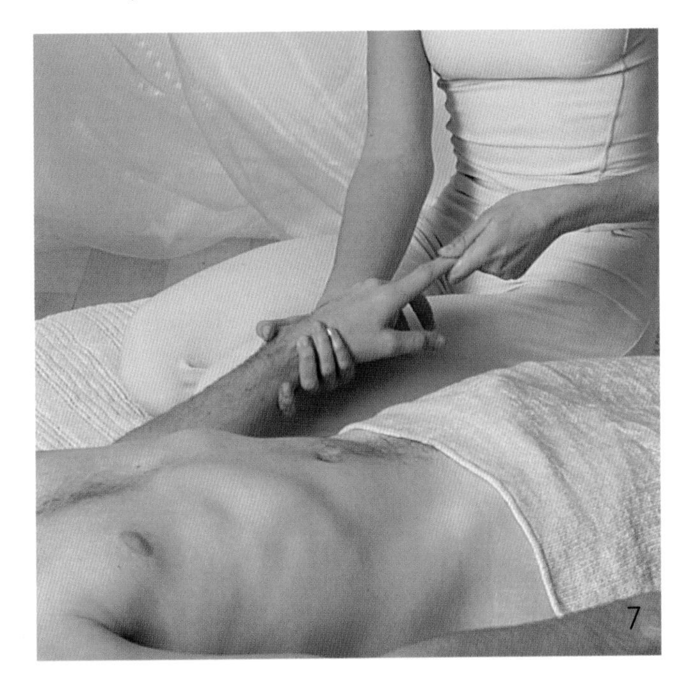
7

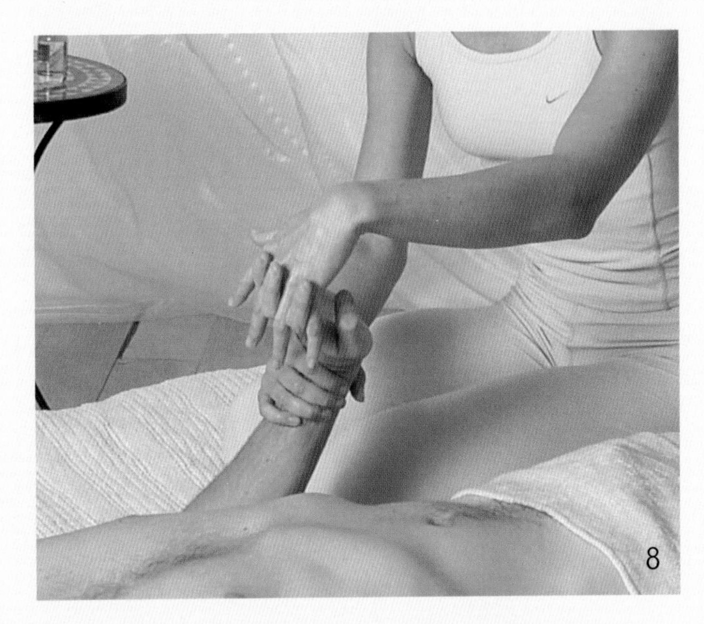
8

8 **Fingers laced:** Hold the wrist with the same hand as the arm you are working on. Lace the opposite hand in your partner's hand loosely so that the palms are facing each other. Slowly circle their entire hand, keeping their wrist still. Circle 3 times in each direction. Then bring their hand forwards and backwards, thinking about loosening up the wrist. Put the hand back down on the table or mat.

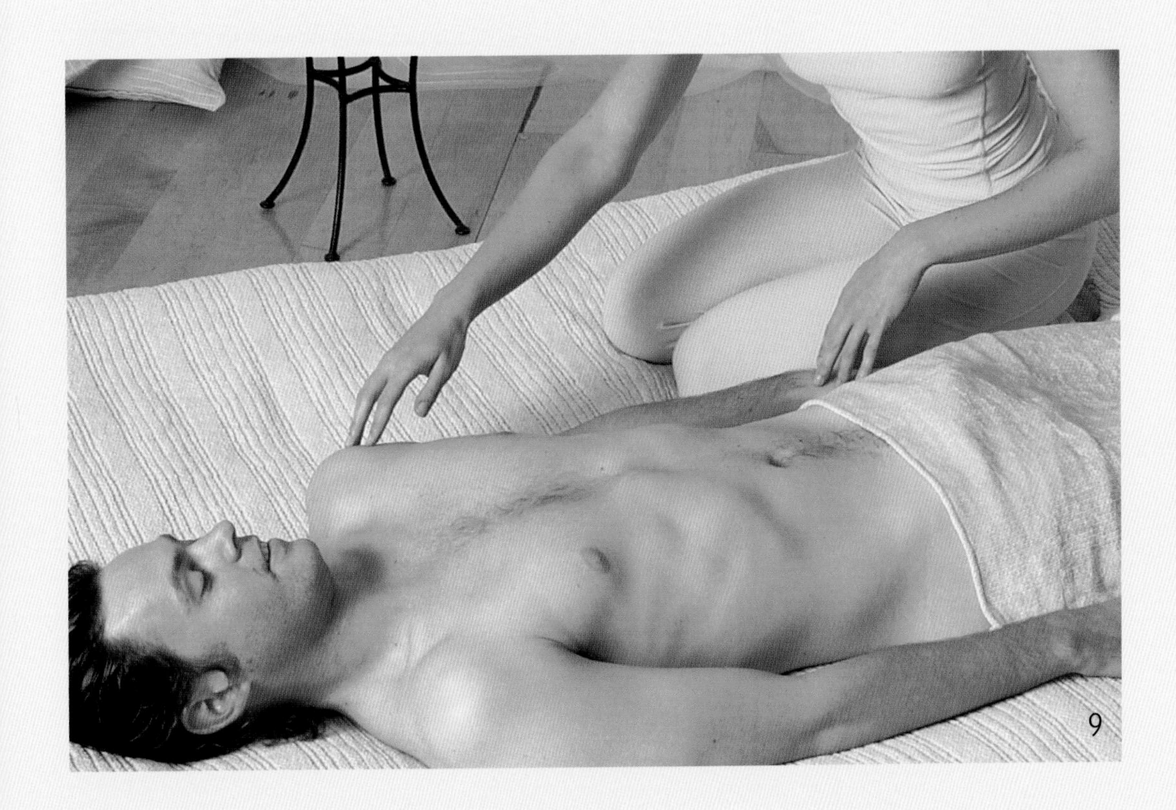
9

9 **Feather stroking:** Touch the top of the arm lightly with the fingertips of one hand. Lightly stroke down the arm to the fingers. Repeat several times, alternating hands.

Ending: Place the arm underneath the towel and repeat to the opposite side.

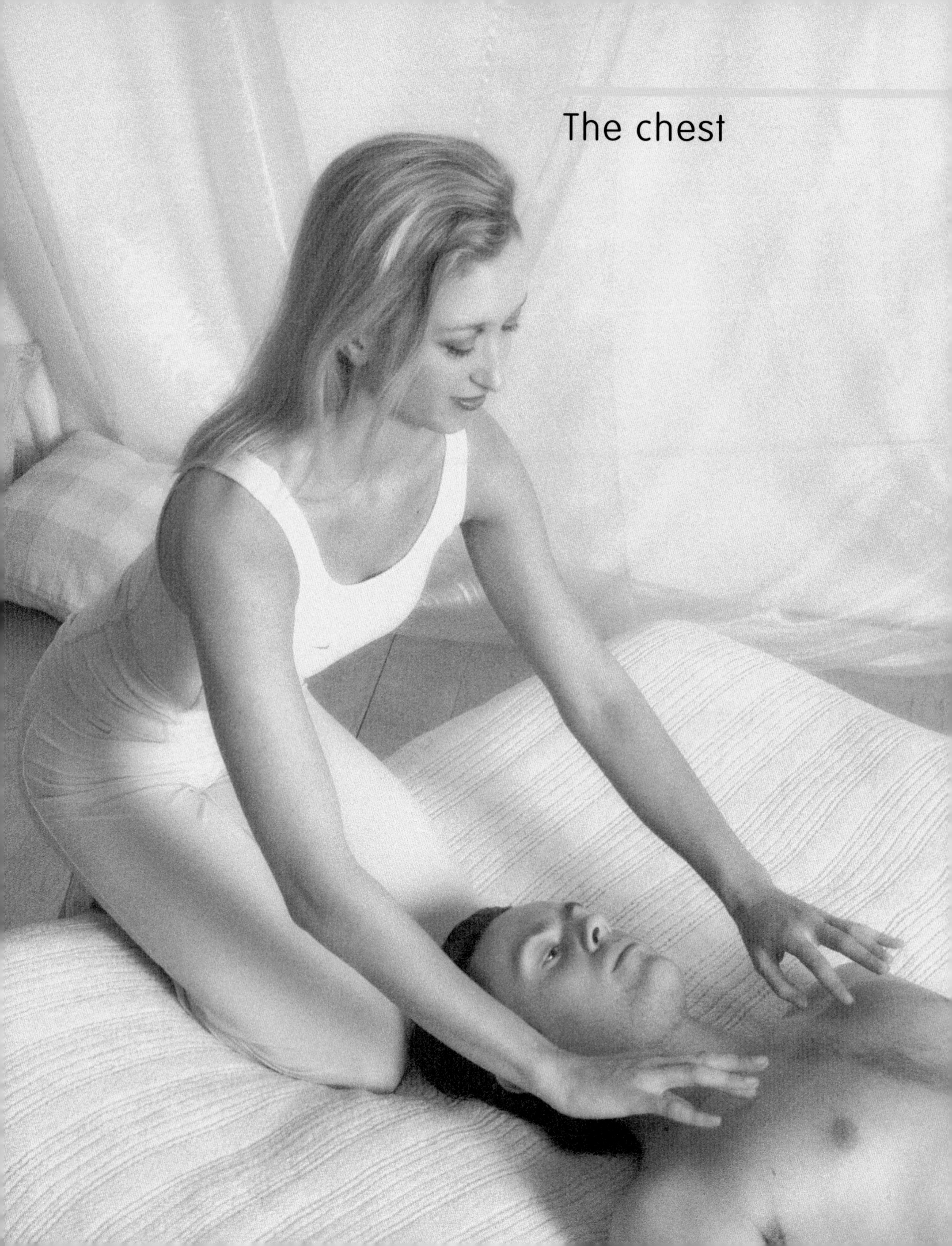

The chest

1 **Rocking:** Sit kneeling or with your legs crossed at your partner's head, facing their feet. Place the palms of the hands on their shoulders with the fingers pointing towards their hands. Put pressure through the palm of one hand, slightly pushing the shoulder down. As you release, press through the other hand. Rock the shoulders gently back and forth. Then spread the oil.

2 **Circling chest, neck and shoulders:** Place the hands in the centre of the chest with the fingertips touching and the elbows out to the sides. Press the hands towards the shoulders. Circle the shoulders and bring the hands across the underneath side of the shoulders. When the hands meet at the bottom of the neck pull them up the neck to the base of the head. Repeat twice.

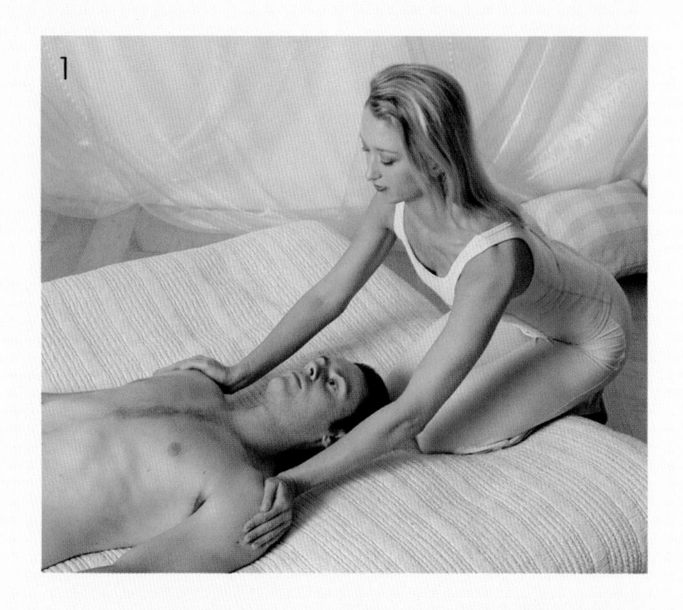
1

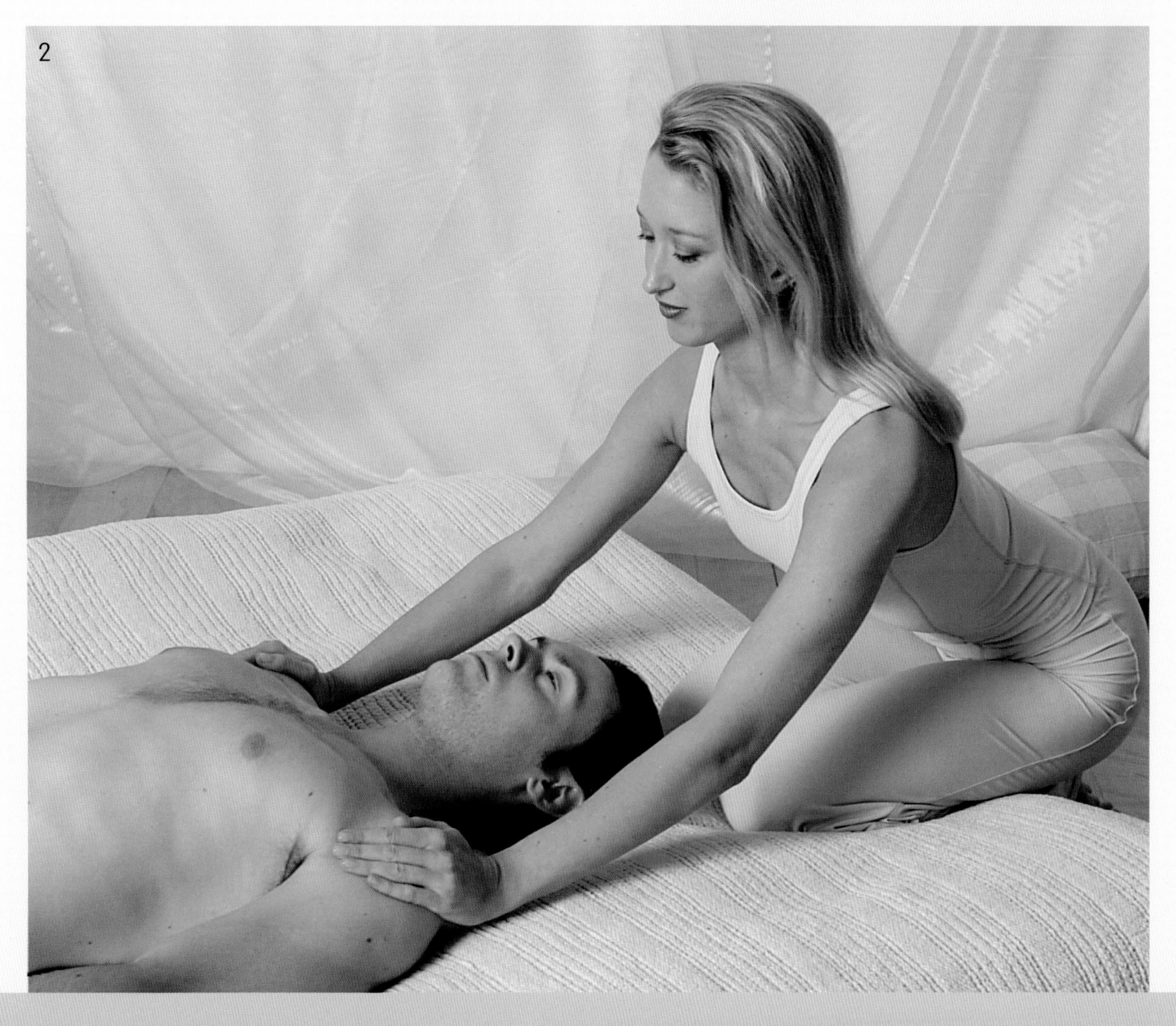
2

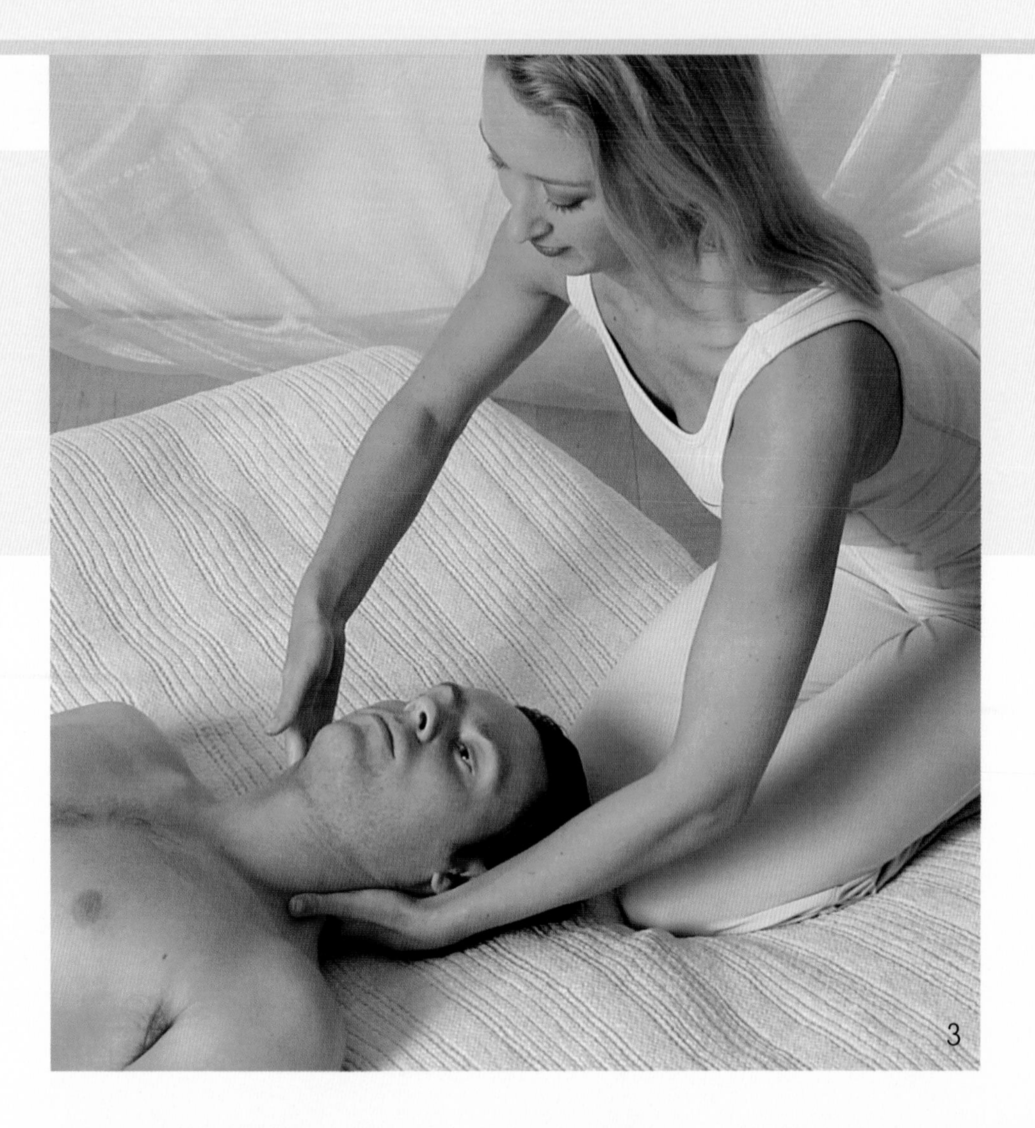

3 Hand-over-hand to neck: Place one hand around the back of the base of the neck. Loosely hold the neck as you slide the hand up to the base of the head. As the hand is moving, replace it with your opposite hand. Keep changing the hands as you massage the neck.

4 Hand-over-hand effleurage: Kneel to the side of your partner. Place one hand on top of the other on the chest with your fingertips facing away from you. Glide the hands out towards the opposite shoulder. Press gently down on the shoulder as you circle the hands around the shoulder and back to their starting position. Repeat this movement a few times. Move to the other side and repeat the whole sequence.

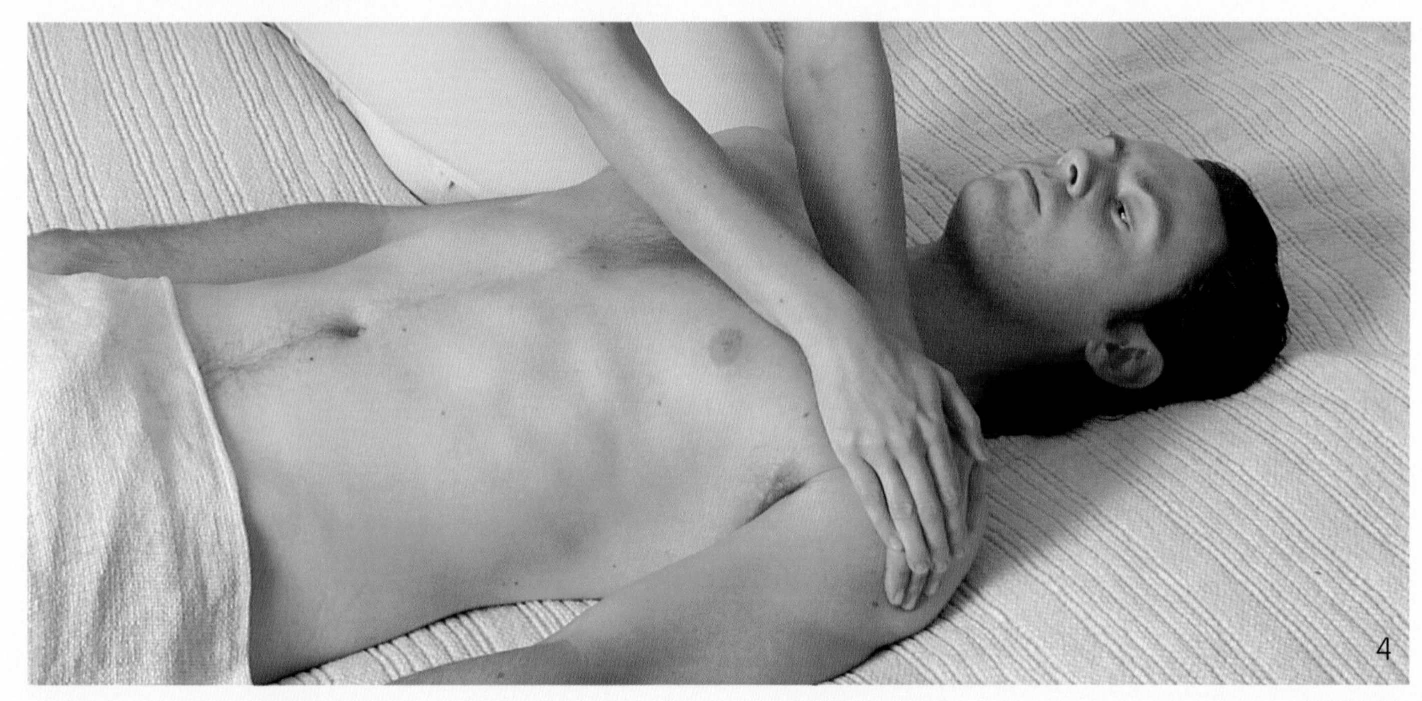

5 Friction to shoulders: Place the thumbs just under the collarbone with the fingers underneath your partner's shoulders. Keeping the thumbs where they are, circle the fingers, massaging the shoulders. Repeat this action with the thumbs underneath and the fingers on top. This time the thumbs are circling and the fingers remain still.

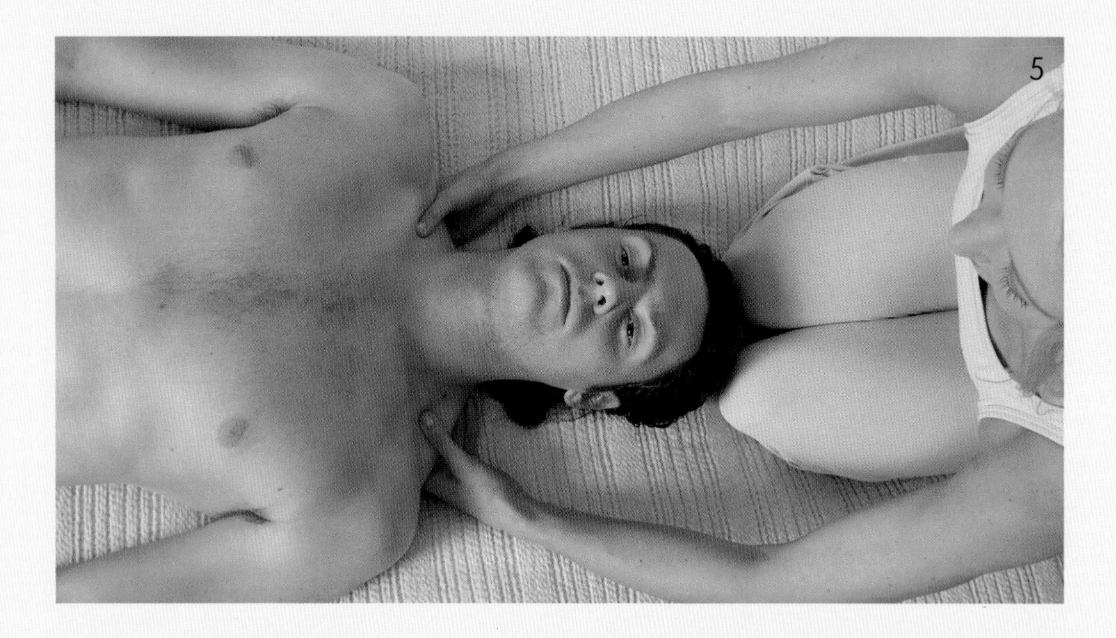
5

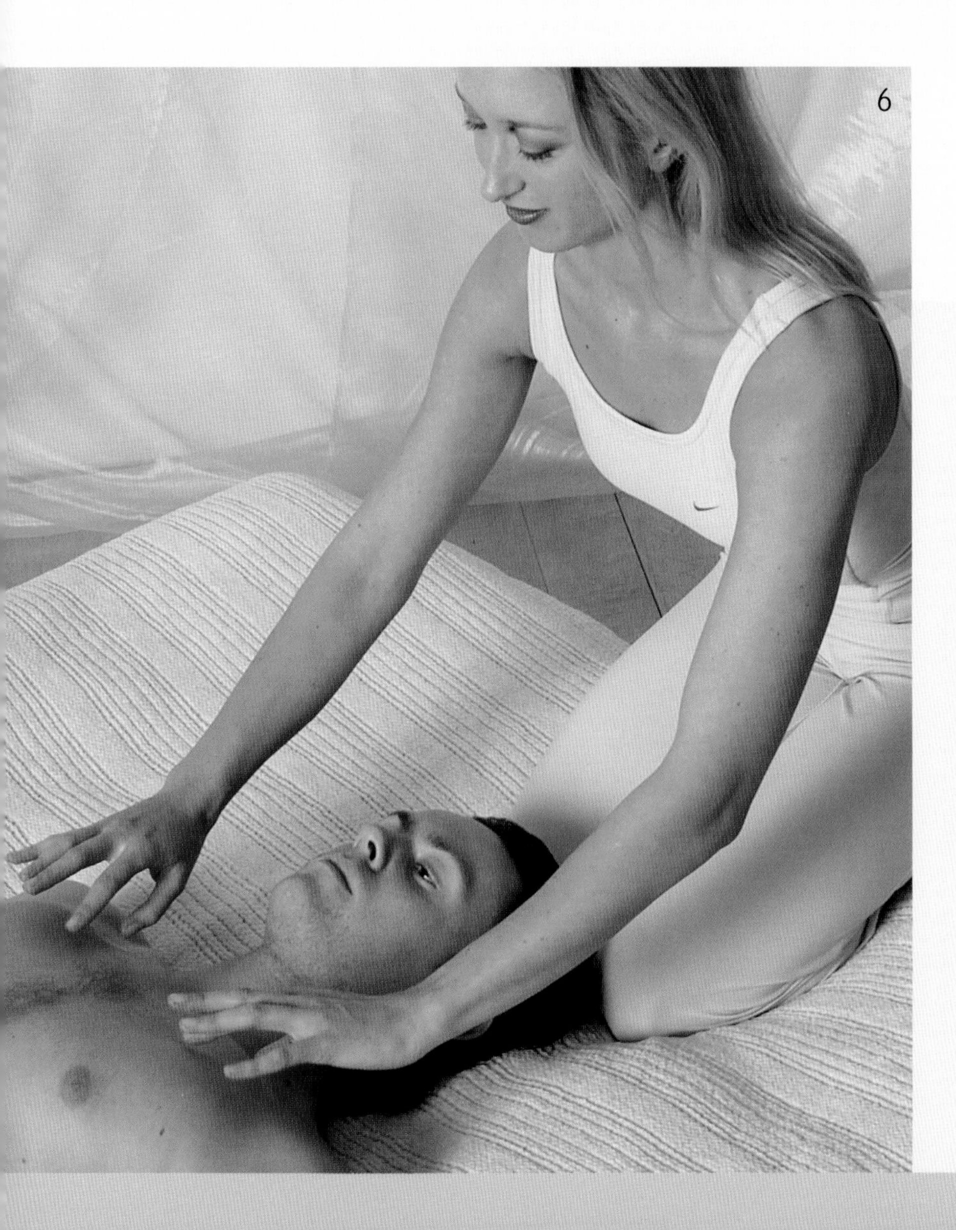
6

6 **Tapoment:** Place the fingertips above the chest area. Lightly tap the chest separately with the fingertips. Move the fingers along the whole chest area. Think of raindrops lightly falling onto the surface of the skin.

7 **Circling the chest, neck and shoulders:** Repeat step 2.

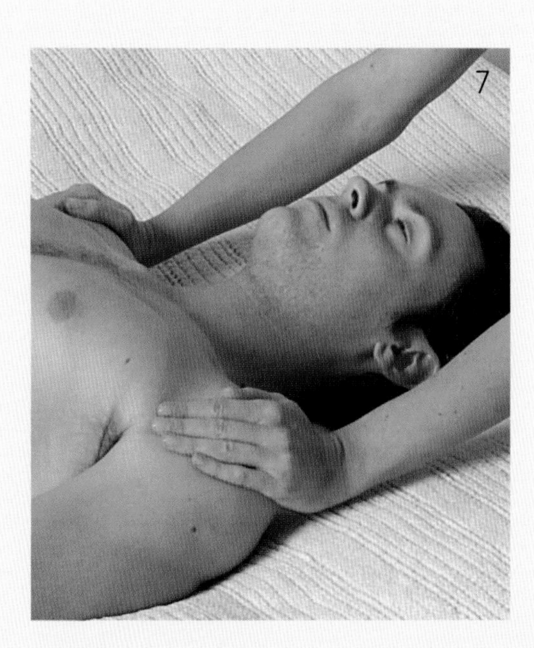
7

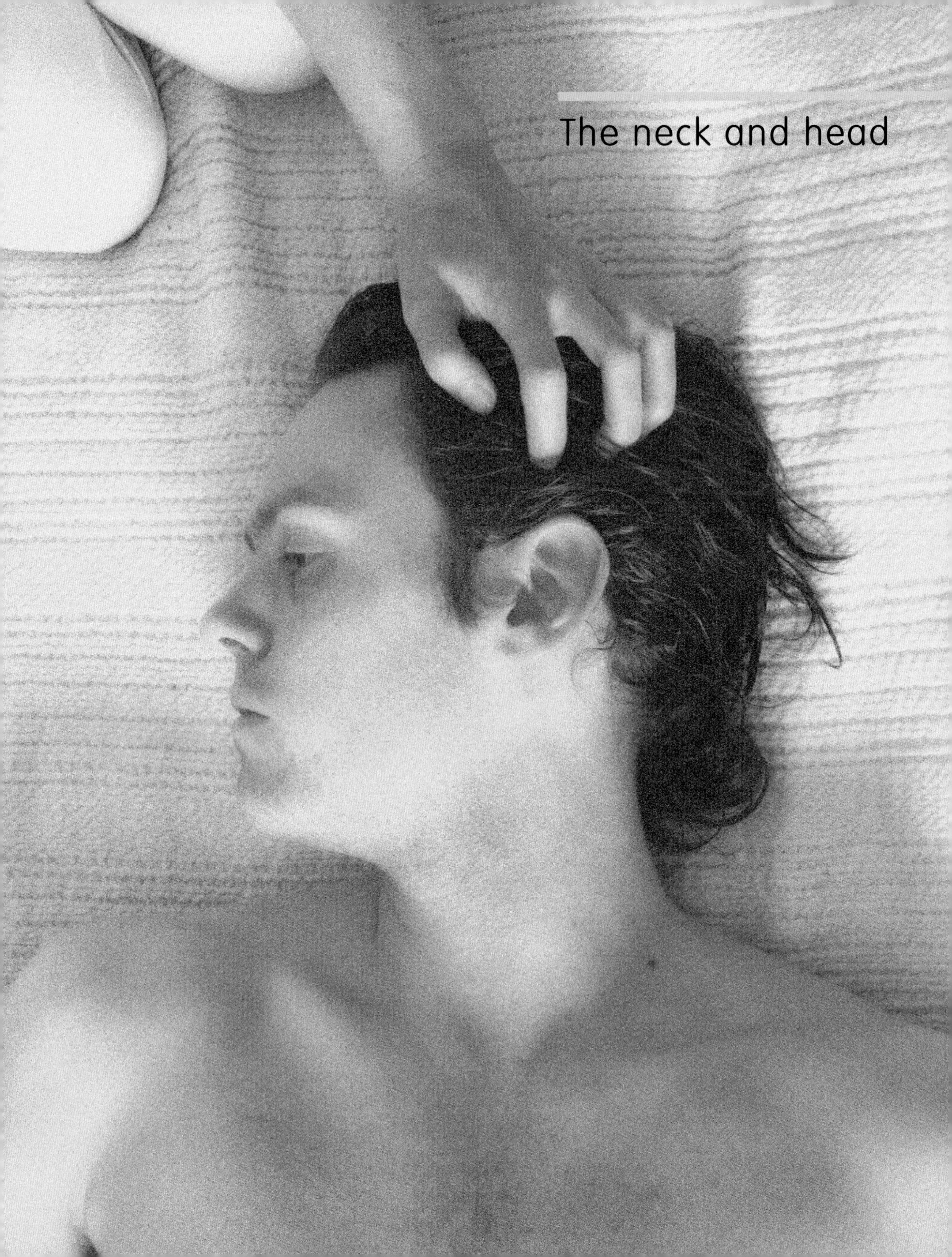

The neck and head

1 Turn head: Gently turn the head to one side to expose the side of the neck.

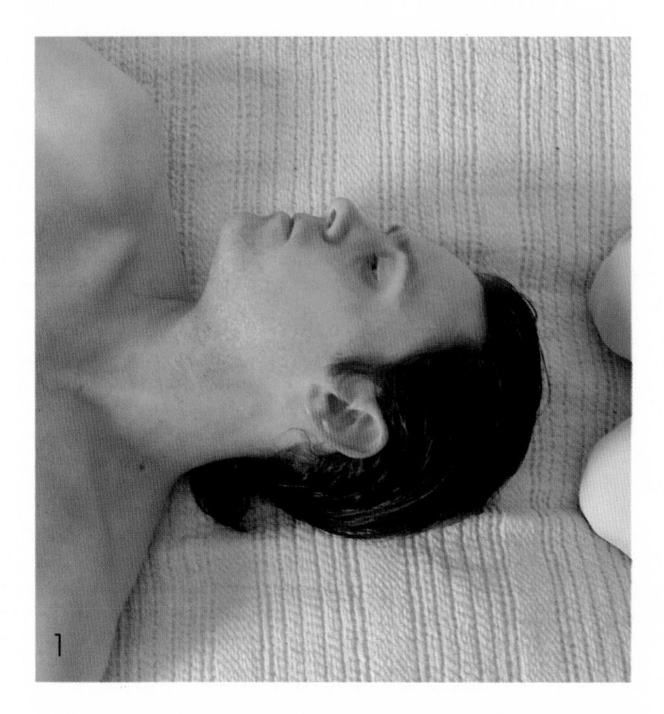

2 One hand effleurage: Place the hand flat against the base of the skull with the fingers facing downwards and the thumb out to the side. Slide the flat part of the hand along the neck to the shoulder, letting the thumb mould to the contour of the body. Wrap your fingers around the shoulder and then reverse, keeping the thumb on top and the fingertips down. Repeat a few times.

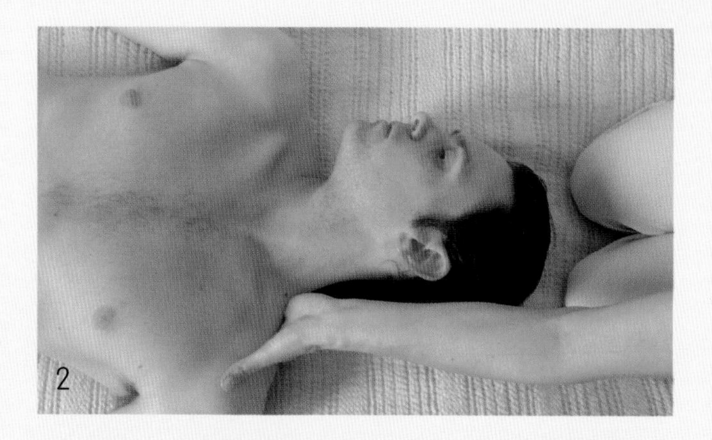

3 Knuckles: Touch the fingertips of the left hand to your palm. Place the knuckles under the neck and shoulders. Keeping your wrist still, circle the arm, massaging the underneath side of the neck and shoulders.

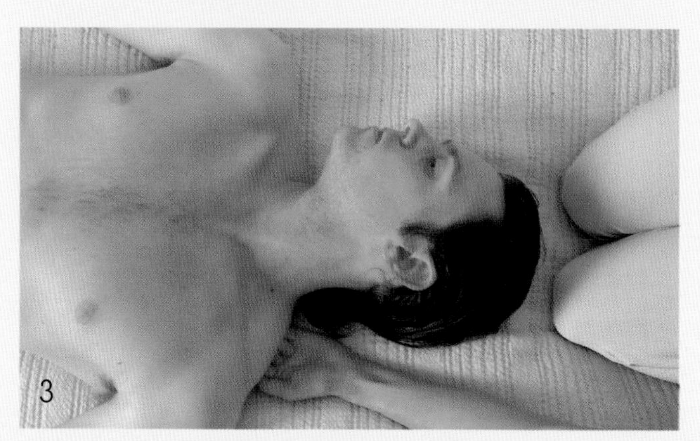

4 Friction to base of head: Place the fingertips of one hand in the base of the skull and form a claw with your hand. Make tiny circles with the hand, being sure to move the scalp. Wipe the oil off your hand before working in the hair.

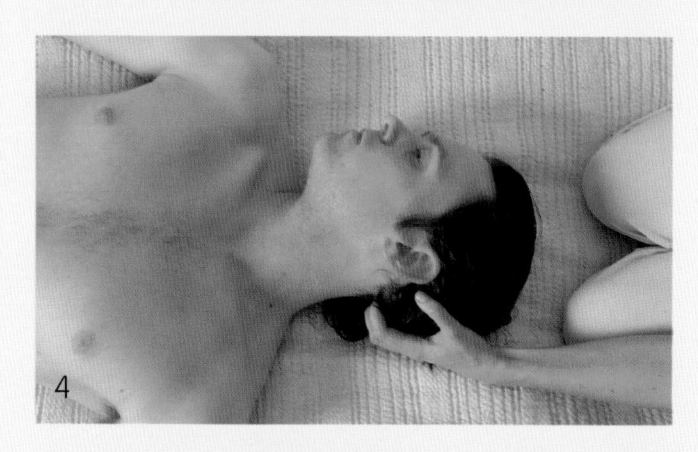

5 Friction to the head: Form a claw with your hand. Place the hand at the base of the skull. Make small circles with the fingers, moving the scalp. Then move the hand a little higher on the head.

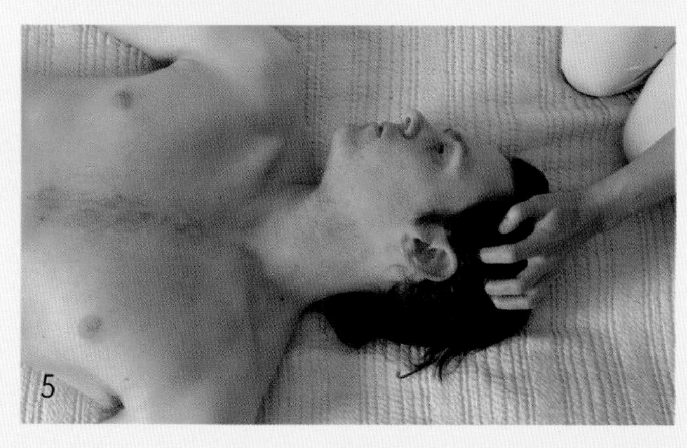

Repeat. Work your way up to the forehead.

Ending: Turn head slowly to the other side to repeat.

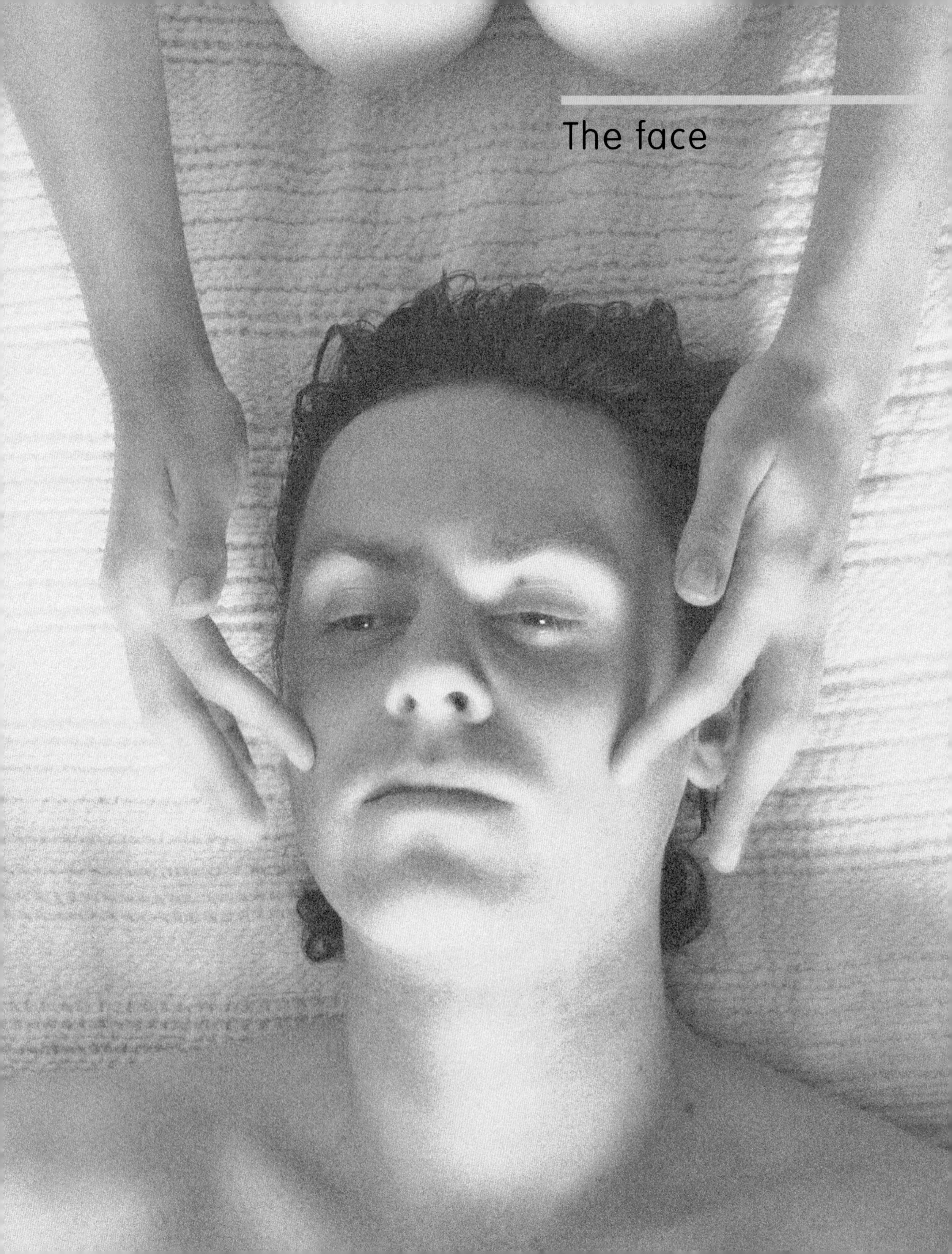

The face

Spreading the oil: Put one or two drops of oil onto your fingers. Rub the fingertips together.

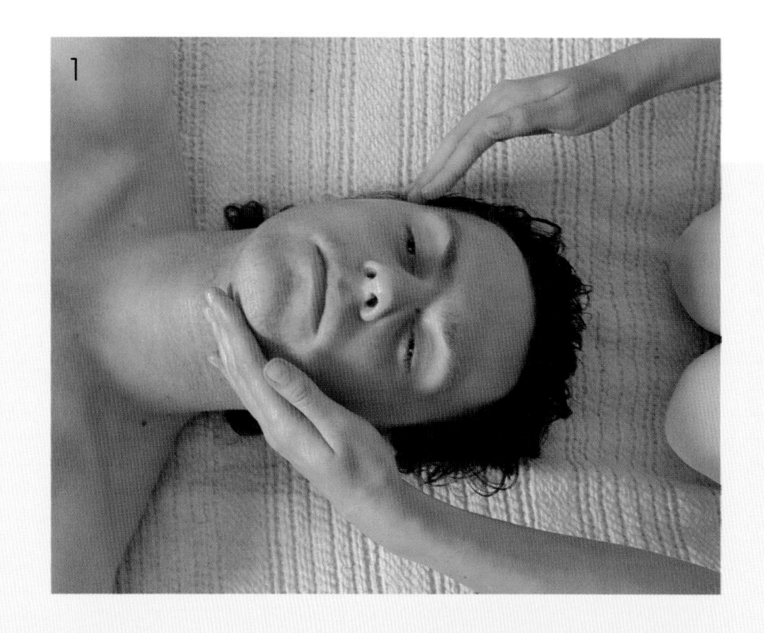

1 **Alternating effleurage to the chin:** Place the fingers together underneath the chin with your elbows out to the sides. Slide one hand gently up to the ear, and then the other hand towards the opposite ear. Repeat a few times. The rhythmic qualities of the movement can be very soothing and relaxing.

2 **Effleurage to the forehead:** Place one hand across the forehead sideways. Gently stroke the forehead as you slide the hand away. Replace the hand with your other hand. Repeat the movement a few times, trying to think of soothing and relaxing the forehead.

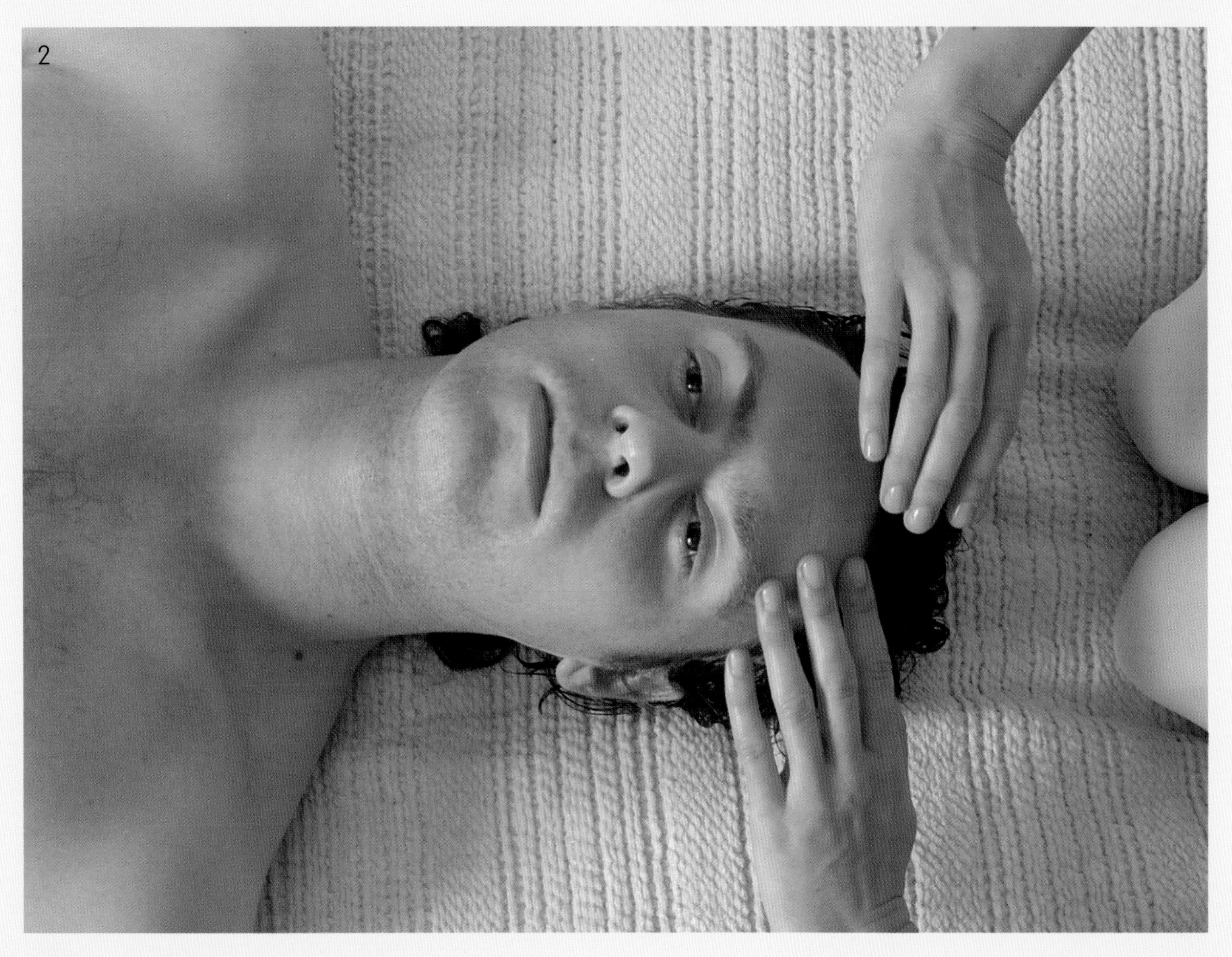

3 **Tapoment:** Place the fingertips lightly over the forehead. Gently tap the forehead with the pads of the fingertips, letting them fall separately. Continue this action with the fingers as you move the hands around the cheeks and chin. Avoid the eyes, nose and mouth for this movement.

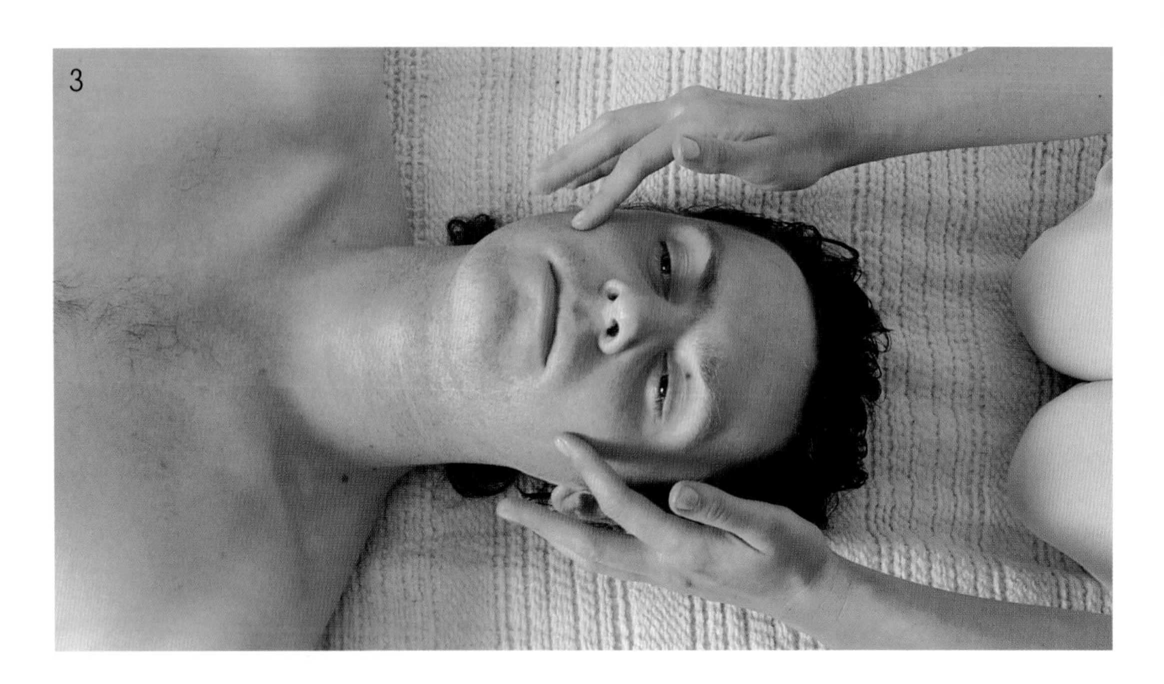

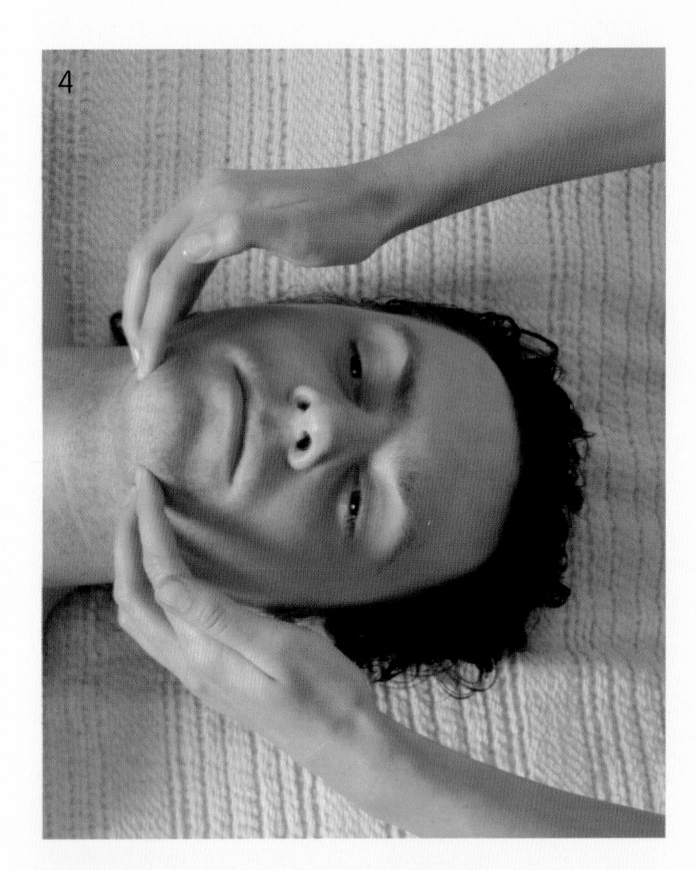

4 **Friction:** Place the fingertips on the jaw line and spread them out. Gently make tiny circles, barely moving the fingers. Move the fingers to the jaw and repeat. Move the fingers to the cheeks.

5 **Squeeze the chin:** Place the thumbs on top of the chin with your first two fingers underneath. Gently squeeze the chin, sliding the fingers towards each other. Repeat this action a few times.

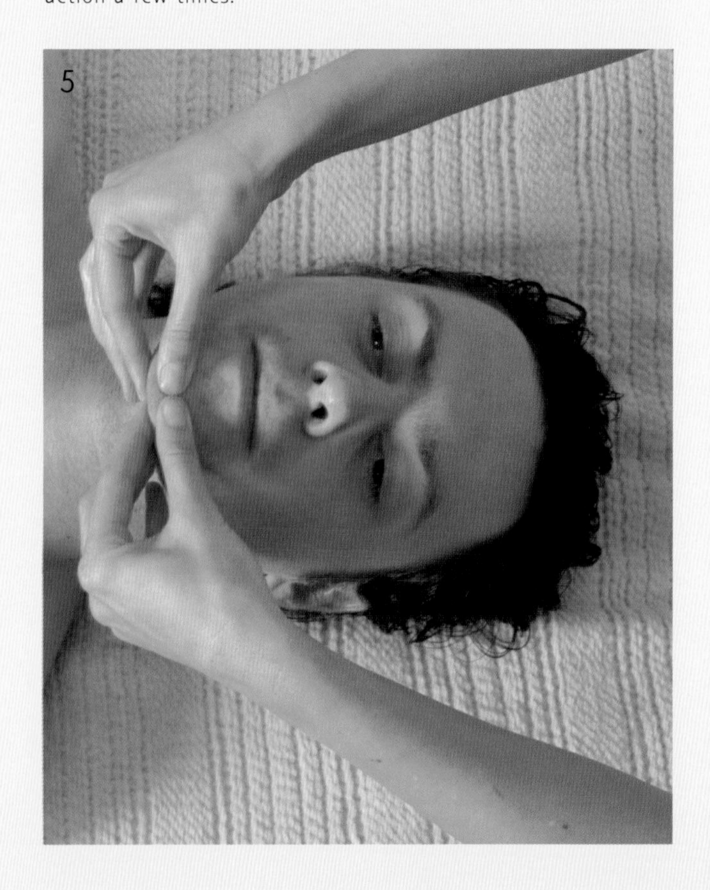

6 Circles to the ears: Place both hands underneath the chin with your fingertips facing each other. Sweep the hands in opposite directions towards the ears. Circle the fingers in front of the ears and then around the back of the ears. Gently pinch the ear lobe between the thumb and forefinger and pull towards the neck, letting the fingers slide away from the ear lobe. Repeat a few times.

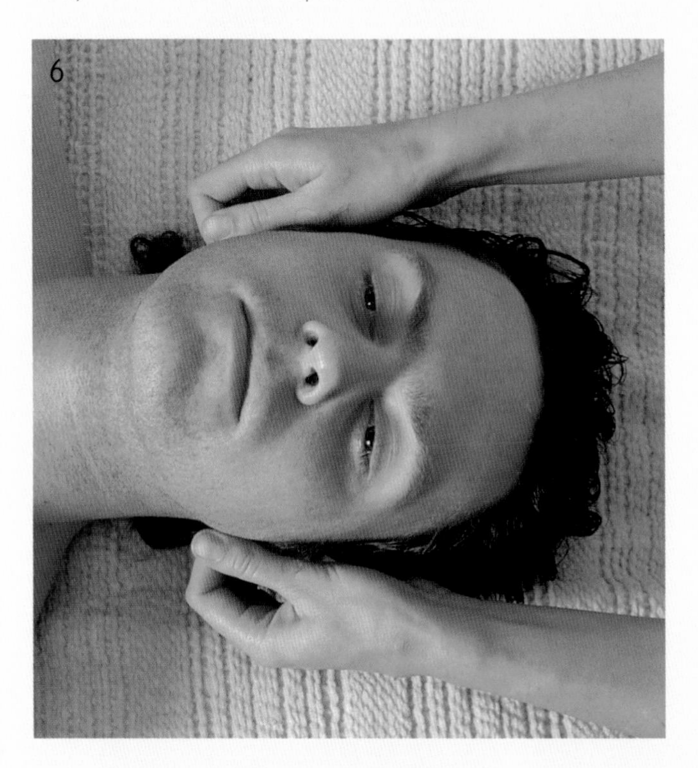

6

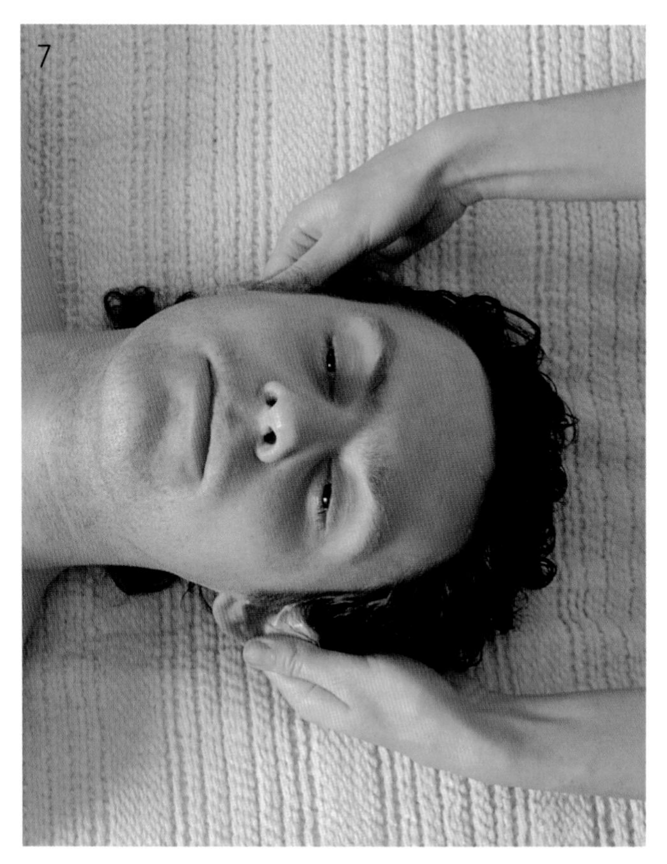

7

7 Massaging the ears: Place the thumb on top of the ear and bend your forefinger underneath the ear. Make circles with the thumb and forefinger, massaging out the ear. Gently pull the ear out and away from the body.

Ending the massage: Hold the head for a moment with the thumbs together on the forehead and the fingertips towards the ears. Move to the side of your partner and squeeze their shoulders. Then place your hands on their hips and gently squeeze. Move down to your partner's knees and squeeze. Move to their feet and hold their feet for a moment.

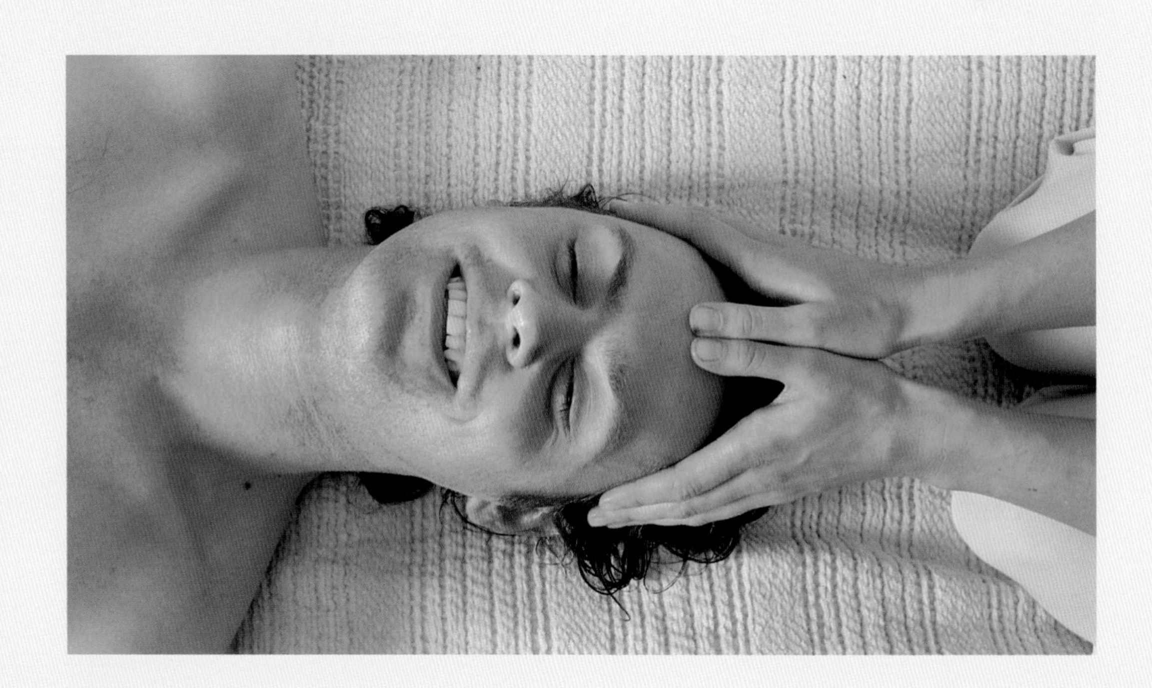

Quick guide – back

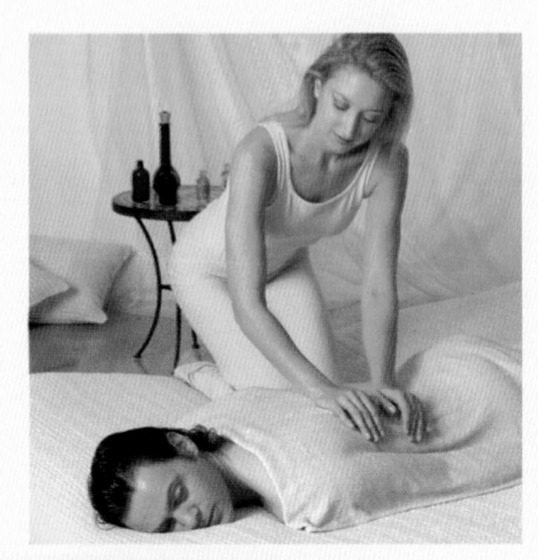

1. Softening

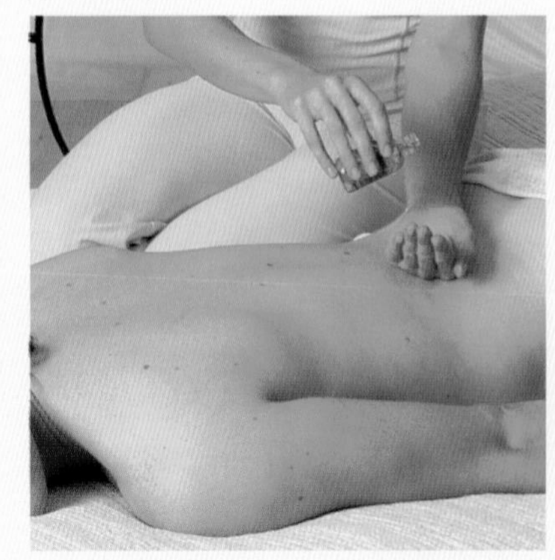

2. Spreading the oil

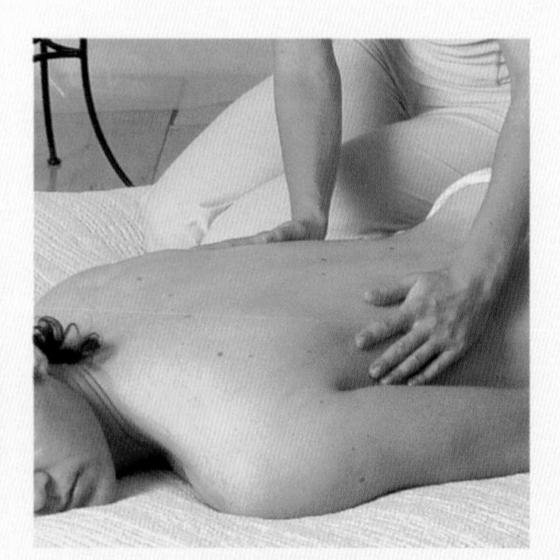

3. Effleurage

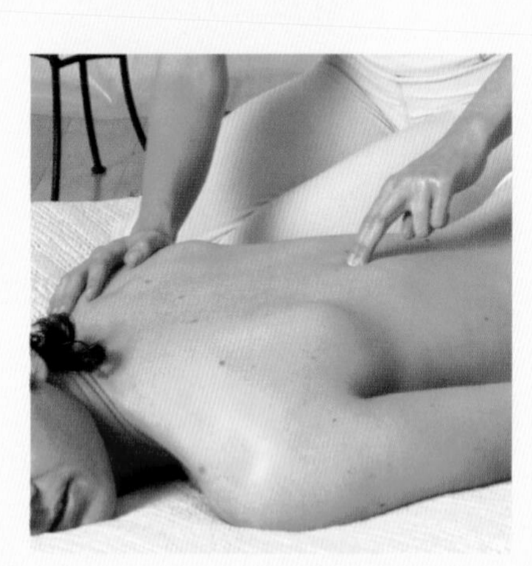

4. Vibration

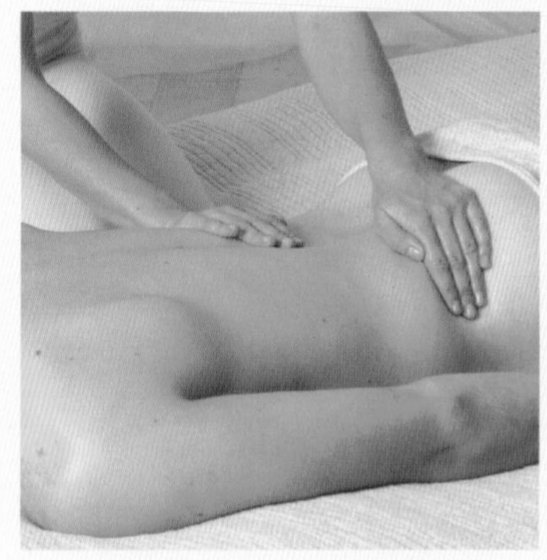

5. Wringing across the back

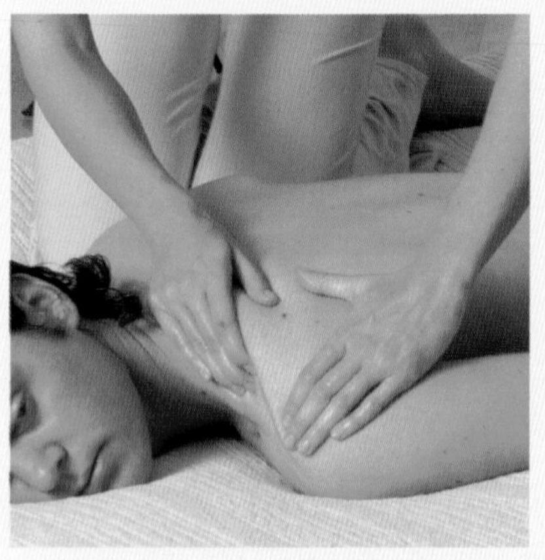

6. Kneading to the shoulders and neck

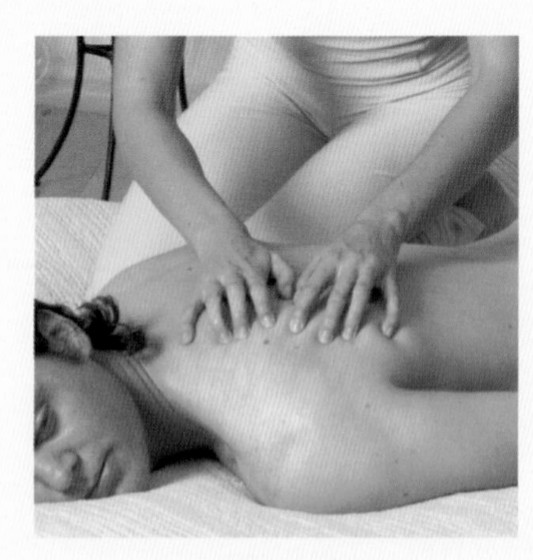

7. Lion claw

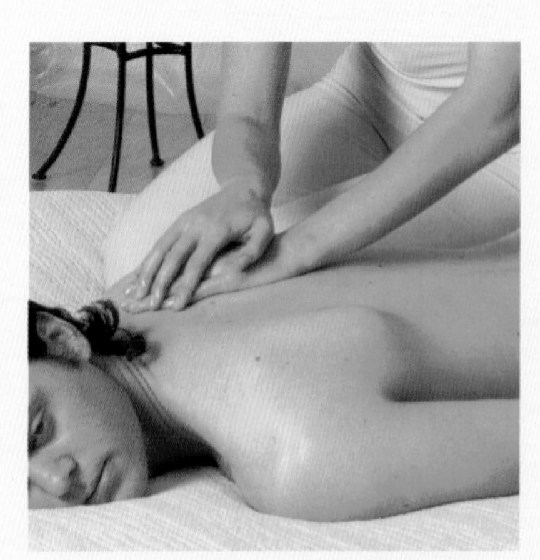

8. Hand-over-hand effleurage to the shoulder

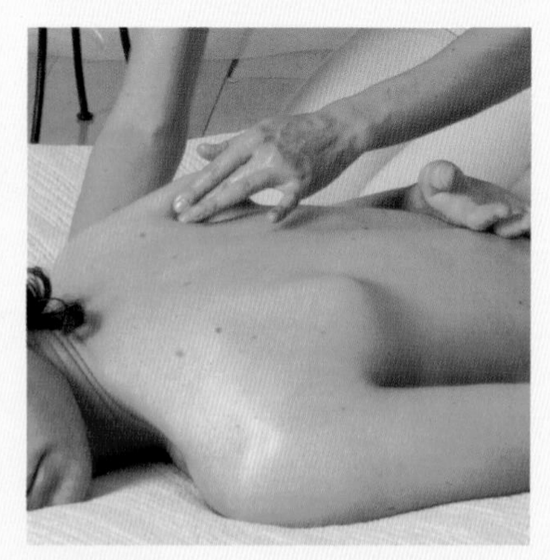

9. Friction to the shoulder blade

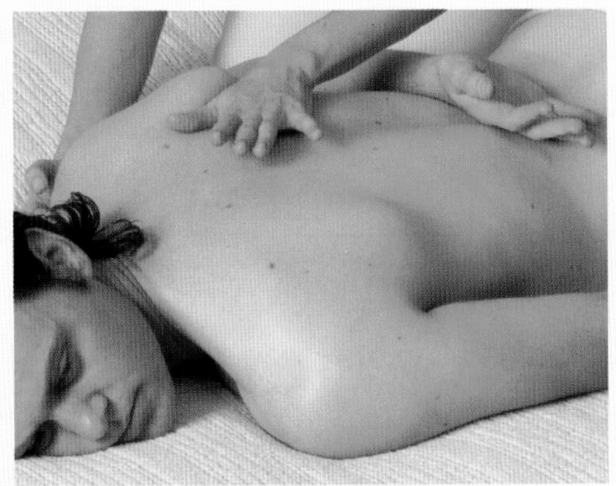

10. Vibration to the shoulder blade

11. Repeat steps 8-10 to the other side

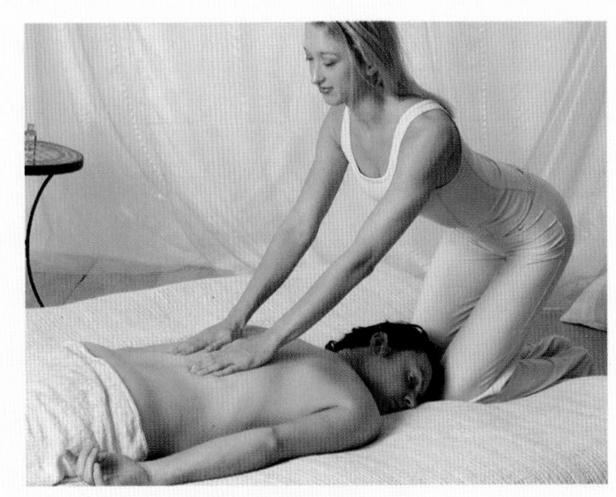

12. Pull-ups

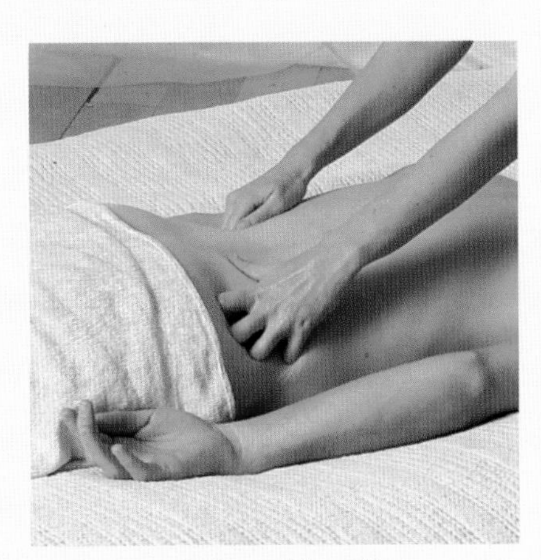

13. Knuckle rolls

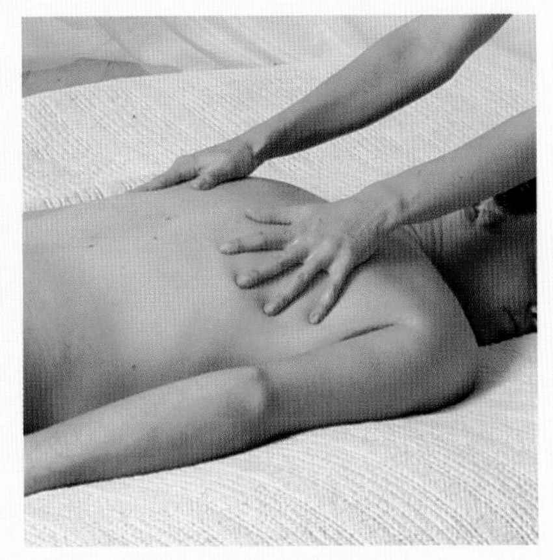

14. Fanning

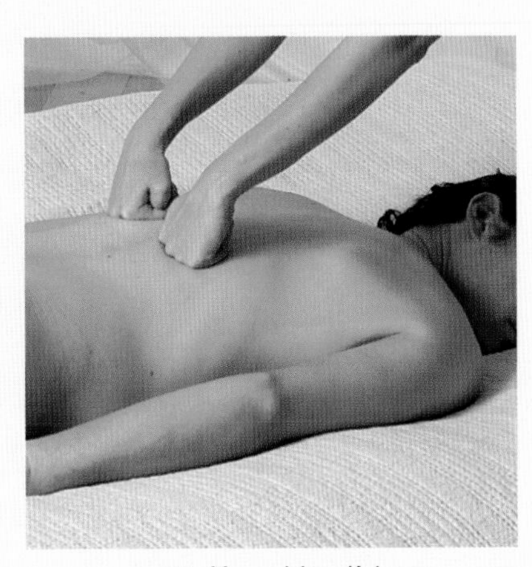

15. Knuckle slide

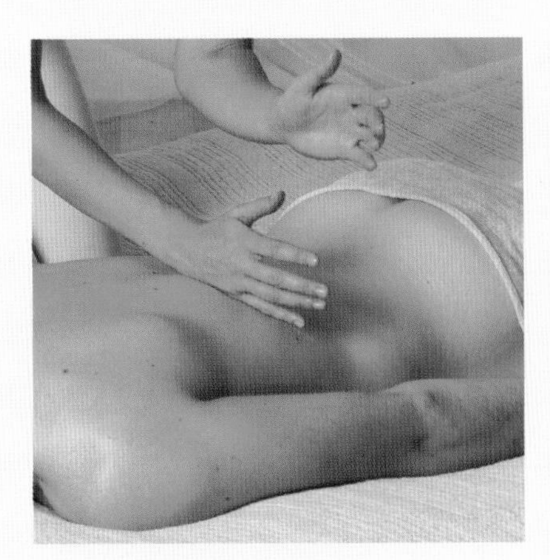

16. Hacking

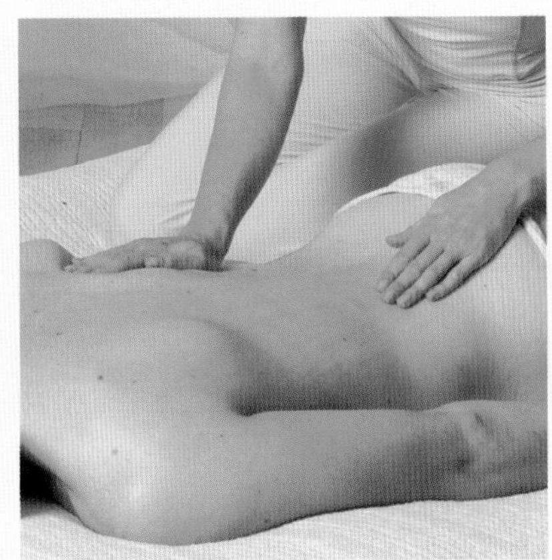

17. Alternating effleurage

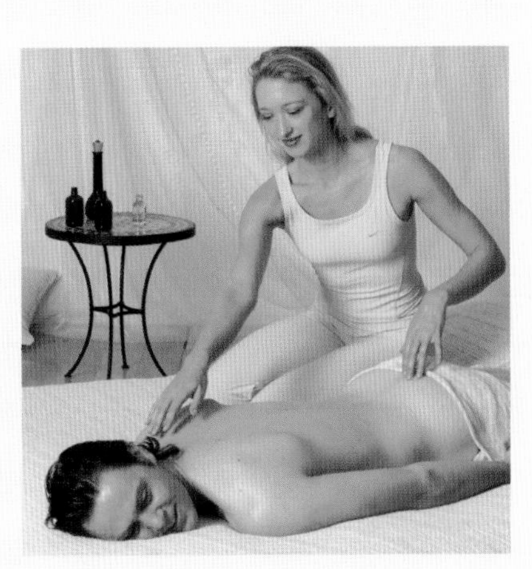

18. Feather stroking

Quick guide – back of the leg

1. Softening

2. Spreading the oil

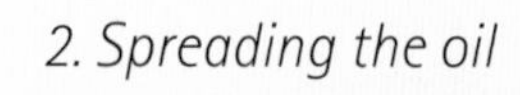

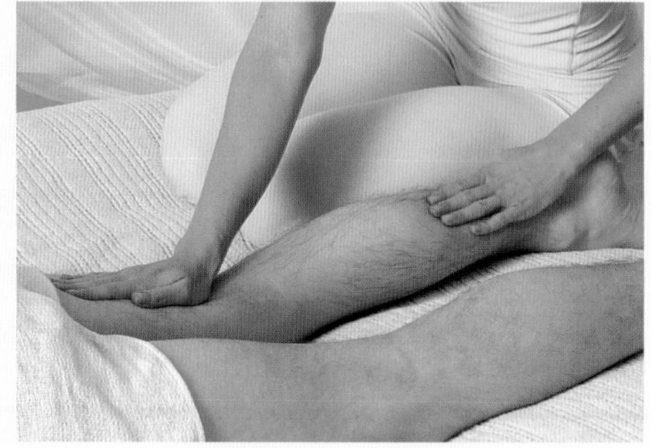

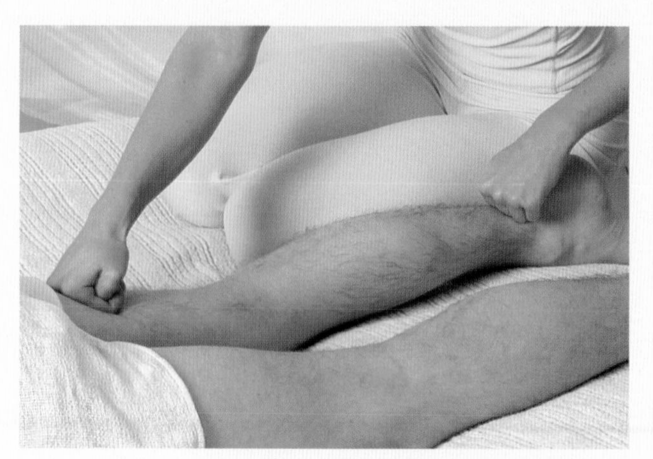

3. Alternating effleurage

4. Knuckle slide

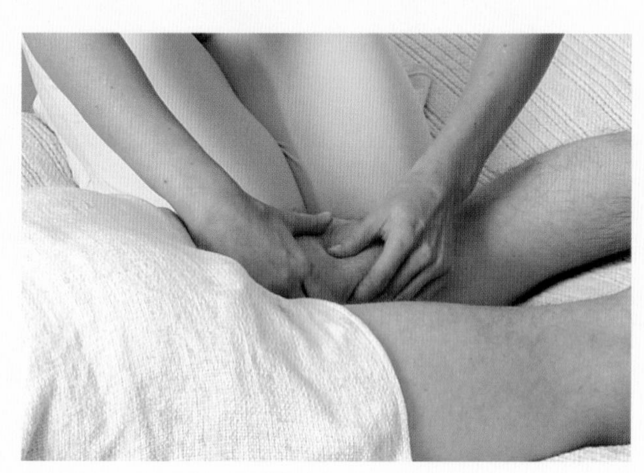

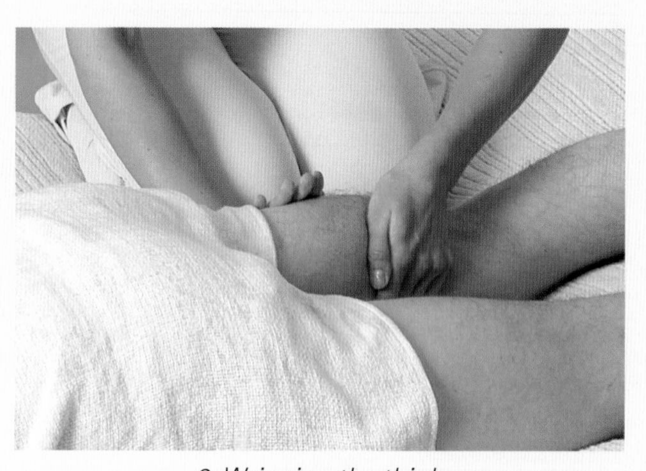

5. Kneading the inner thigh

6. Wringing the thigh

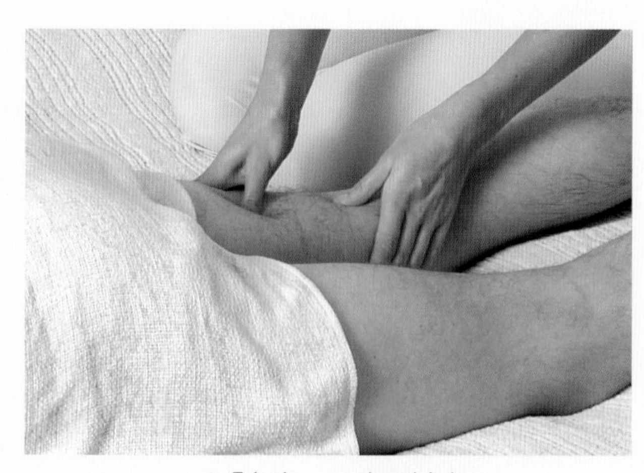

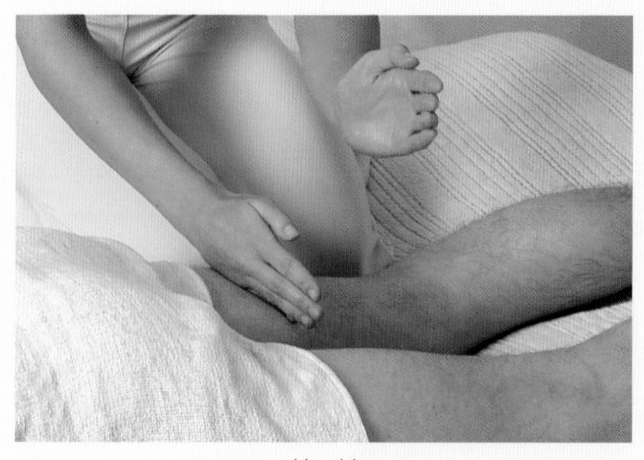

7. Friction to the thigh

8. Hacking

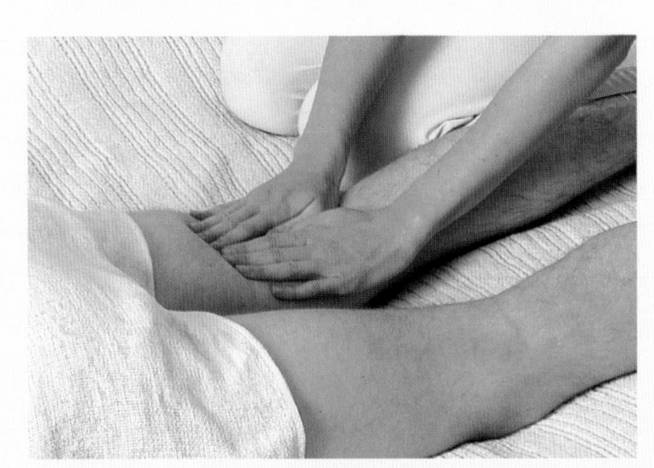

9. *Basic effleurage*

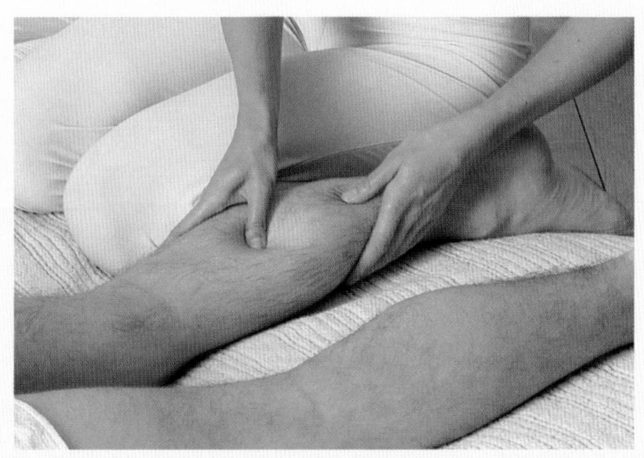

10. *Friction to the calf*

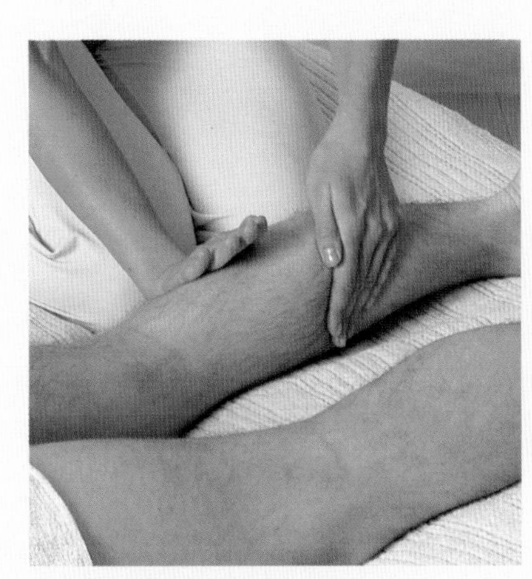

11. *Wringing the calf*

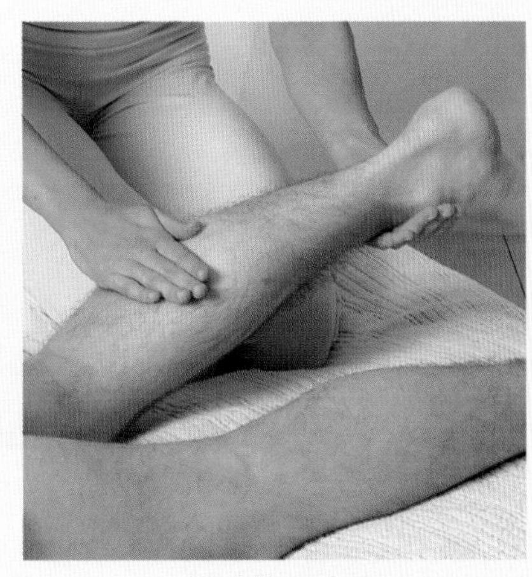

12. *Vibration*

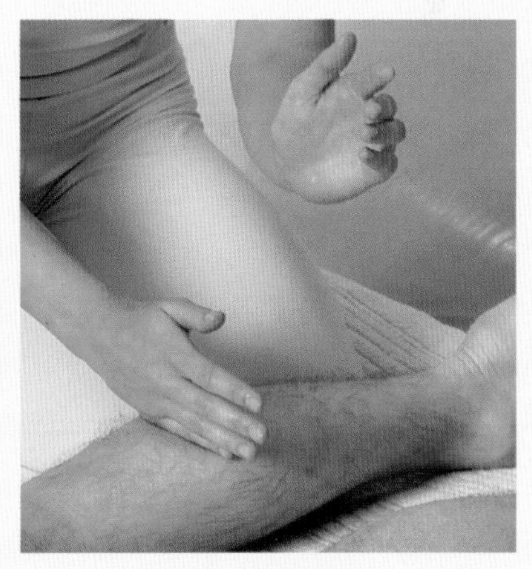

13. *Hacking*

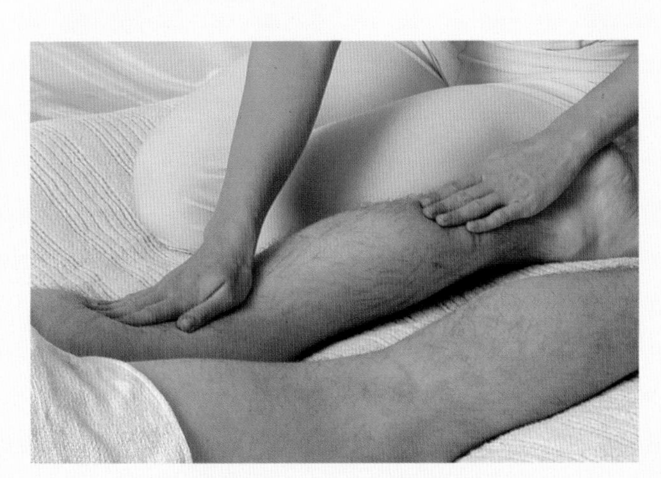

14. *Alternating effleurage*

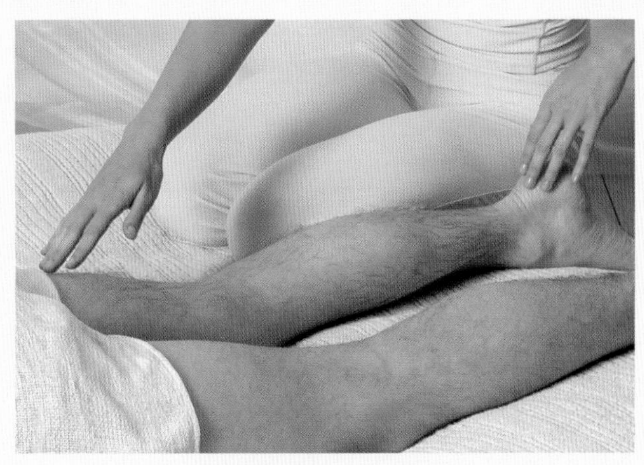

15. *Feather stroking*

Quick guide – front of the leg

1. Softening

2. Spreading the oil

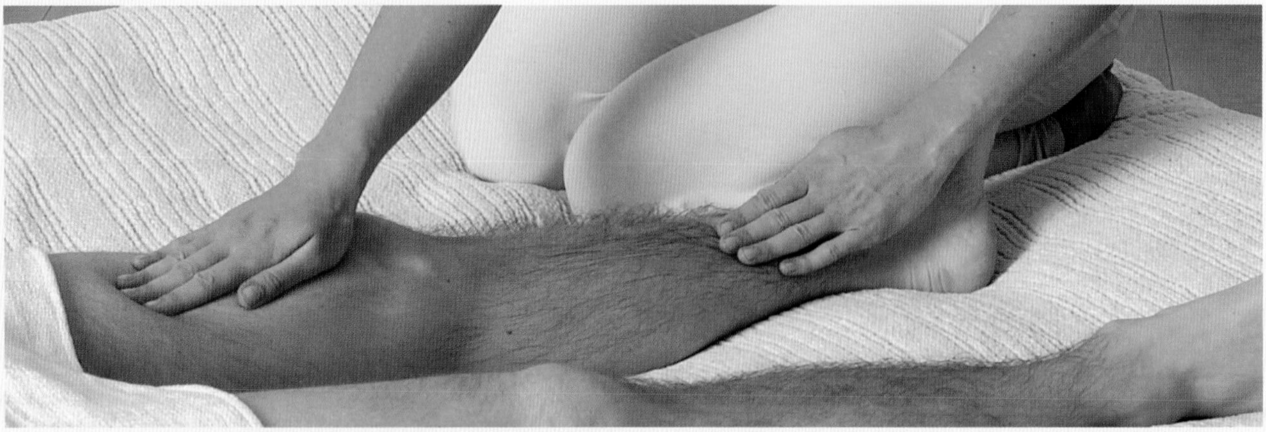

3. Alternating effleurage

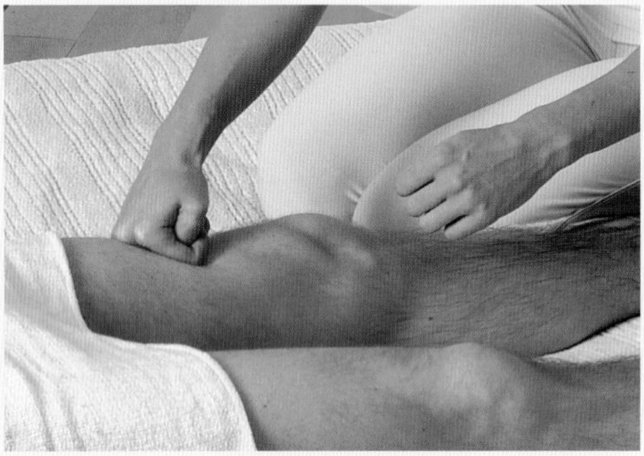

4. Knuckles up thigh

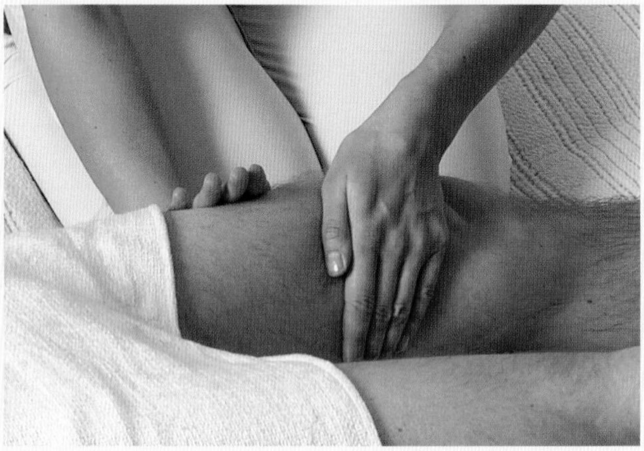

5. Wringing the thigh

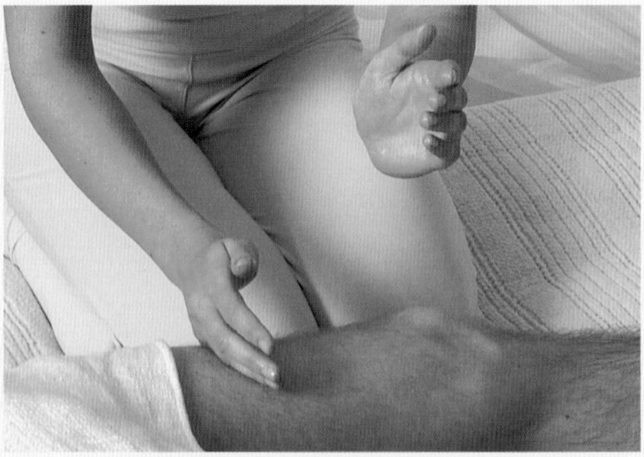

6. Hacking

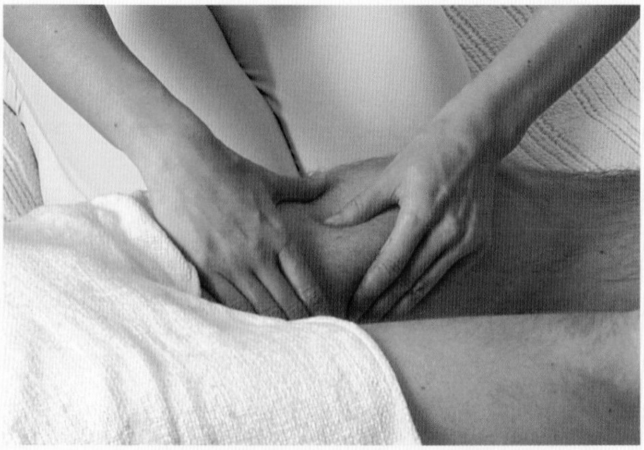

7. Kneading the inner thigh

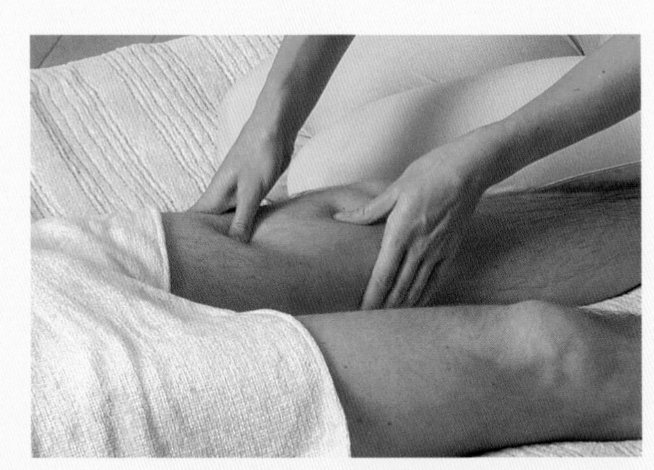

8. Friction to the thigh

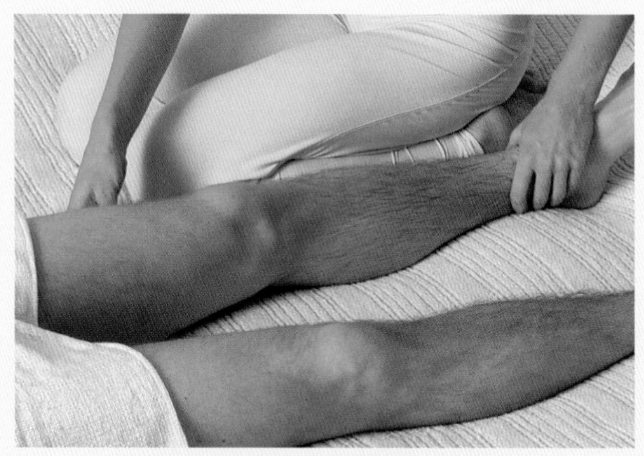

9. Friction to the outside of the leg

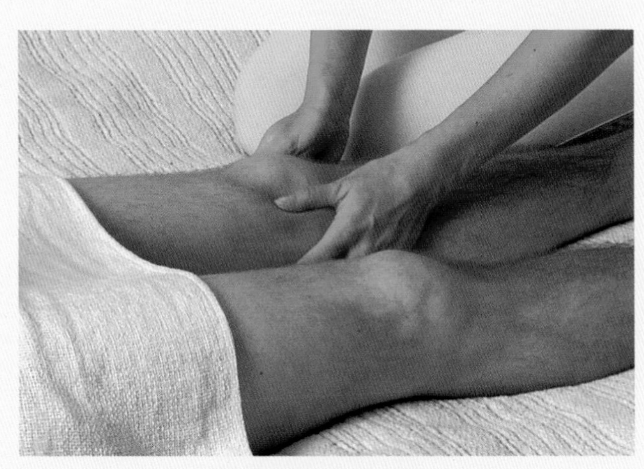

10. Opening the knee

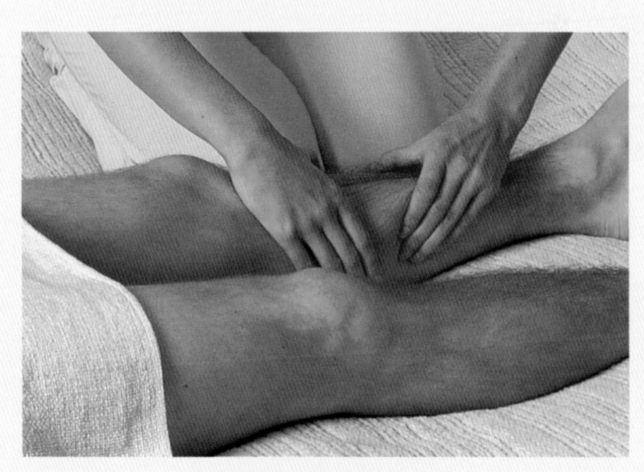

11. Kneading the calf

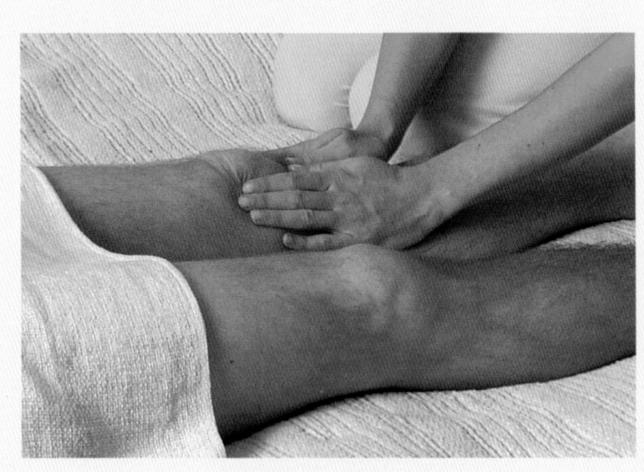

12. Basic effleurage

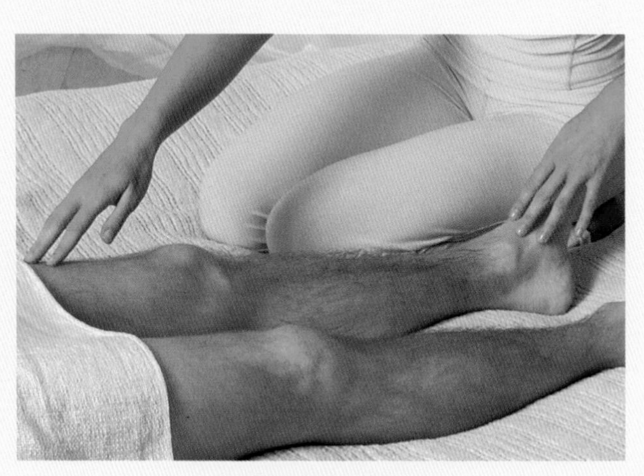

13. Feather stroking

Quick guide – foot

1. Spreading the oil

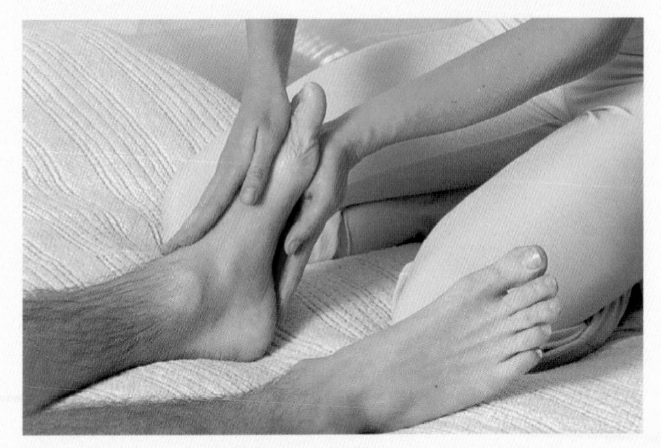

2. Sandwiching

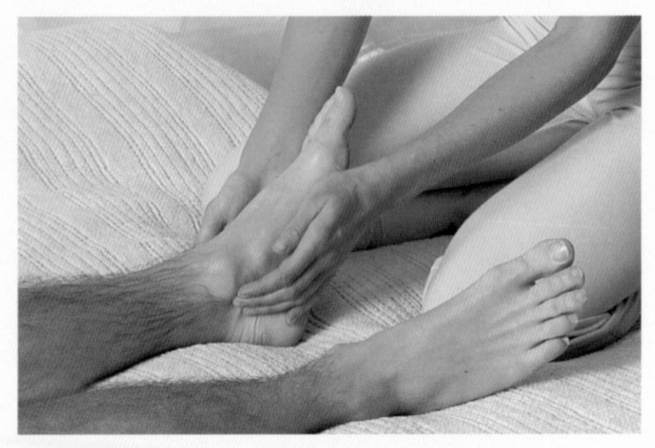

3. Circling anklebones

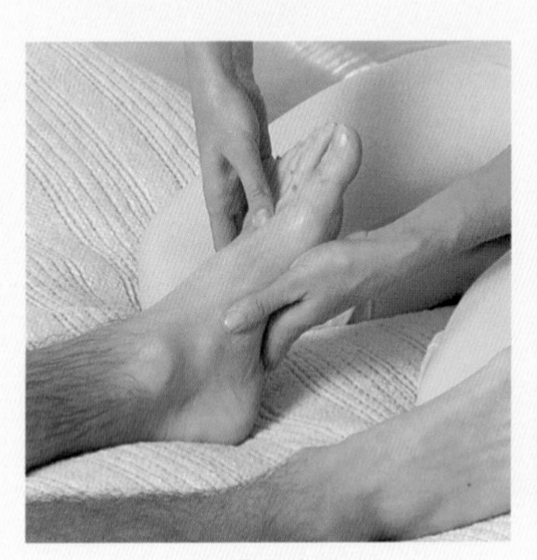

4. Friction

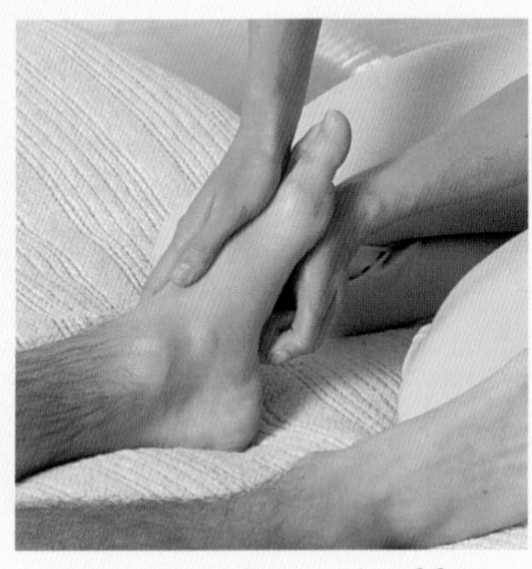

5.Knuckle rolls to sole of foot

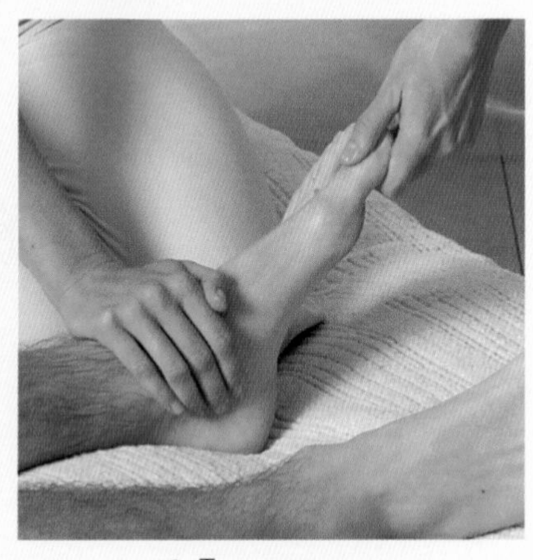

6. Toe massage

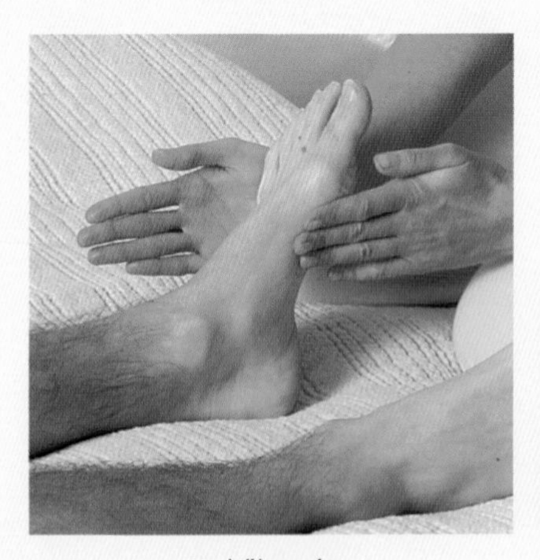

7. Vibration

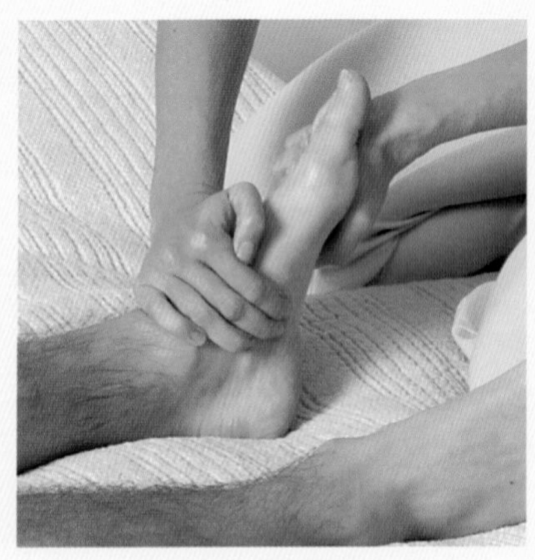

8. Squeeze foot

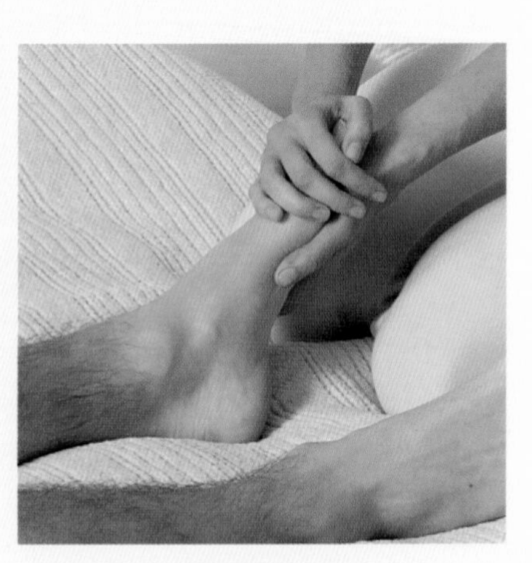

9. Holding

Quick guide – arm

1. Softening

2. Spreading the oil

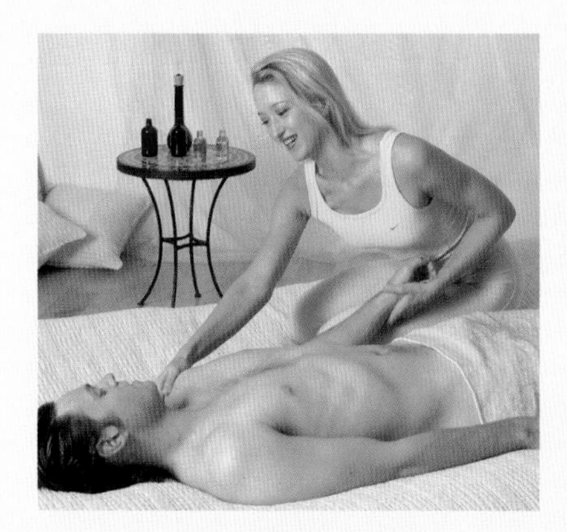

3. Alternating effleurage

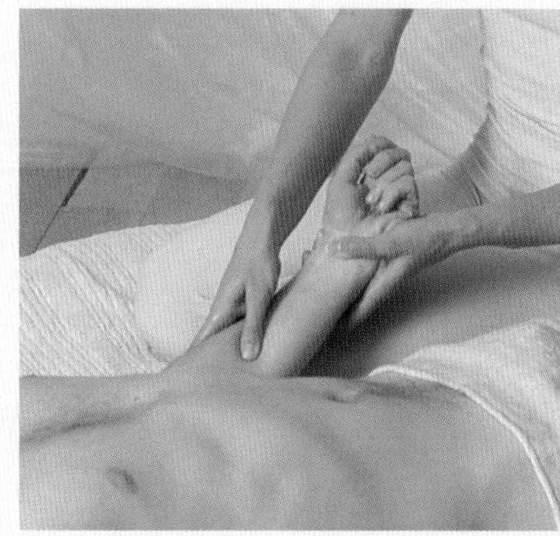

4. Friction to the forearm

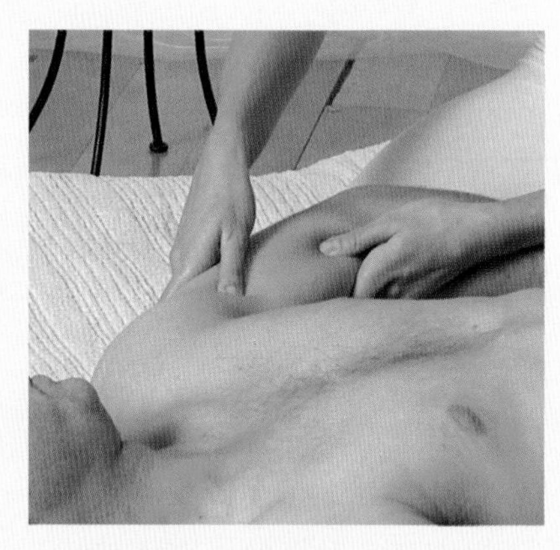

5. Friction to the upper arm

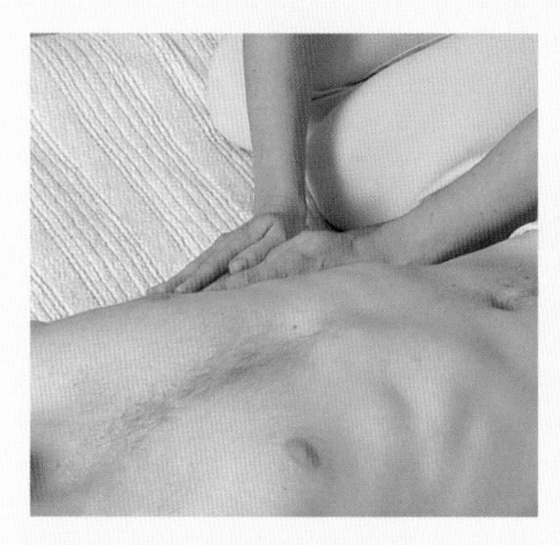

6. Basic effleurage

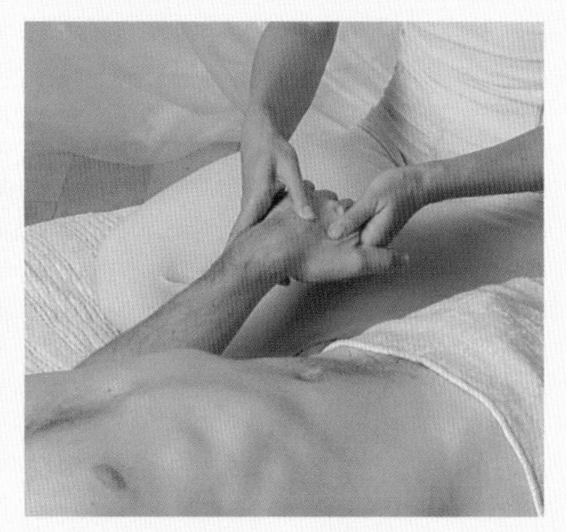

7. Friction to the hand

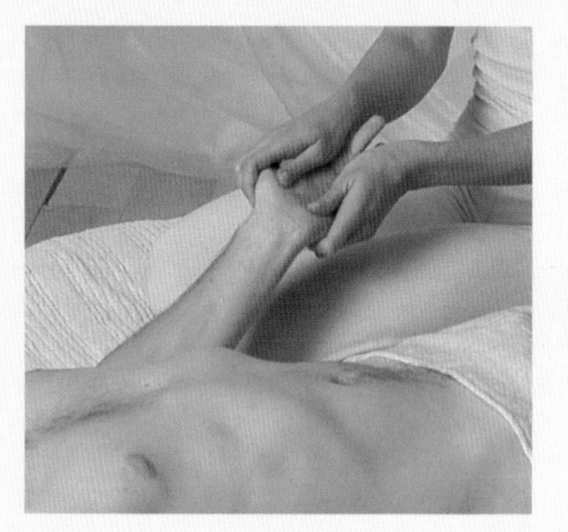

8. Opening

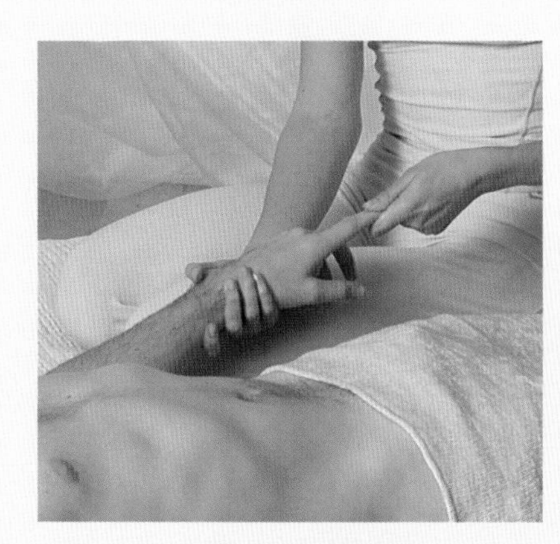

9. Finger massage

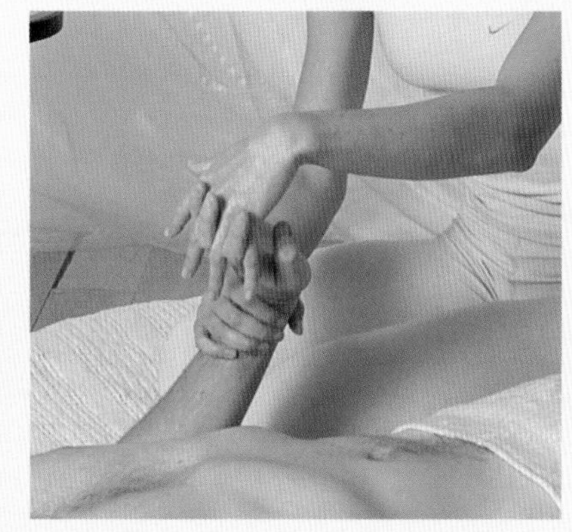

10. Fingers laced

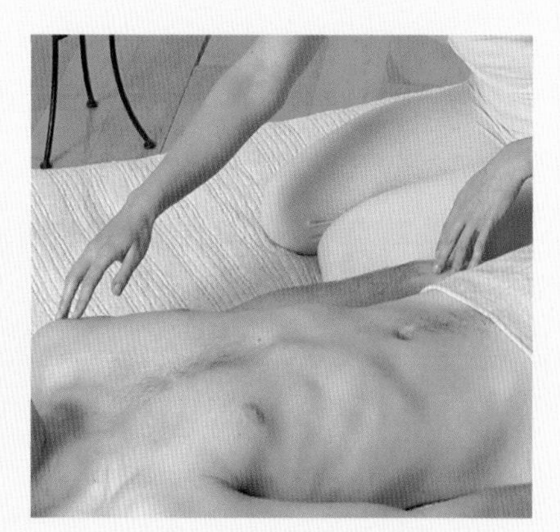

11. Feather stroking

Quick guide – stomach

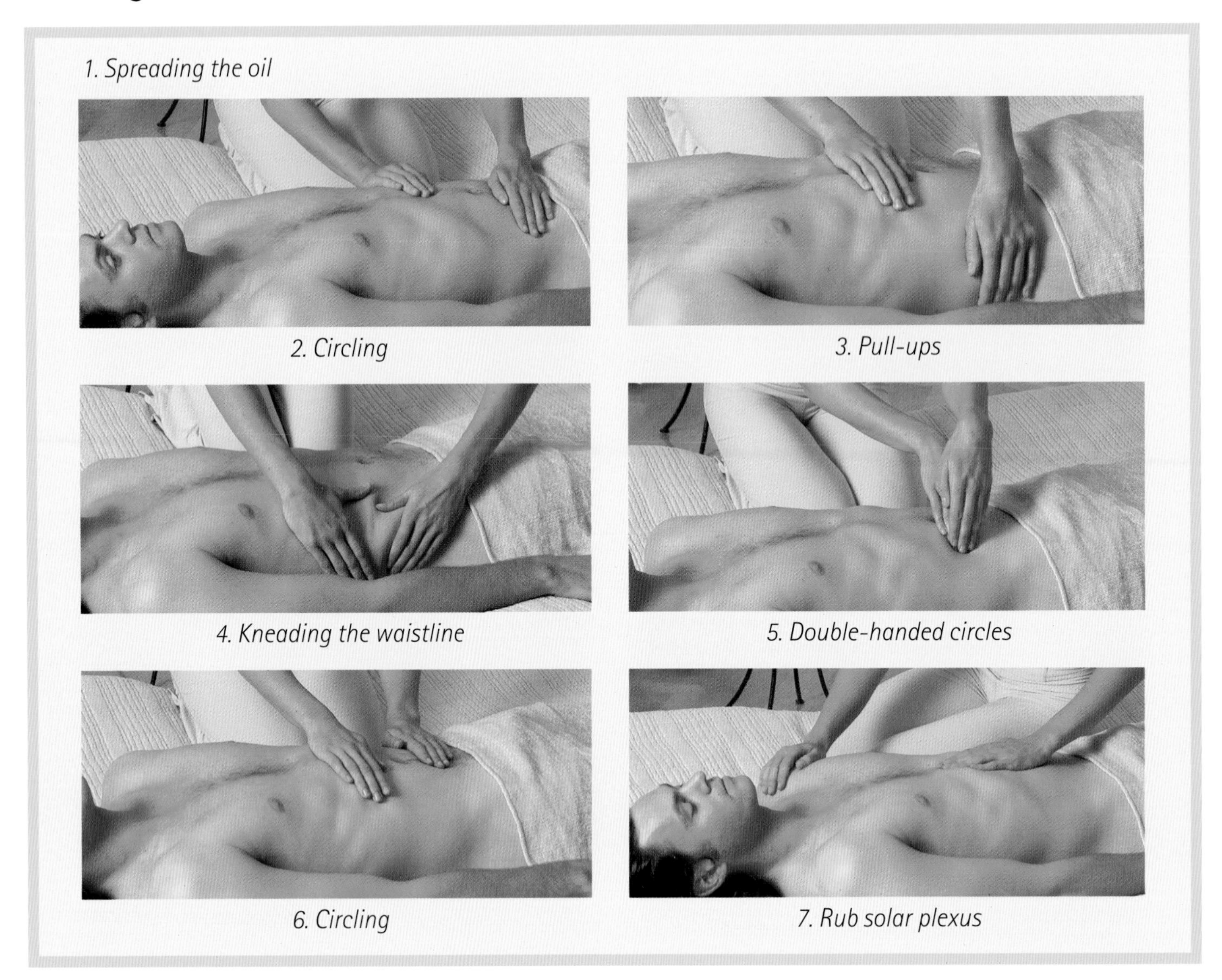

1. Spreading the oil

2. Circling

3. Pull-ups

4. Kneading the waistline

5. Double-handed circles

6. Circling

7. Rub solar plexus

Quick guide – chest

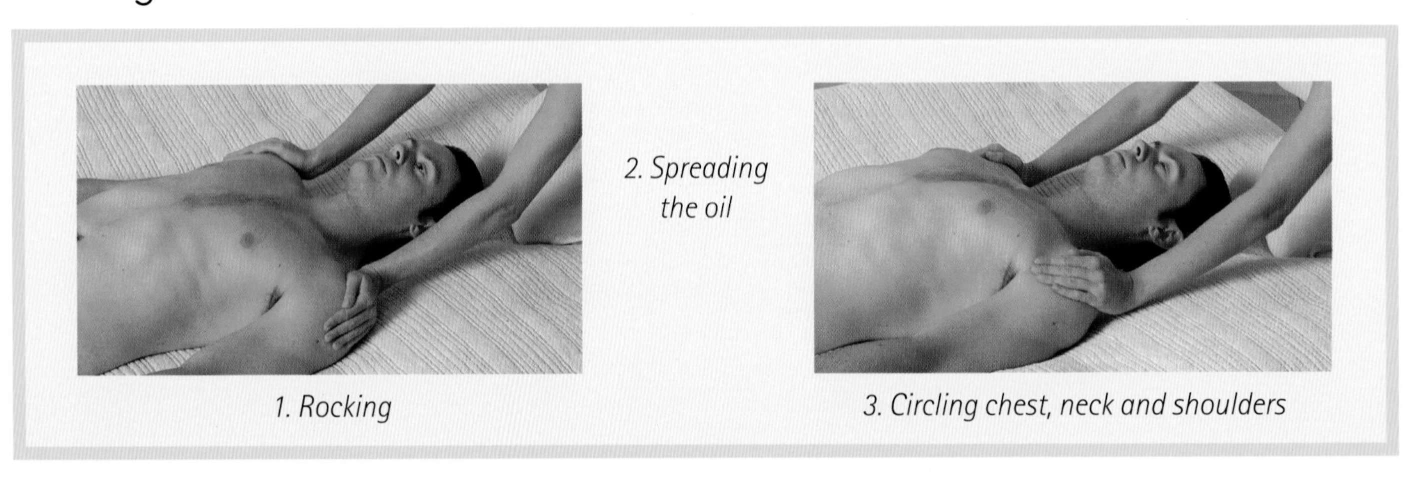

1. Rocking

2. Spreading the oil

3. Circling chest, neck and shoulders

Quick guide – chest cont.

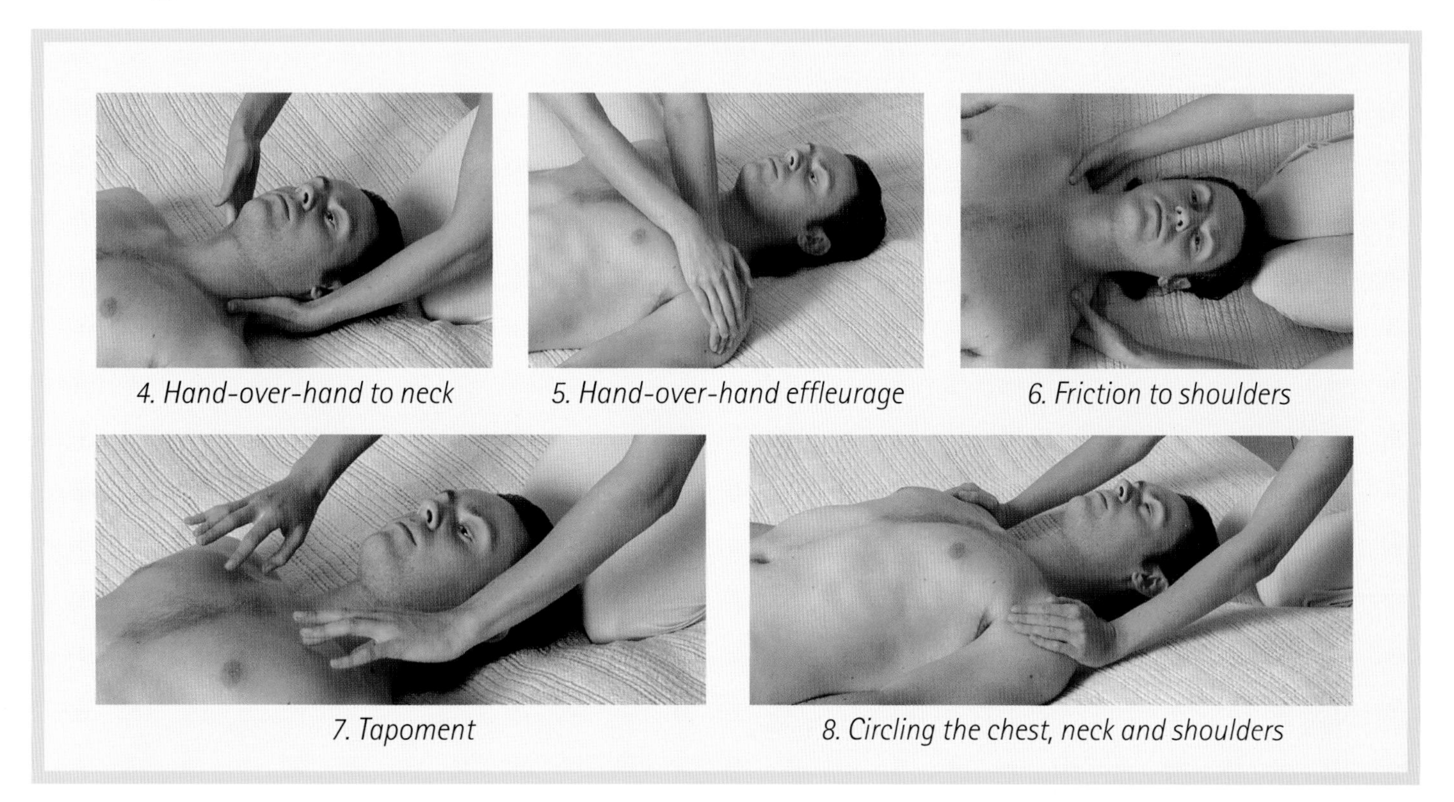

4. Hand-over-hand to neck
5. Hand-over-hand effleurage
6. Friction to shoulders
7. Tapoment
8. Circling the chest, neck and shoulders

Quick guide – neck and head

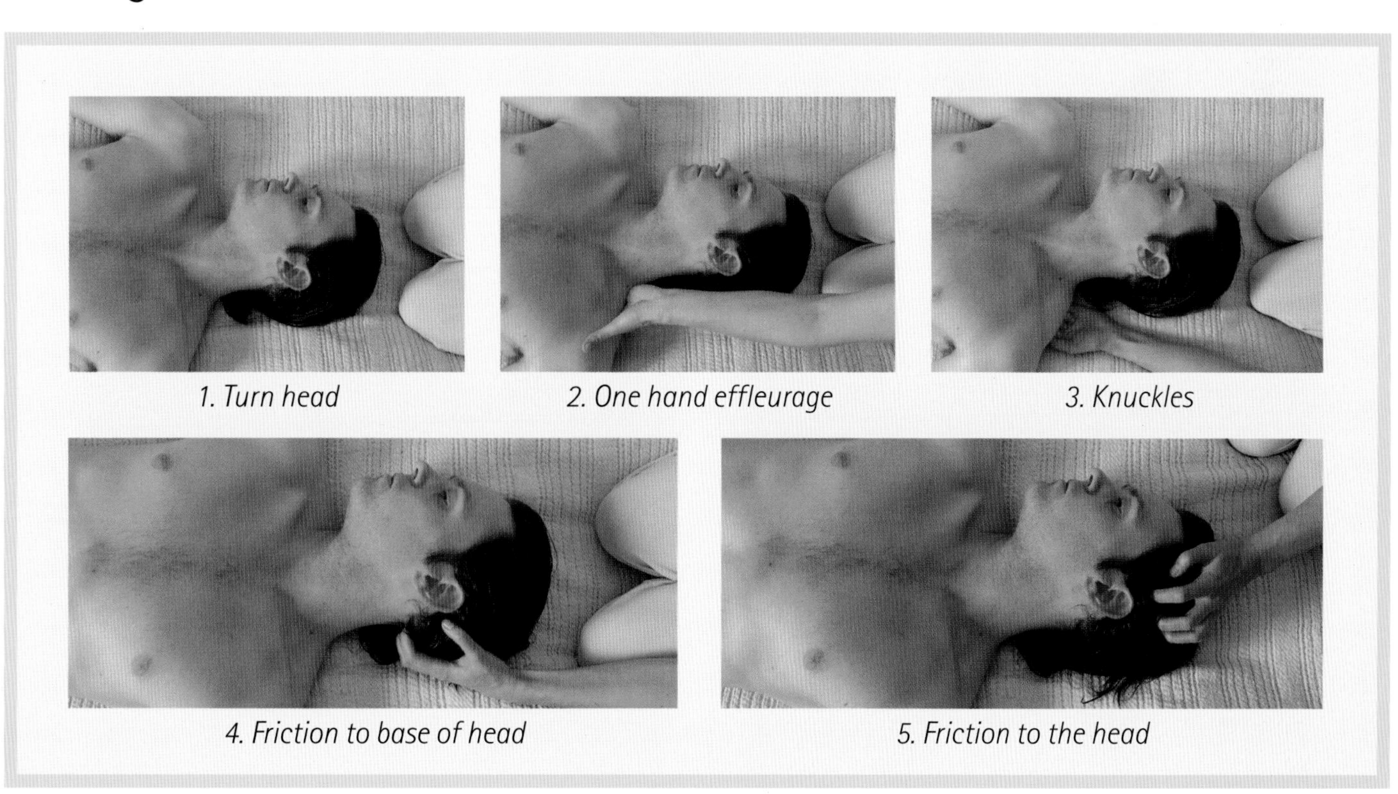

1. Turn head
2. One hand effleurage
3. Knuckles
4. Friction to base of head
5. Friction to the head

Quick guide – face

1. Spreading the oil

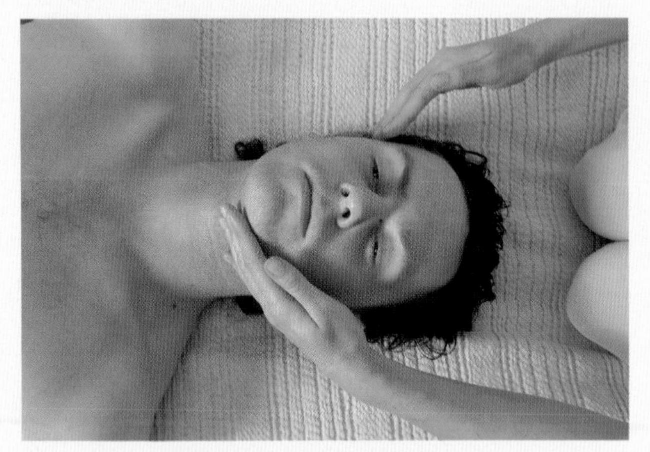

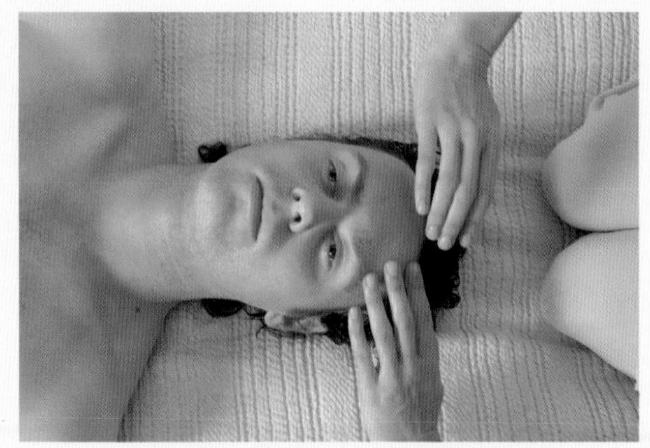

2. Effleurage to the chin

3. Effleurage to the forehead

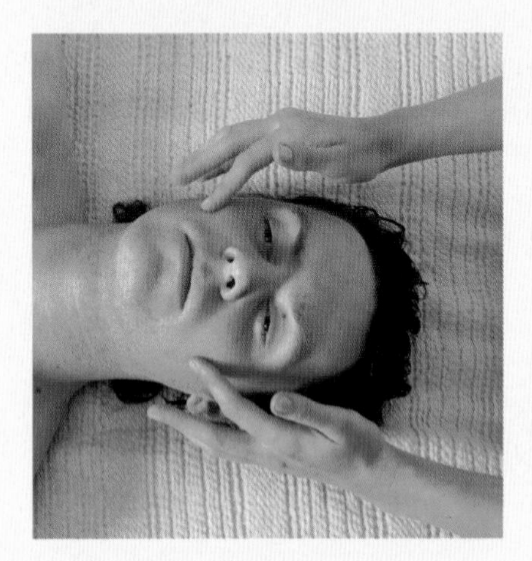

4. Tapoment

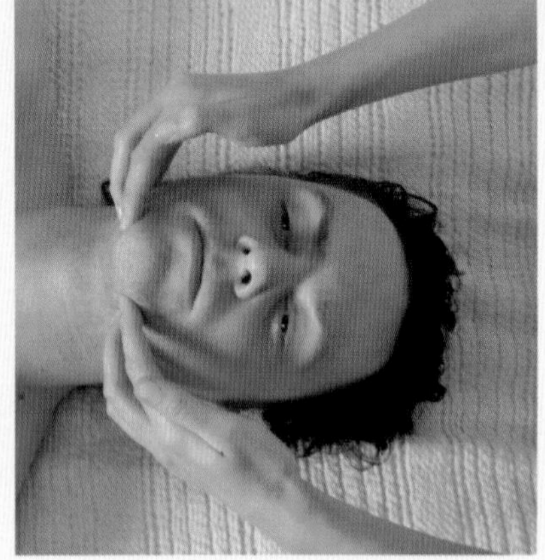

5. Friction

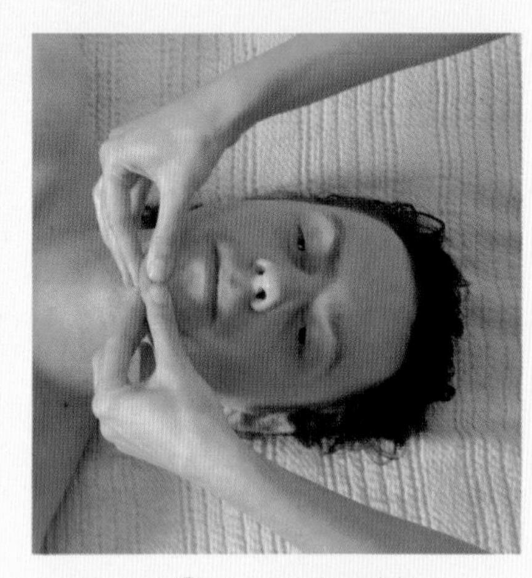

6. Squeeze the chin

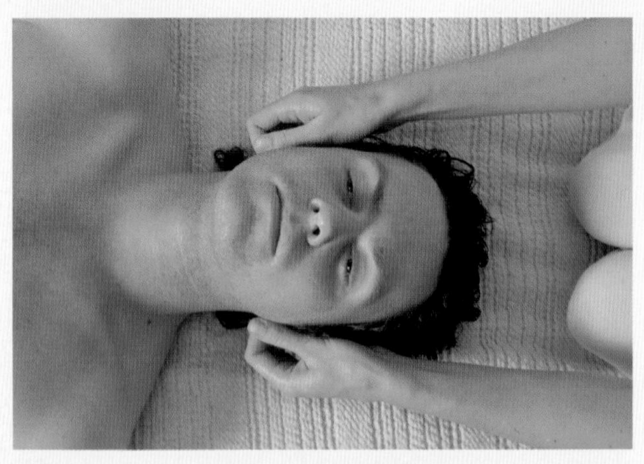

7. Circles to the ears

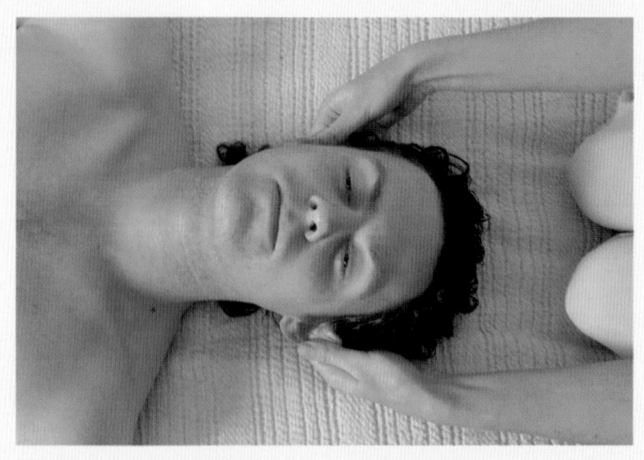

8. Massaging the ears

Advanced techniques

This section looks at more advanced massage strokes, and then demonstrates a sequence using these strokes. The techniques in this section are slightly more difficult than those in the previous sections. Be sure you have mastered the first two sections before moving on to the Advanced techniques. By now you should be comfortable giving a massage and may want to add more techniques to your repertoire.

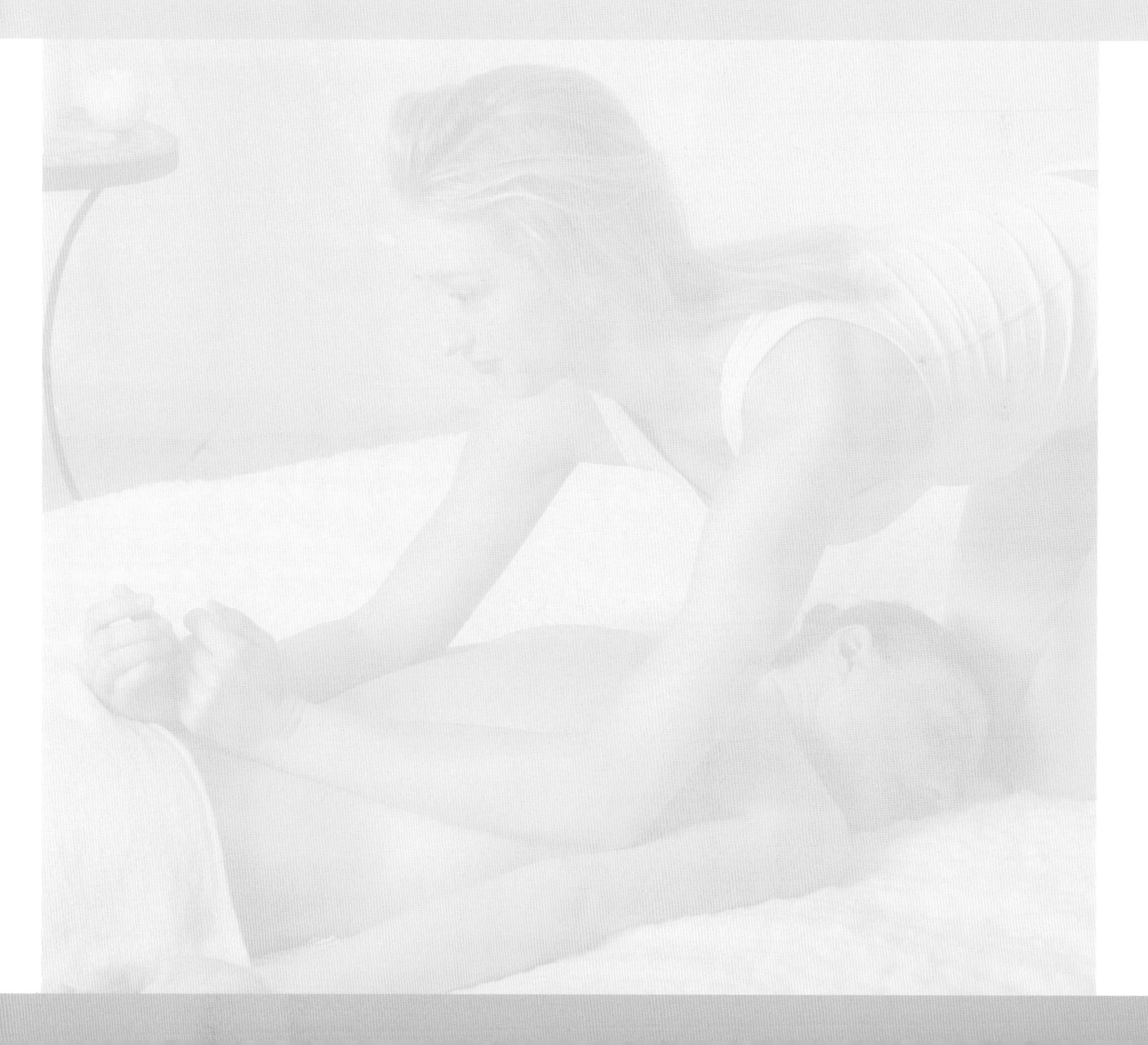

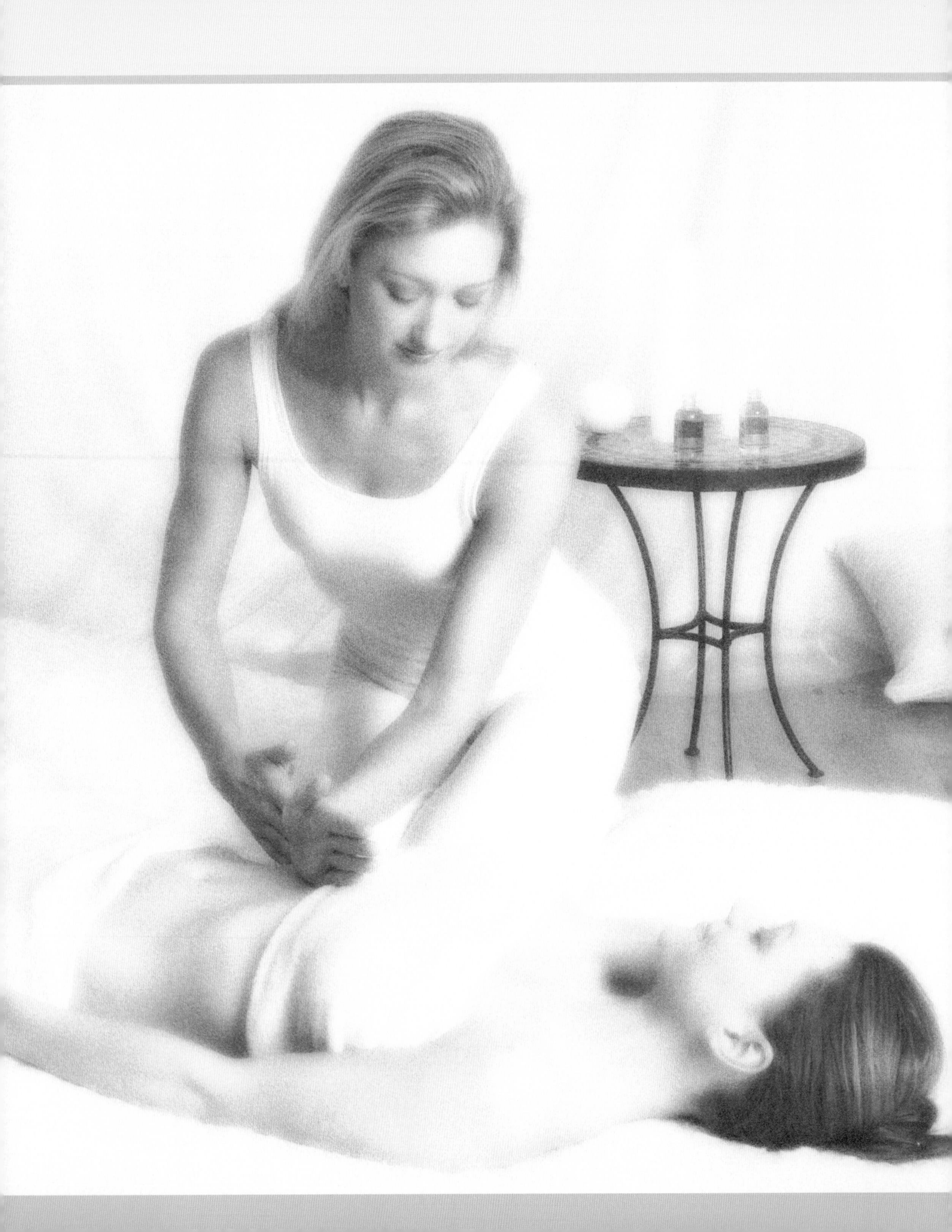

Strokes

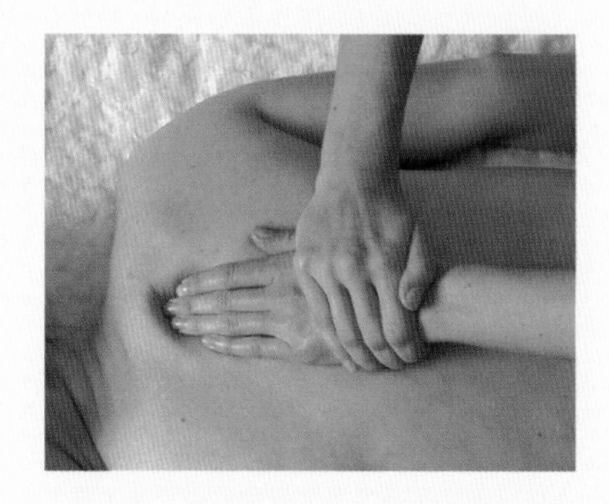

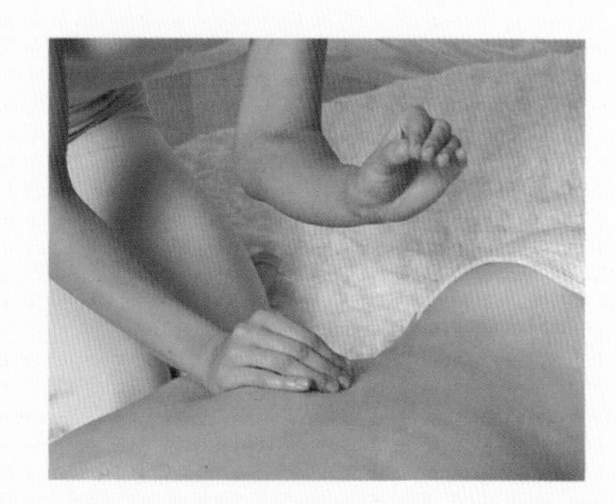

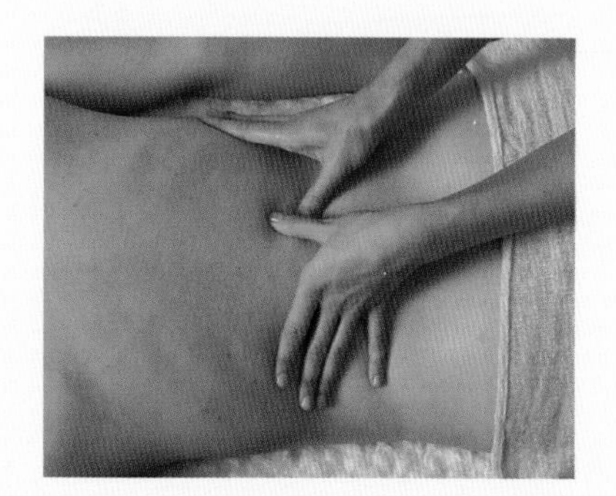

The techniques in this section either work more deeply into the muscles of the body, or are slightly more complex than the techniques in previous sections. Work slowly and read through the technique for each stroke first. Practice it several times before incorporating it into a massage.

Figure-of-eight

This stroke is a development of the basic effleurage movement. Start off in the exact same way as for effleurage.

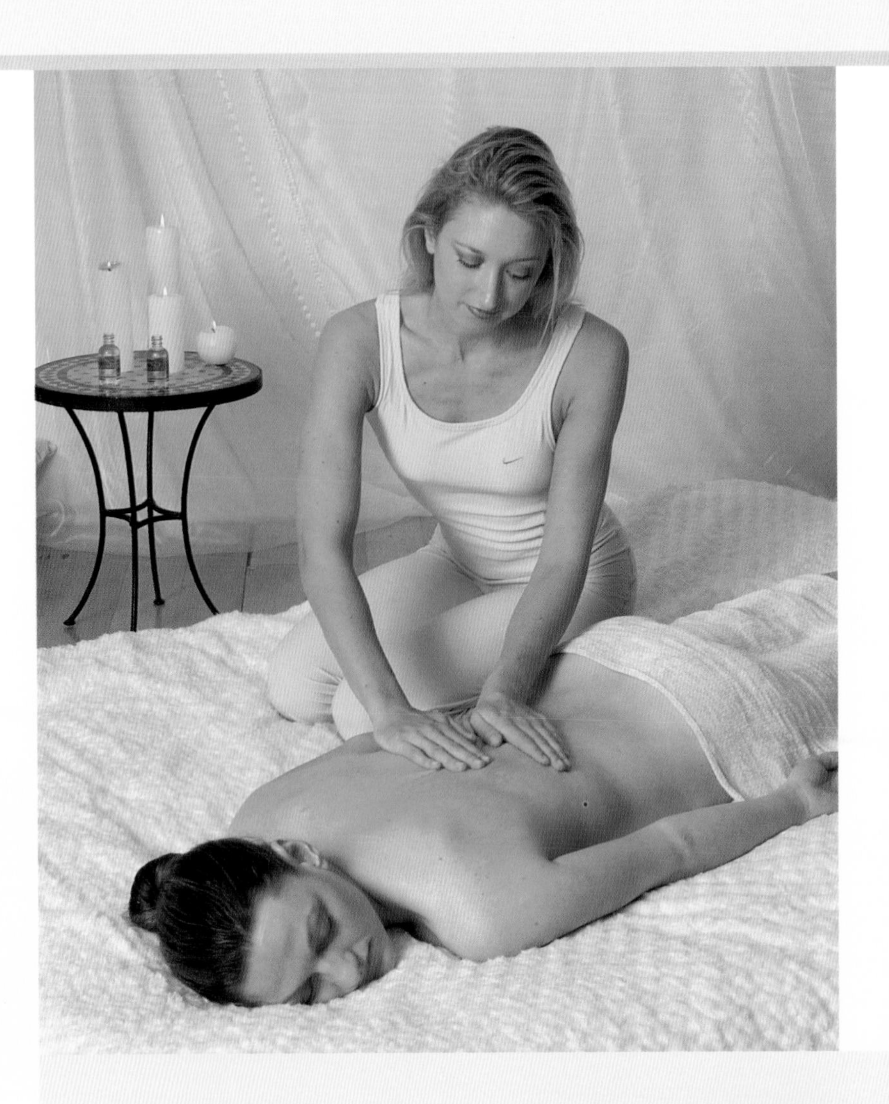

To the back

1 Place the hands flat on either side of the base of the spine with the fingertips facing the head.

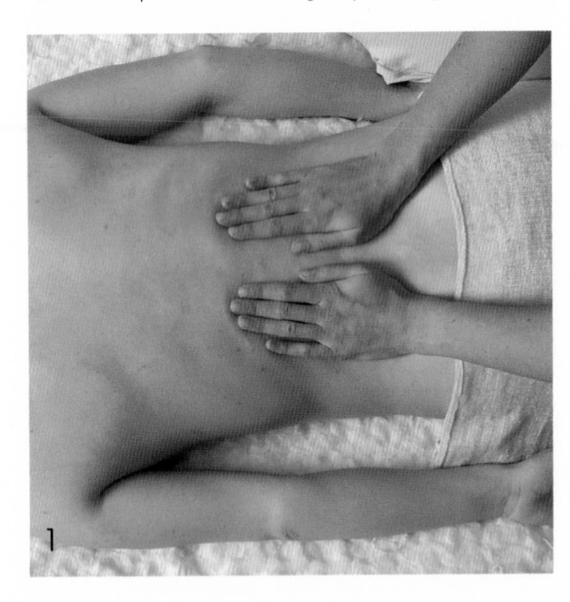

1

2 The pressure is even as you go up to the neck and across the shoulders.

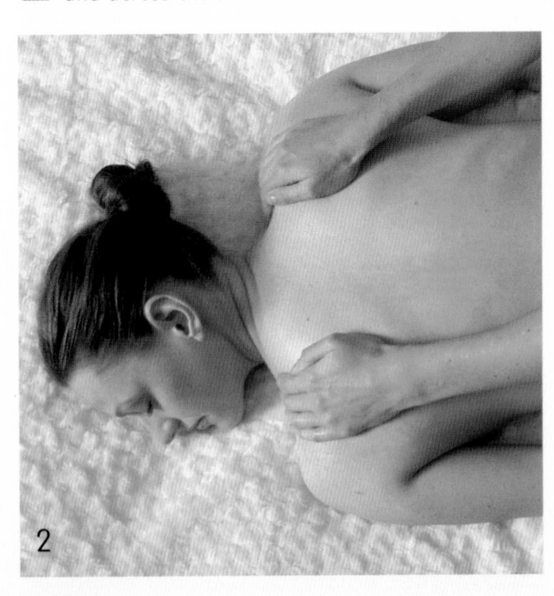

2

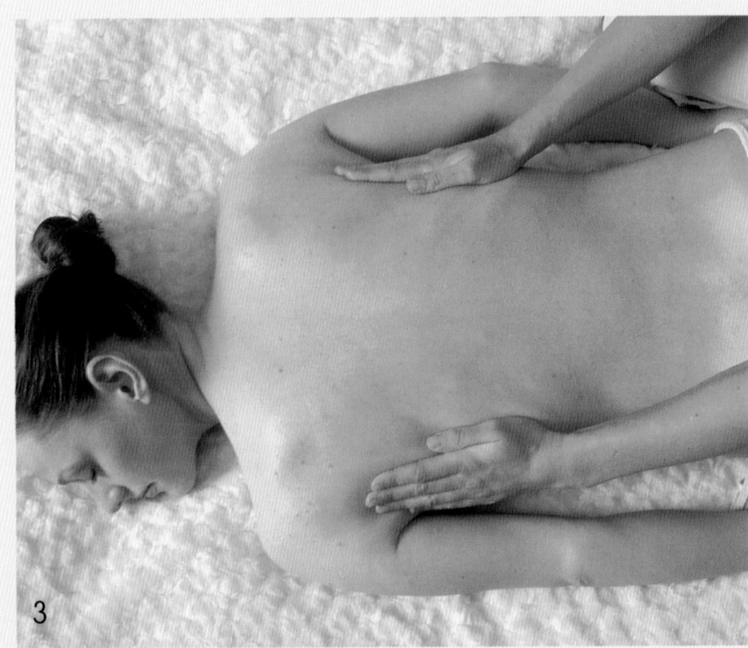

3

3 Let your hands slide halfway down the spine to the lower ribs.

4 Keeping contact with the spine, slide the hands across the ribs. . .

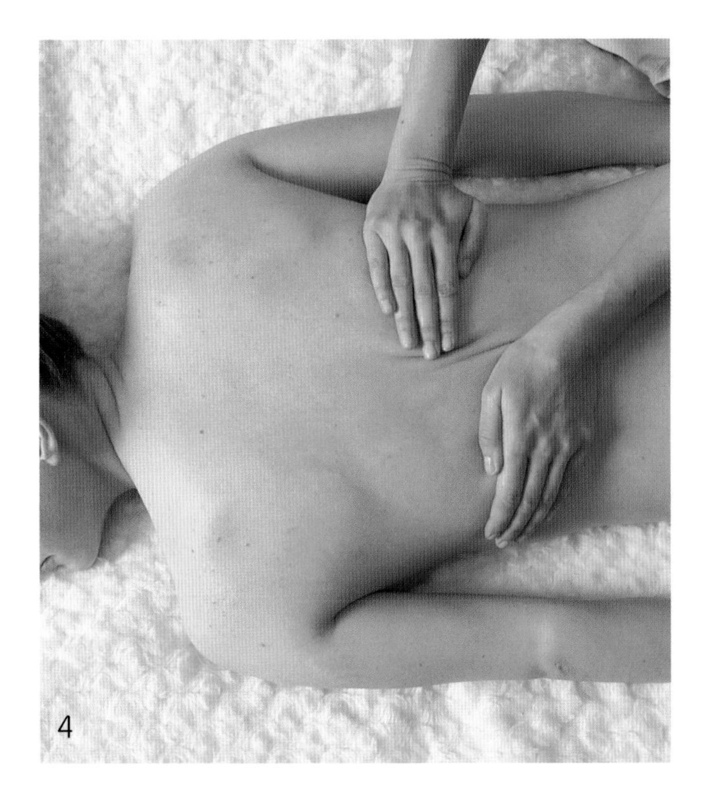

5 . . . .so that they end up on opposite sides.

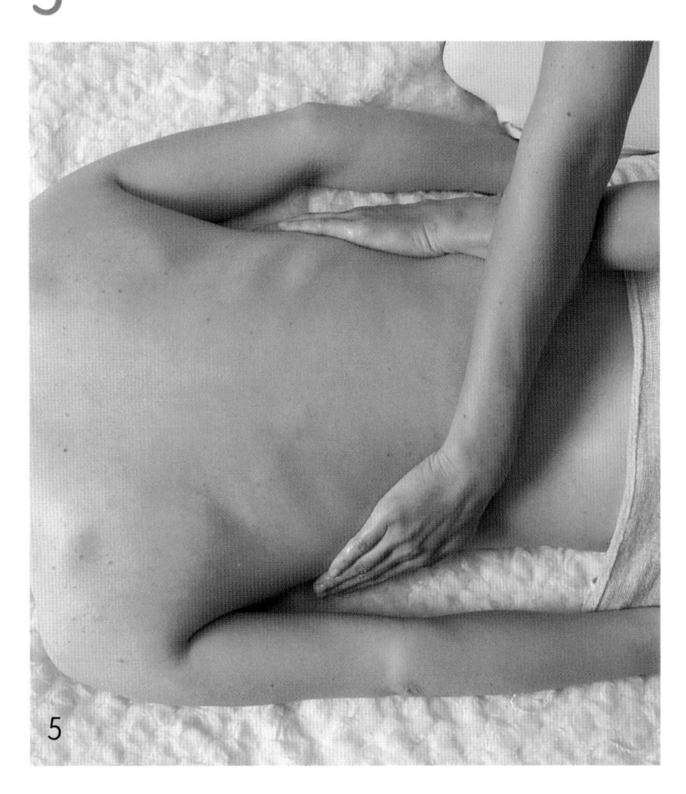

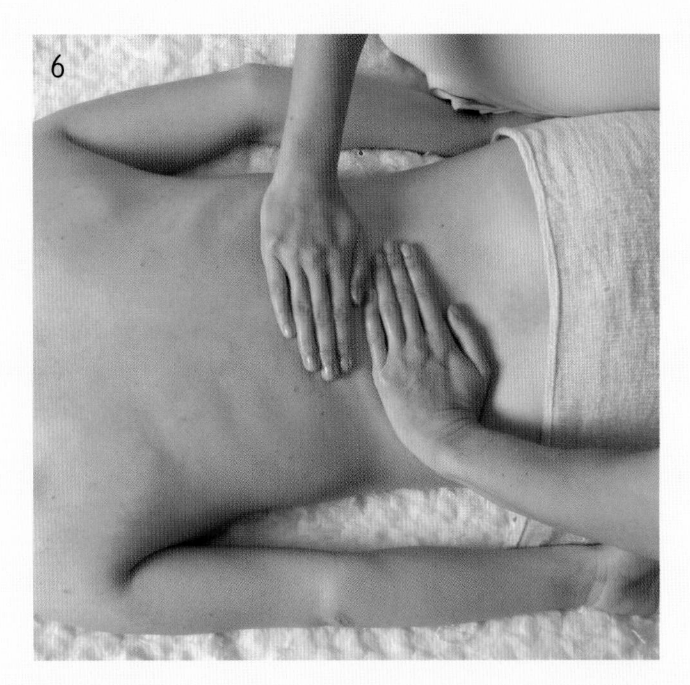

6 Continue sliding the hands down the back and repeat the motion of the hands sliding across, completing the figure-of-eight. Your hands should be slightly higher than the hips.

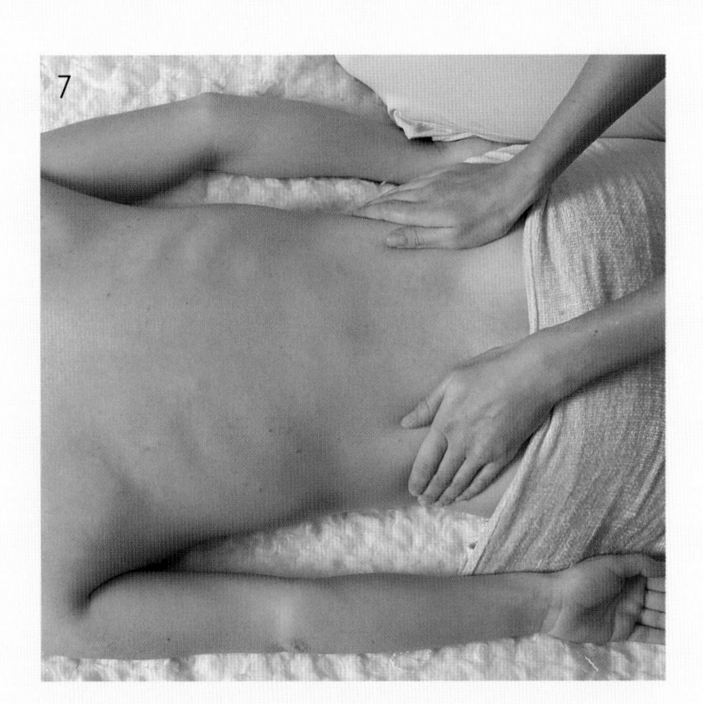

7 As you bring them back to the base of the spine to repeat, lift up slightly.

Note: the pressure should be even and continuous throughout the movement and the rhythm should be slow and controlled.

Thumb walking

This stroke releases toxins. Your partner should feel a lovely rolling motion with the thumbs.

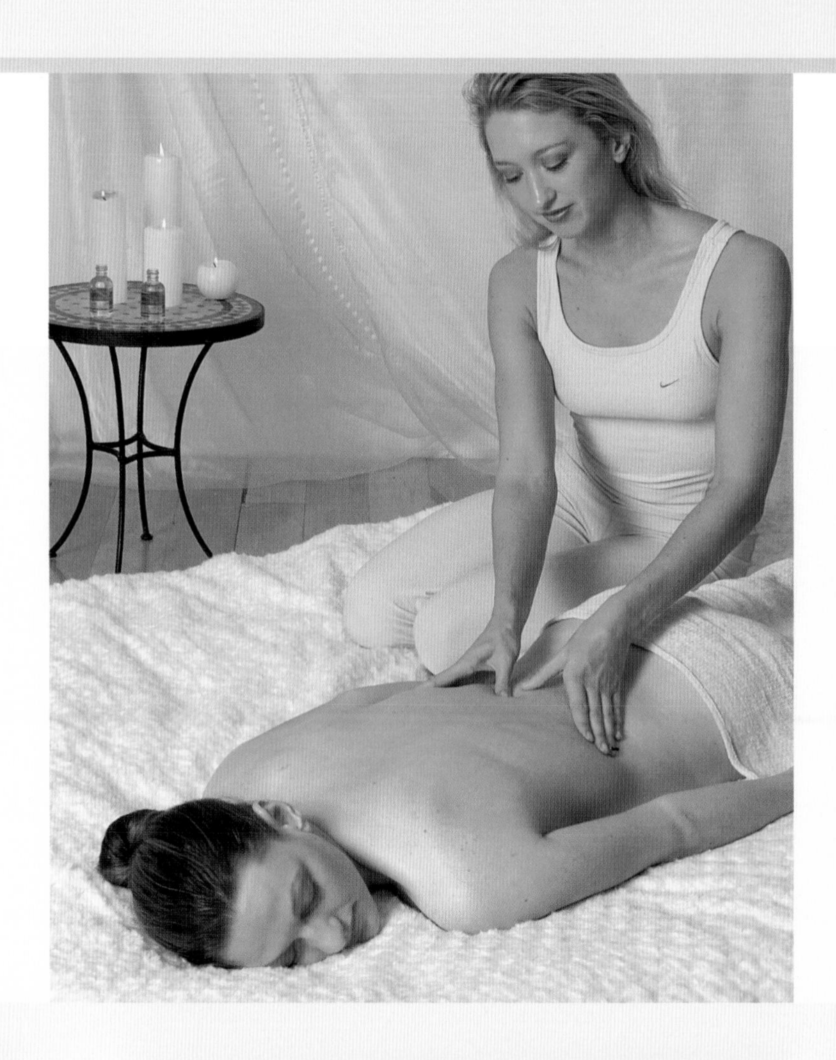

Across lower back

1 Start with the hands at the base of the spine. Think of four lines running along either side of the spine up to the beginning of the ribs.

2 Walk the thumbs up one line by pressing down with one thumb as the other thumb lifts off to replace it. The thumbs should continuously circle each other as they travel up towards the ribs. When you finish one of your imaginary lines, start at the base of the pelvis for the next one.

Repeat until all four lines are complete, then move to the other side and repeat.

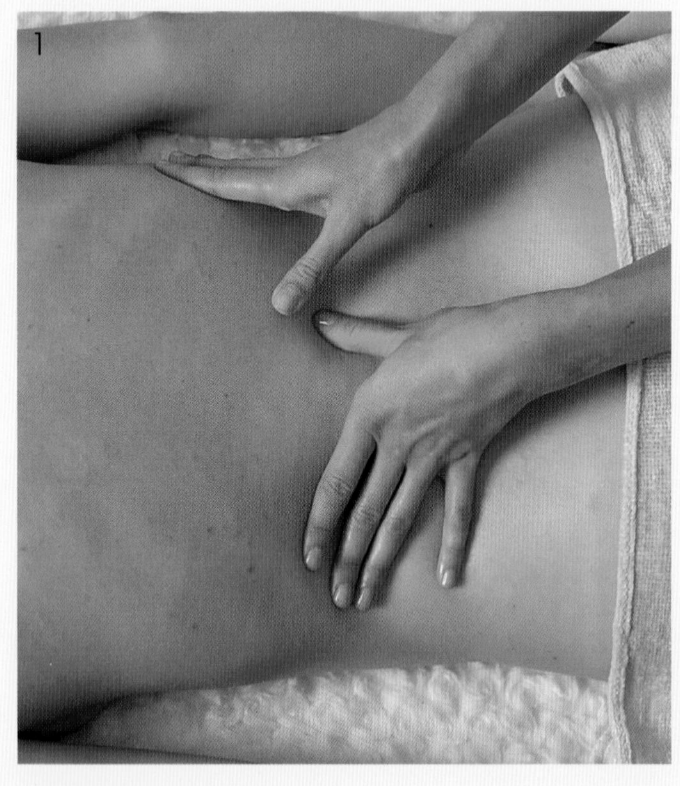

1

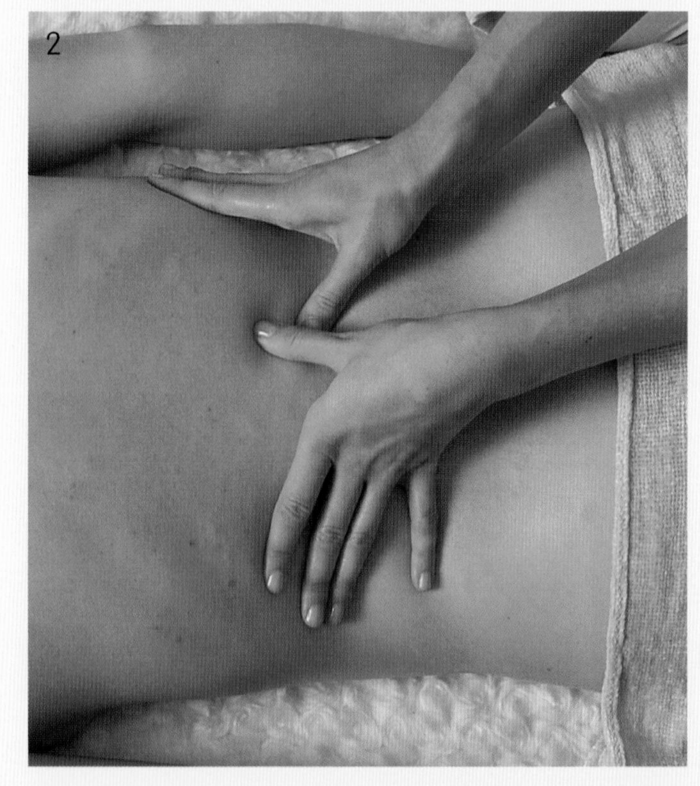

2

Digital pressure

This is a deep pressure stroke.

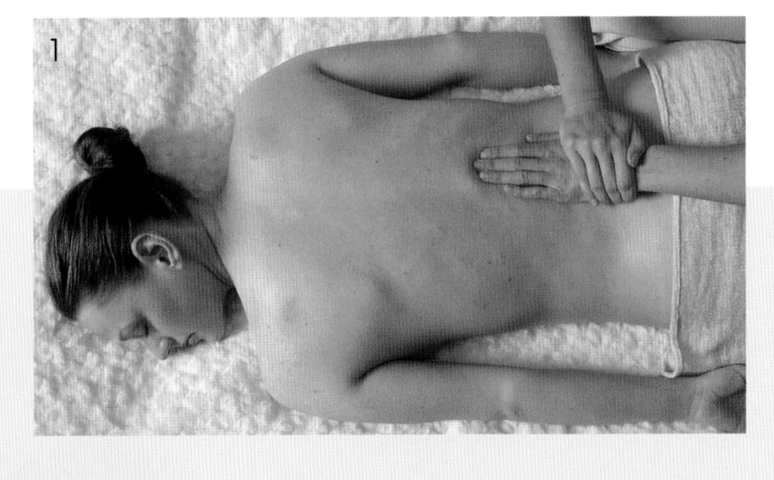

To the back

1 Kneel on the side of the back that you will be working on. Start with the fingers of one hand flat, and the other holding your wrist. Place the flat fingers at the base of the back with the fingertips towards the head.

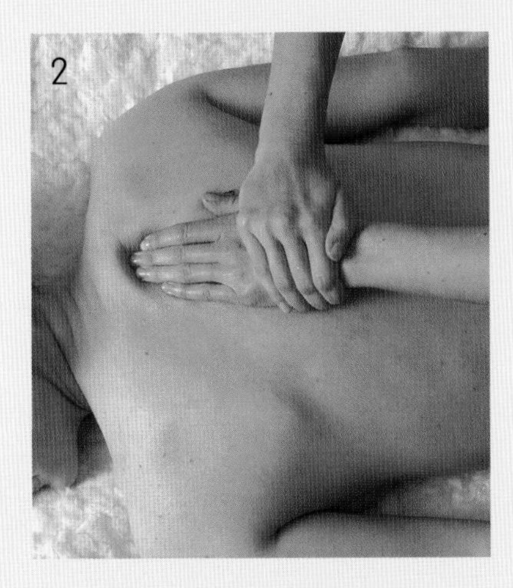

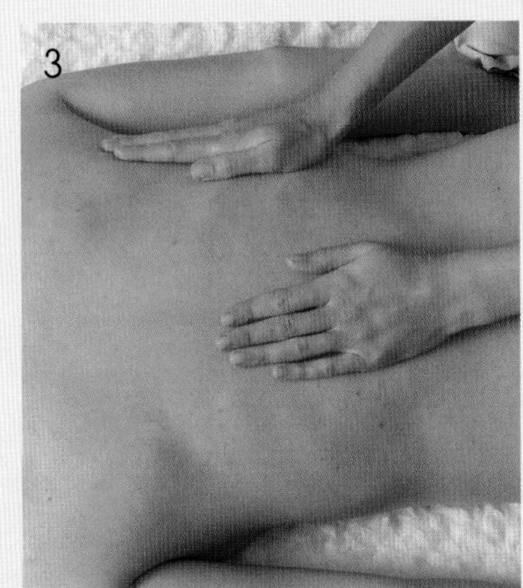

2 Using both arms, press and slide the fingers slowly up towards the neck.

3 Release the hands and slide them in opposite directions across the shoulders and down the outside of the back, moulding to the contour of the body. Put your fingers in a different place on the lower back and repeat. Make sure you are staying on the side of the back that you are on.

Repeat, covering that side, and being careful not to work directly on the spine.

Move to the other side and repeat.

To the legs

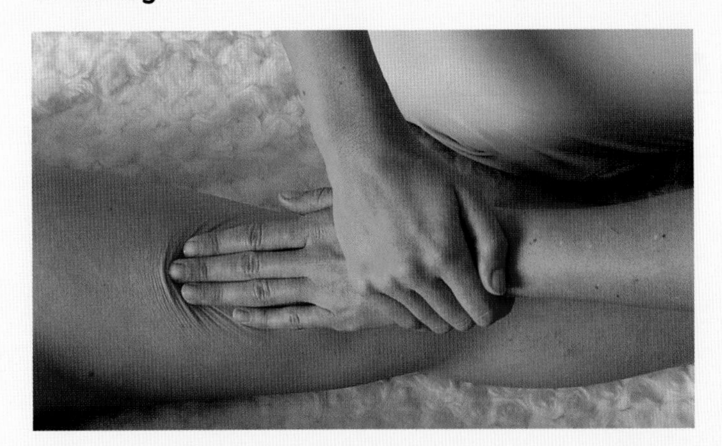

1 Start with the fingers of one hand flat, and the other holding your wrist. Place the flat fingers against the thigh, above the knee. Using both hands, slide the fingers up to the knee. You can use the forearm of the opposite arm as a guide along the leg.

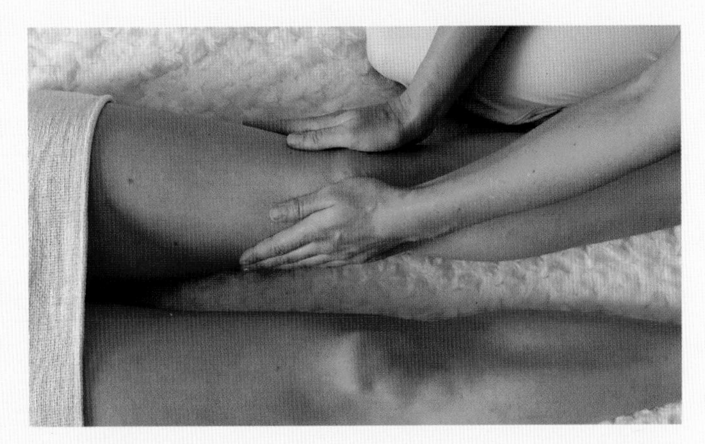

2 Separate the hands and glide them down the outside of the thigh back to the knee.

Move to a different part of the thigh. Repeat until you have covered the entire area. Repeat the whole sequence to the thigh, being careful to avoid the knee area.

Stroking down rib cage 1

This is a very relaxing drainage stroke, performed by the outside of your hands. Imagine a soft rolling motion as you move the edge of your fingertips up and down.

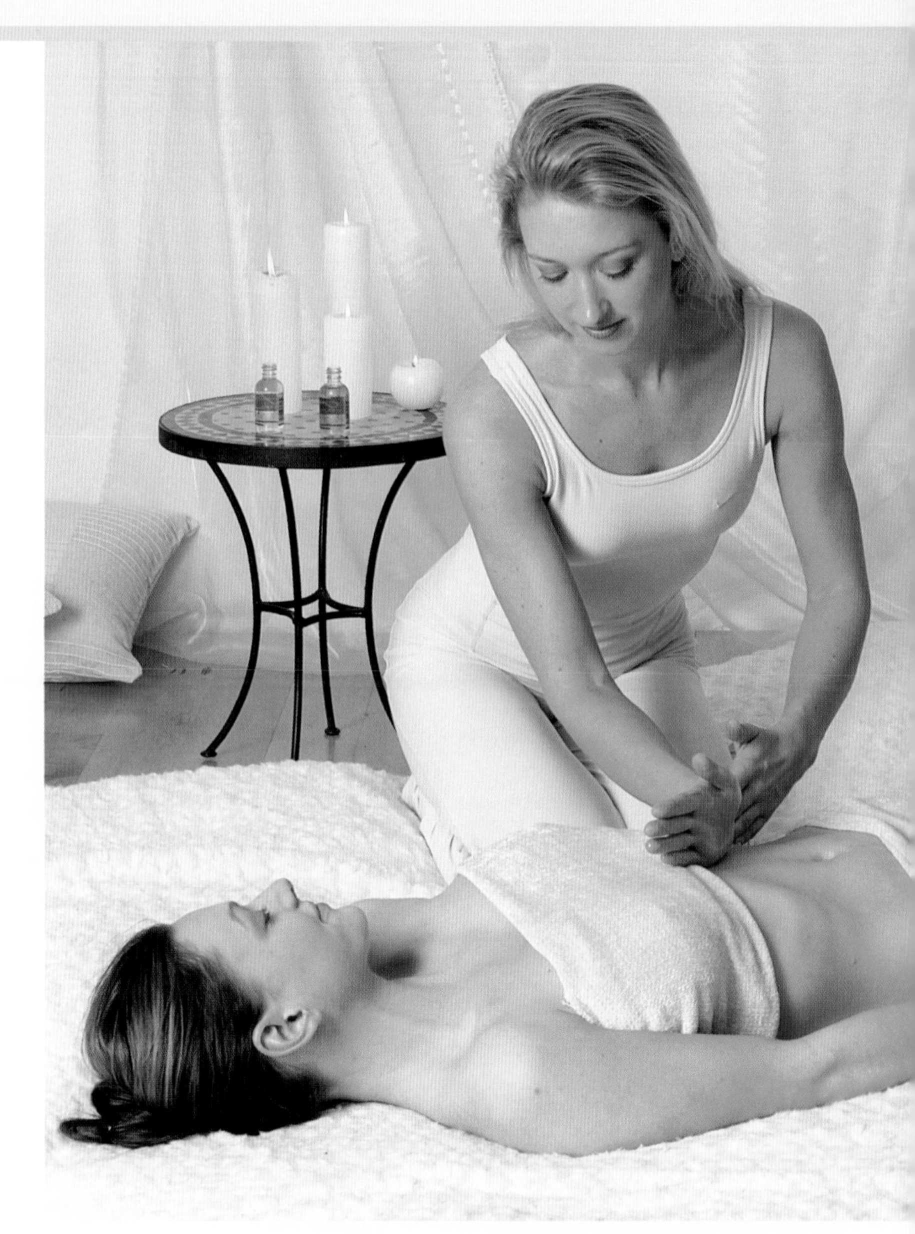

Hand-over-hand

1 Flatten both hands, with the palms facing each other. Think of a gentle slicing motion when performing this stroke. Start on the side of the rib cage nearest to you. Place one hand on the inside edge of the rib cage closest to the breast bone. Slowly drag that hand down the inside line of the rib cage.

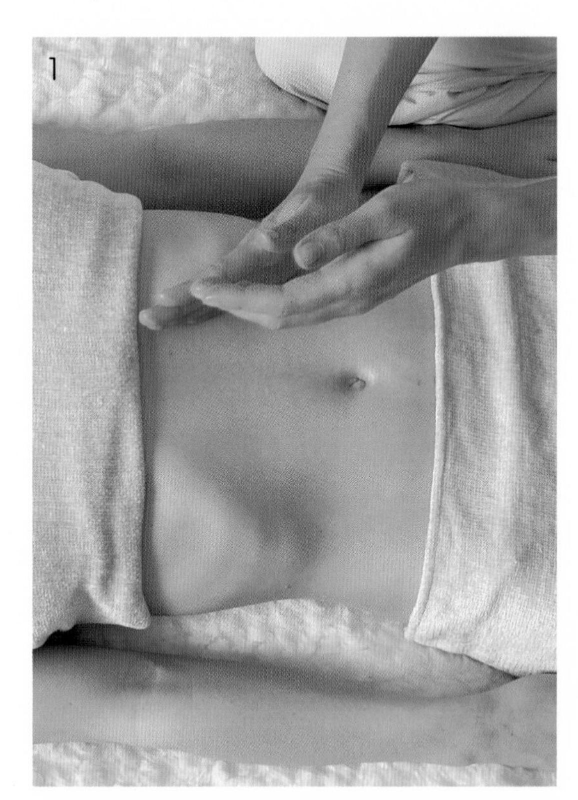

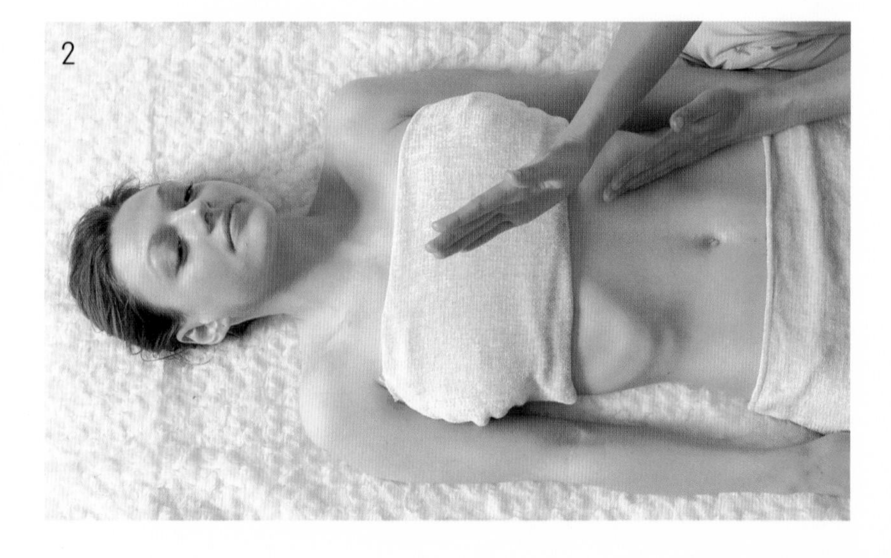

2 As your first hand drags down the inside line of the rib cage, immediately replace it with your other hand. Continue alternating hands along the rib cage in a gently rolling motion. Move to the other side of the body and repeat on the other side.

Stroking down rib cage 2

This is a little more complex than the previous stroke. Remember to work lightly on the stomach as it is a very sensitive area. Imagine making a diamond shape around your partner's stomach.

Two hands

1 Put your fingertips together with your flat hands like two sides of a triangle.Place your hands just below your partner's breastbone on the inside edge of the rib cage.

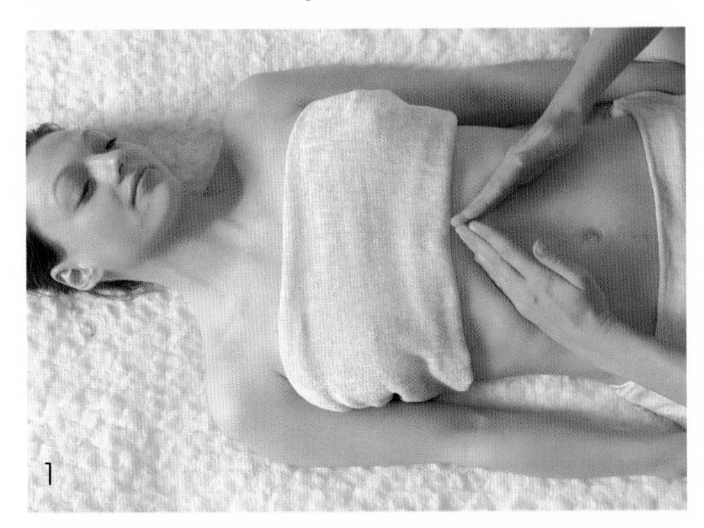
1

2 Slide the hands down the inside of the rib cage. Let your hands roll to the waistline and place them either side of the hips.

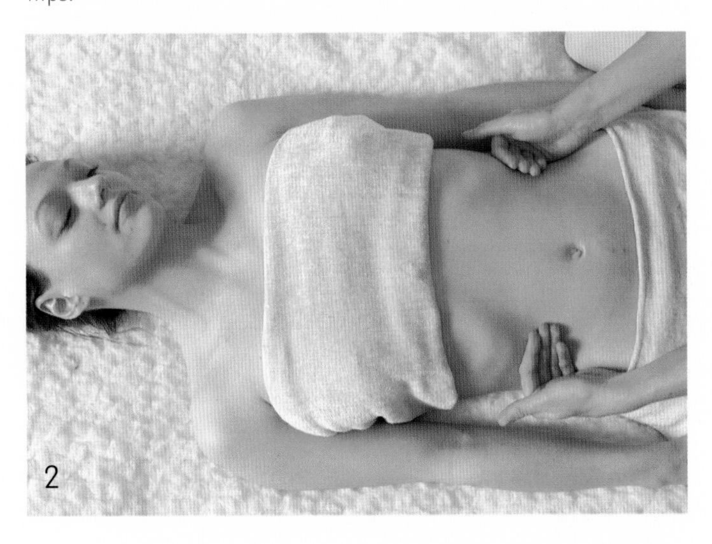
2

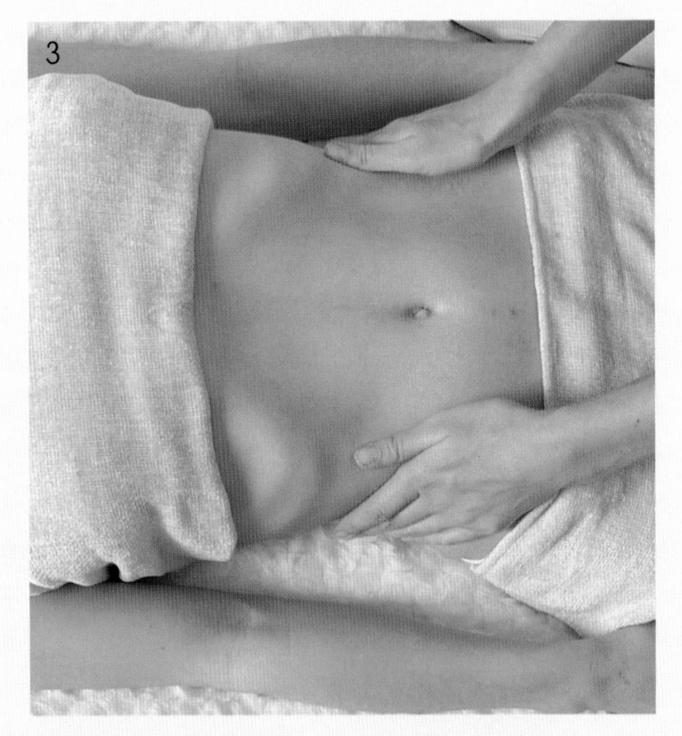
3

3 Lift up with both hands gently on the waistline.

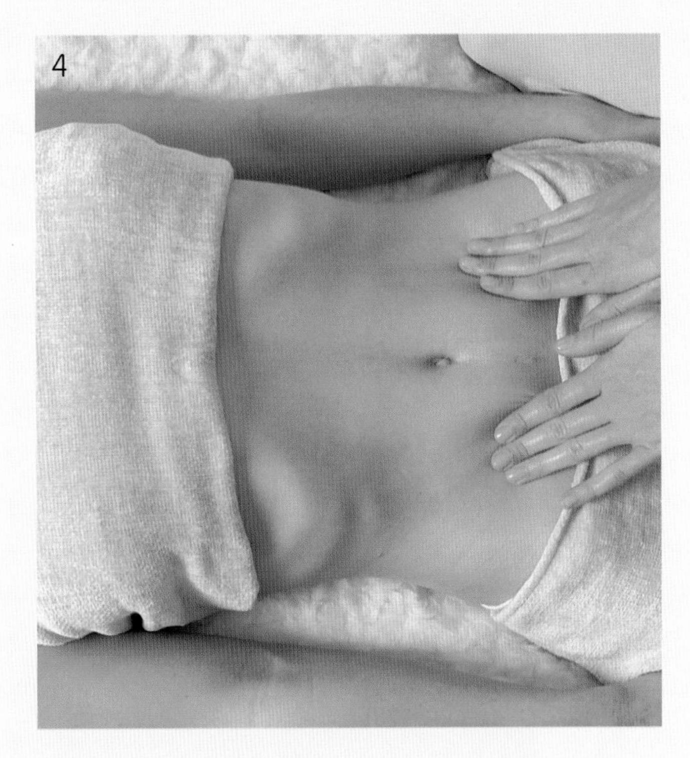
4

4 Lightly drag the fingertips from the waistline to about 5 cm below your partner's navel.

Repeat the entire sequence three times.

Train tracks

This movement works deeply into the muscle, releasing toxins and breaking up lactic acid. It is usually performed on the legs, and is the same whether you are working on the front or back of the upper leg or the calf.

1 Start at the base of the area you are working on. Place your thumbs together in the centre of the area.

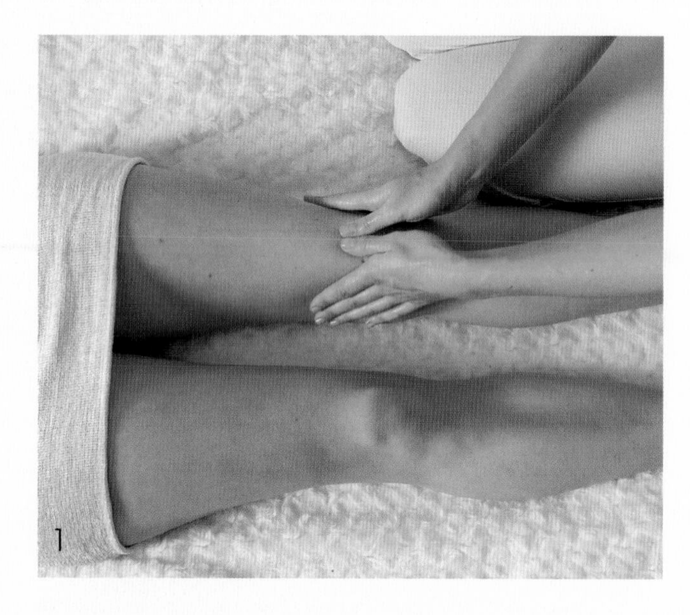

2 Pressing firmly, slide the thumbs up the whole length of the muscle, and then bring the hands out to the sides.

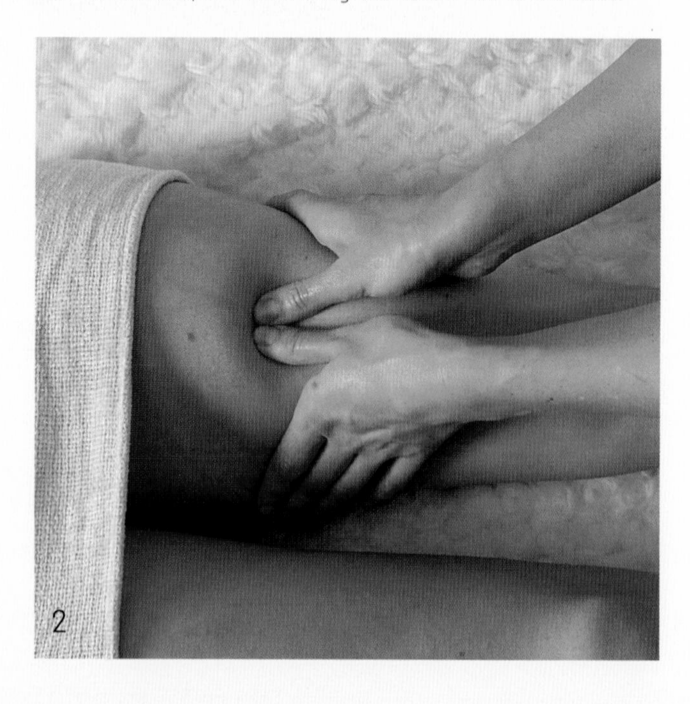

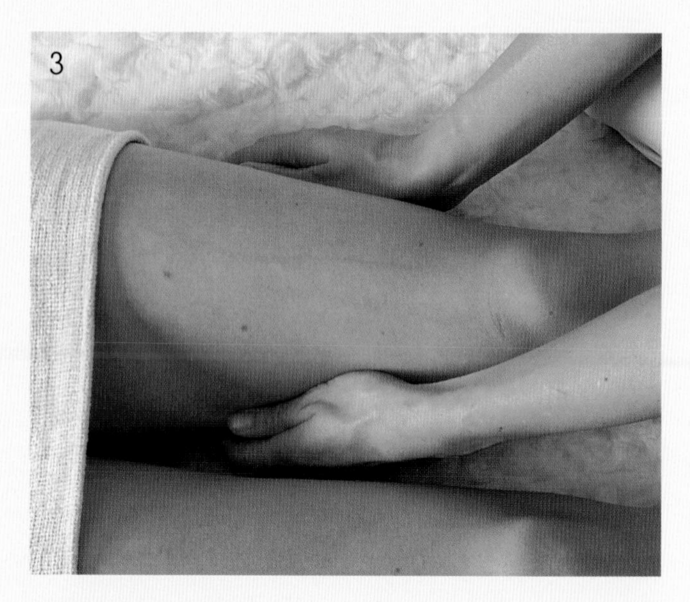

3 Slide the hands halfway down the length of the muscle. Press the palms into the sides and lift up as you bring the palms together.

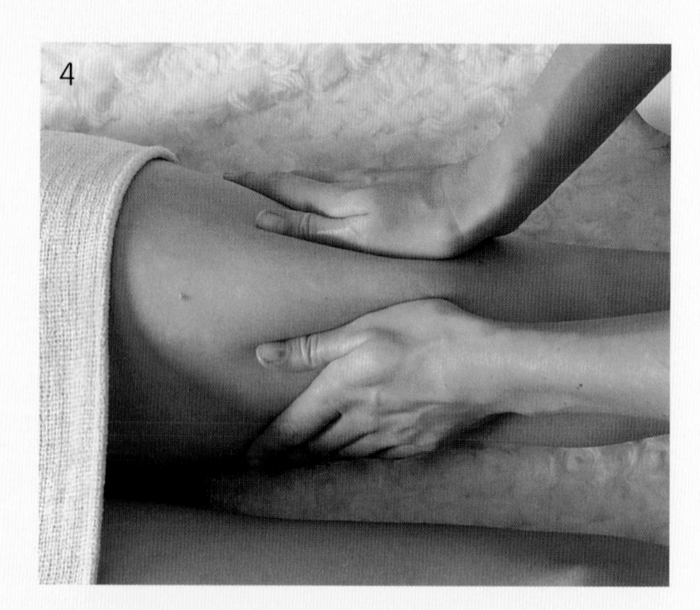

4 Slide the hands lightly back to the original position. Repeat, bringing the thumbs a couple of centimetres apart.

Repeat again with the thumbs 5 cm apart.

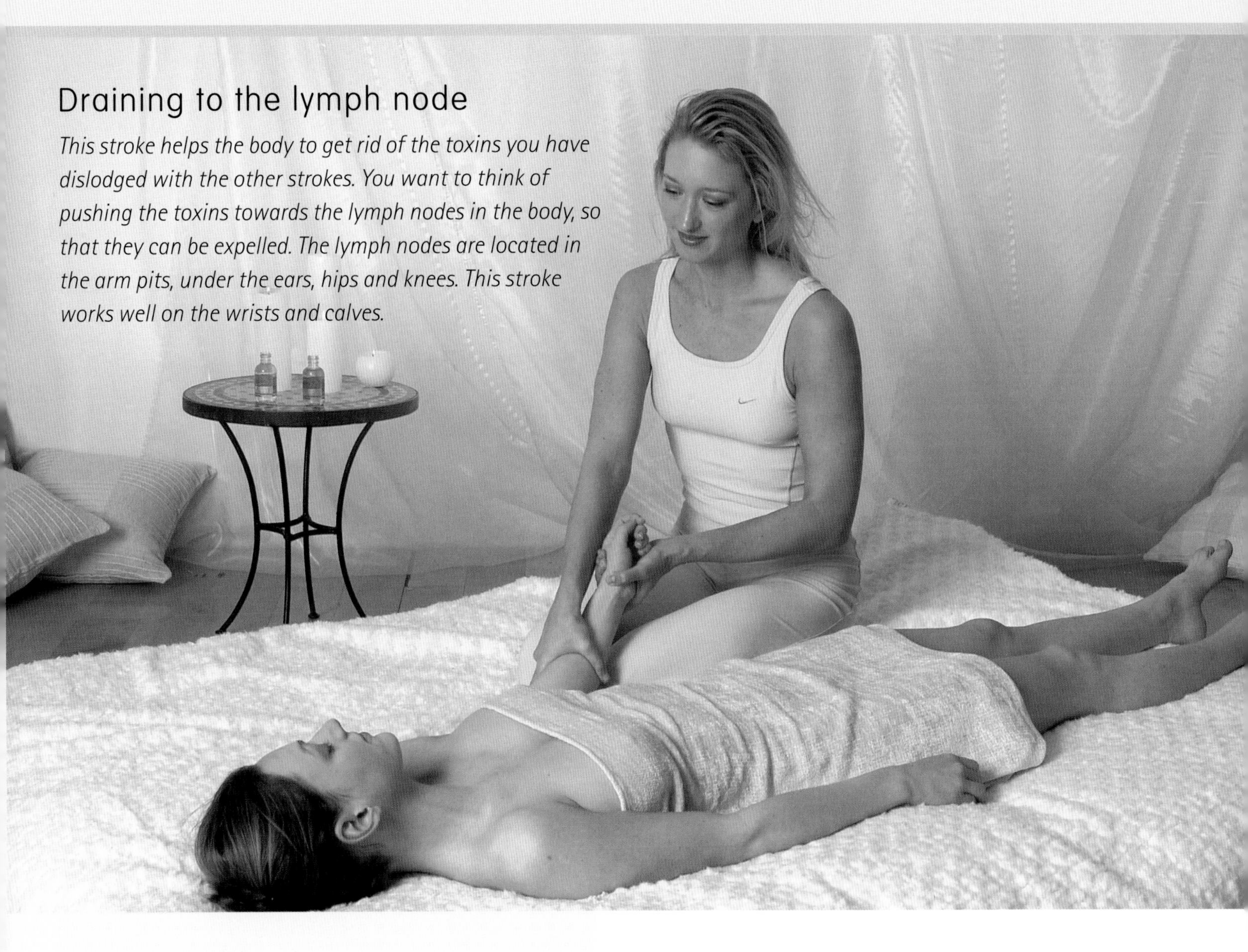

Draining to the lymph node

This stroke helps the body to get rid of the toxins you have dislodged with the other strokes. You want to think of pushing the toxins towards the lymph nodes in the body, so that they can be expelled. The lymph nodes are located in the arm pits, under the ears, hips and knees. This stroke works well on the wrists and calves.

On the leg

If you are working on the calf, lift the ankle up with one hand, and place the palm of the other hand across the ankle. Using short, sweeping motions, work your way down to the knee. The pressure should be firm and controlled.

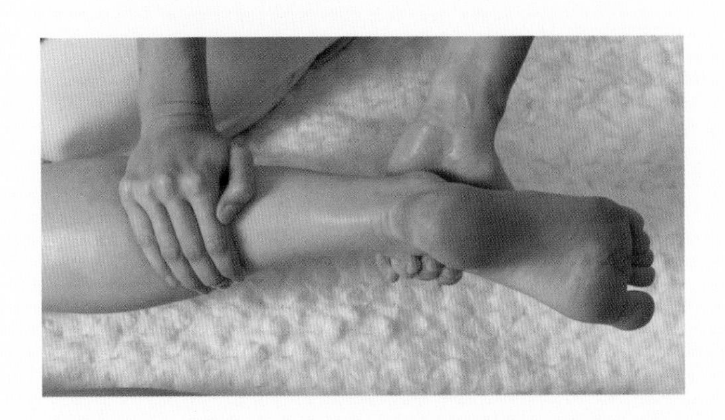

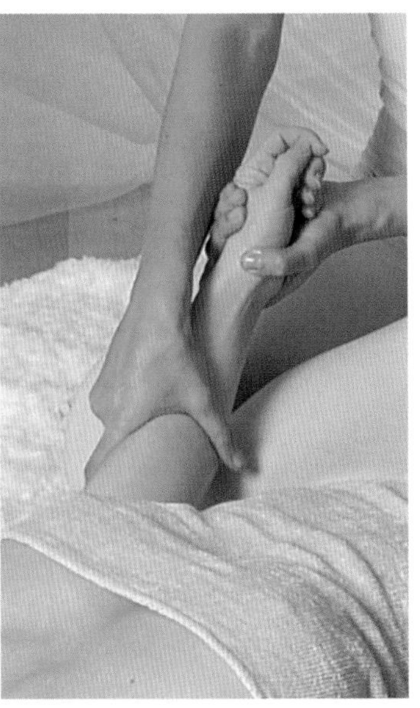

On the arm

Hold the hand slightly lifted up. Take your opposite hand, and place the wedge between the thumb and finger onto the wrist. In short sweeping motions, work your way down to the elbow. Repeat three times.

Forearms

Forearms can be used in several ways and are great to use in a massage if your hands are getting tired.

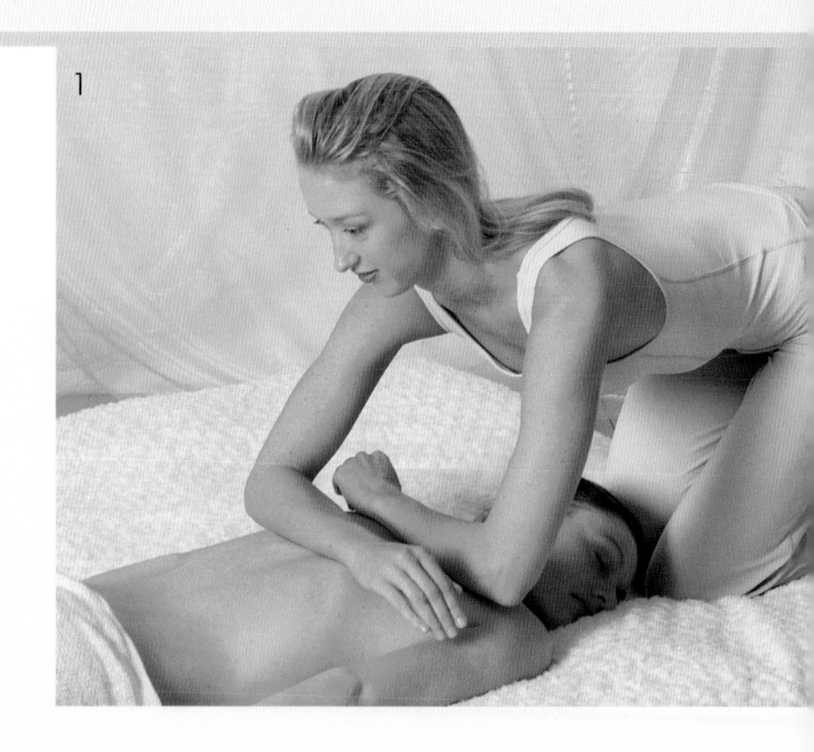

On the back

1 Kneel at the head of your partner facing their feet. Place the fleshy part of your forearms in a parallel line across the shoulders.

2 Lean your weight into your arms and slowly drag your forearms down to the pelvis.

3 Bend your elbows out to the sides so the arms form a loose diamond shape.

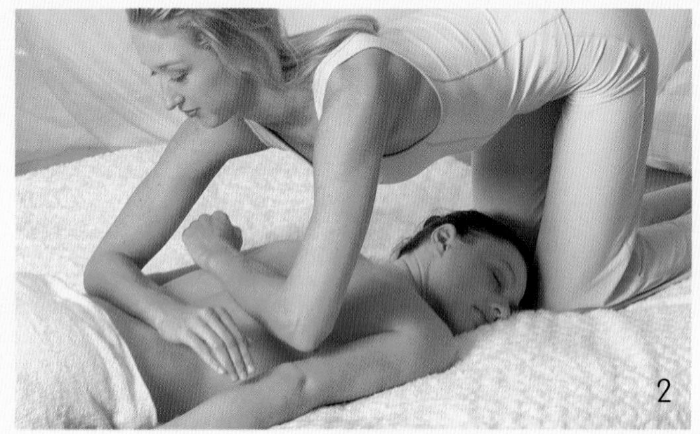

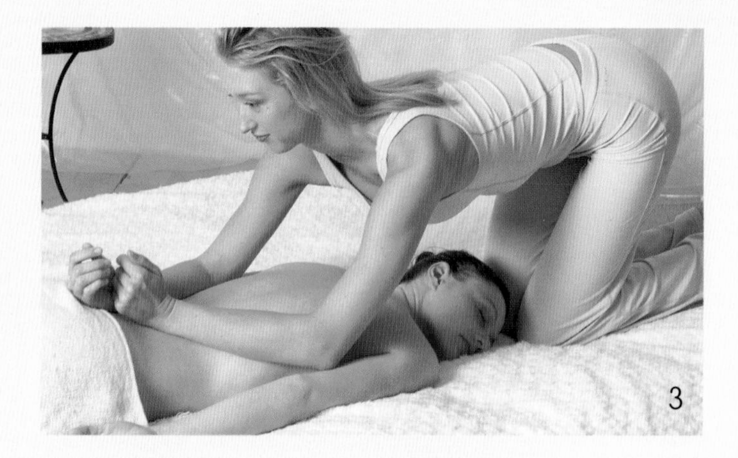

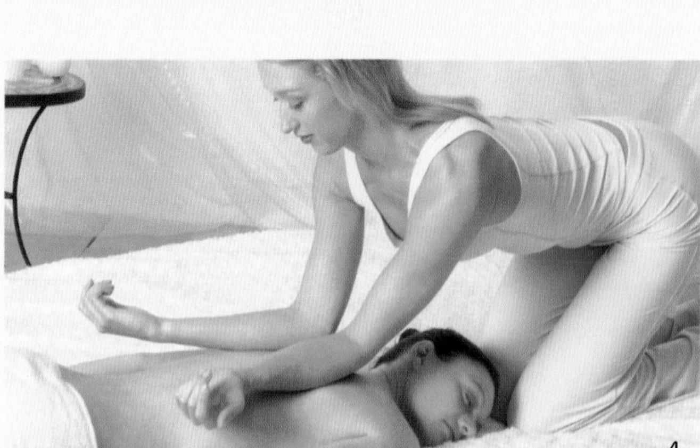

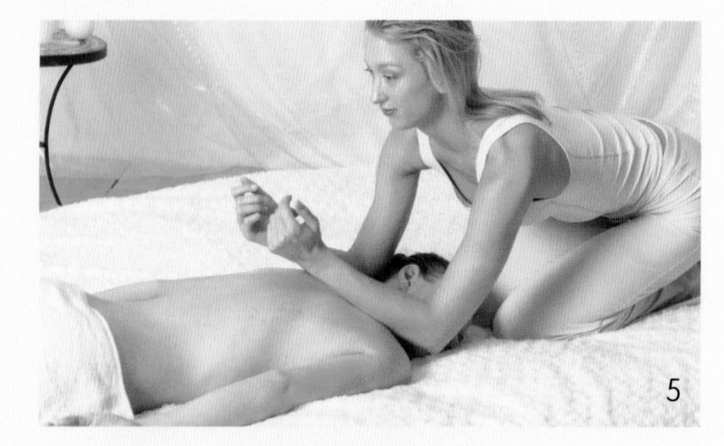

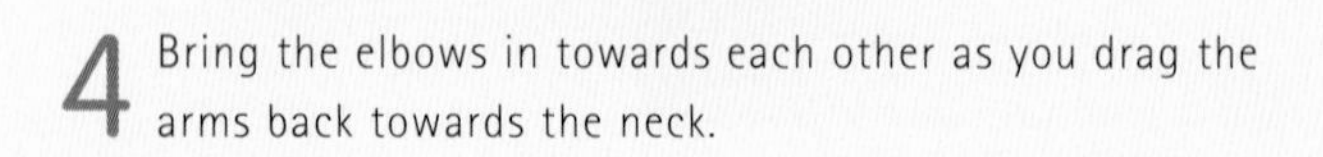

4 Bring the elbows in towards each other as you drag the arms back towards the neck.

5 Slide your forearms across either side of the neck. Bring your forearms back into a parallel line across the shoulders to start again.

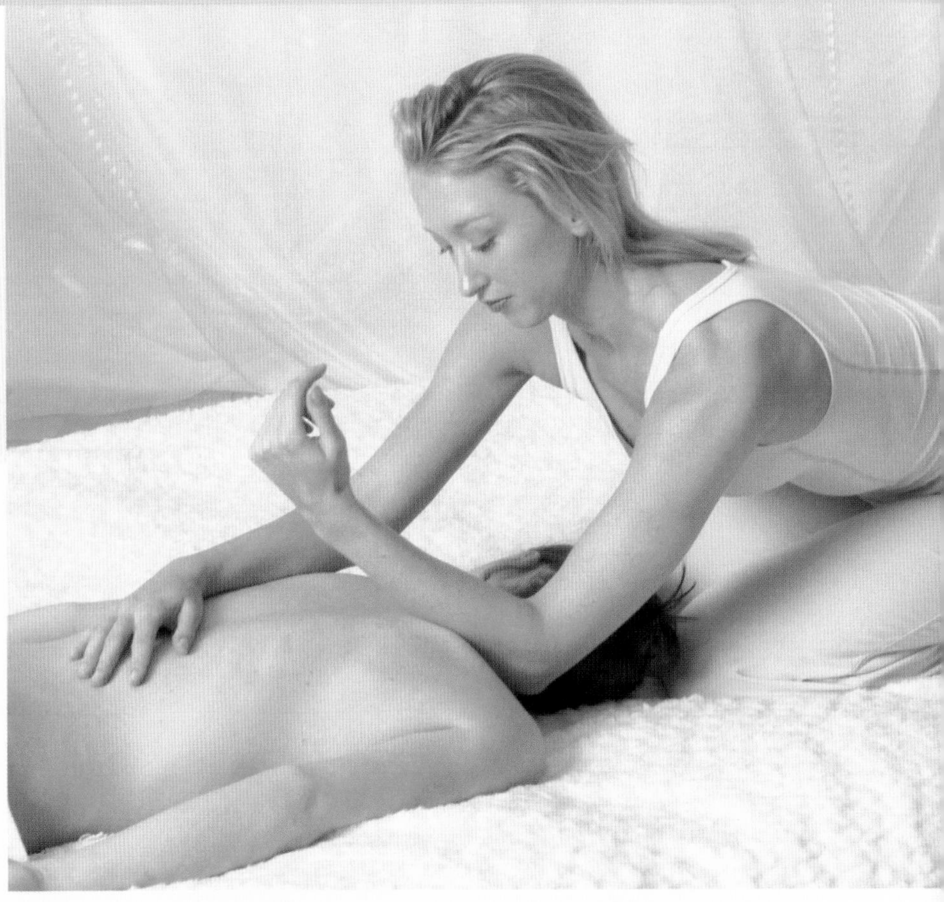

To the neck – one arm

Continue kneeling at your partner's head facing their feet. Have your partner turn their head to the opposite side of the side you are working on. Place one forearm in the groove of their neck with the palm facing you. Slide the forearm up and down from the wrist to the elbow, releasing any tension.

To the lower back

1 Kneel to the side of your partner and place one wrist against their waistline.

2 Press the wrist into their waist as you slide the forearm up. Turn the palm over as you slide the forearm back down. Think of a saw or violin action as you do this.

Repeat several times.

Repeat to the other side.

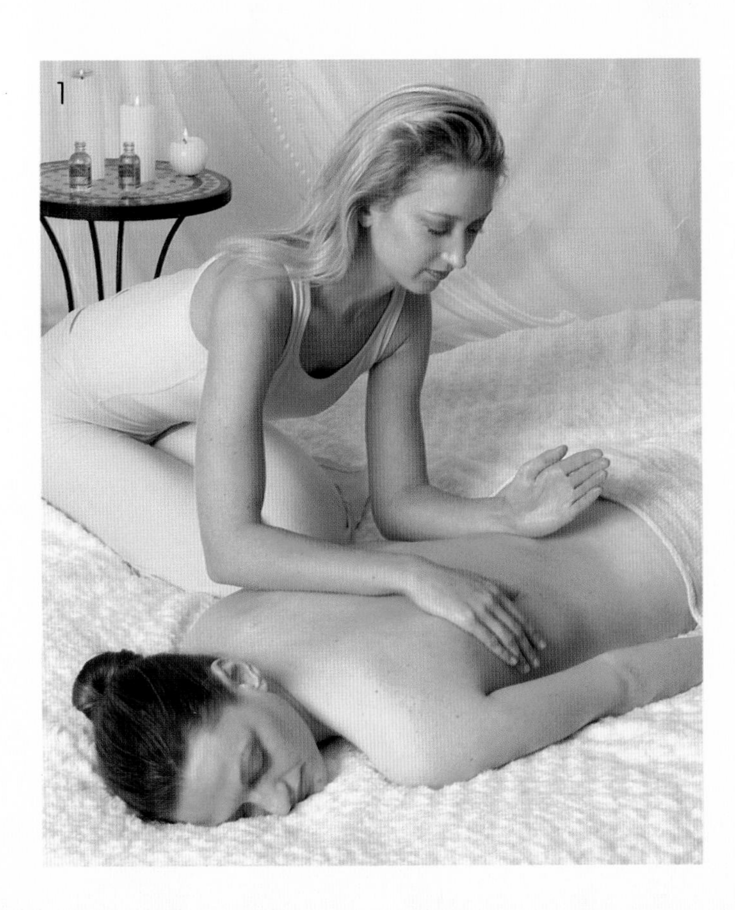

1

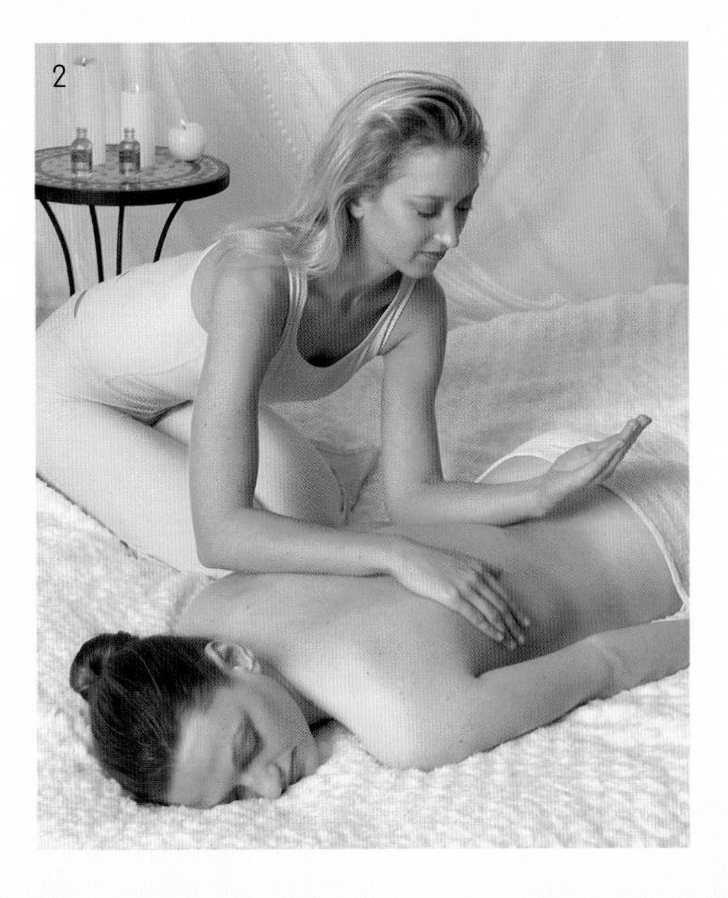

2

Arch back

This stroke is performed with your partner lying on their back.

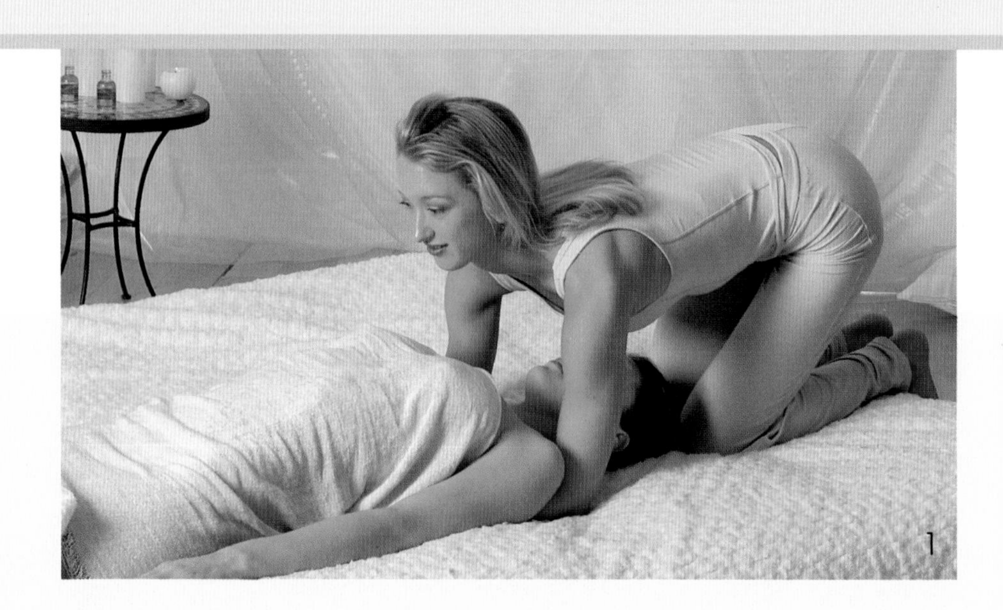

1 Kneel at your partner's head facing their feet. Ask your partner to lift their shoulders slightly and arch their back. While they do this, slide your hands underneath them as far down either side of the spine as you can comfortably reach.

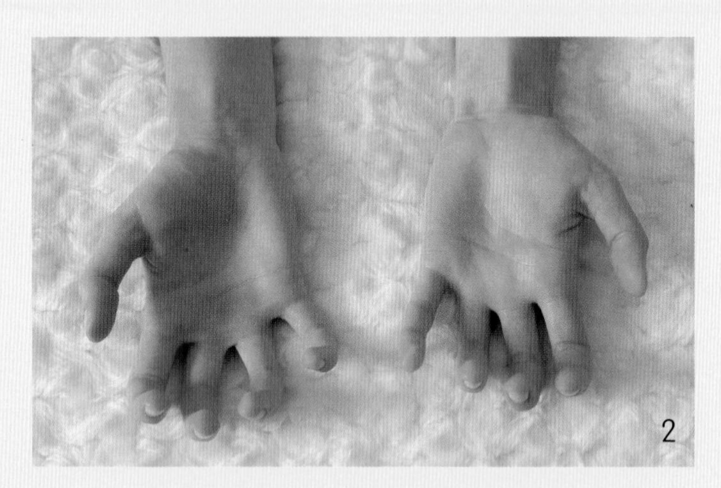

2 Form claws with both of your hands.

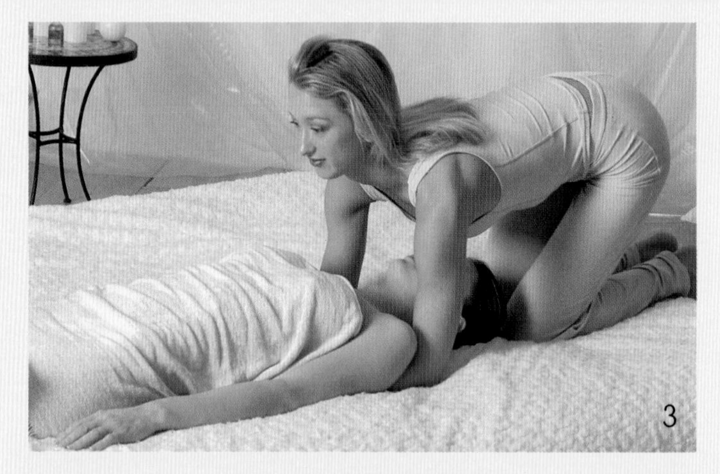

3 Ask your partner to relax their weight onto your fingertips.

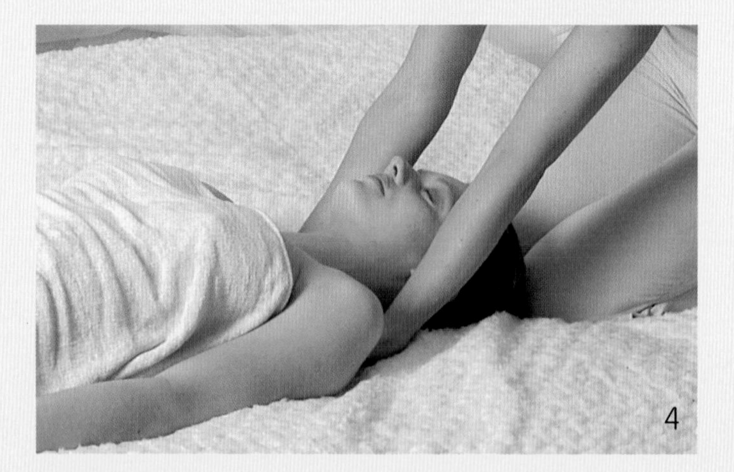

4 Drag your hands up either side of the spine towards the neck, pressing firmly into the flesh with your fingertips.

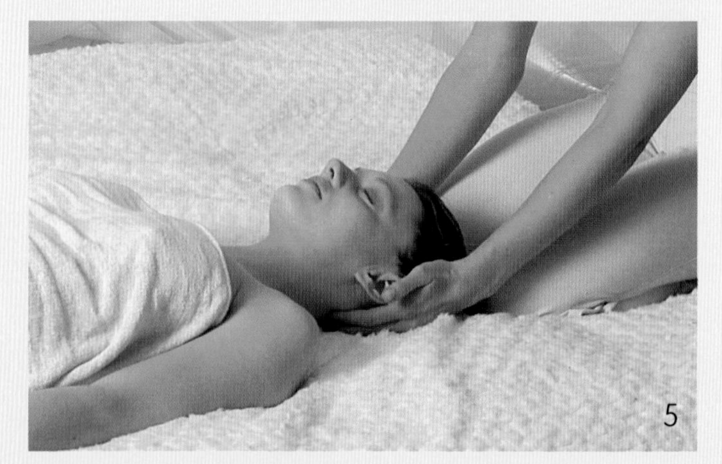

5 Keep sliding the hands along the neck to the head. When you reach your partner's hair, gently pull the hair towards you. Repeat this about three times.

Arm stretch

1 Hold your partner's wrist with one hand and bring the arm above their head. Place your opposite hand under the towel towards their waist.

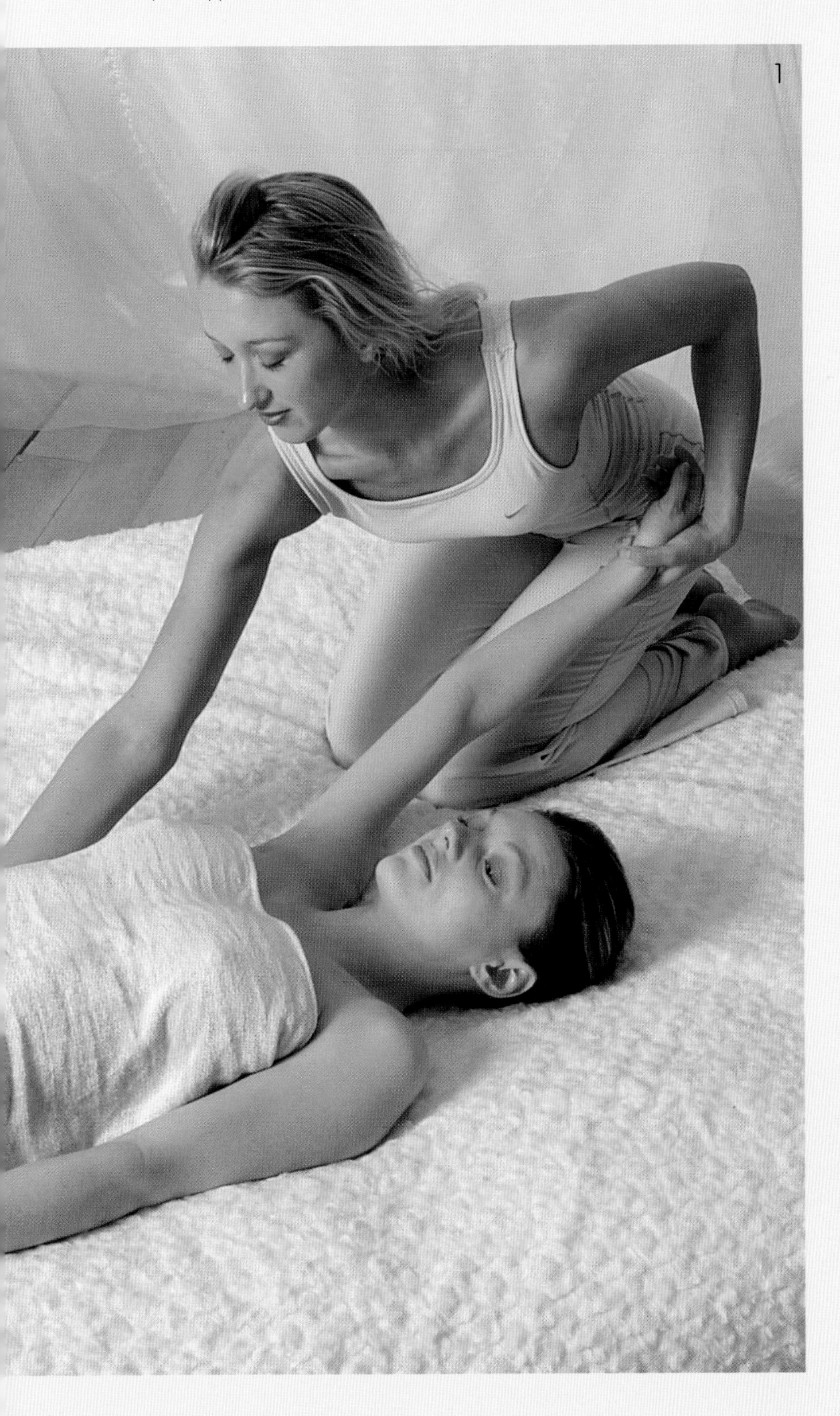

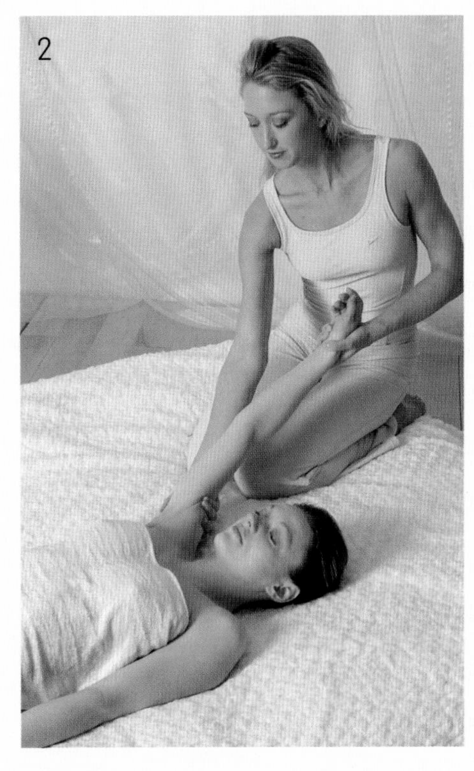

2 Glide your hand along their waistline and up to the shoulder cuff.

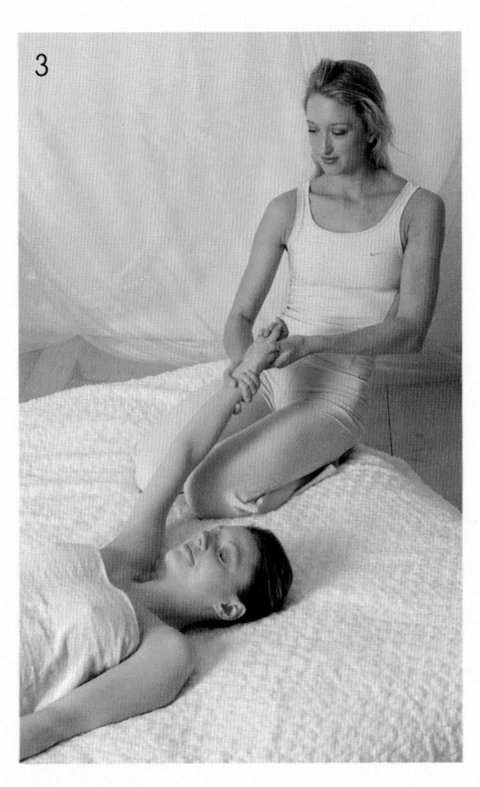

3 Continue up to the wrist. Gently pull the arm and repeat a few times.

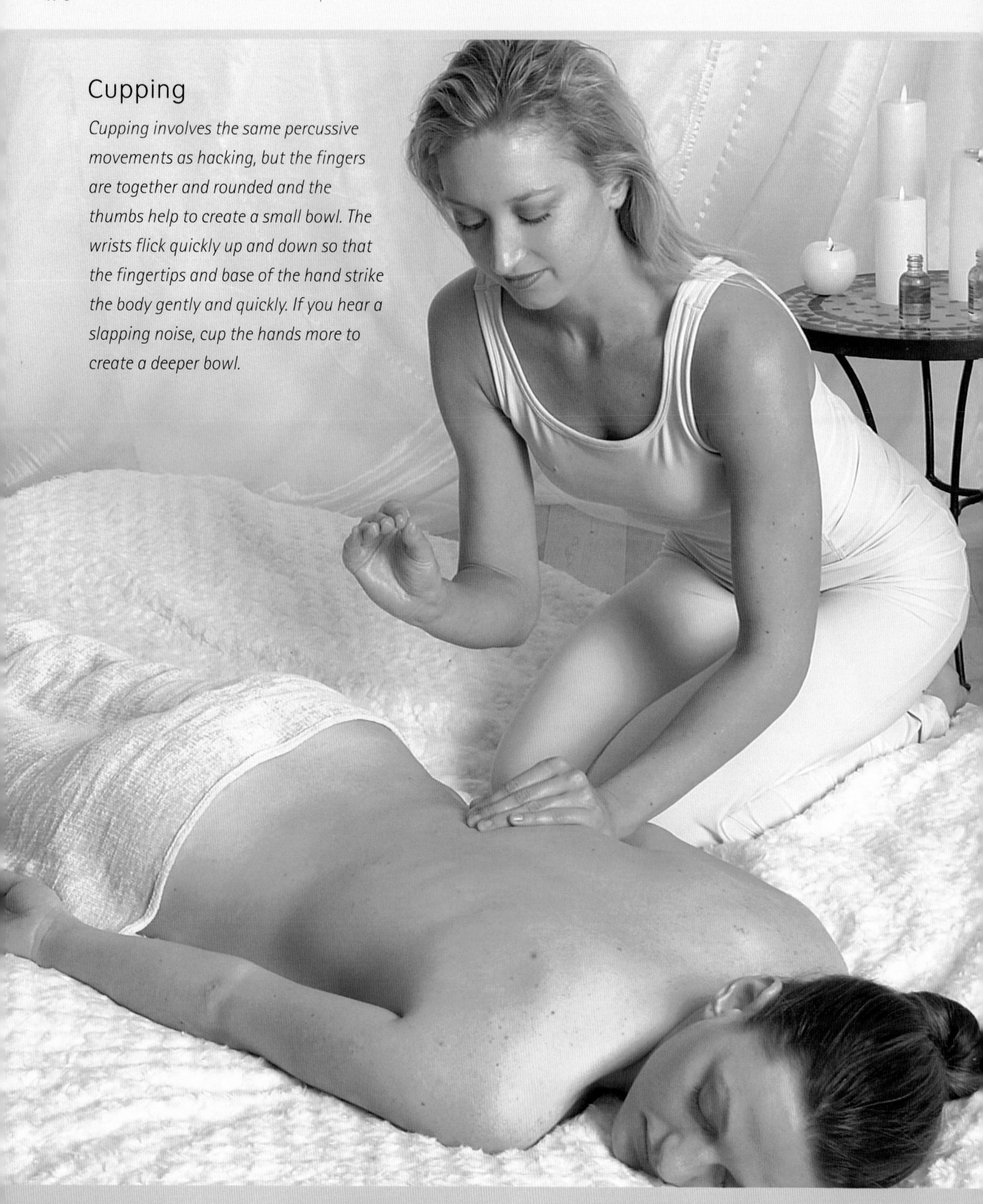

Cupping

Cupping involves the same percussive movements as hacking, but the fingers are together and rounded and the thumbs help to create a small bowl. The wrists flick quickly up and down so that the fingertips and base of the hand strike the body gently and quickly. If you hear a slapping noise, cup the hands more to create a deeper bowl.

On the back

1 Kneel at your partner's side facing their back. Place the fingers together and round the hands to create a bowl shape. Pretend you are trying to hold water in your hands.

2 Turn the hands over above the back. Quickly strike the back, using the wrists to create fast, rhythmic movements and covering the whole of the back, avoiding the kidneys.

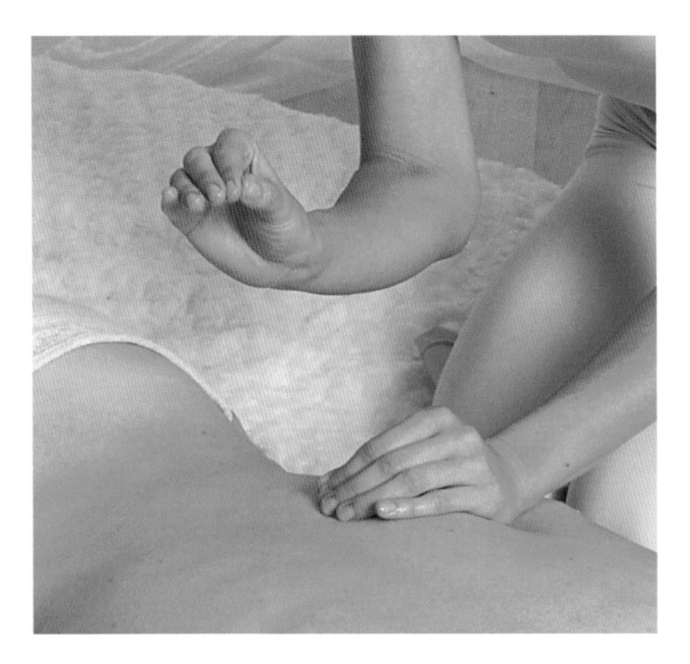

On the legs

Kneel facing the thigh, with your knees bent and your hands in a small bowl shape just above the thighs. Quickly strike the thighs with fast, percussive movements.

Repeat to the calves.

Note: avoid the back of the knee.

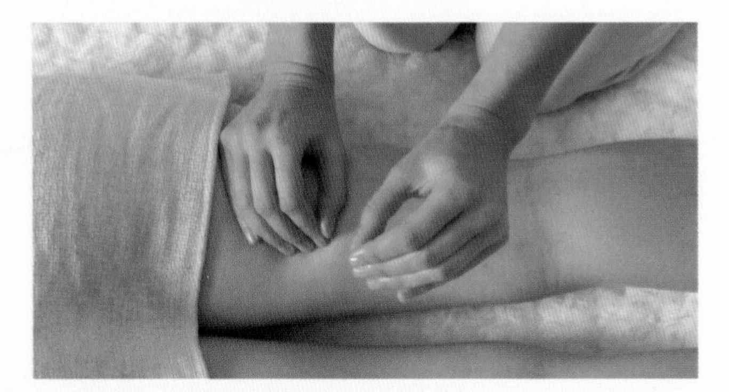

Fists

This is a percussive stroke, which is useful for the buttocks.

Leave the buttocks covered with a towel. Kneel to the side, facing the buttocks. Form loose fists with your hands. Strike the buttocks lightly with your fists, alternating your hands. Cover the entire area.

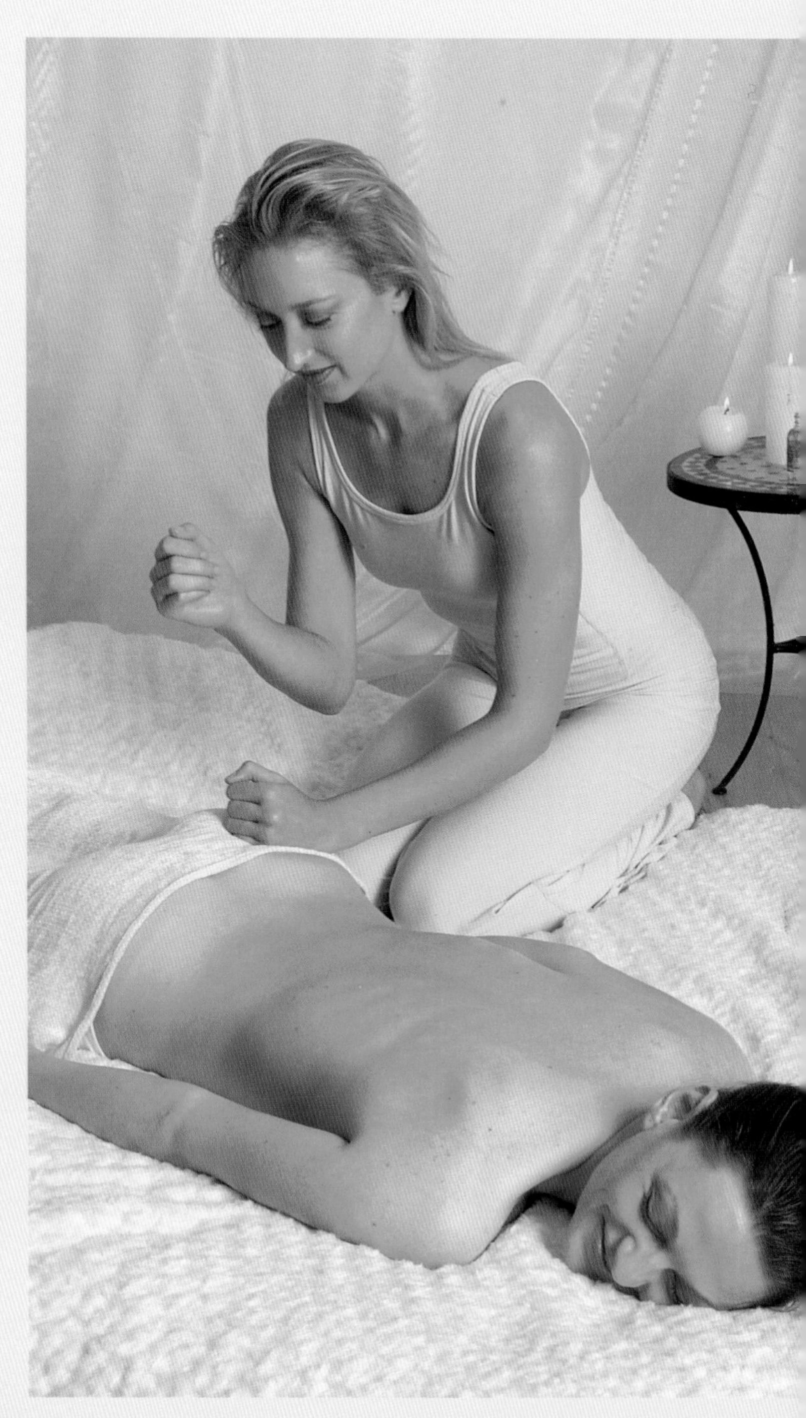

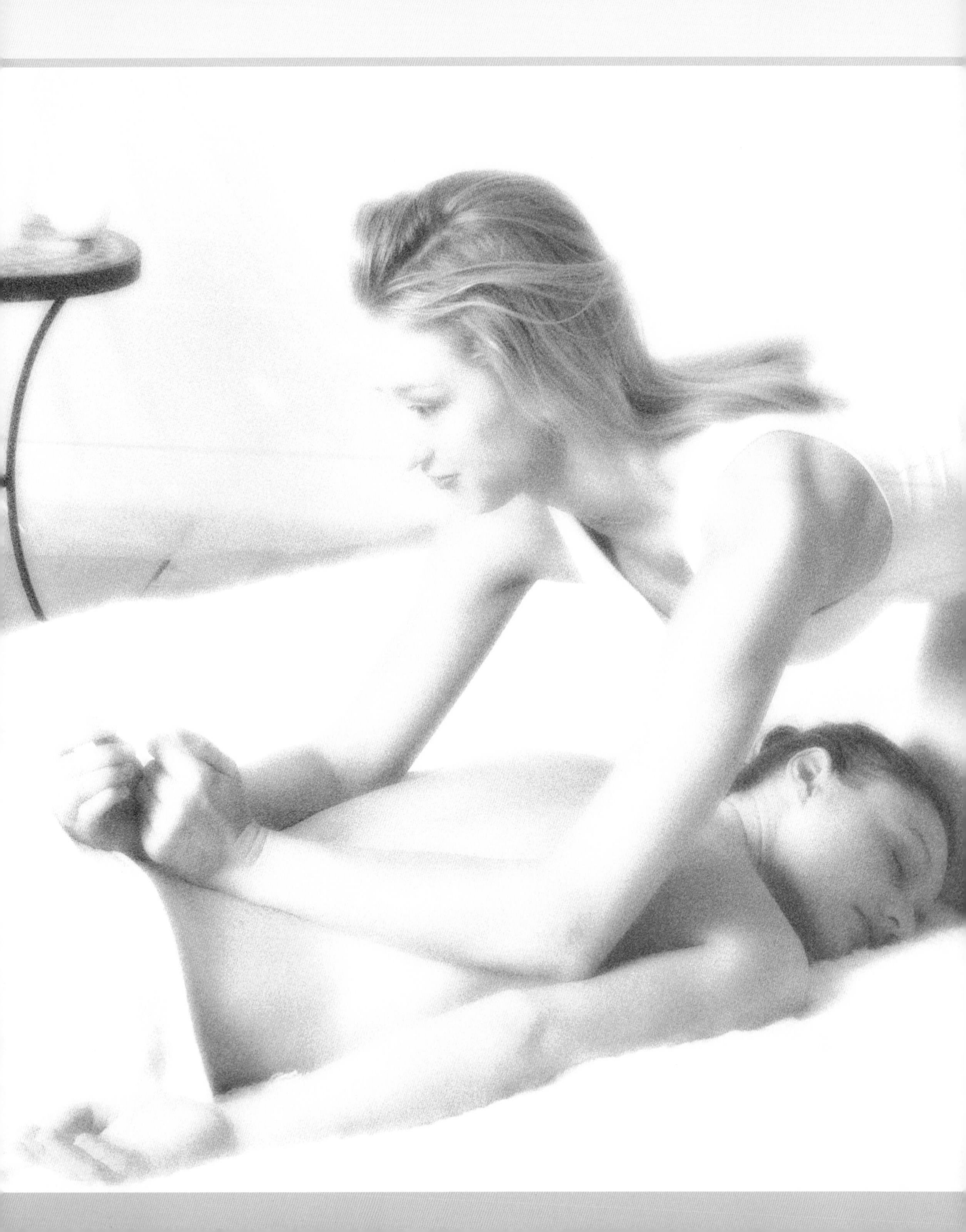

Advanced massage

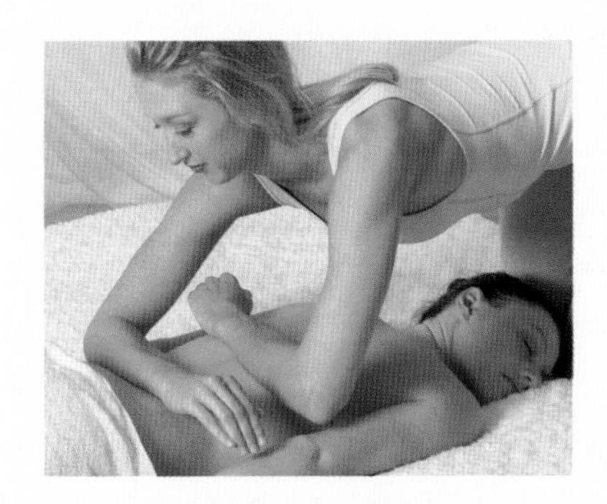

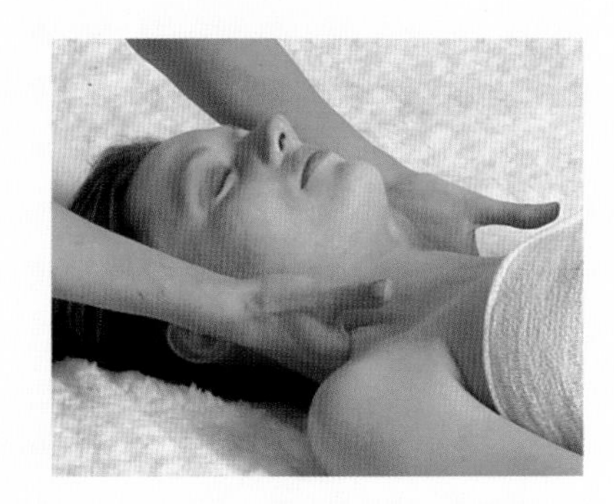

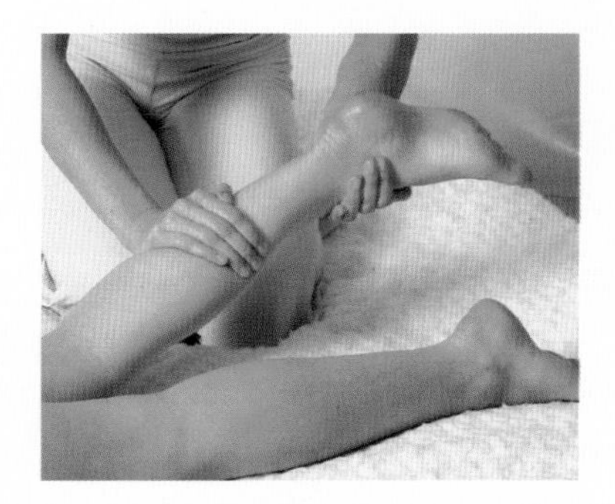

This massage incorporates some of the strokes from the previous sections. It does not contain all the strokes or the massage would simply last for hours. Try to think about everything you have learned from the previous sections. Concentrate on your posture, the pressure of your hands, the transitions between strokes, and feeling the reaction of your partner's muscles.

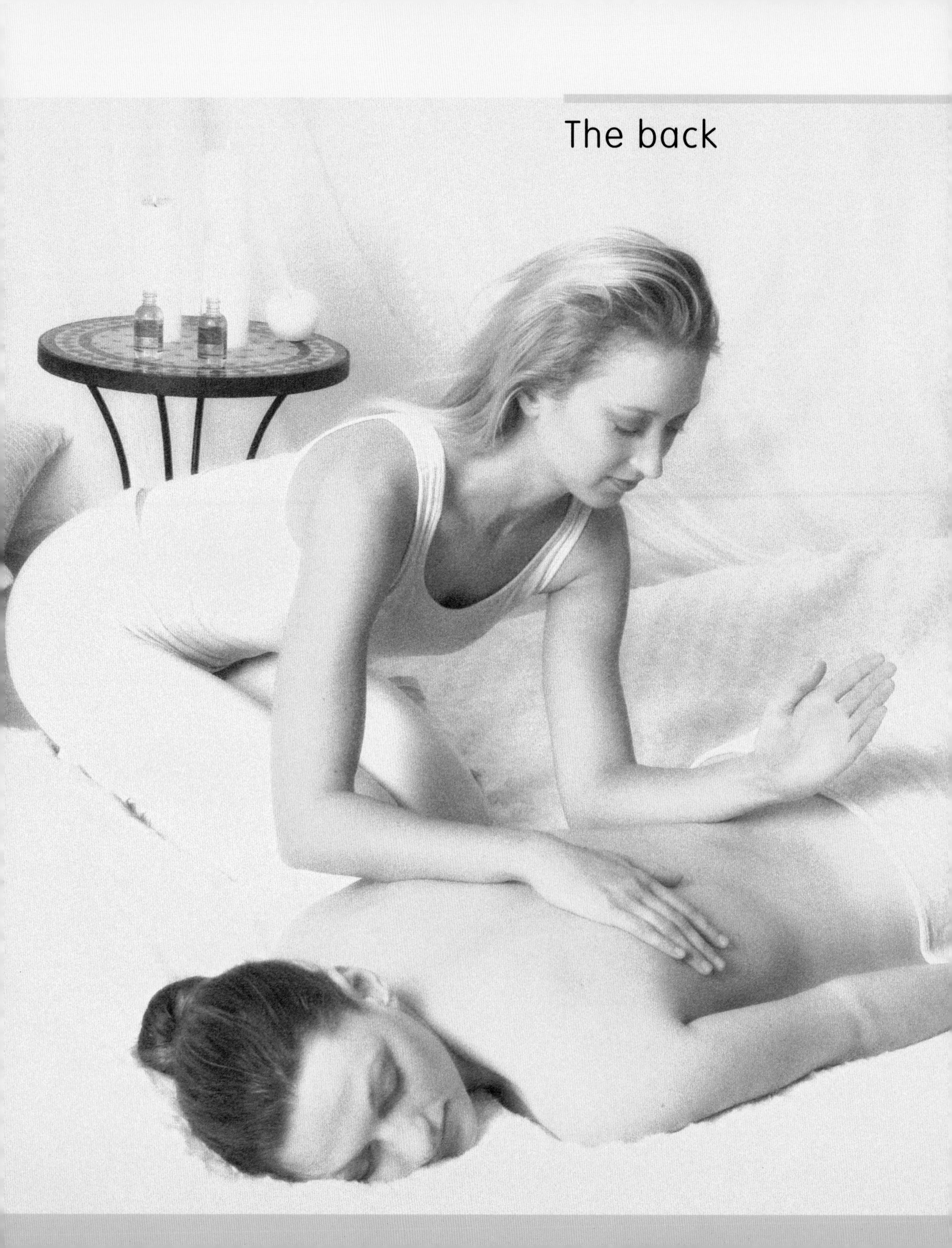

The back

Softening: Kneel to one side of your partner. Place the palms of your hands on one side of the fleshy part of the spine. Gently press into the flesh and release. Repeat along both sides of the spine. Vigorously rub over the entire back.

1 **Spreading the oil:** Uncover the entire back. Place a small amount of oil in the palm of one hand. Rub your hands together and spread the oil up the back.

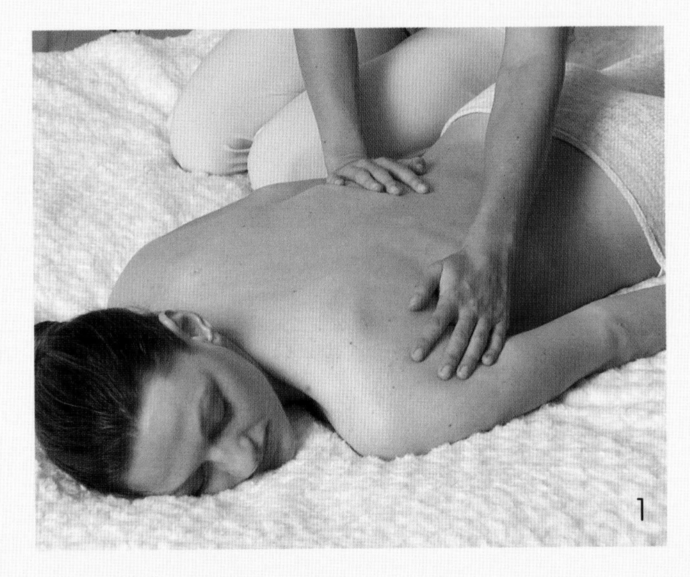
1

3 **Friction:** Place the thumbs on the outside of the base of the spine. Make circles up the spine, using the whole arm to make the circles and not the thumb joint. Flatten the hands across the shoulders and back down the outside of the back. Maintain contact the whole time. Repeat 3 times.

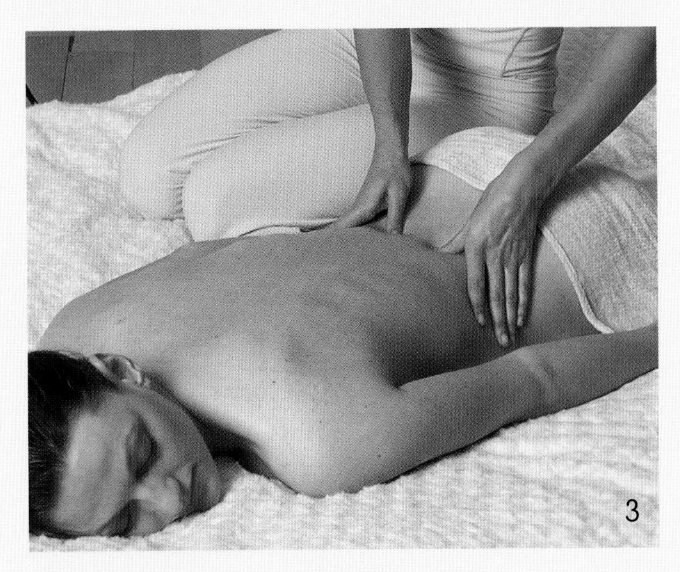
3

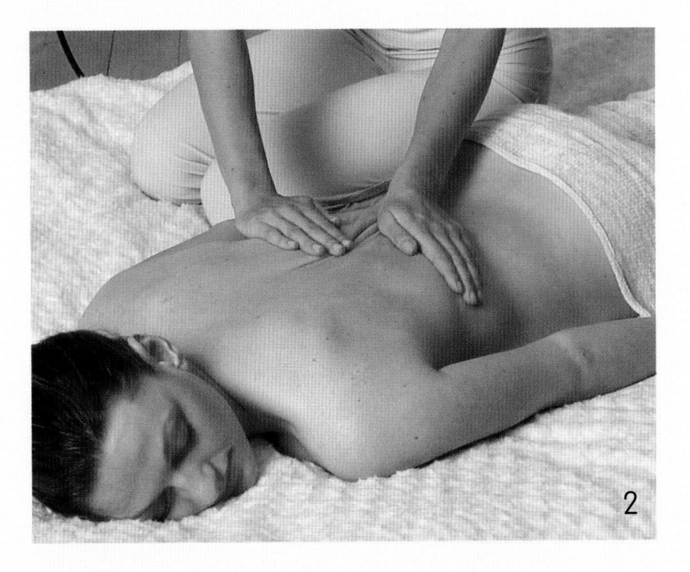
2

2 **Effleurage figures-of-eight:** Kneel to the side of your partner, facing their head. Place the hands on either side of the base of the spine. Press firmly through the whole hand as you glide the hands up the back to the nape of the neck. Slide the hands out along the shoulders and half way down the back. Keeping both hands on the body, cross the hands over to the opposite side. Continue sliding the hands down the back keeping the arms crossed. Uncross the hands by sliding them across the back and down towards the hips. Slightly lift up on the hips as you return the hands to the original position. Repeat this movement twice more.

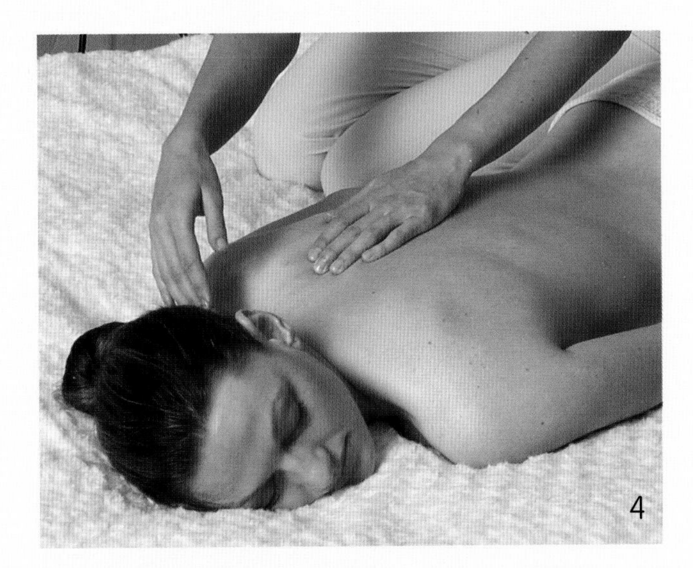
4

4 **Pull-ups to shoulders:** Place one hand underneath the shoulder. Gently pull the shoulder up and back as you slide your hand towards your partners shoulder blade. Replace the first hand with your other hand and repeat, thinking of waves rolling across the shoulder.

5 Kneading to shoulders and neck: Place the hands on one shoulder. Pinch the flesh with one hand as you drag it across to the other hand. As you release the flesh, pick it up with the other hand. Repeat to both shoulders, and then use one hand to do the back of the neck.

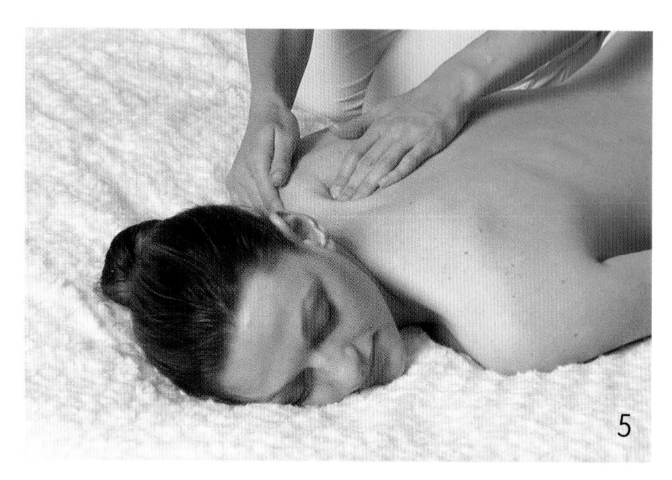

5

6 Knuckle slide: Kneel at your partner's head facing their feet. Form fists with your hands and place the flat part on either side of your partner's spine near the neck. Apply light pressure as you slide your fists down their back towards the base of their spine. Uncurl your hands and glide them along the hips towards the waist. Now, pull the hands up the outside of their back to start again. Repeat twice more.

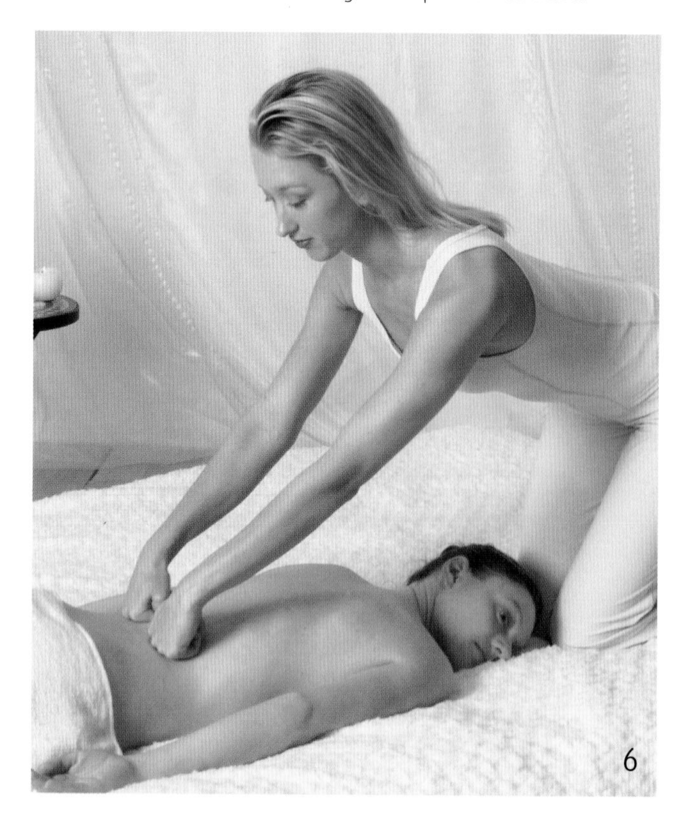

6

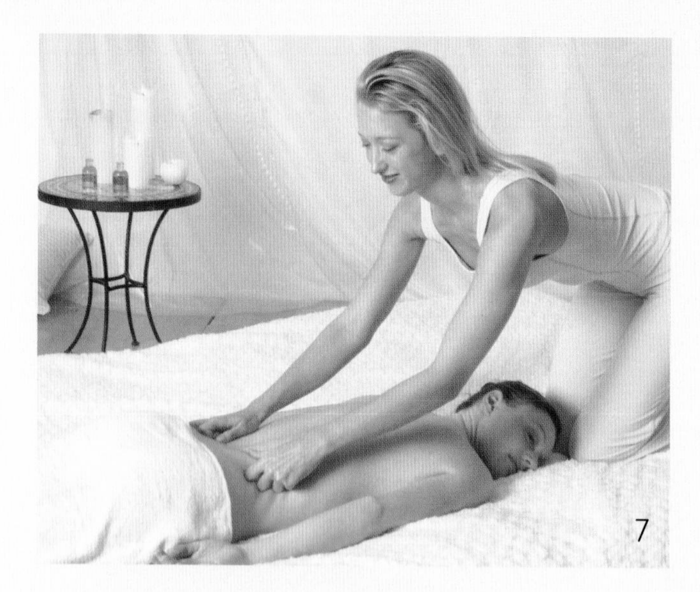

7

7 Knuckle roll: On the last knuckle slide, leave your hands in fists and massage the hips and waist by rolling the knuckles in small circles across the entire area.

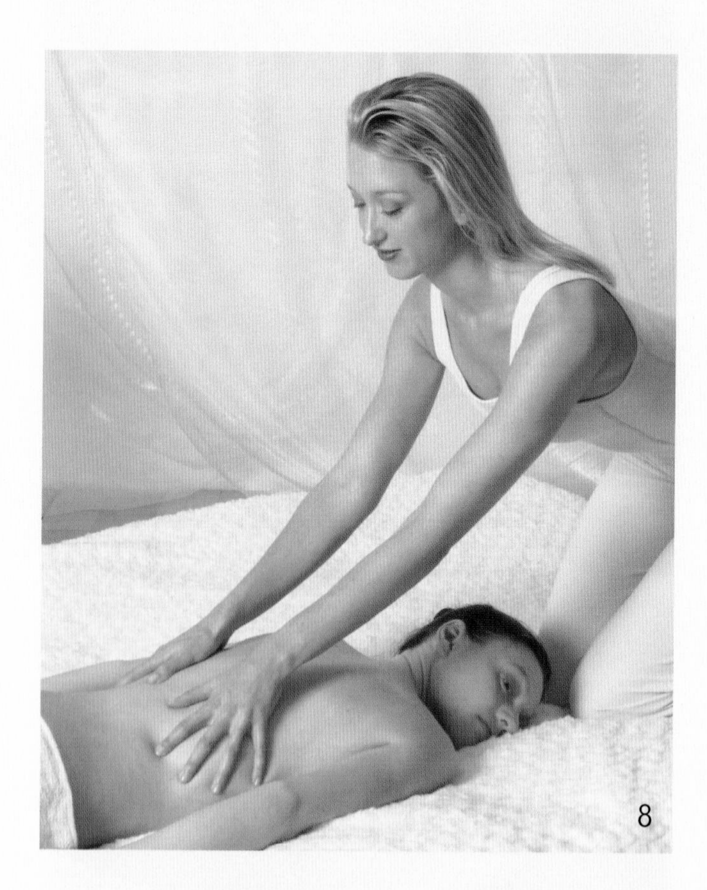

8

8 Fanning: Place your fingers at the base of your partners spine. Circle the fingers three times, covering the lower back and top of the buttocks. Move the hands up to the ribs and repeat. Move the hands up to the shoulders and repeat one more time.

9 Forearms: Continue kneeling at your partner's head. Place your forearms in parallel lines across the top of their back. Press your weight into your arms as you slide them down the back towards the base of the spine. Now let the elbows relax and form a diamond shape as you slide the elbows towards the ribs. Bring the elbows slightly together as you glide the elbows down the sides of the neck. Repeat twice.

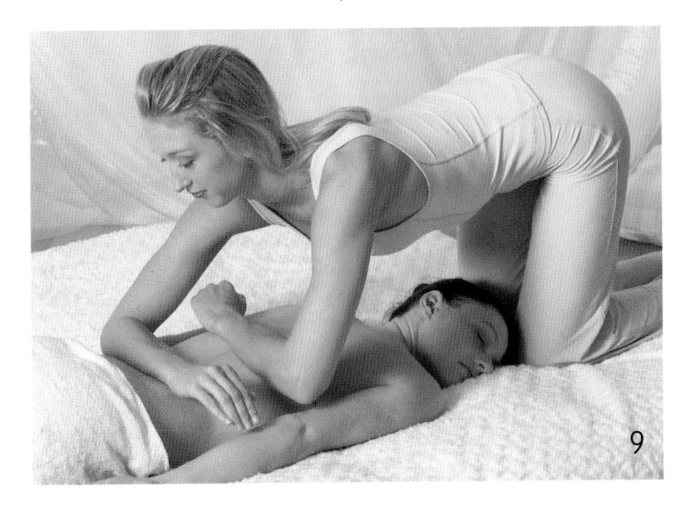
9

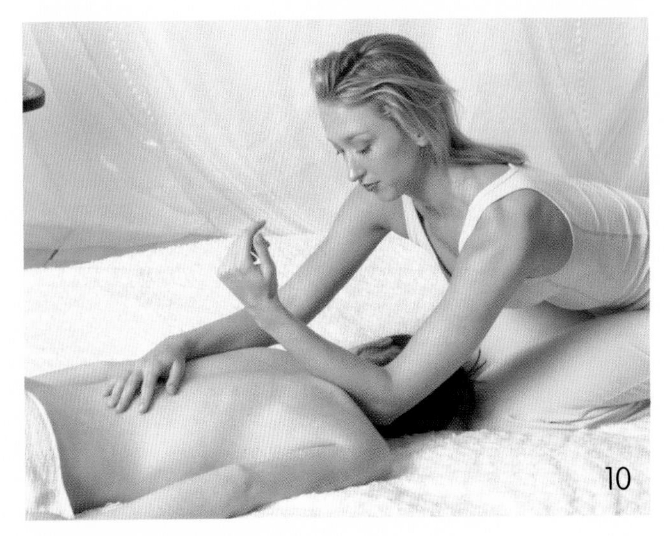
10

10 Forearm to the neck: Place one forearm across the opposite shoulder of your partner, with the palm towards you. Slide the arm up and down along the shoulder from the wrist to the elbow. Repeat a few times, thinking of a violin or saw. Have your partner look in the opposite direction and do the other side.

11 Forearm to the back: Move so that you are kneeling at your partner's side facing their lower back. Place one forearm to their waist with your palm facing you. Slide the forearm up and down the waist, trying to release tension in the lower back.

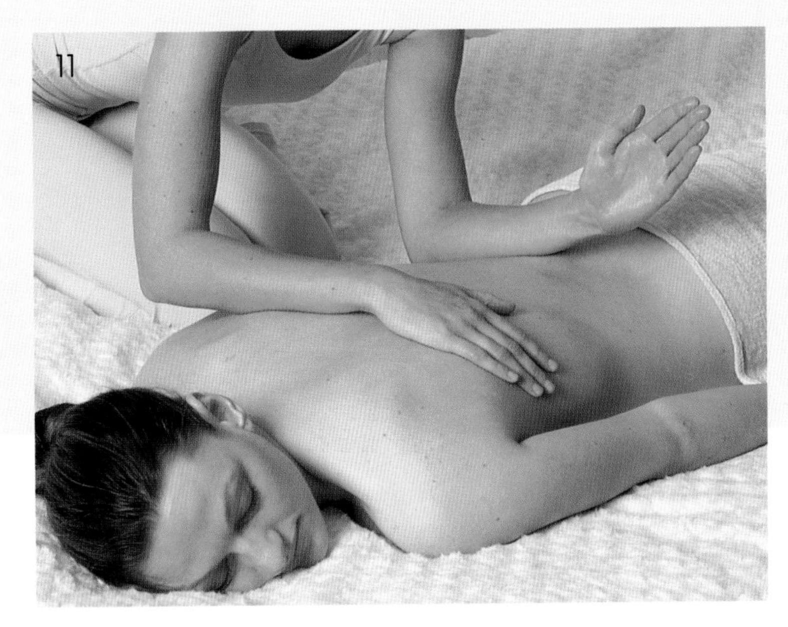
11

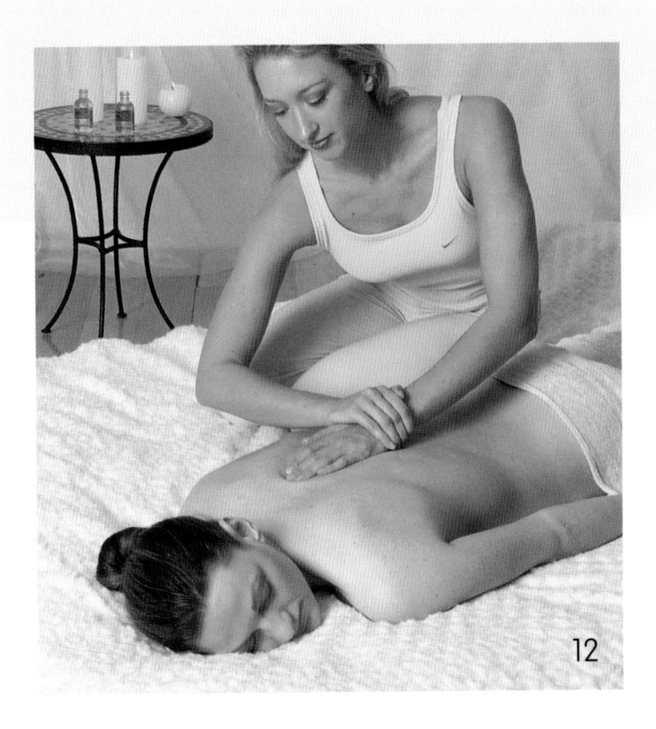
12

12 Digital pressure: Place the fingers of one hand flat at the base of the back. Hold the wrist with your opposite hand. Press firmly as you drag the fingers up the back to the neck. Release the wrist and slide both hands in opposite directions along the shoulders and down the outside of the spine. Repeat until you have covered both sides of the spine.

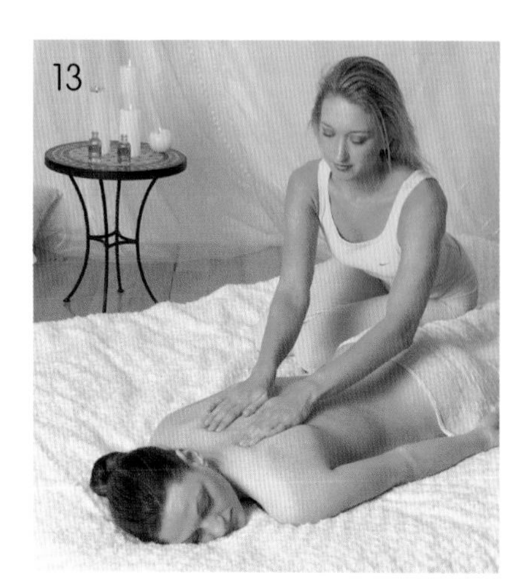

13 Basic effleurage: Place both hands flat at the base on either side of the spine. Slide both hands up the spine to the nape of the neck. Glide the hands along the shoulders and back down either side of the back to repeat.

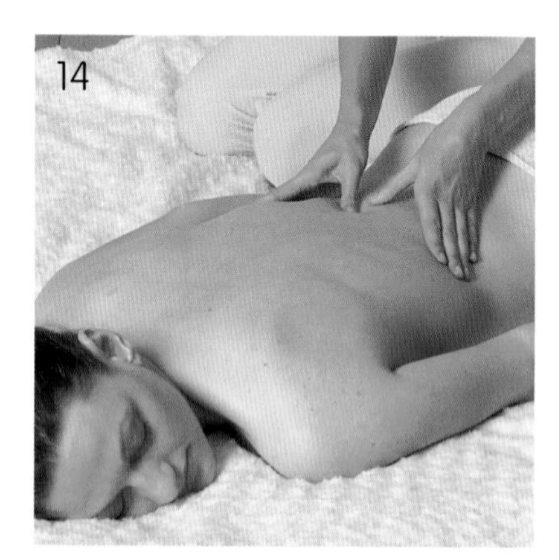

14 Thumb walking: Start by imagining four parallel lines on either side of the spine running from the pelvis up to just below the ribs. Place the thumbs at the base of one of the lines closest to the spine. Walk the thumbs up the line by pressing first one thumb and then the other into the flesh. The thumbs should circle each other to create a rolling effect. When you reach the ribs start at the base of the next line slowly working your way out towards the hip. After completing one side, start on the other side closest to the spine and work your way out to the opposite hip.

15 Cupping: Move to the side of your partner and switch your hands to cupping. Close the fingers and form a bowl with both of your hands. Strike the surface of the skin with the pads of your fingers and the palms of your hands only. Try not to stay in one place. Move along the length and breadth of the back, while avoiding the kidney area.

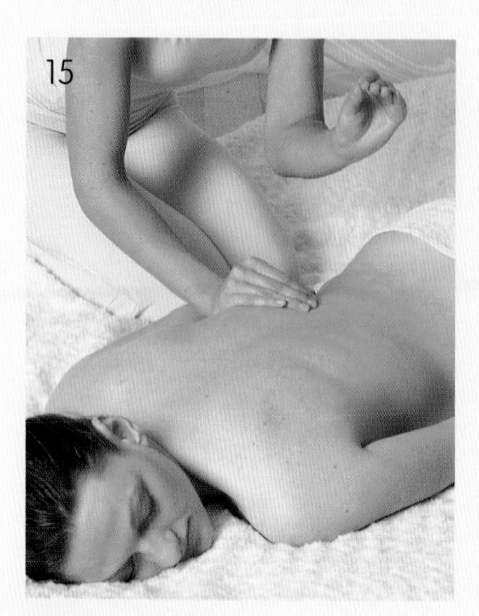

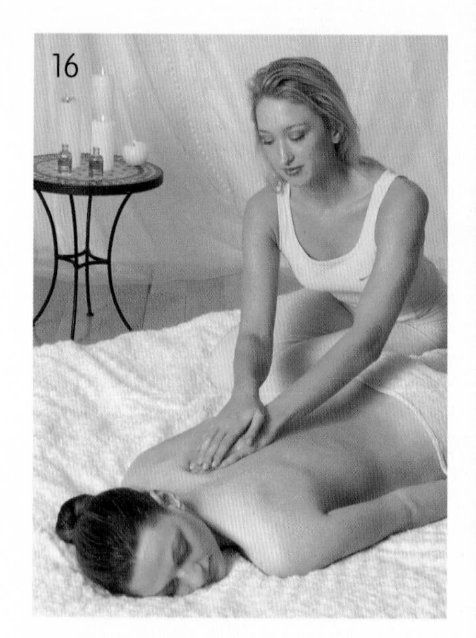

16 Hand over hand effleurage: Place one hand on top of the other on the outside of the spine. Pressing through the palm of the hand, slide the hand up to the neck, across the shoulder and back down the outside of the back. Repeat a few times and then move to the other side and repeat.

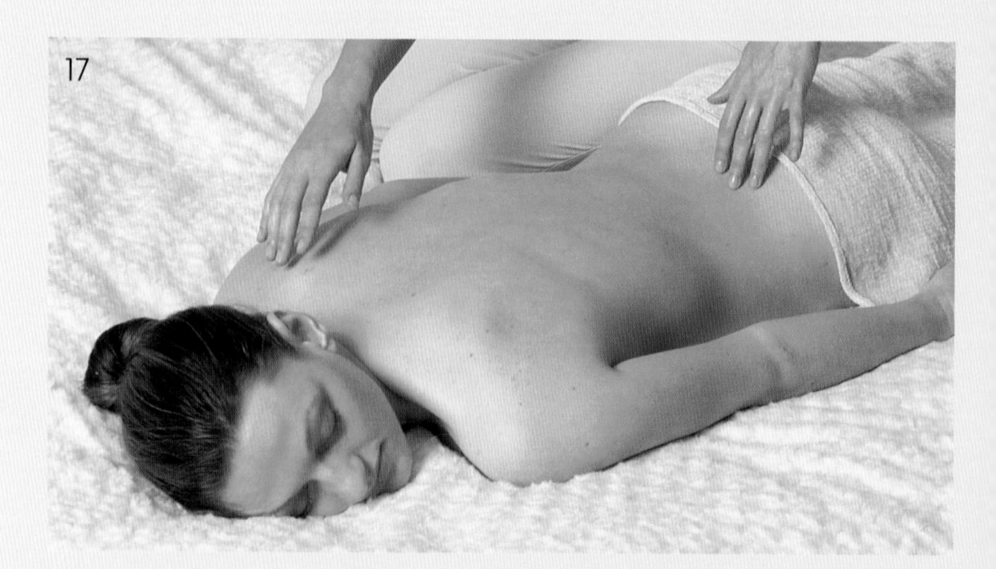

17 Feather stroking: Touch the fingertips of one hand to the top of the back. Lightly stroke down the back. When that hand reaches the base of the spine, start the other hand stroking down the back.

Ending: Cover the back with the towel.

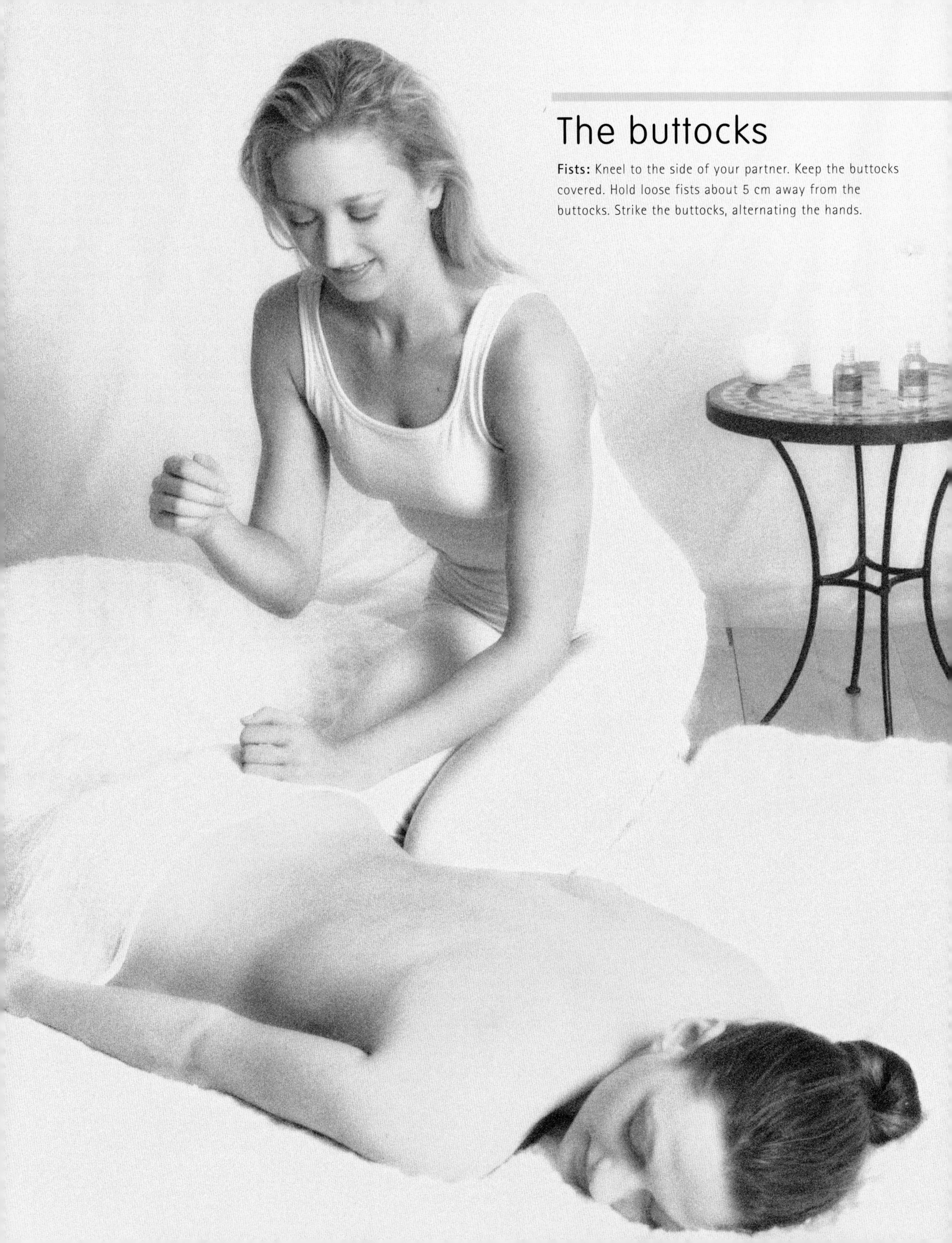

The buttocks

Fists: Kneel to the side of your partner. Keep the buttocks covered. Hold loose fists about 5 cm away from the buttocks. Strike the buttocks, alternating the hands.

Back of the leg

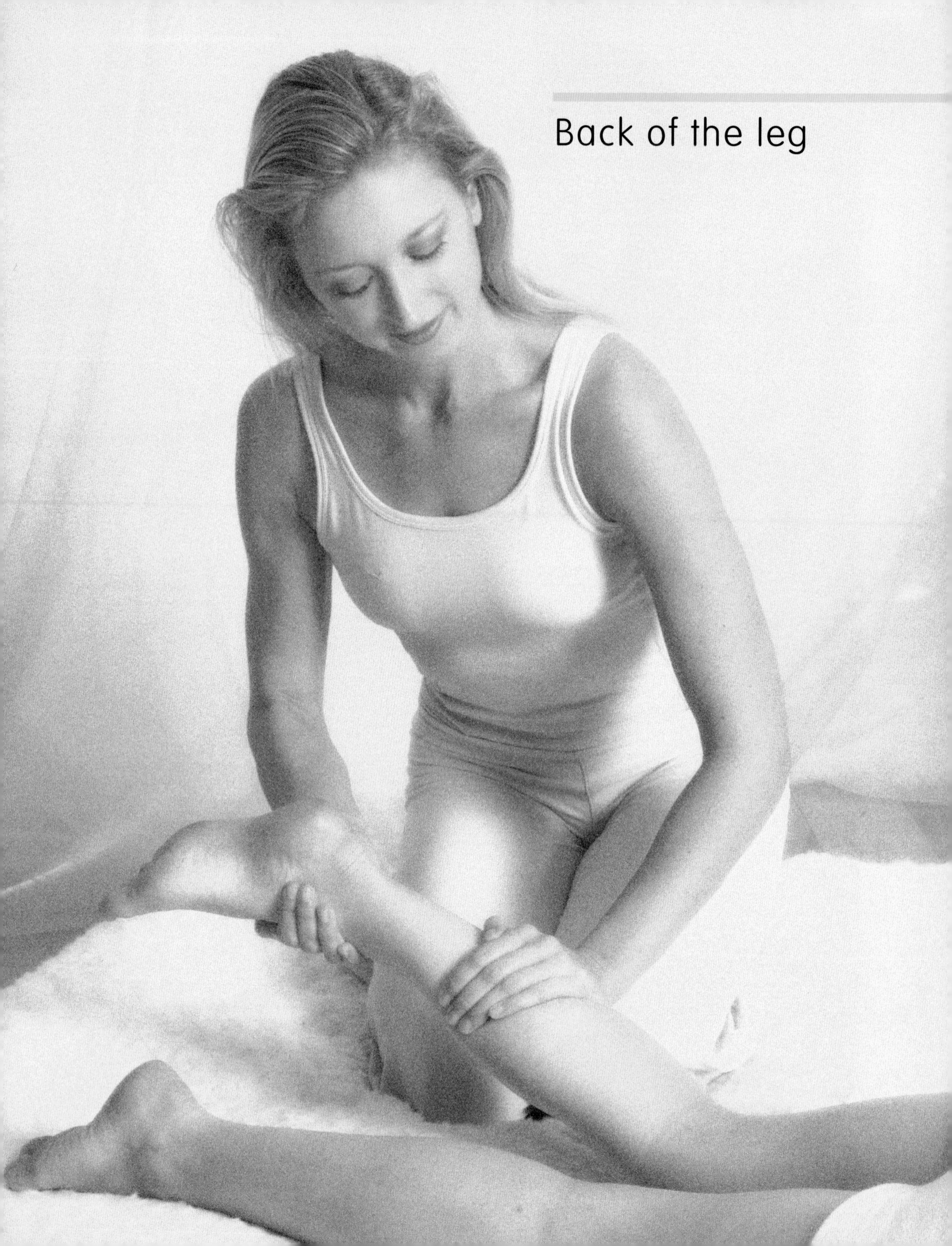

Softening: Place the hands on top of the towel with the fingers on one side of the leg and the palms on the other. Gently squeeze the flesh underneath the towel. Release and repeat, moving the hands so that you cover the entire length of the leg. Rub the whole leg vigorously.

Spreading the oil: Uncover the leg so that you can see your partner's hip while still retaining their modesty. Pour a small amount of oil into the palm of your hand. Rub your hands together and spread the oil, starting at the ankle and working your way up to the hip.

1 **Alternating effleurage:** Place both hands at the ankle. Slide one hand up the leg to the hip, being careful to avoid the back of the knee. Slide the hand down the outside of the leg. As that hand returns, start the other hand sliding up.

2 **Friction to the thigh:** Start with the thumbs just above the knee. Make circles across the whole thigh area with the whole arm, not just the thumb joint.

3 **Kneading the inner thigh:** Kneel facing your partner's thigh. Place both hands on the inside of the leg with the fingers facing down. Pick up the flesh with one hand. Pinch it as you slide it across to the other hand. As you release the flesh, pick it up with your opposite hand. Think of kneading dough as you pass the flesh back and forth between your hands.

4 **Wringing:** Place one hand on each side of the thigh. Press the palms in as you lift the flesh while crossing the hands over the top to the opposite sides. Make sure the hands are at least 5 cm apart. Repeat a few times, working over the entire thigh.

5 **Train tracks up the thigh:** Place the thumbs together just above the knee with the fingers out to the side. Press the thumbs into the belly of the thigh, sliding them up towards the hip. Open the thumbs at the top of the hip and slide the hands halfway down the thigh. Lift the muscle up from the sides, bringing the hands back together. Float the hands down to the starting position and repeat with the thumbs 3 cm apart. Repeat one more time with the thumbs 5 cm apart.

6 **Digital pressure to the thigh:** Place the fingers of one hand flat just above the knee. Hold your wrist with your opposite hand. Slide the fingers up to the buttocks. Let go of the wrist and slide the hands back down to above the knee along the outside of the thigh. Repeat, covering the whole area.

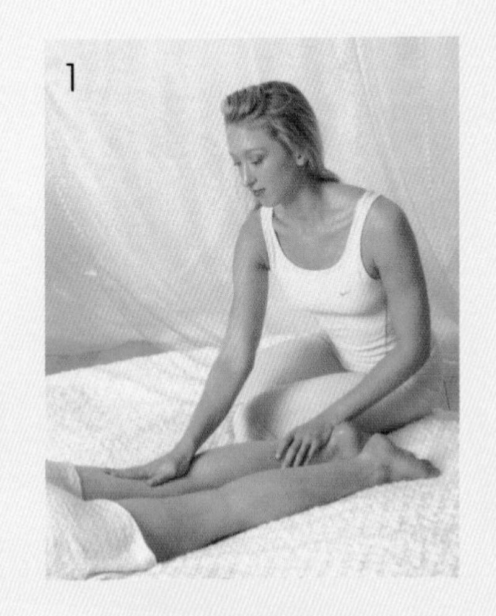
1

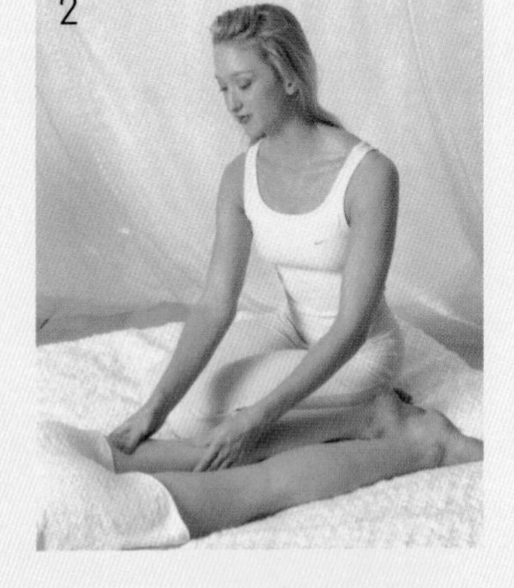
2

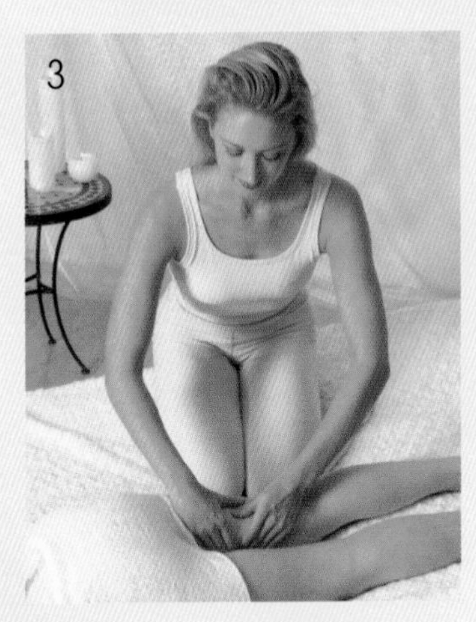
3

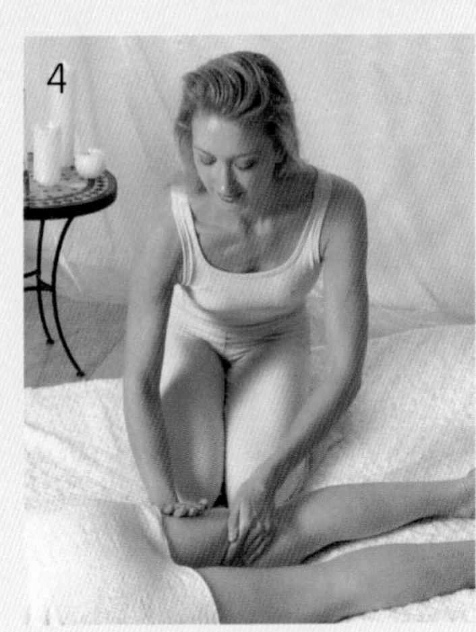
4

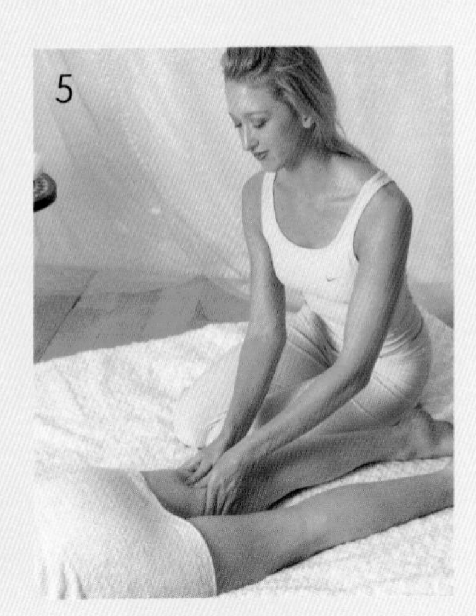
5

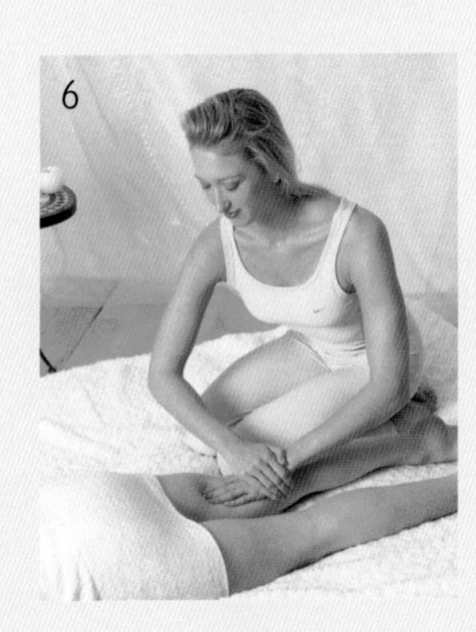
6

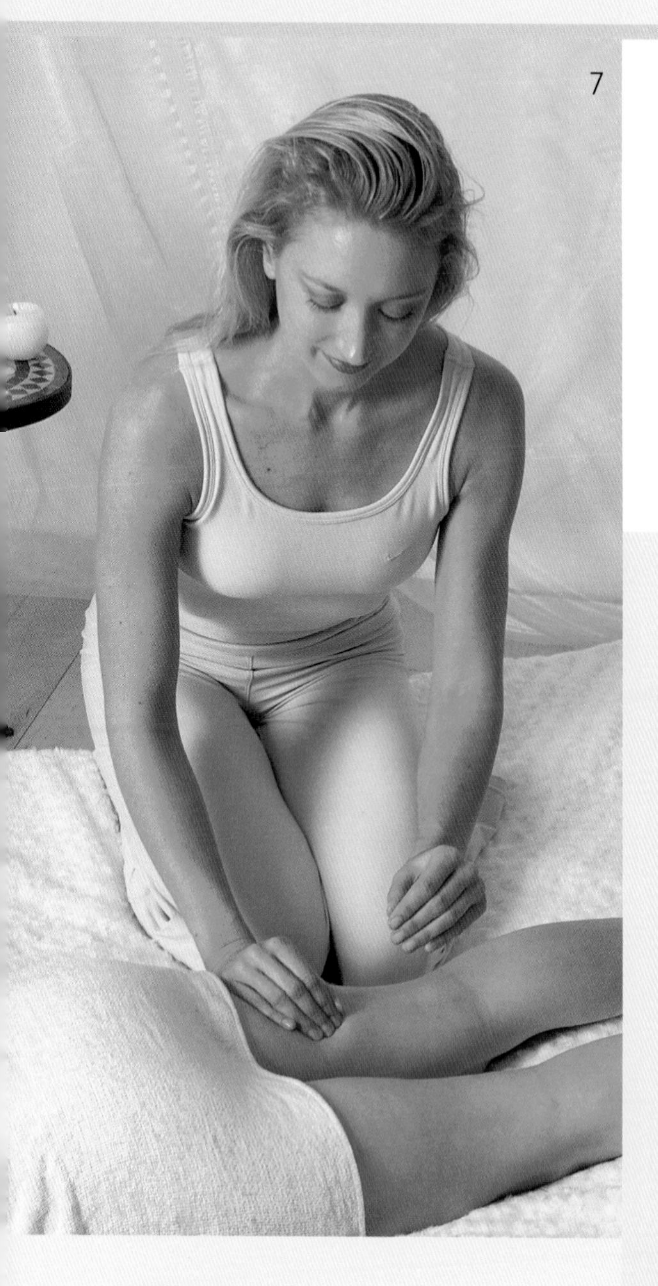

7 **Cupping:** Form the hands into bowls with the fingers tight together and the palms facing down. Strike the thigh with the pads of the fingers and the palms only. Be sure to use precise, rhythmic movements.

8 **Basic effleurage:** Place both hands above the knee with the fingertips facing the hip. Slide the hands together up to the hip, open them out to the sides and glide them back down to above the knee. Repeat, effleuraging the whole leg. Repeat again just to the calf.

9 **Friction to the calf:** Place the thumbs on the ankles. Make circles, using the whole arm to cover the calf.

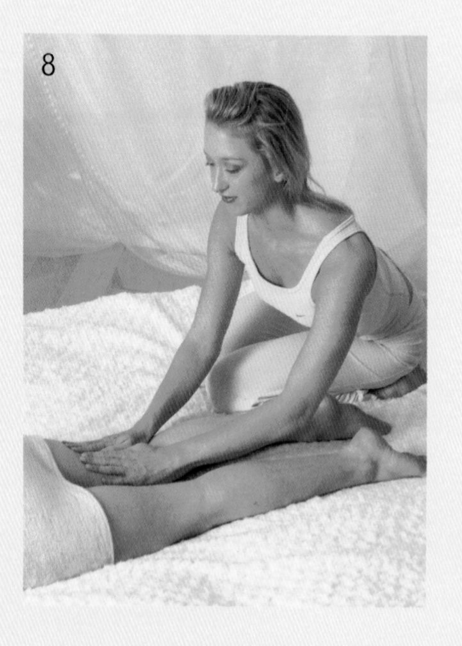

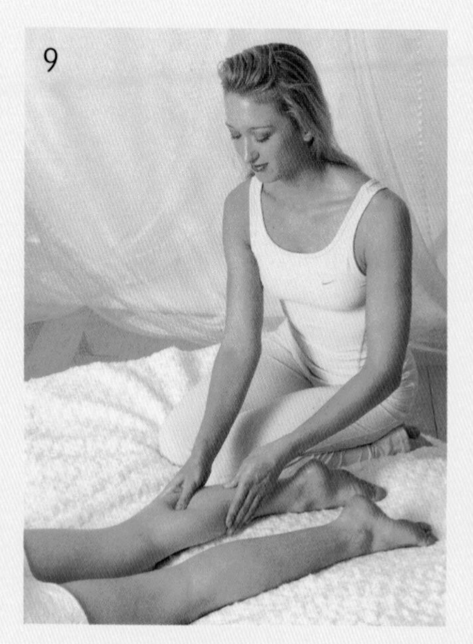

10 **Wringing:** Place one hand on each side of the calf. Press in as you slide the hands past each other to the opposite side. Keep repeating, making sure there is a space between your hands as they cross.

11 **Digital pressure to the calf:** Place the fingers of one hand flat at the ankle with the fingertips facing the hip. Hold the wrist with your opposite hand to help glide the fingers up towards the knee. Let go of the wrist and slide the hands back along the outside of the calf. Repeat, covering the entire calf.

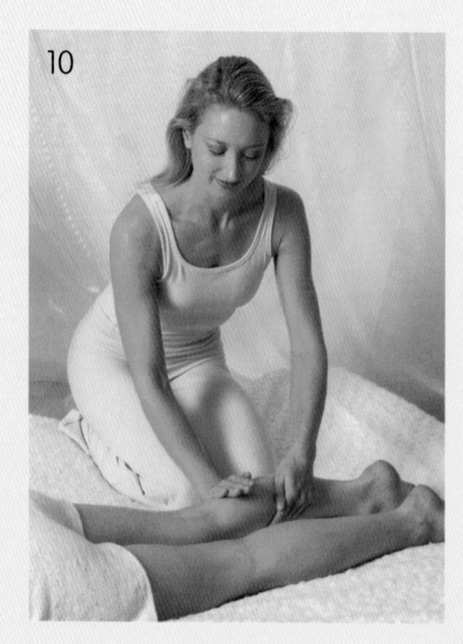

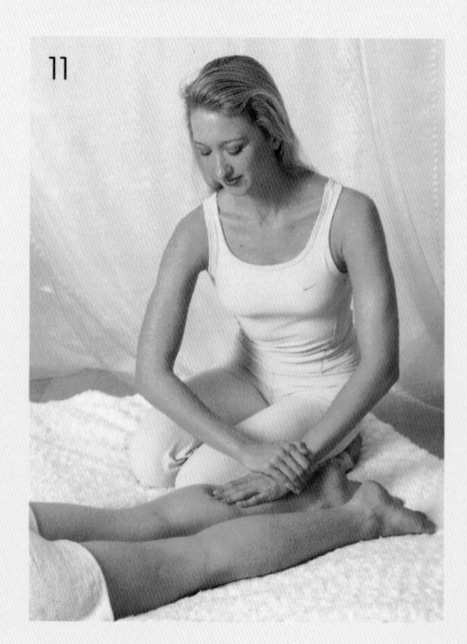

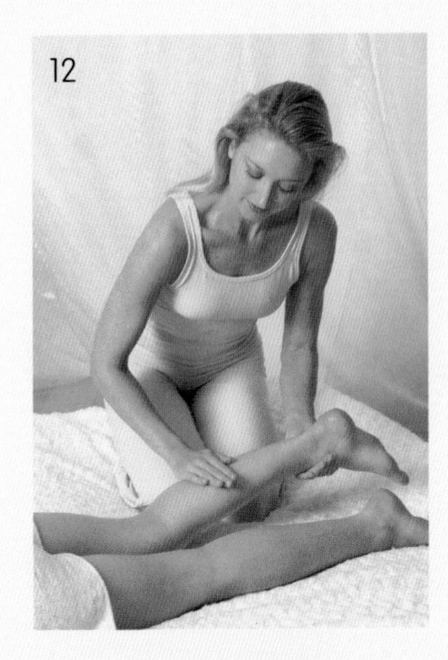

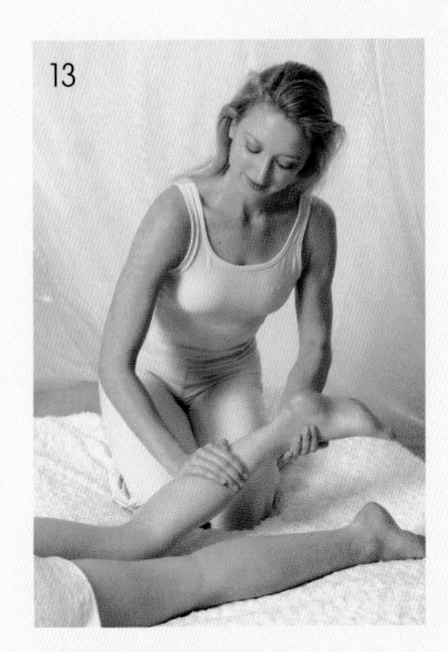

12 Vibration: Lift the ankle and place one hand flat across the calf. Rub vigorously back and forth, shaking the calf muscle for about 10 seconds.

13 Lymph draining: Holding the ankle slightly off the ground, place your top hand around the ankle. With short, sweeping movements, brush the hand down towards the back of the knee. Repeat this action a few times, thinking of draining the toxins towards the lymph nodes. Place the leg back on the mat.

14 Cupping: Form the hands into little bowls with the fingers together. With quick, alternating movements, strike the calf with the pads of the fingertips and the base of the palms. You should hear a suction noise, rather than a slapping sound.

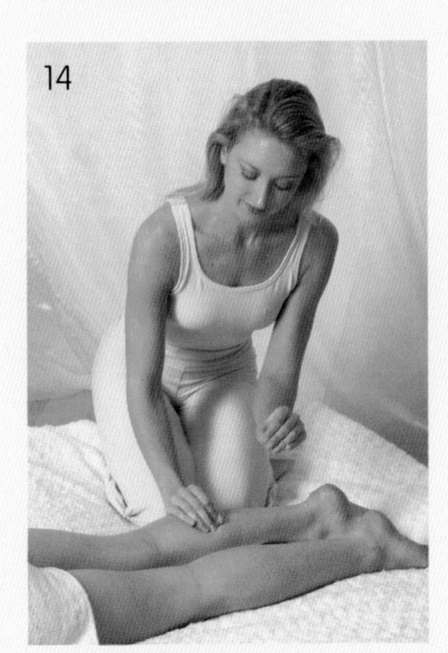

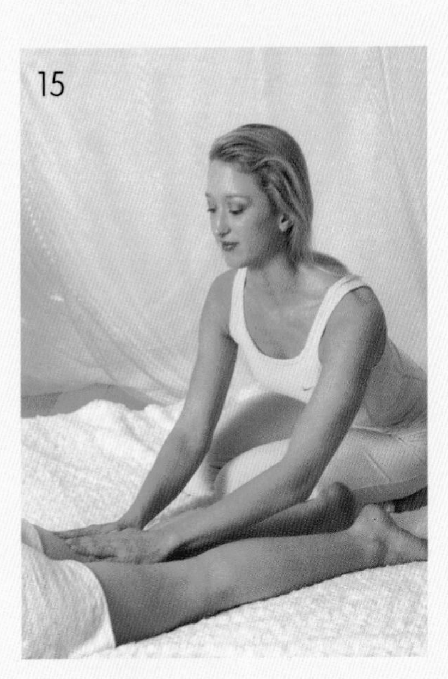

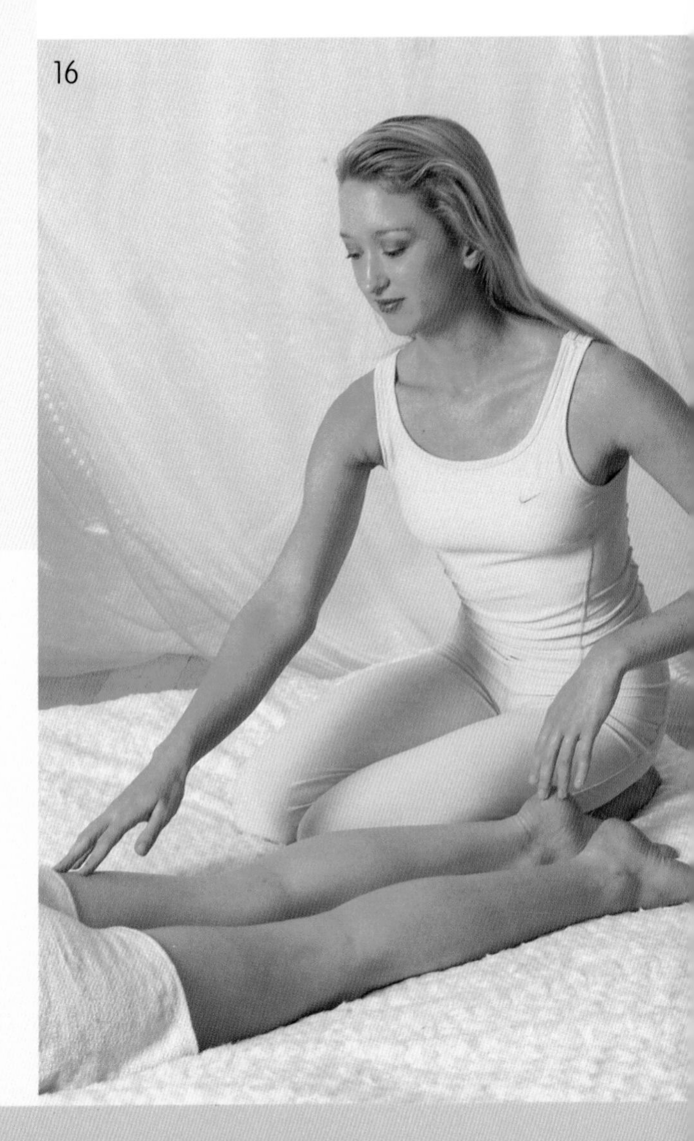

15 Basic effleurage: Place the hands on the ankle with the fingertips facing the hip. Slide the hands up towards the hip, avoiding the back of the knee. Bring the hands to the sides of the leg and slide them back down to the ankle. Repeat, thinking of pressing firmly on the way up and gently on the way back down.

16 Feather stroking: Lightly touch the top of the leg with the fingertips of one hand. Gently stroke down the leg. Repeat alternating hands.

Ending: Cover the leg and repeat to the other side. Lift the towel slightly away from you to allow your partner to turn over onto their back while retaining their modesty.

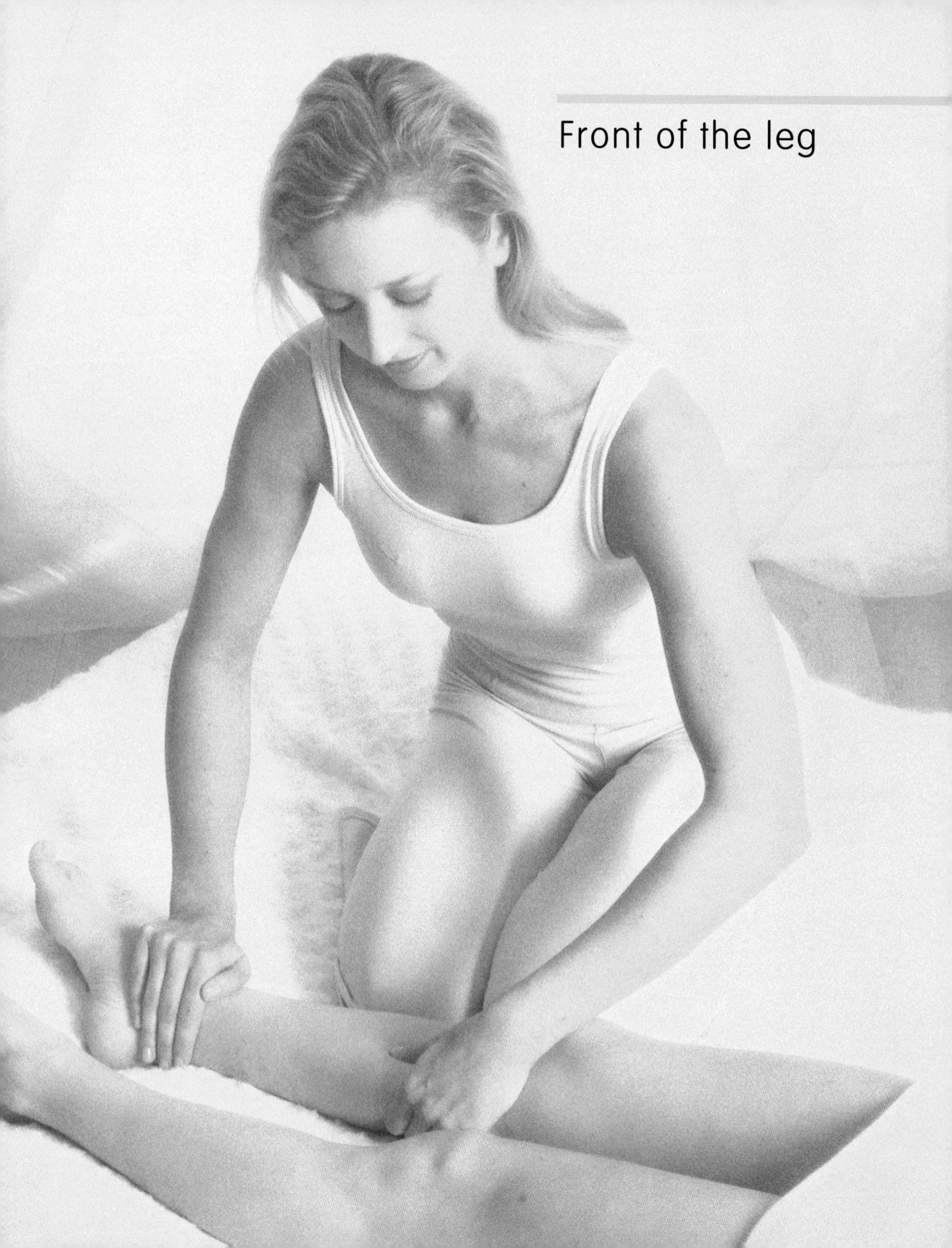

Front of the leg

Softening: Place the hands on the leg above the towel with the fingers on one side and palms on the other. Gently squeeze the flesh. Repeat until you have covered the entire length of the leg. Place the hands flat and rub vigorously up and down the leg.

Spreading the oil: Uncover the leg so that you can see the hip joint while still retaining your partner's modesty. Pour a small amount of oil into your hand. Rub your hands together to warm the oil and spread the oil up your partner's leg.

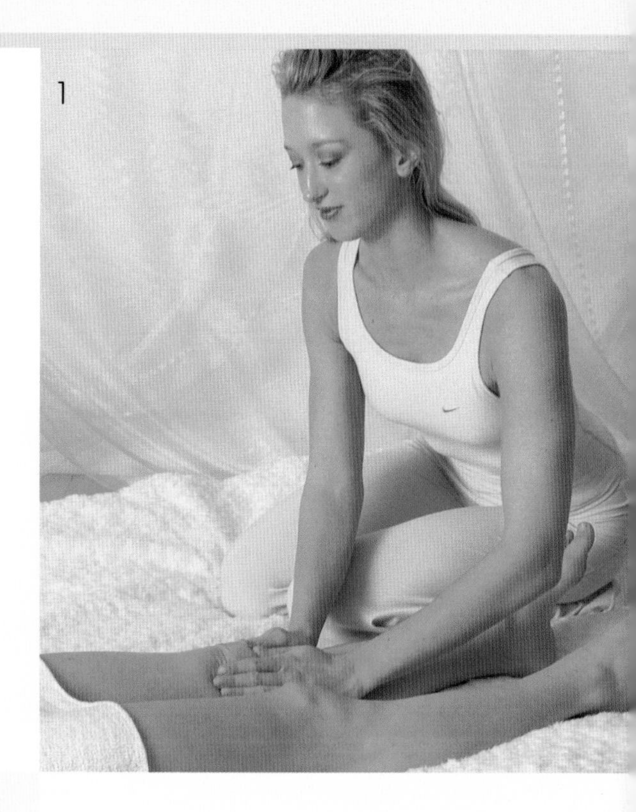

1 **Basic effleurage:** Place both hands on the ankles, with the fingertips facing the hip socket. Slide the hands up the leg, avoiding the knee. Separate the hands at the hip and glide them back down the outside of the leg. Repeat a few times.

2 **Forearms:** Place the forearms in an x shape across the ankle. Gently glide the fleshy part of the forearms up the leg to the hip, avoiding the knee. When you reach the hip, pull the arms back down the leg, slightly leading with the elbows.

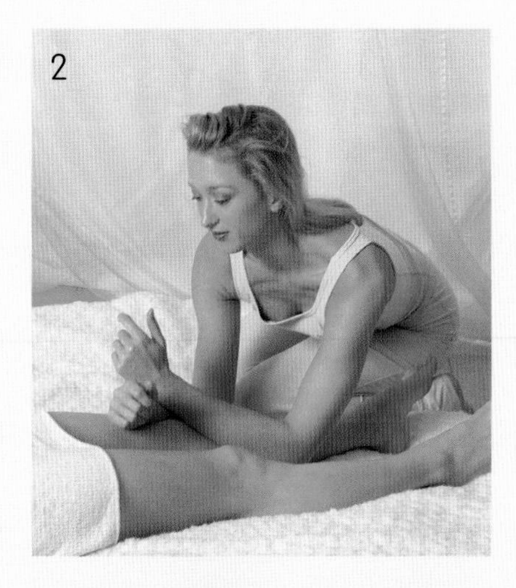

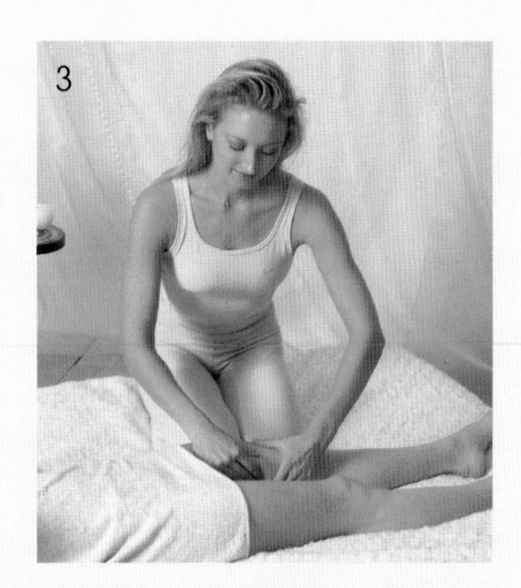

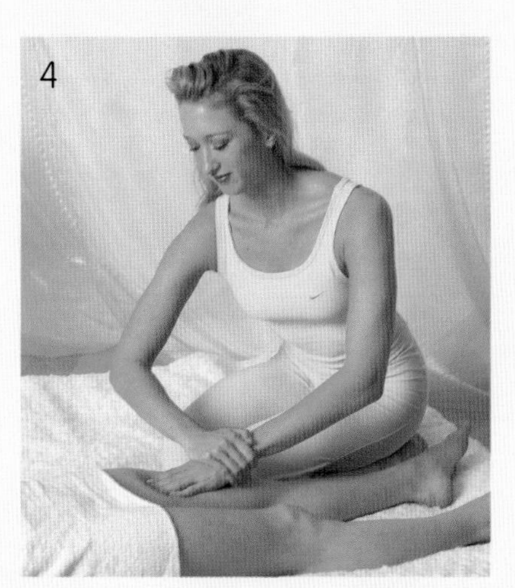

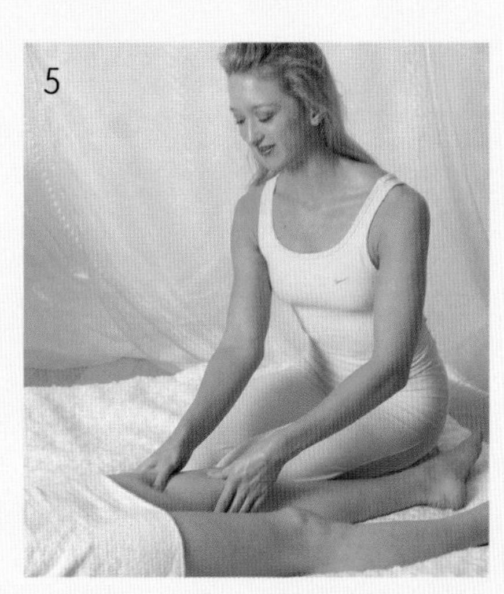

3 **Kneading to the thigh:** Kneel facing your partner's leg. Place your hands on their inner thigh with the fingers facing down and the thumbs and elbows out. Pick up the flesh and squeeze it as you slide it over to the other hand. As you release the flesh, pick it up with your opposite hand. Repeat, and imagine kneading dough, as you move your body back and forth with the movement. Slowly cover the entire thigh area.

4 **Digital pressure:** Place the fingers of one hand flat on the thigh just above the knee. Hold the wrist with your opposite hand. Press firmly with the fingers as you glide the fingers up towards the hip socket. Open the hands to the outside of the leg and bring them back to just above the knee. Move the hands to a slightly different starting position and repeat. Repeat until you have covered the entire thigh area.

5 **Friction to the thigh:** Place the thumbs just above the knee. Lock the thumb joint and make circles, using the whole arm and covering the entire thigh.

6 Train tracks to the thigh: Start with both thumbs together just above the knee and the fingers out to the sides. Press the thumbs into the muscle as you slide them up to the hips. Separate the hands and glide them halfway down the thigh. Lift up the thigh as you bring the hands together. Float the hands back down to start again. Repeat with the thumbs a couple of centimetres apart. Repeat one more time with the thumbs 5 cm apart.

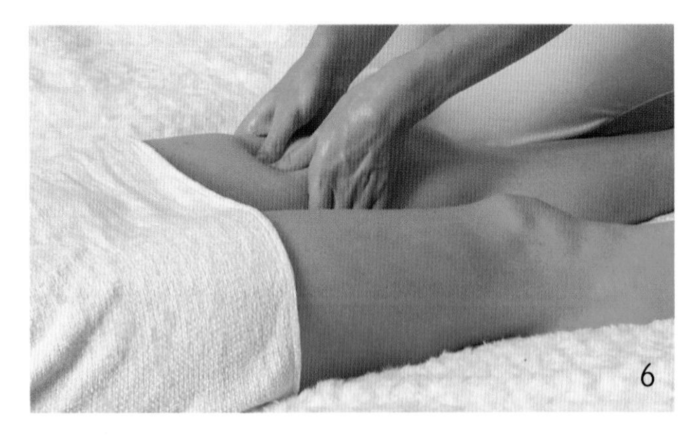
6

7 Cupping: Form the hands into bowls with the fingers tight together and the palms facing down. Strike the thigh with the pads of the fingers and the palms only. Be sure to use precise, rhythmic movements.

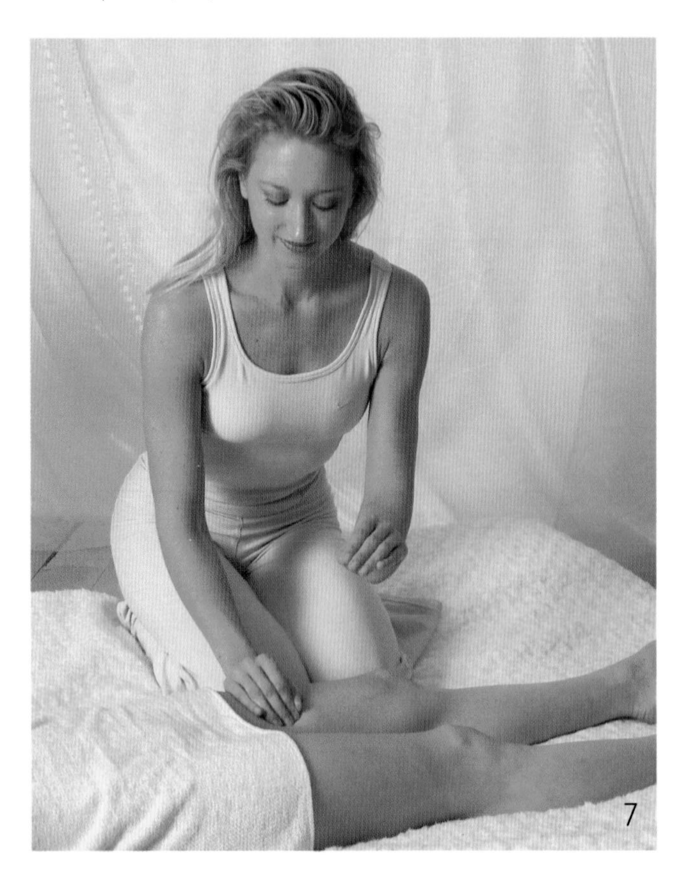
7

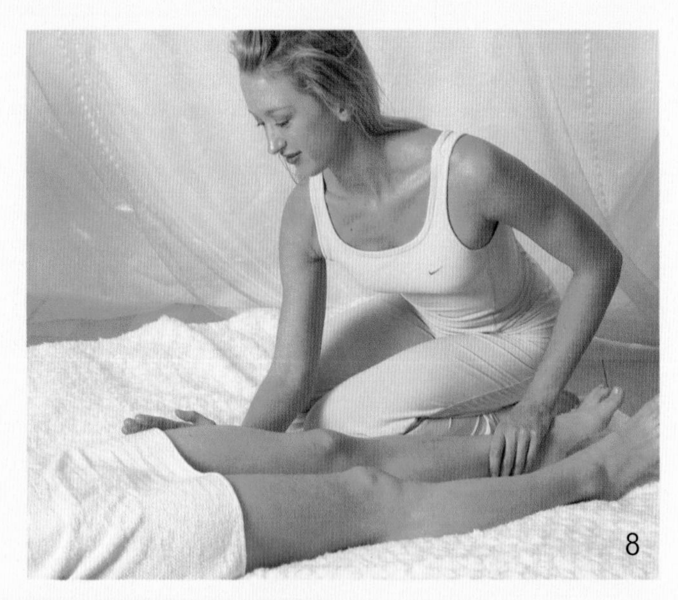
8

8 Heel of hand: Place the palm of one hand on the outside of the leg above the knee. Press firmly with the heel of the hand as you go up towards the hip socket. Repeat a few times.

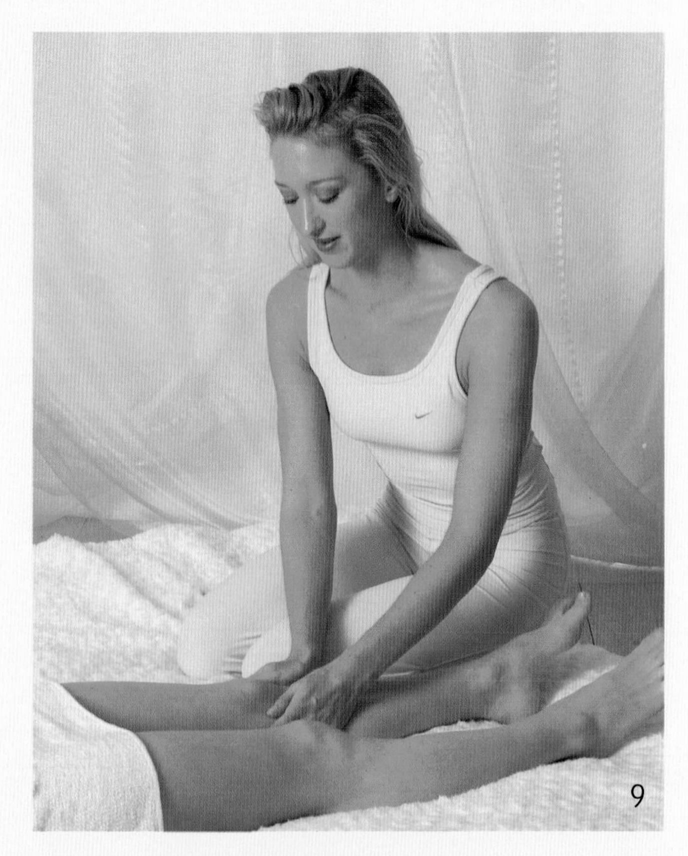
9

9 Opening: Place the length of the thumbs together on top of the knee with the fingers out to the sides. Press out and down as you circle the knee with the tips of the thumbs. Repeat twice.

10 **Kneading to the calf:** Sit or kneel to the side of your partner. Place the fingertips on the calf with thumbs out. Squeeze the flesh and slide it over to your opposite hand. Release it as you pick it up with your other hand.

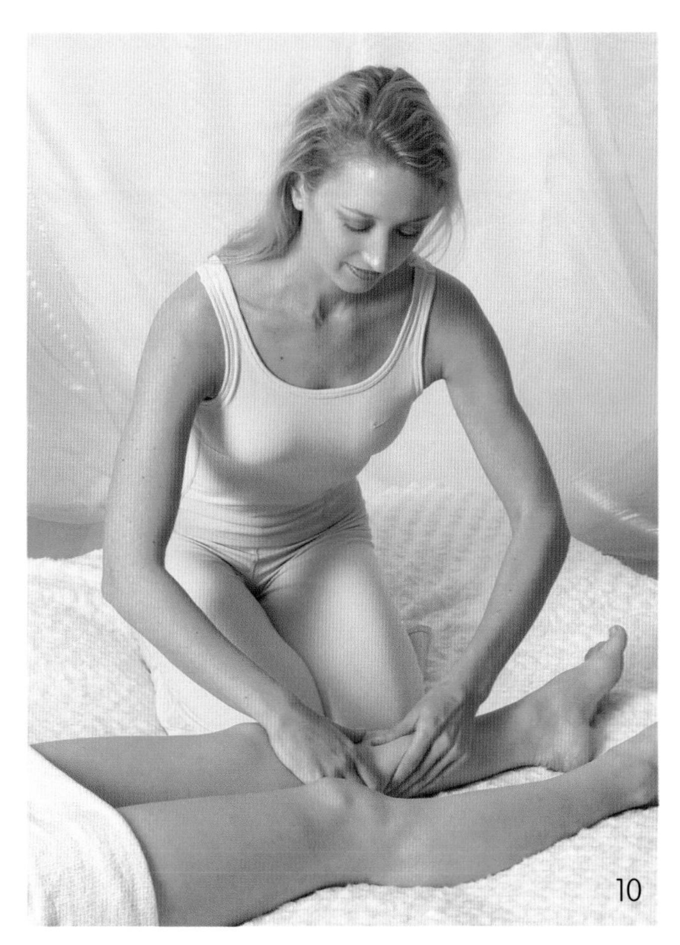
10

11 **Friction:** Hold the ankle with one hand. Start with the thumb just below the knee facing the foot. Circle the thumb down the shin towards the ankle. When you reach the anklebone circle it 3 times with your thumb. Repeat twice.

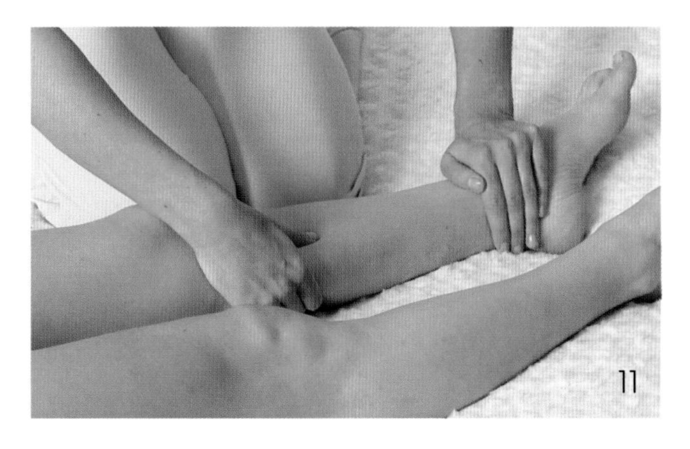
11

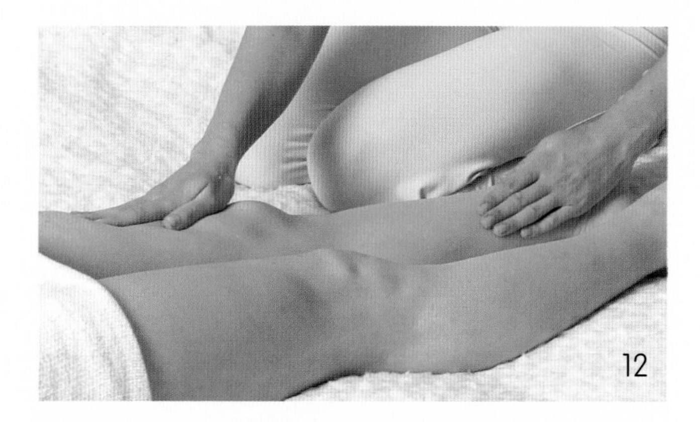
12

12 **Alternating effleurage:** Place the hands on the ankle with the fingers facing the hip joint. Slide one hand up the leg, avoiding the knee area. Glide the hand to the side and back down the outside of the leg. Repeat with the other hand, remembering to press firmly on the way up and gently on the way back.

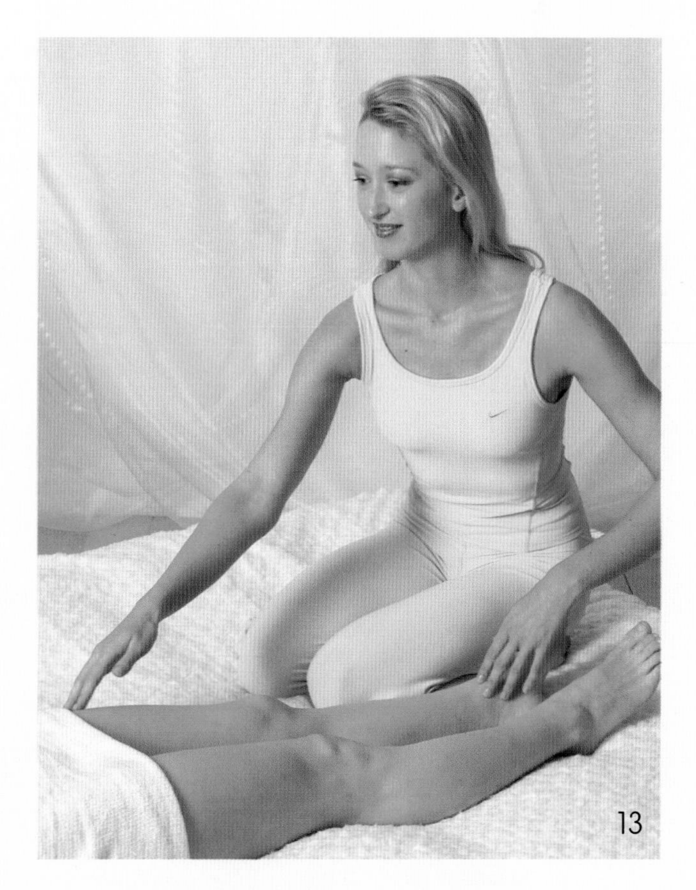
13

13 **Feather stroking:** Lightly touch the top of the leg with one hand. Gently stroke down the leg, letting the fingertips mould to the contour of the leg. Repeat, alternating hands.

Ending: Cover the leg and repeat the sequence to the other leg.

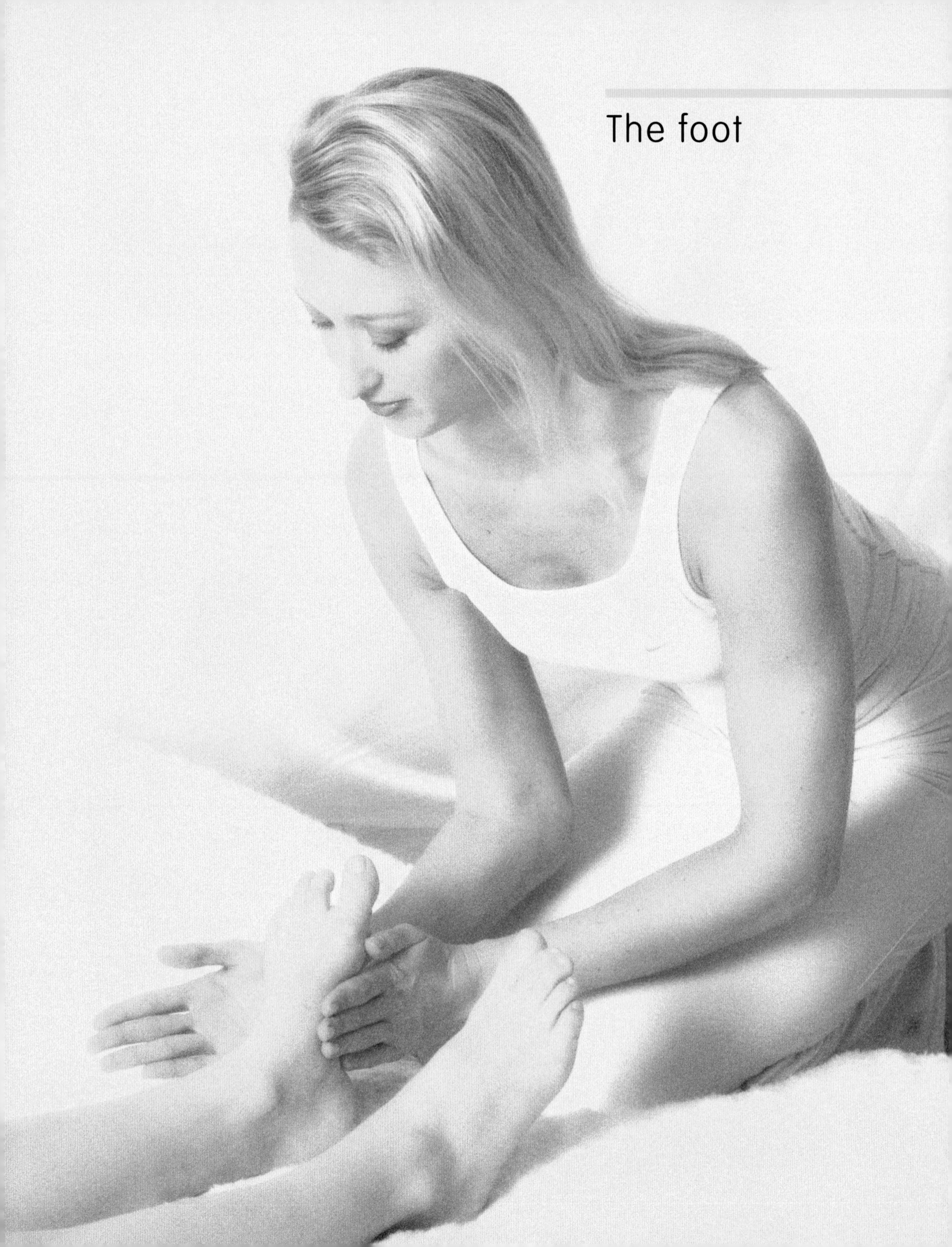

The foot

Spreading the oil: Uncover the foot and place a small amount of oil in the palm of your hand. Rub your hands together and spread the oil over the entire foot area.

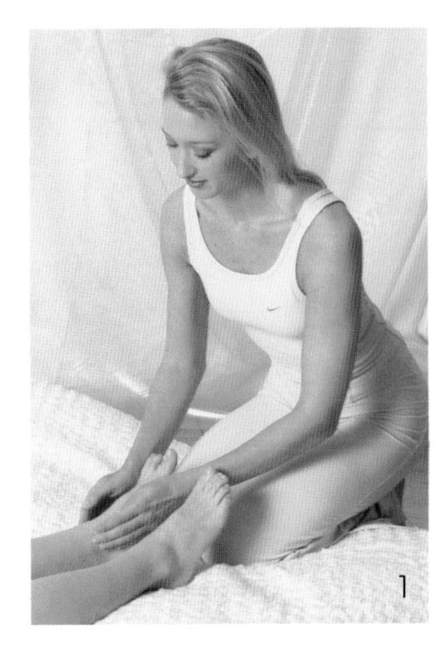

1

1 **Circling:** Place the fingertips of both hands on either side of your partner's anklebones. Make small, slow circles around the anklebones.

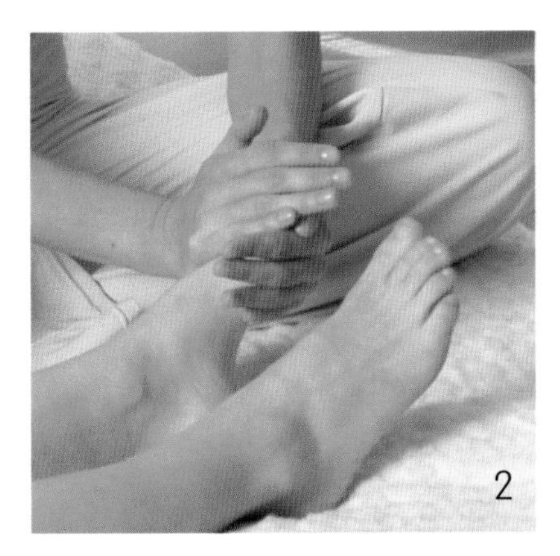

2

2 **Rolling foot in palms:** Sit with your legs crossed to the side of the foot you are working on. Place the top of the foot between the palms of your hands with your fingers facing away from you. Roll the foot and toes between your hands. This is done by circling the palms around each other.

3 **Friction:** Place the thumbs on the top of the foot. Making circular motions, cover the entire area. Then repeat to the bottom of the foot.

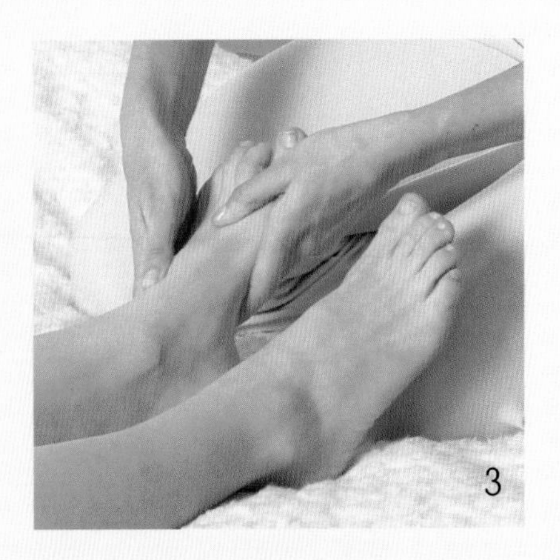

3

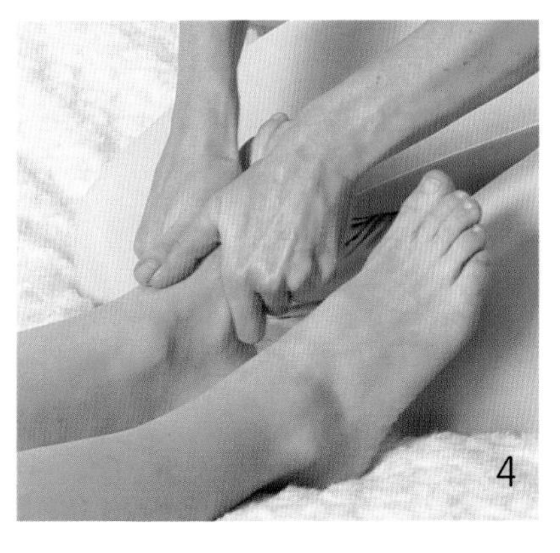

4

4 **Opening:** Place the palms of your hands together on the top of the foot with the fingers wrapped around to the bottom. Press the palms into the foot as you pull back with the fingers.

5 **Knuckle roll:** Touch the fingertips of one hand to the palm. Place the knuckles on the bottom of the foot. Make circles, rolling the knuckles across the bottom of the foot.

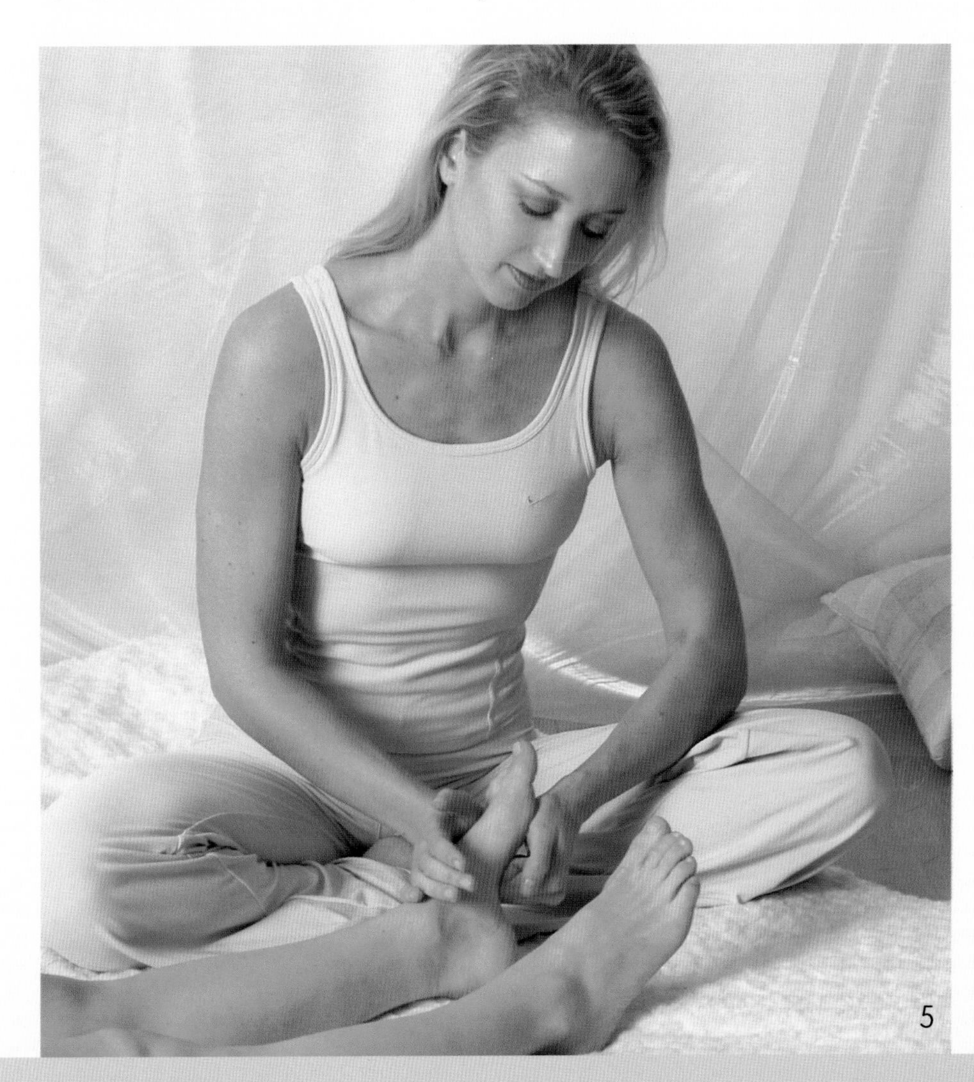

5

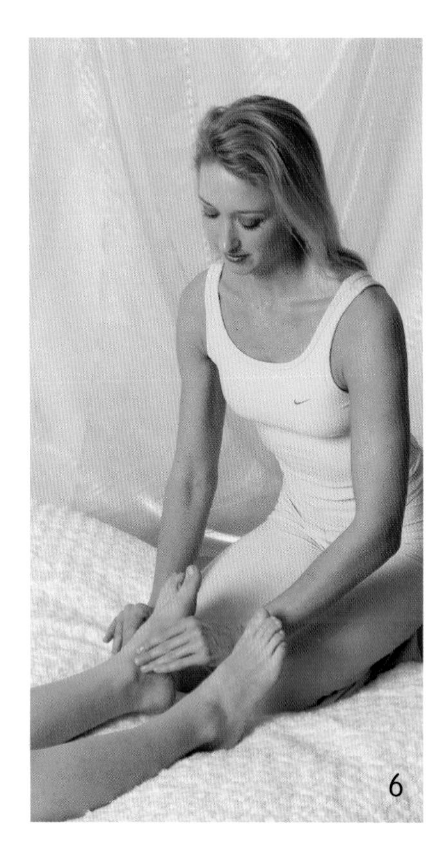
6

6 **Thumbs up:** Place the thumbs together on the heel with the fingers holding the foot. Press the thumbs into the foot as you slide them up to the toes. Repeat twice.

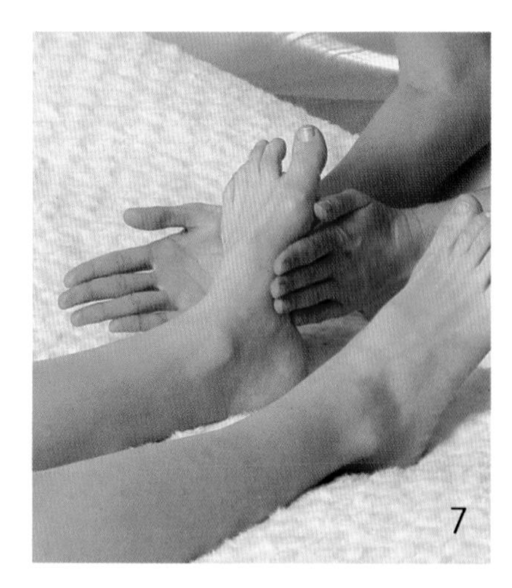
7

7 **Vibration:** Place the hands flat, facing each other, on the sides of the foot. Shake the foot vigorously back and forth.

8 **Sandwiching:** Place one hand on the top of the foot and one hand on the bottom of the foot with the fingertips of both hands facing the ankle. Press the palms together and slide the hands up towards the toes. Repeat, changing the side of the foot that the hands are on. Repeat a few times.

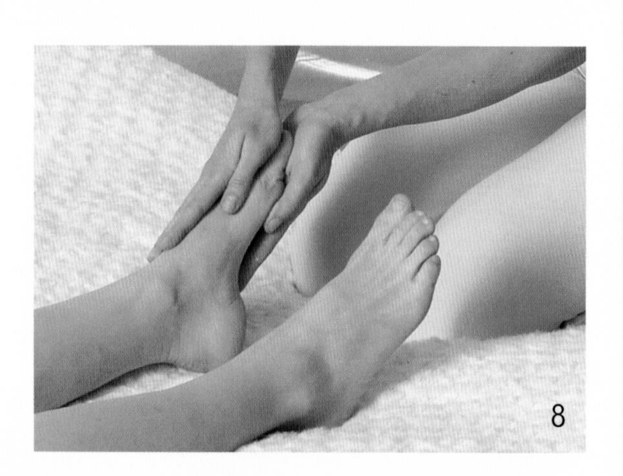
8

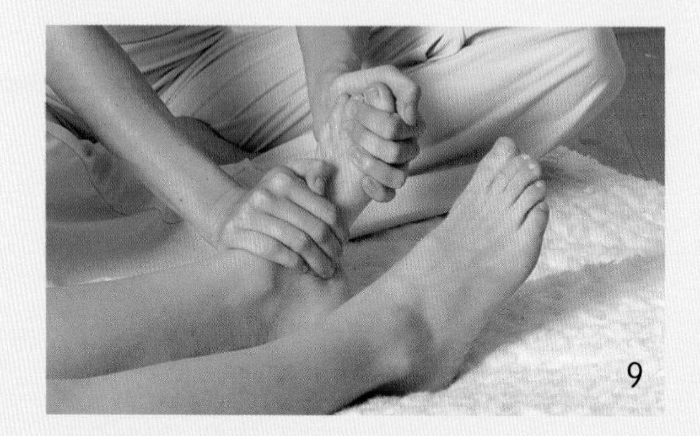
9

9 **Squeezing:** Wrap your hands around the foot. Squeeze the foot with both hands. Change the position of your hands and repeat. Change your hands one more time and repeat again.

10 **Holding:** Place both hands gently around the foot and hold for a few moments.

Ending: Cover the foot and repeat the sequence to the other side.

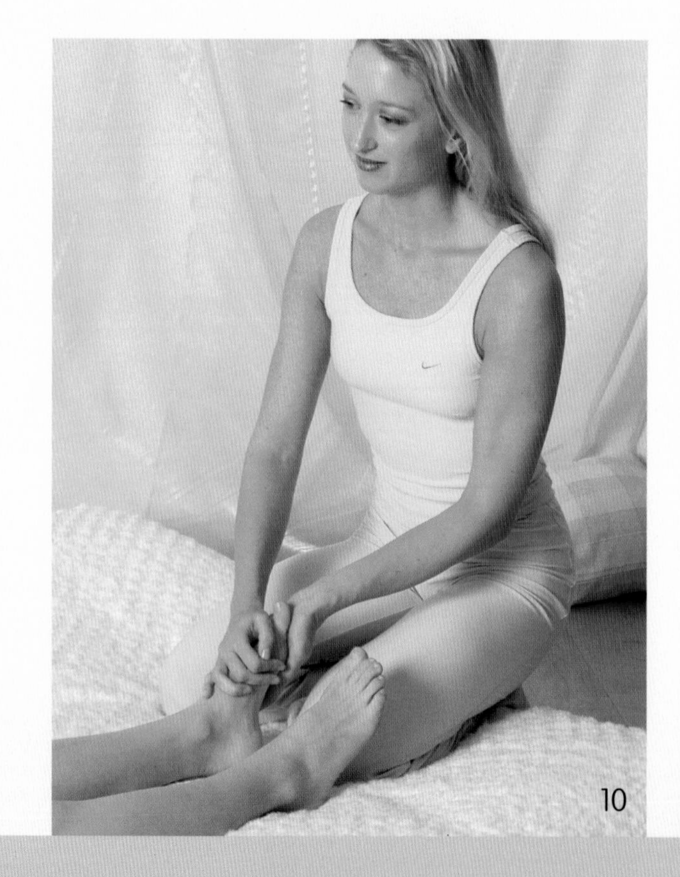
10

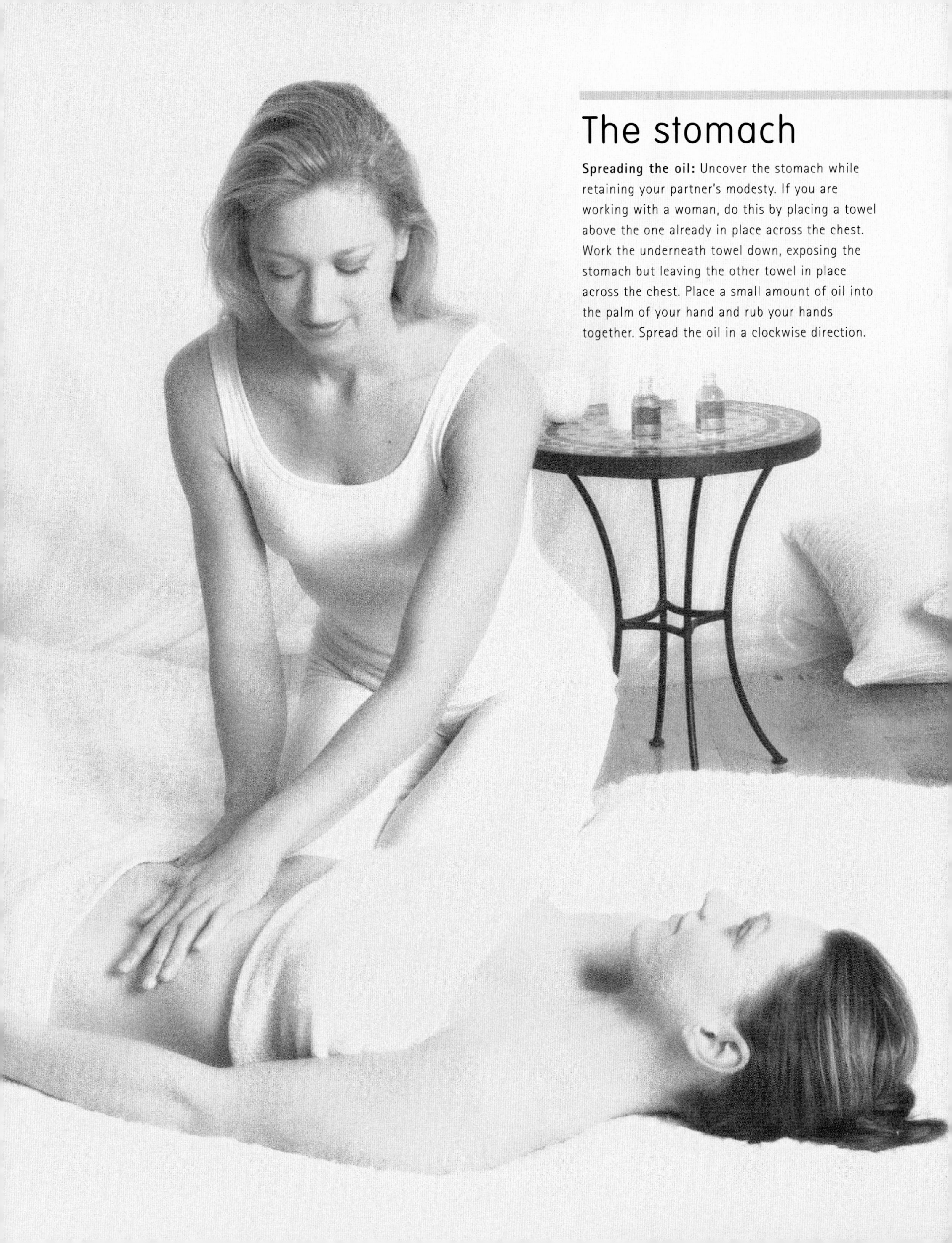

The stomach

Spreading the oil: Uncover the stomach while retaining your partner's modesty. If you are working with a woman, do this by placing a towel above the one already in place across the chest. Work the underneath towel down, exposing the stomach but leaving the other towel in place across the chest. Place a small amount of oil into the palm of your hand and rub your hands together. Spread the oil in a clockwise direction.

1 Circling: Place the hands flat on the stomach. Make circles around the belly button in a clockwise direction. Pick up the hands and put them back down as necessary.

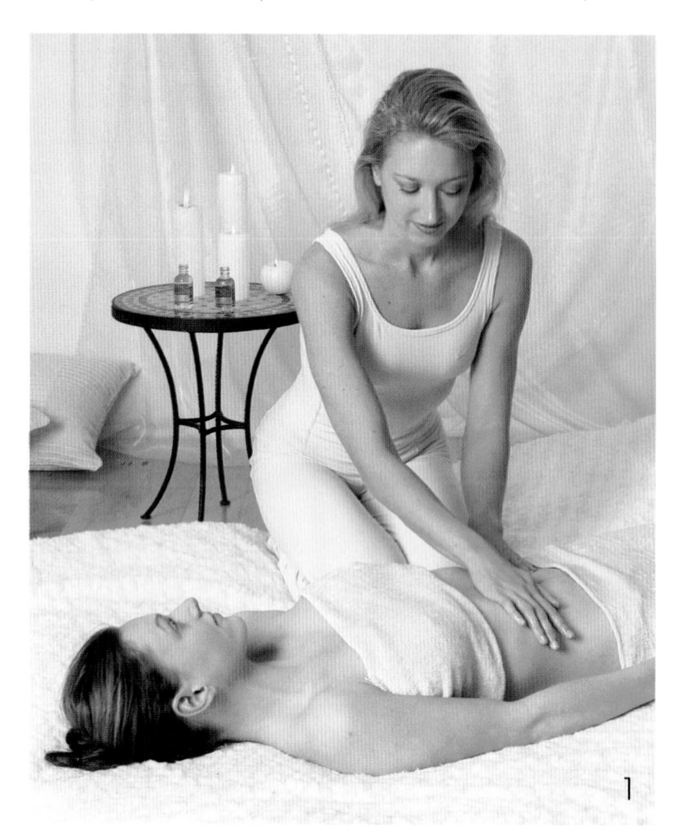
1

2 Flat hands along the rib: This stroke uses the outside of both of your hands. Flatten them and place the outer edge of one hand along the bottom of the ribs closest to you. Drag the hand towards you along the line of the rib. As the hand gets to the end, start the other hand dragging towards you. Repeat several times and then cross over to the other side to repeat.

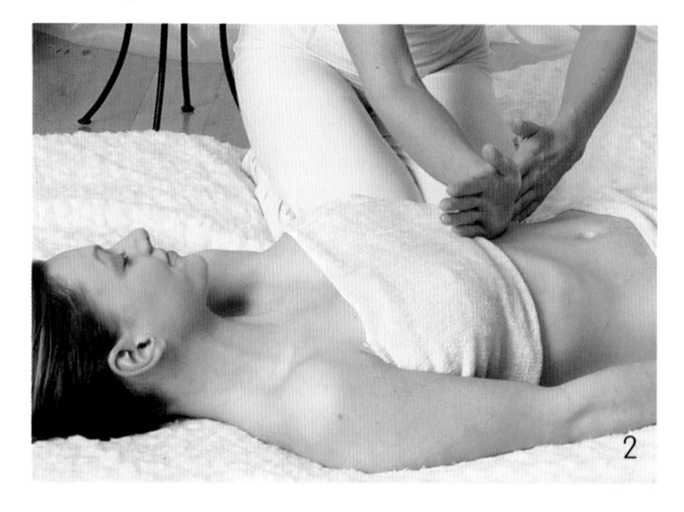
2

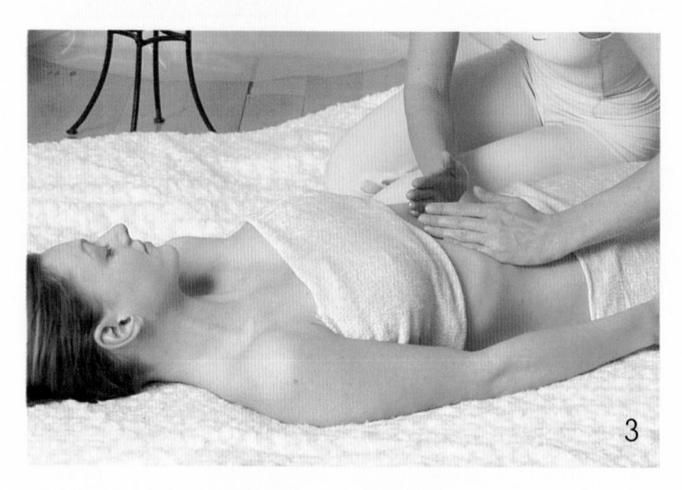
3

3 Both hands along the ribs: Kneel at your partner's hips facing their head. Place your fingertips together, hands flat and elbows out. Your arms should be in a V position similar to the ribs. Place the flat edges of the hand under the ribs. Separating the fingertips, slide the hands out along the line of the ribs. Float the hands down to the waist. Gently pull up on the waist and bring the hands together just underneath the belly button. Repeat twice.

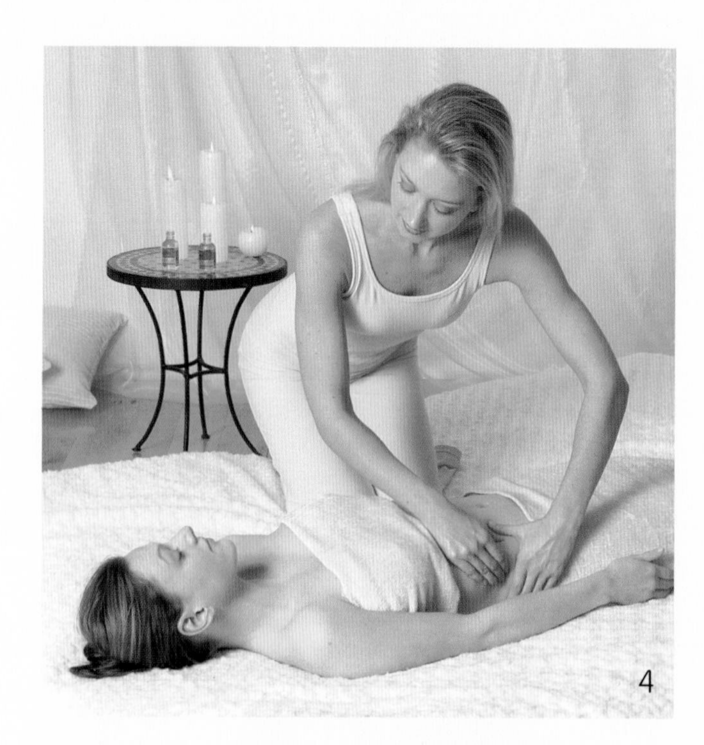
4

4 Kneading: Place the hands on the opposite side of your partner with the fingertips facing down and your thumbs out to the sides. Pick up the flesh with one hand and squeeze it as you slide it over to your other hand. As you release the flesh, pick it up with your other hand. Repeat a few times, shifting your weight with the movement. Repeat to the other side.

5 **Double-handed circles:** Kneel on the right side of your partner. Place one hand on top of the other with the fingertips just below the belly button on the right side. Imagine a square around the belly button. You are going to make tiny circles on three sides of the square. Circle up towards the ribs, across towards the other side, and down the other side only. Repeat the action three times. This stroke massages the digestive tract.

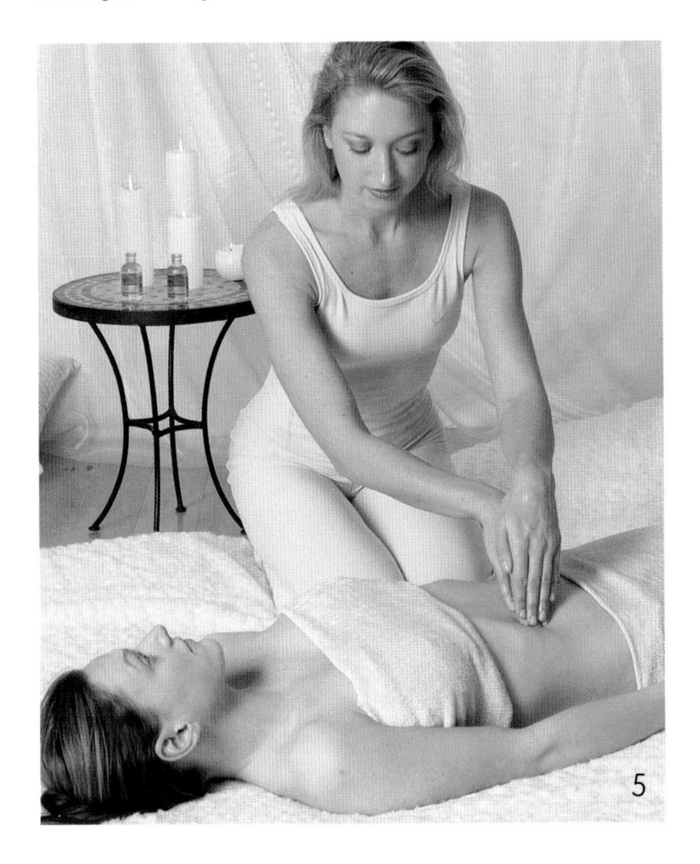

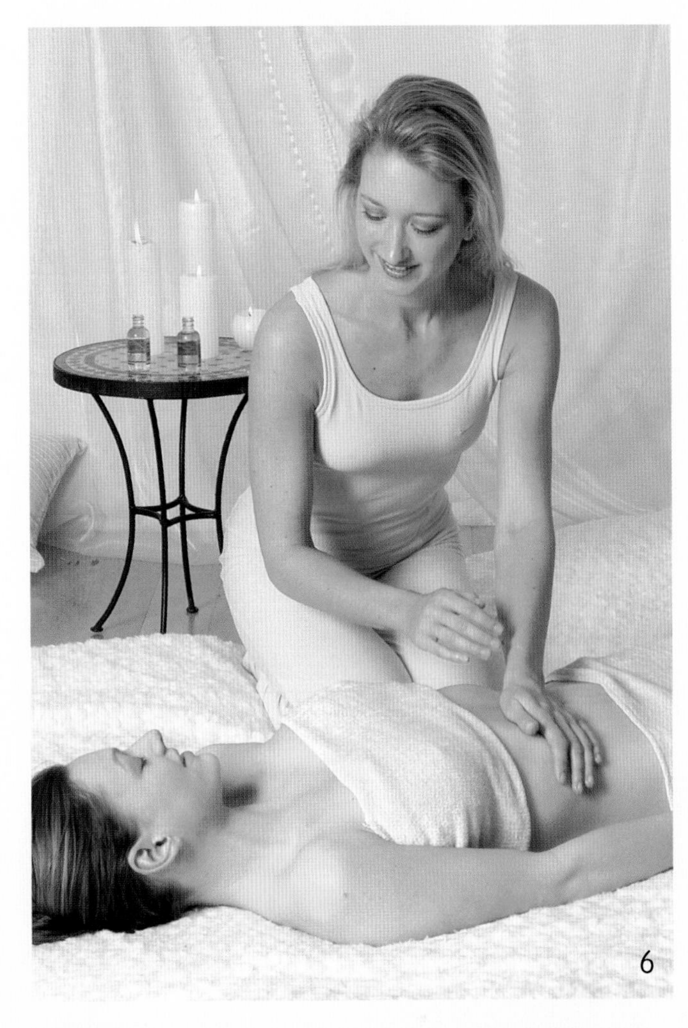

6 **Circling:** Place the hands flat on the stomach. Make circles around the belly button in a clockwise direction. Pick up the hands and put them back down as necessary.

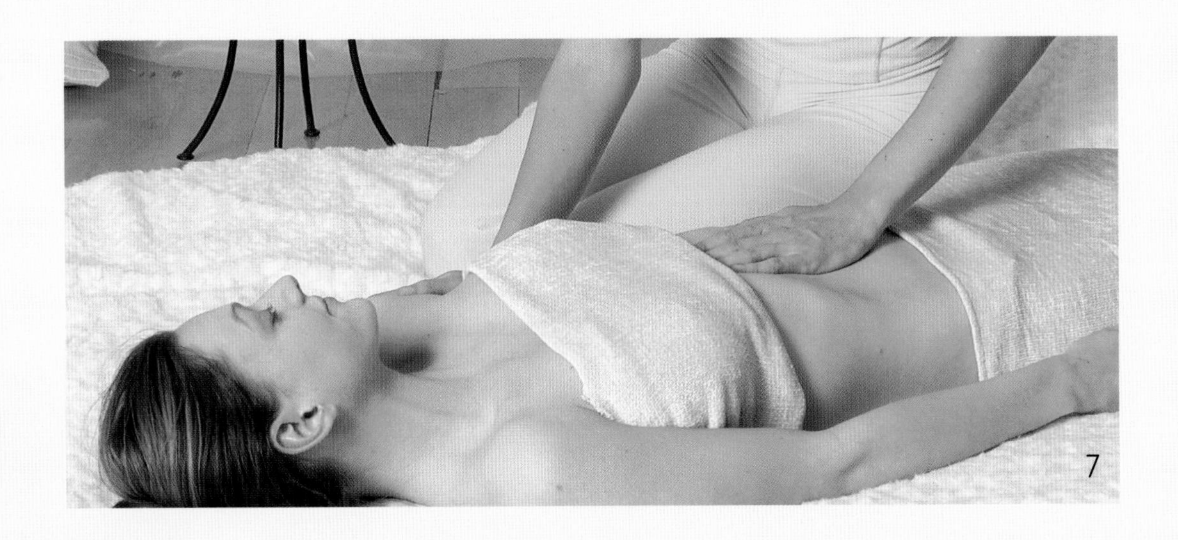

7 **Rub solar plexus:** Place one hand on the stomach with the fingers facing your partner's head just below the chest. Rub the fingers in a clockwise direction with the palm of the hand remaining still.

Ending: Cover the stomach and chest with the bottom towel. Slowly work the chest towel out from underneath the top towel.

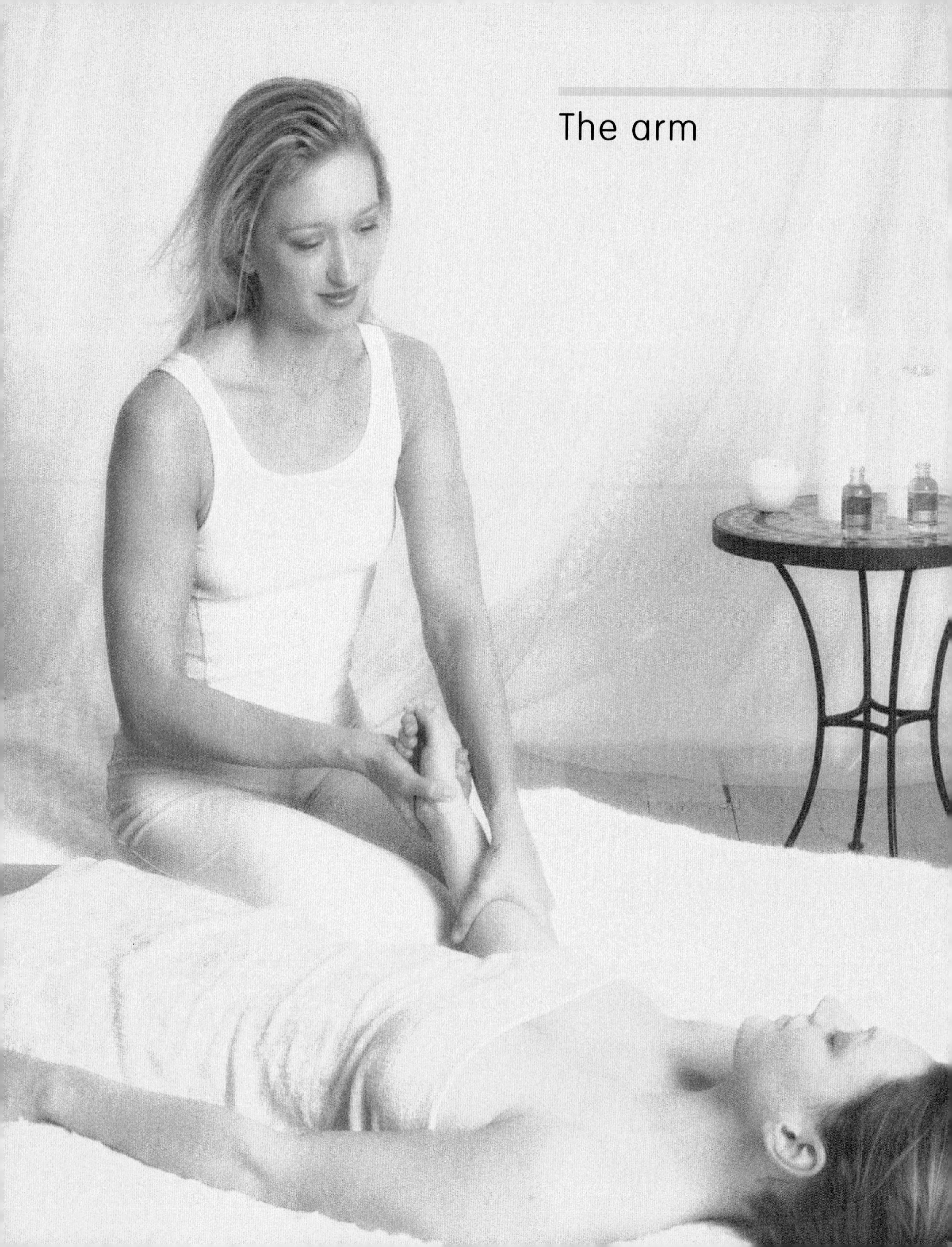

The arm

Softening: Place the hands above the towel with the fingers on one side of the arm and the palms on the other. Gently squeeze the flesh underneath the towel and release. Move the hands to a different place on the arm and repeat. Repeat, covering the whole arm.

Spreading the oil: Uncover the arm and pour a small amount of oil into the palm of one hand. Rub your hands together and spread the oil, starting at the wrist and working your way up to the shoulder. Be sure to cover the entire arm.

1 **Alternating effleurage:** Hold the wrist with one hand. Slide the other hand up from the wrist to the shoulder, avoiding the elbow. Bring the hand to the outside of the arm and glide the hand back down. Change hands and repeat. Repeat a few more times.

2 **Friction to the lower arm:** Turn the palm upwards. Hold the wrist with one hand. Place the thumb of your opposite hand on the wrist. Make small circles with the thumb up to the elbow. Repeat twice, covering the whole inner arm. Turn the wrist over and repeat to the top of the forearm.

3 **Draining to the lymph node:** Hold the wrist up at a slight diagonal. Place the wedge between the thumb and forefinger on opposite sides of their arm at the wrist. Making short, sweeping motions, push down the arm towards the elbow. Repeat this a few times.

4 **Friction to the upper arm:** Place the thumbs on top of the arm with the fingers underneath. Circle the thumbs while squeezing the flesh underneath with your fingers. Cover the whole upper arm.

5 **Digital pressure:** Hook your inside arm through your partner's elbow. Place the fingertips of your other hand on their upper arm just above their elbow. Press deeply as you slide the fingertips up to their shoulder. Circle the shoulder and press the fingers into the flesh underneath their arm as you glide the fingers back down the upper arm to repeat.

6 **Arm stretch:** Hold the wrist with one hand. Bring the arm up over the head. Place the other hand underneath the towel towards the waist. Drag the hand up the waist to the shoulder. Wrap the fingers around the shoulder and slide the hand up to the wrist. Give a gentle pull to the arm at the wrist. Repeat twice.

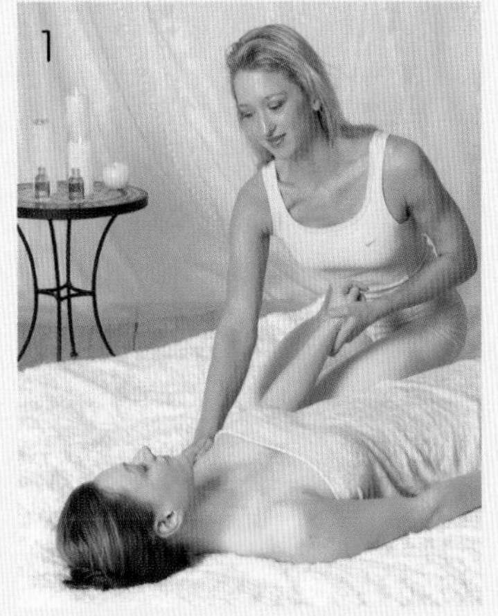

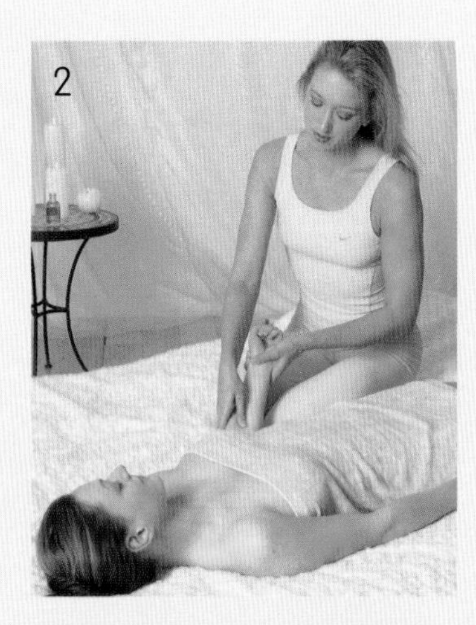

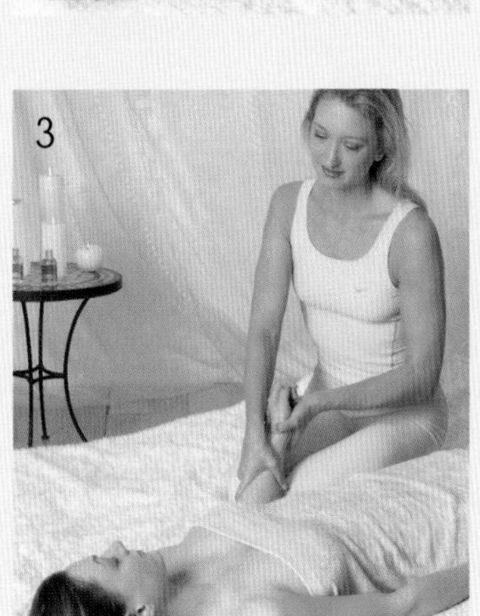

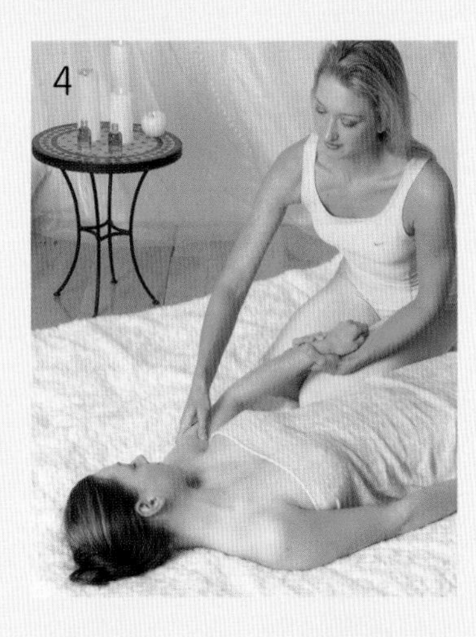

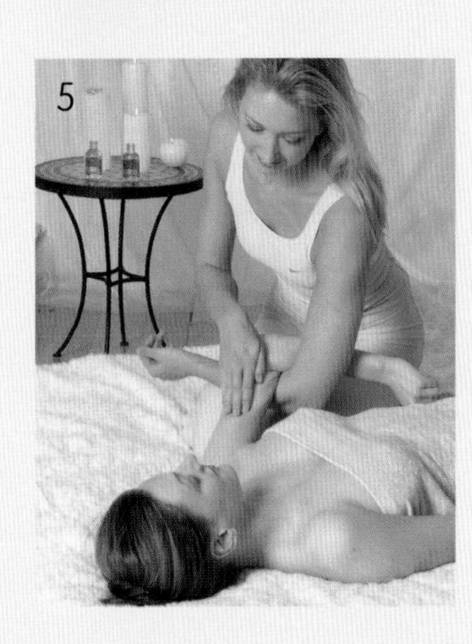

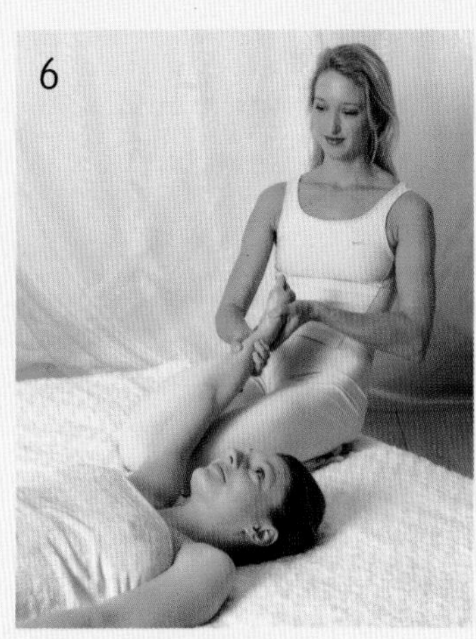

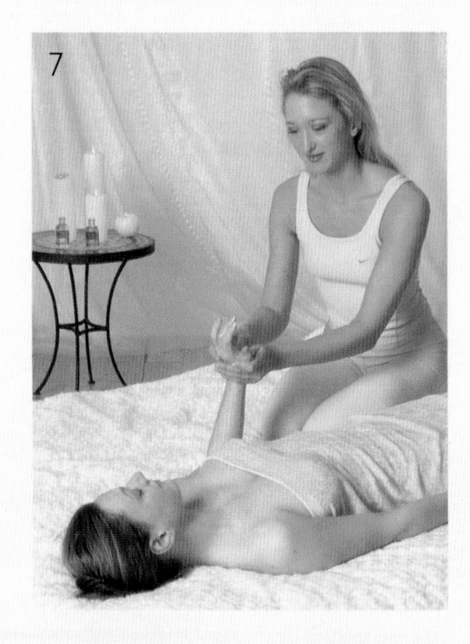

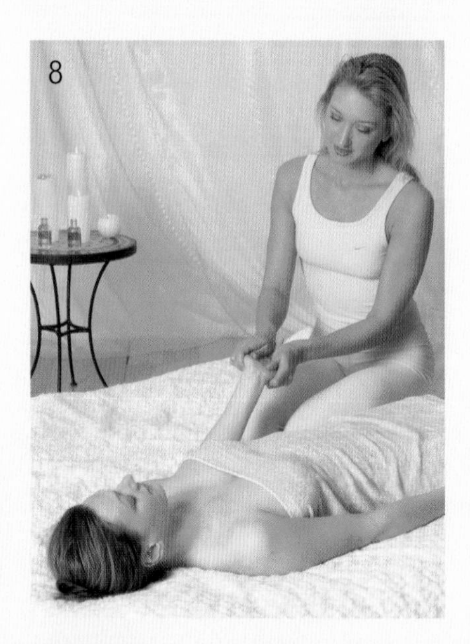

7 Friction to the wrist and hand: Bring the arm back down by your partner's side. Place the thumbs on the wrist. Make circles covering the wrist and hand. Turn the palm over and repeat the circles to the palm.

8 Opening: Lace your pinkies in your partner's thumb and pinkie. Place the thumbs lengthwise on the palm. Press the hand out and open your partner's hand as you drag the thumbs away from each other across the palm. Repeat a few times.

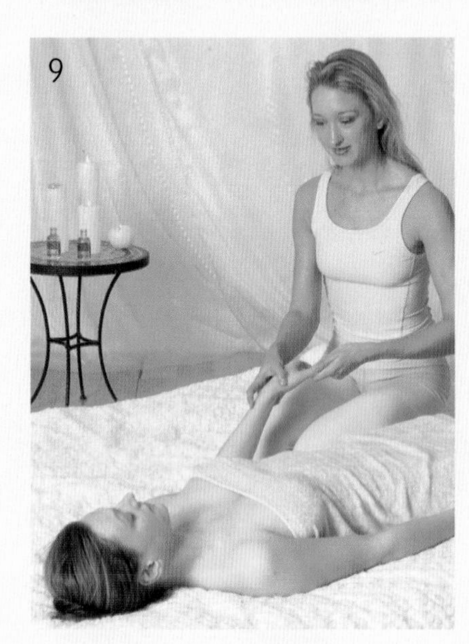

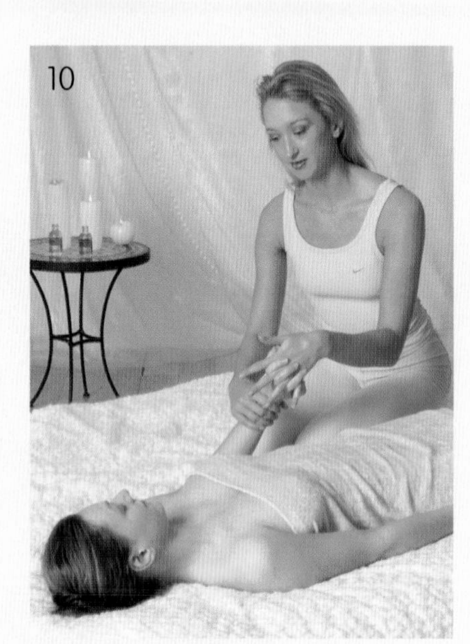

9 Finger massage: Hold the pinkie with the thumb and forefinger. Circle the finger from the base of the finger to the tip and give a gentle pull. Repeat to each finger.

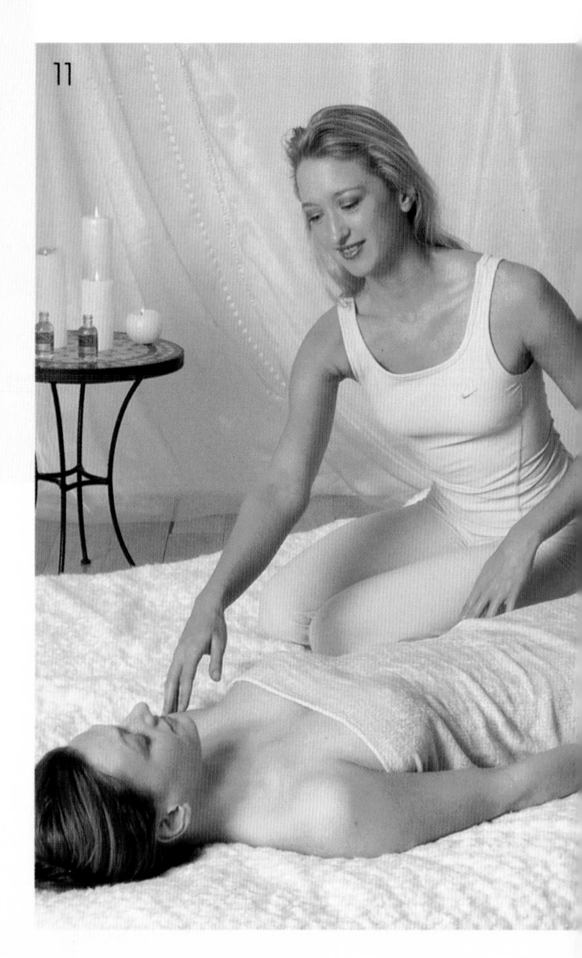

10 Fingers laced: Lace the fingers of one hand in your partner's. Hold the wrist with your other hand and make loose circles. Repeat three times in each direction. Gently move your partner's hand forwards and backwards. Place the hand back down on the table.

11 Feather stroking: Place the fingertips of one hand on the shoulder. Gently glide the fingertips down to the wrist. As the hand reaches the wrist, start the other hand at the shoulder and repeat.

Ending: Cover the arm and repeat to the other side.

The chest

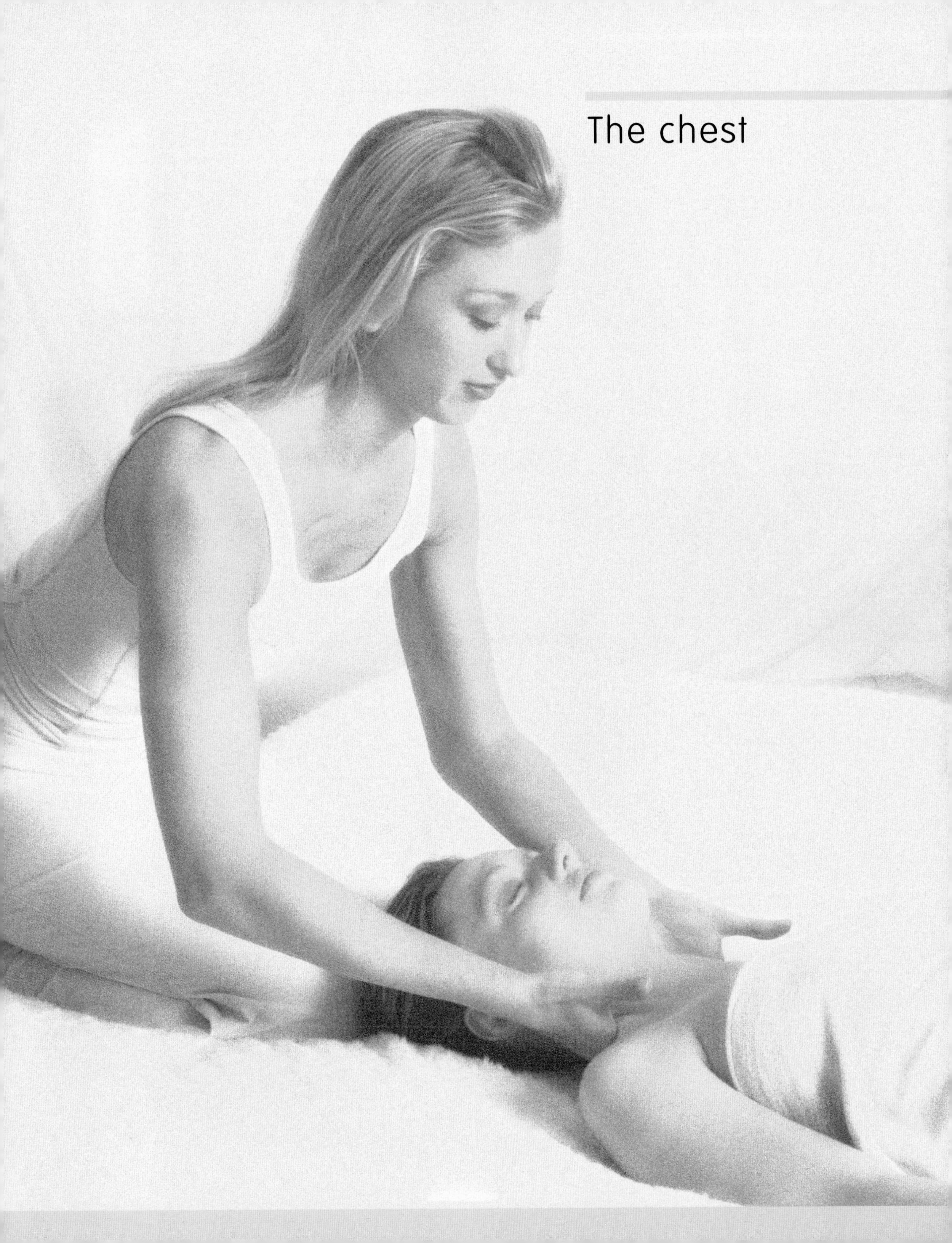

1 Rocking: Sit or kneel at your partner's head facing their feet. Place your hands on the outside of their shoulders with the fingers facing outwards. Press into one palm, and then into the other, gently rocking your partner back and forth.

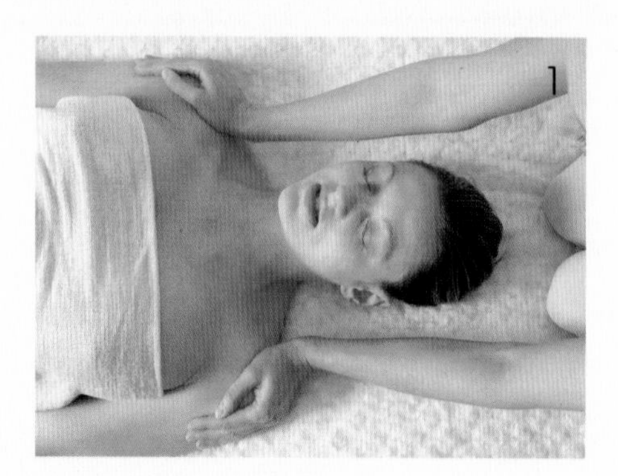

2 Spreading the oil: Uncover the chest while retaining your partner's modesty. Pour a small amount of oil into the palm of your hand and rub your hands together. Place the hands in the centre of your partner's chest with the fingertips together and the palms out to the sides. Slide the hands across the chest to the shoulders, spreading the oil. Then bring the hands around to the back of the neck with the fingertips together. Slide the hands across the back of the neck towards the shoulders. Repeat this sequence a few times, covering the chest, shoulders and neck with the oil.

3 Alternating effleurage: Place one hand sideways in the centre of the chest. Drag the hand across to the shoulder. As that hand reaches the shoulder, place the other hand sideways in the centre of the chest. Repeat, alternating the hands.

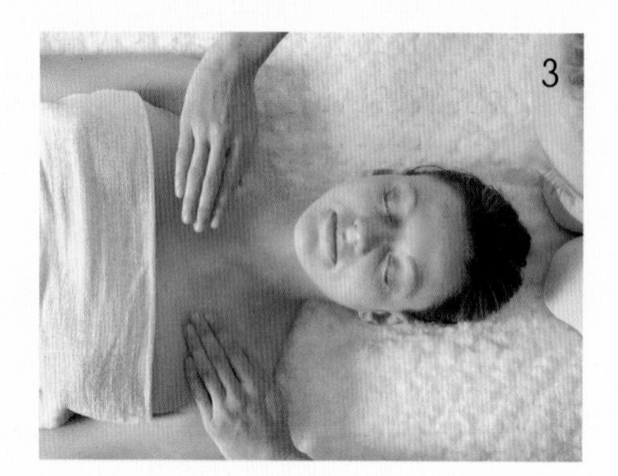

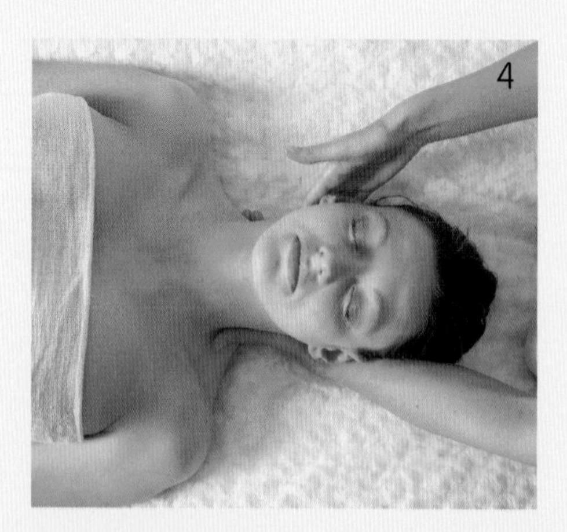

4 Hand over hand to the neck: Place one hand at the base of the neck with the fingers on one side and the palms on the other. Slide the hand up to the base of the skull. Replace that hand with the opposite hand on the base of the neck and repeat. Change hands quickly and smoothly while massaging the neck.

5 Friction to the shoulders: Place the thumbs in the groove of the collarbone. Place the fingers underneath the shoulders. Keeping the thumbs still, circle the fingers. Repeat, placing the thumbs under the shoulders and the fingers in the groove of the collarbone. Circle the thumbs on the shoulders.

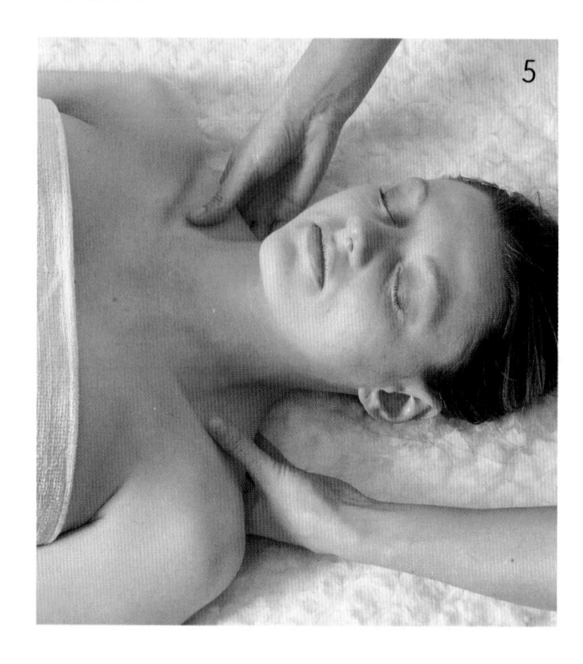

6 Friction to the pecs: Place the fingertips on the shoulder where the arm meets the chest. Make small circles with the fingers in opposite directions.

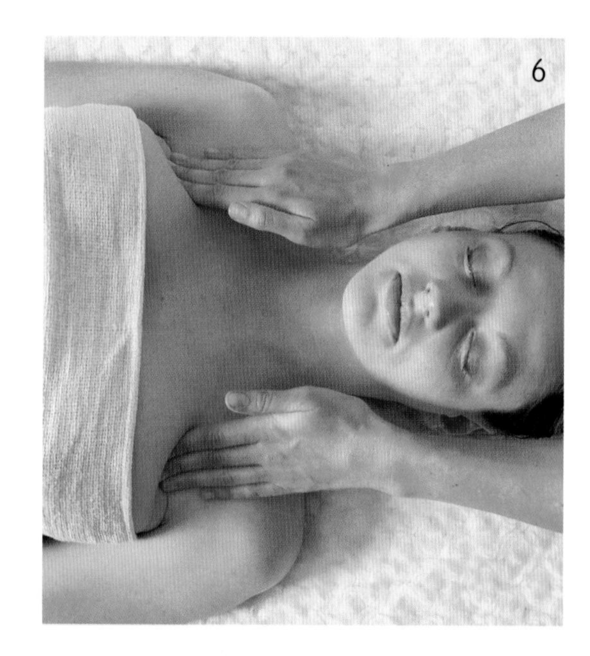

7 **Lymph drainage:** Place the thumbs in the centre of the chest. Slide them out towards the shoulders. Repeat twice.

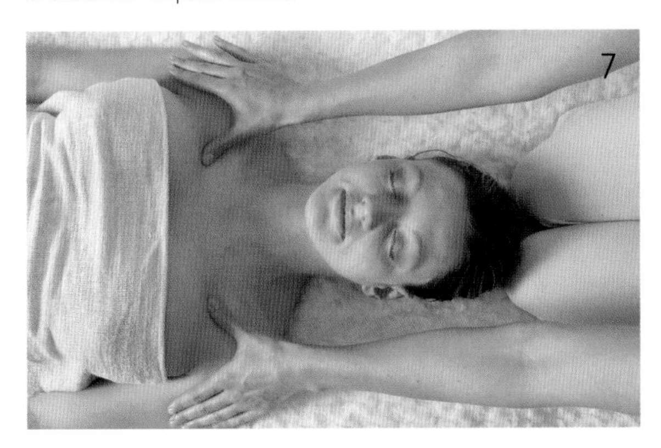

8 **Tapoment:** Lightly place the fingertips above the chest. Let them tap the chest like raindrops hitting the skin individually.

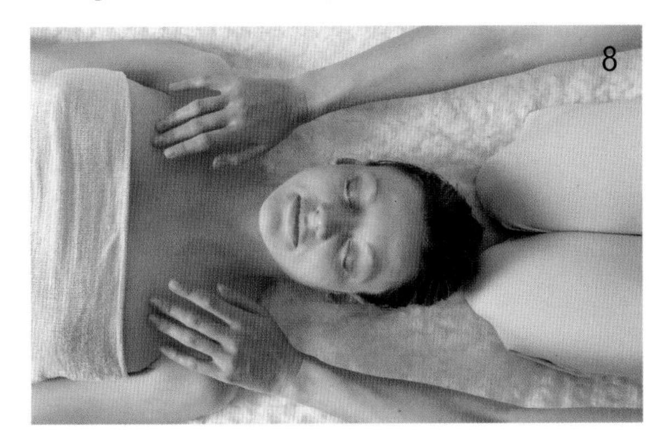

9 **Circling:** Place both hands sideways in the centre of the chest with the fingertips touching. Slide the hands across the chest to the shoulders. Circle the shoulders and bring the hands together at the back of the neck. Pull gently on the head with the fingertips in the groove of the bottom of the skull. Repeat a few times.

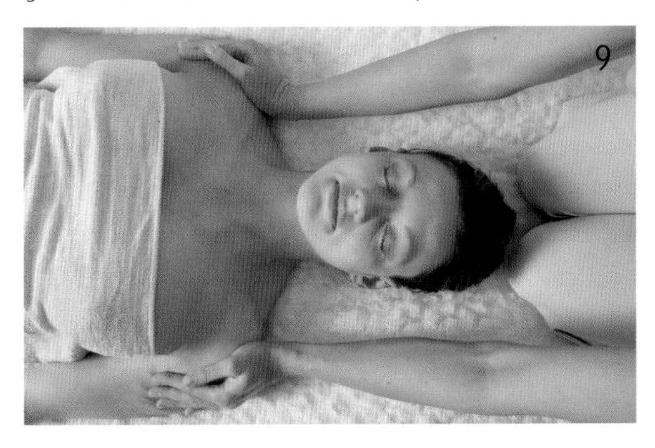

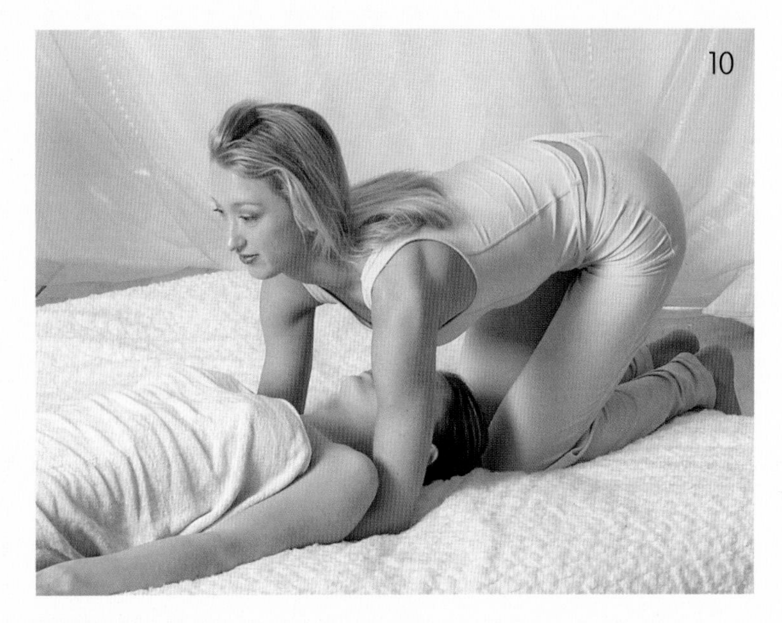

10 Arch back: Kneel at the head of your partner facing their feet. Ask them to lift their shoulders and then arch their back as you slide your hands underneath them. Place your hands as low on their back as is comfortable, with your hands forming a claw on either side of their spine. Ask them to relax back onto your hands. Slide your hands up either side of their spine while firmly holding the claw position with your hands. Slide the hands up to the nape of the neck and gently pull with your fingers on the base of the skull. Repeat a few times.

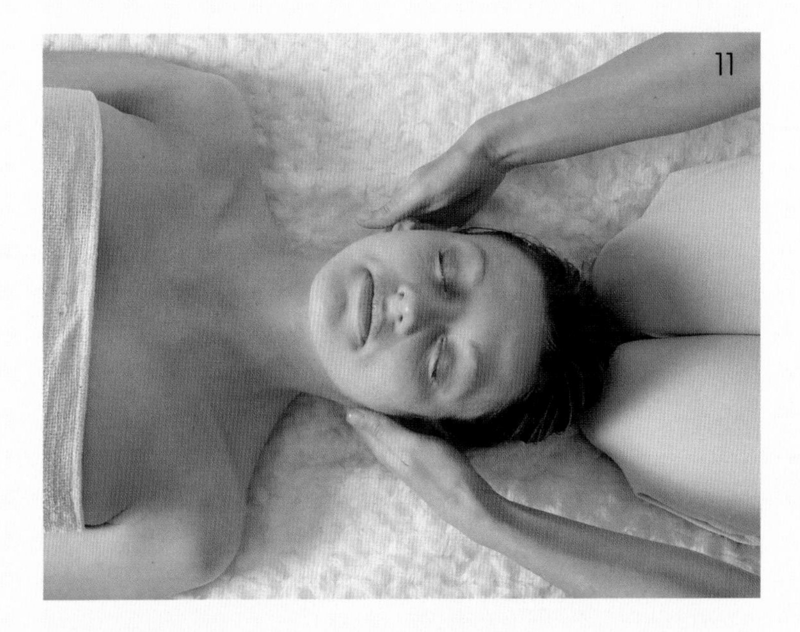

11 Circling: Place both hands sideways in the centre of the chest with the fingertips touching. Slide the hands across the chest to the shoulders. Circle the shoulders and bring the hands together at the back of the neck. Pull gently on the head with the fingertips in the groove of the bottom of the skull. Repeat a few times.

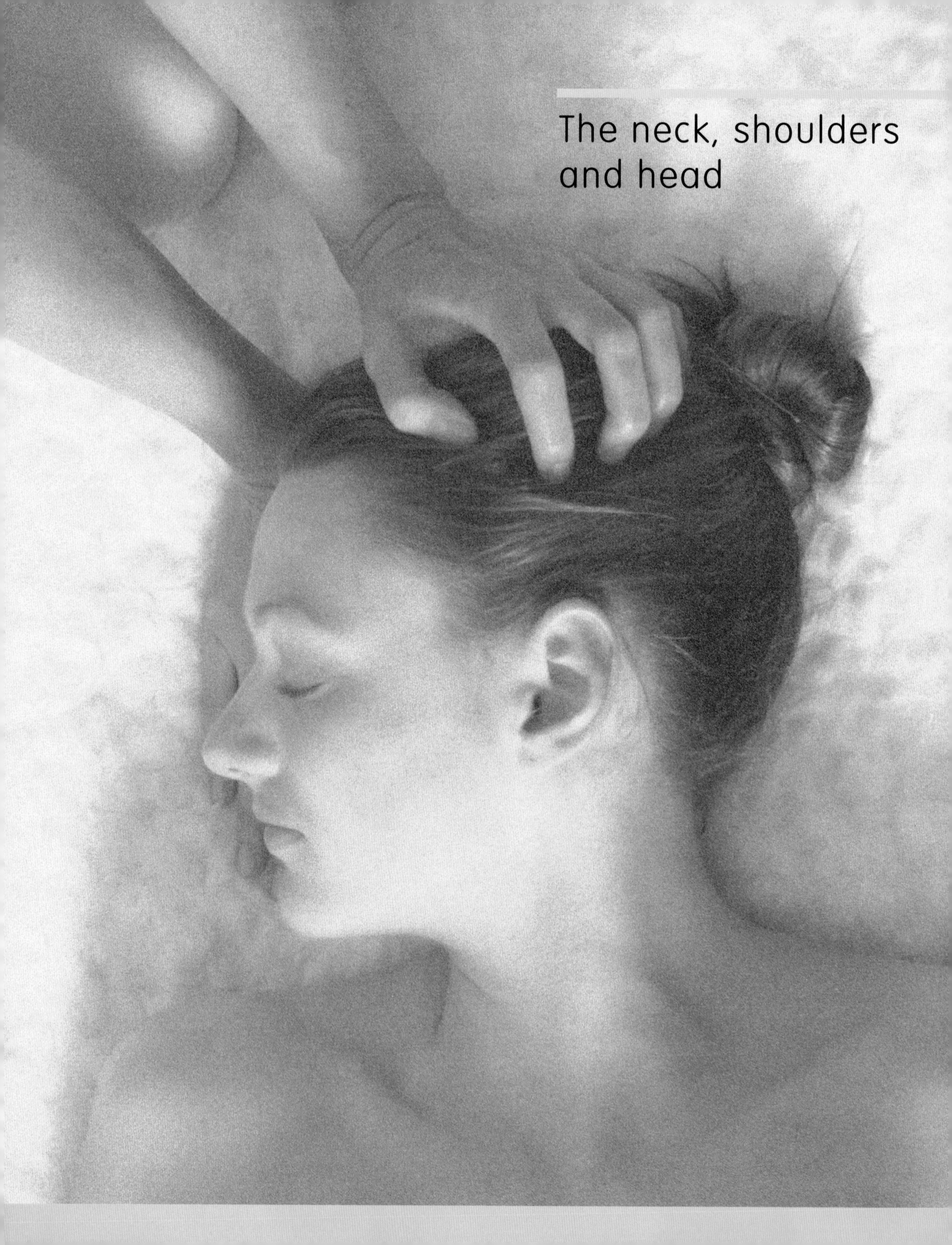

The neck, shoulders and head

1 **Turn head:** Gently turn your partner's head to the right. Place your right hand on the surface in front of their forehead for stability.

2 **One handed effleurage:** Place your left hand flat with the thumb out and the fingertips touching the table by the base of the skull. Run the inside of the fingers along the ridge of the neck to the shoulder letting your thumb mould to the contour of the skin. Wrap your hand around the shoulder and then return back to the base of the skull in the exact same way (with the thumb on top and the flat part of the fingers stroking the neck and shoulders). Repeat, finding any areas of tension.

3 **Knuckling:** Touch the fingers to the palm of your left hand. Place the knuckles underneath the left shoulder. Make circles with the whole arm along the shoulders and neck.

4 **Friction points:** Slide your thumb along your partner's neck. Feel if there is any tension or areas of tightness. If you find a knot, place your thumb directly over the area. Press the thumb into the knot and make a small, slow circle. Release.

5 **Friction to base of head:** Form a claw with your left hand. Place the tips of the fingers in the base of the skull. Make small circles with the fingertips, being sure to move the skin over the bone. Wipe oil off: Be sure to wipe your hands before working on your partner's hair.

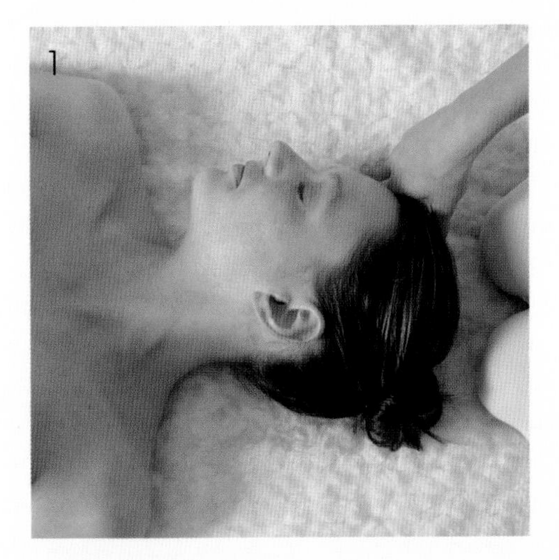

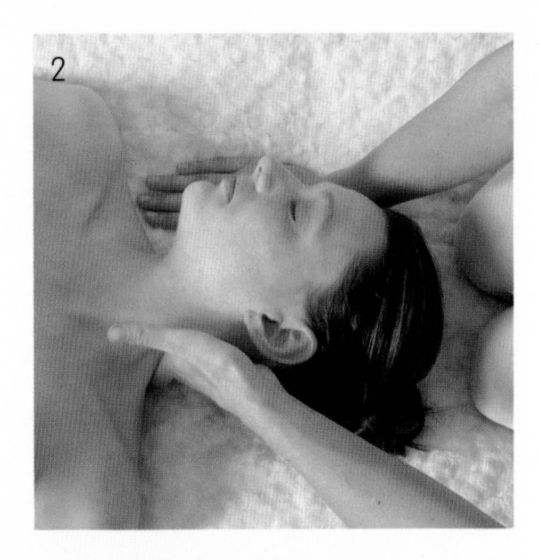

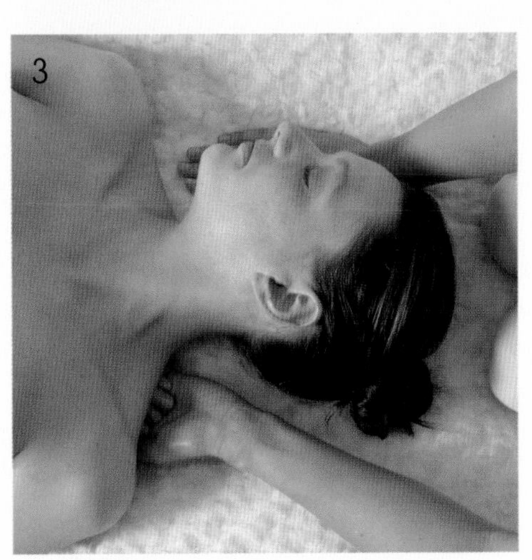

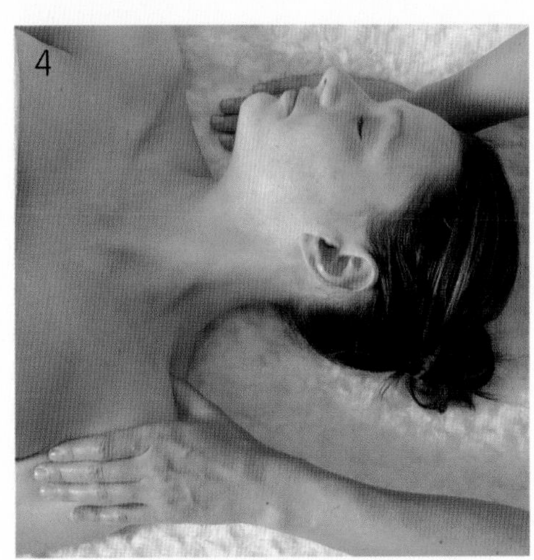

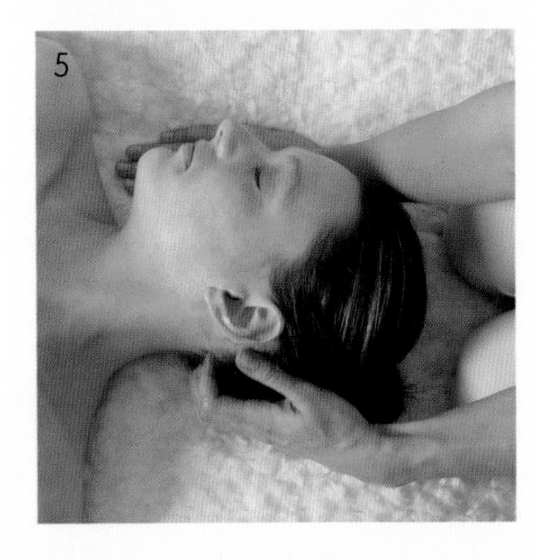

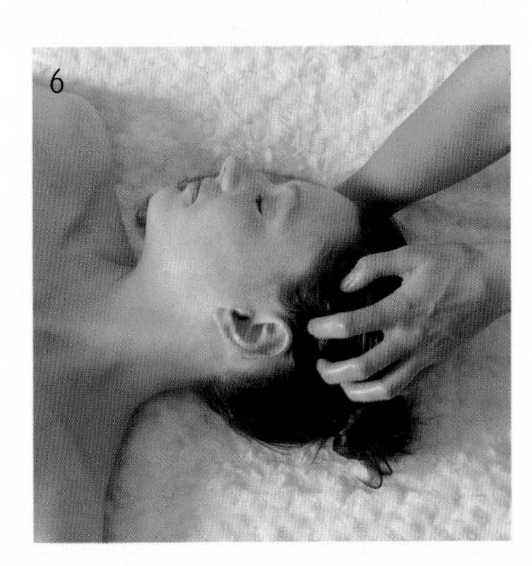

6 **Friction to head:** Again form a claw with your hand. Place the fingers just above the base of the skull. Make small circles, moving the skin over the bone. Raise your fingers a little higher and repeat. Repeat, covering the whole left side of the skull.

Gently turn the head to the left and repeat the whole sequence.

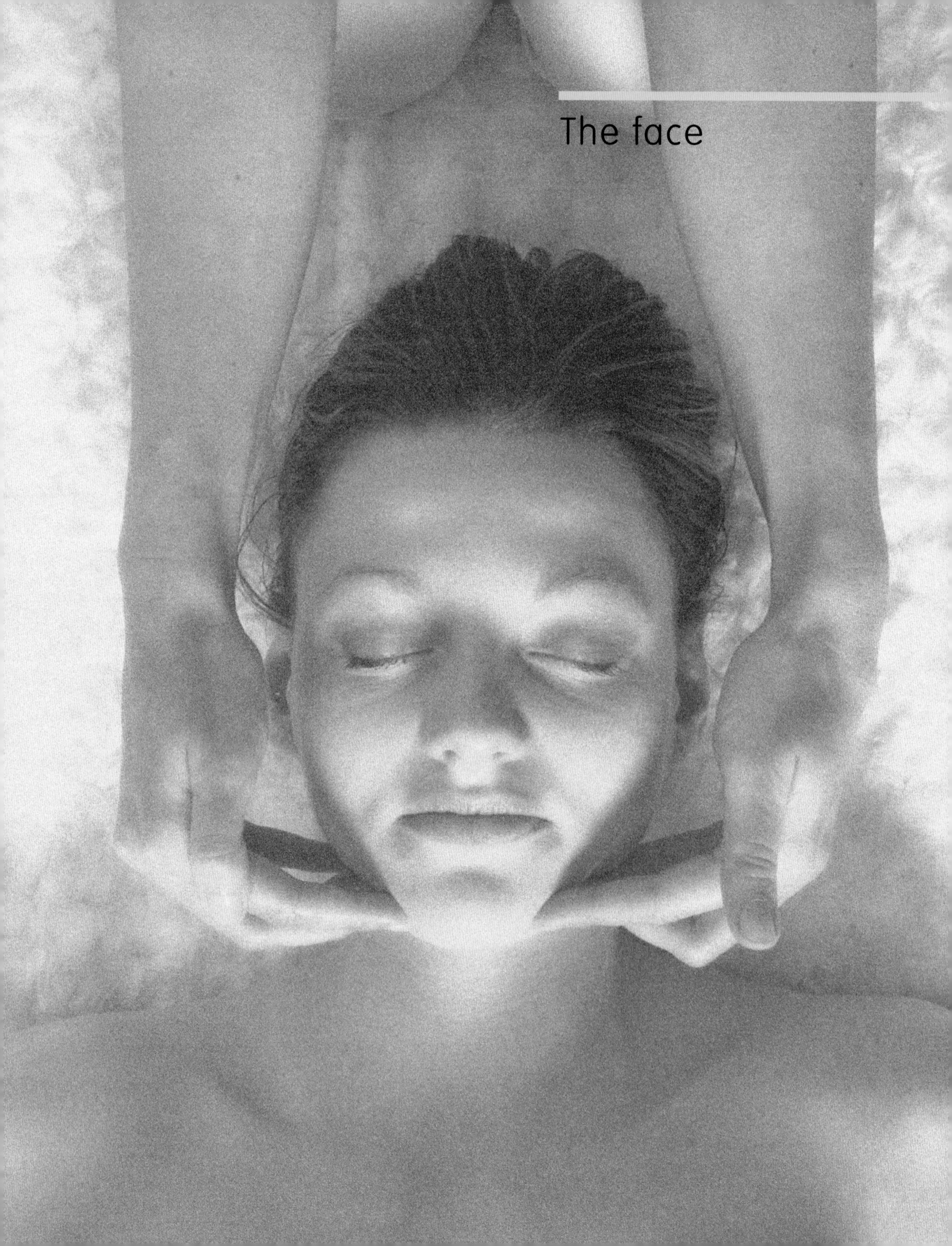

The face

Spreading the oil: Put 2–3 drops of oil onto your fingertips. Start at the chin and spread the oil up to the forehead, avoiding the eyes, nose and mouth.

1 **Effleurage to the chin:** Place the fingertips underneath the chin with the fingers together and the palms out to the sides. Gently stroke one hand across the chin to the ear. Then stroke the other side. Repeat slowly and gently. Place both hands on one side of the chin and stroke hand over hand to the ear. Repeat to the other side.

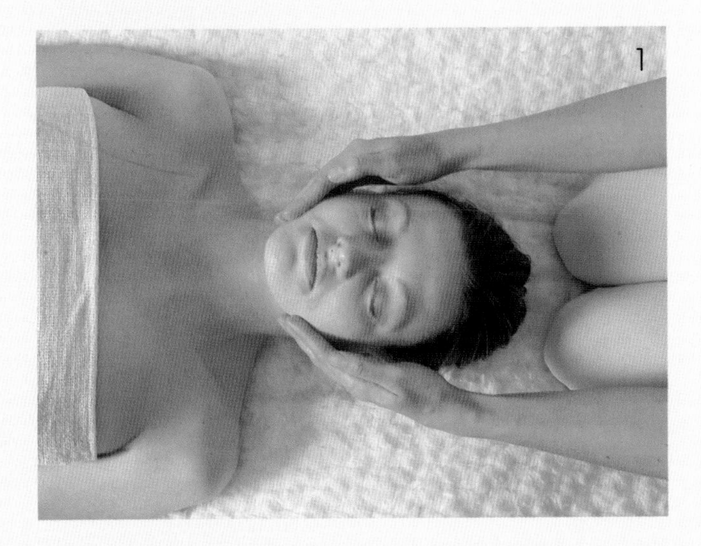

2 **Effleurage to the forehead:** Place one hand sideways across the forehead. Slide the hand across the forehead and immediately replace it with your other hand. Repeat this a few times.

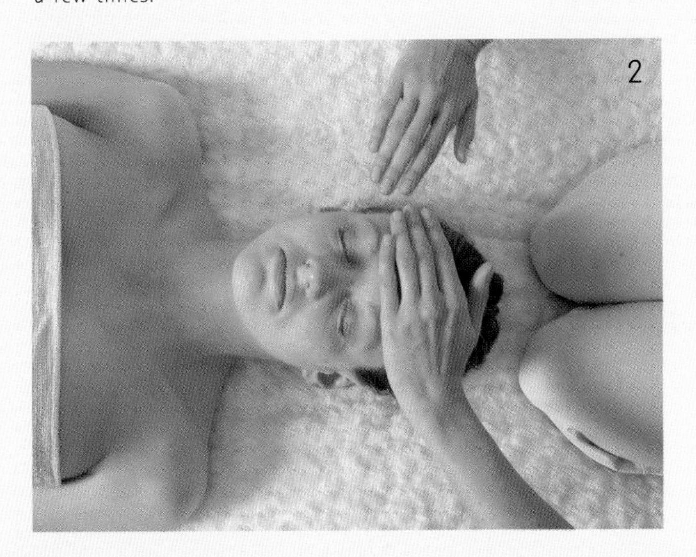

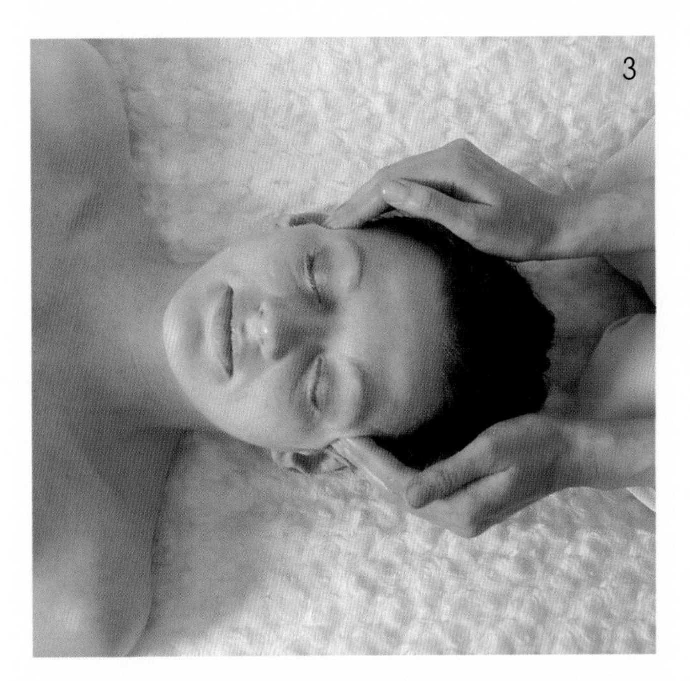

3 **Circling temples:** Start with the pads of the fingertips across the top of the forehead in one line. Press gently as you slide the hands away from each other to the temples. Gently circle the temples with the fingers. Repeat twice more, moving the hands slightly down towards the eyebrows each time.

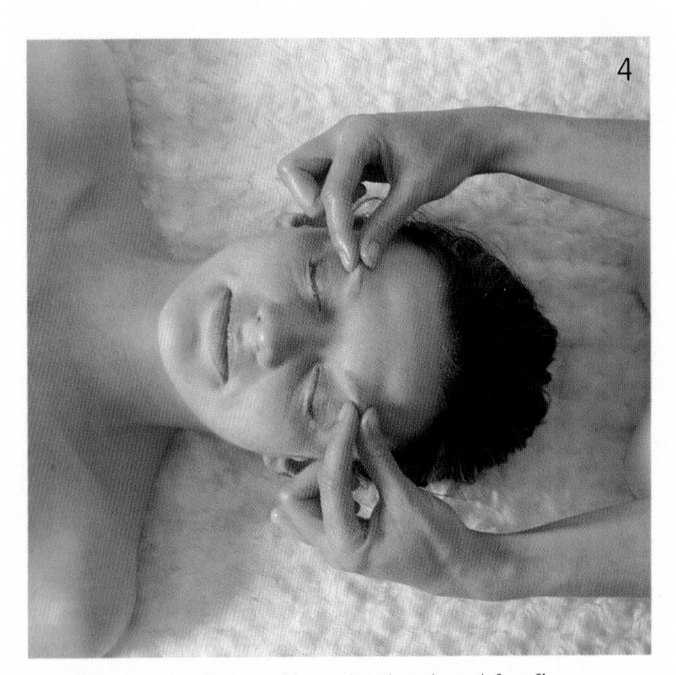

4 **Squeeze eyebrows:** Place the thumb and forefinger gently on the inside of both eyebrows. Squeeze the eyebrow gently and then move the fingers outwards a little to repeat. Repeat, covering the whole eyebrow.

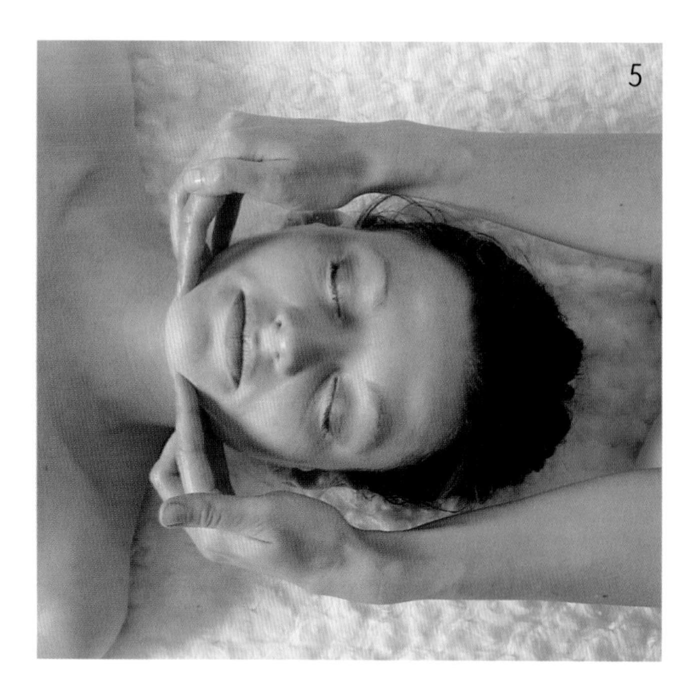

5 Friction: Place the fingers in a line across the chin. Make small circles. Repeat into the jaw.

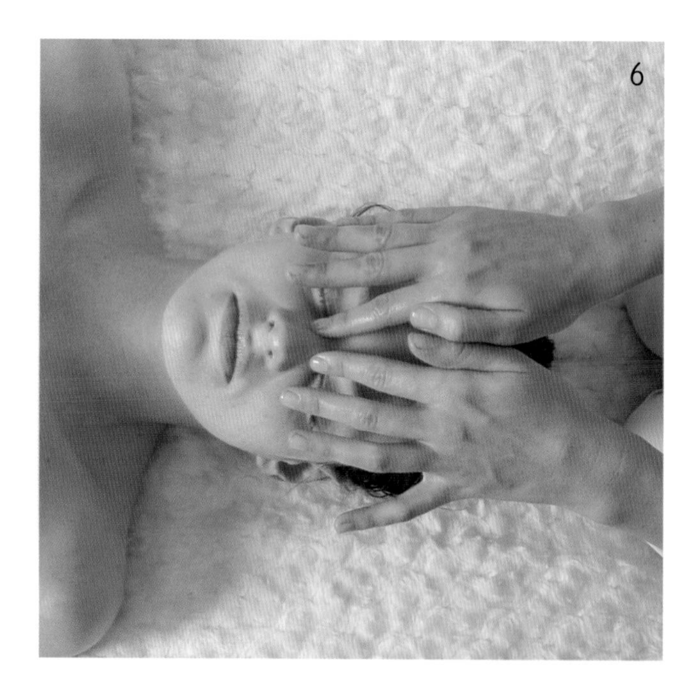

6 Circling the whole face: Using only your two forefingers, start at the chin. Lightly circle the mouth and bring your fingers onto the bridge of the nose. Draw the fingers up to the bridge of the nose, in between the eyes and onto the forehead. Separate the fingers, sliding them across the forehead and back down the cheeks to the chin. Repeat twice, keeping the circles soft and fluid.

7 Tapoment: Hold the fingertips above the forehead. Lightly tap the forehead, alternating the fingers as they fall onto the skin. Slowly bring the fingers around the cheeks and chin, being sure to avoid the eyes, nose and mouth.

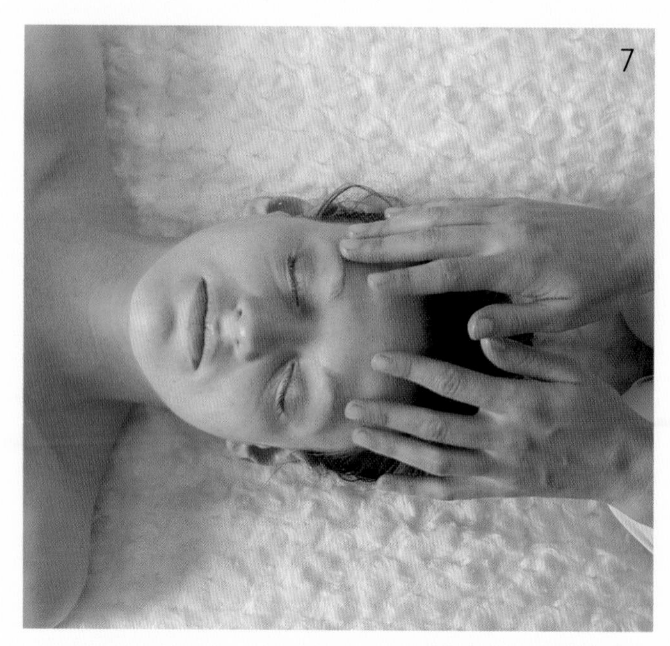

8 Circles to the ears: Place both hands underneath the chin with your fingertips facing each other. Sweep the hands in opposite directions towards the ears. Circle the fingers in front of the ears and then around the back of the ears. Gently pinch the ear lobe between the thumb and forefinger and pull towards the neck, letting the fingers slide away from the ear lobe. Repeat a few times.

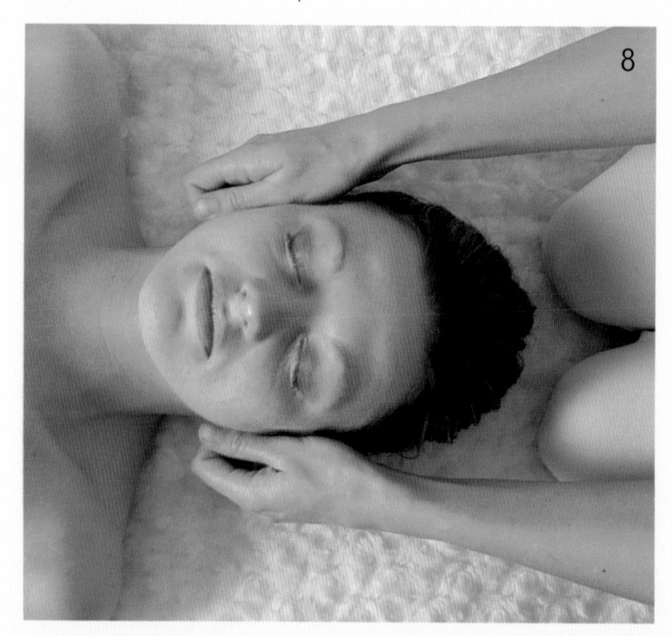

9 **Massaging the ears:** Place the thumb on top of the ear and bend your forefinger underneath the ear. Make circles with the thumb and forefinger massaging out the ear. Gently pull the ear out and away from the body.

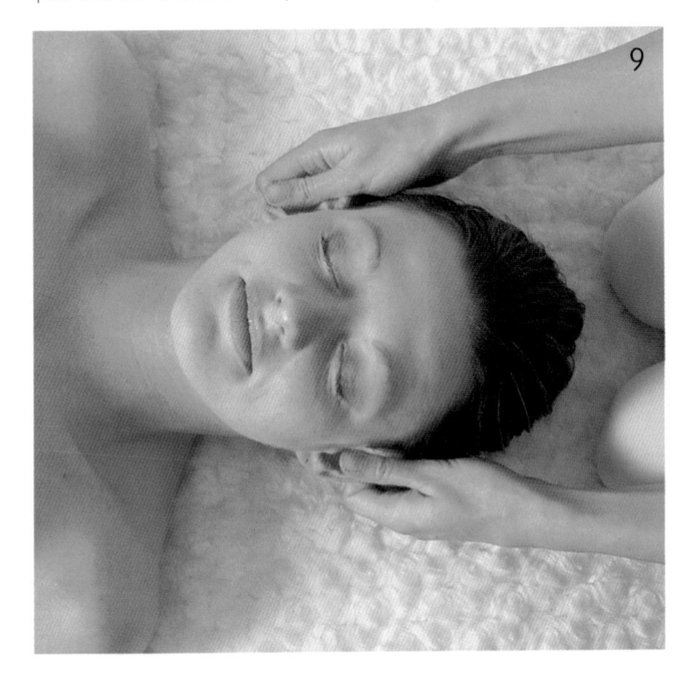

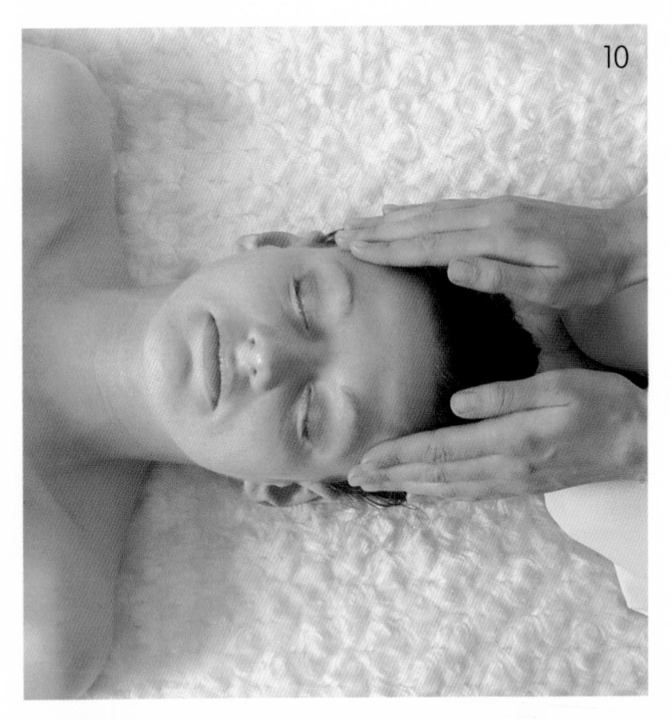

10 **Effleurage the whole face:** Place the fingers together at the base of the chin. Slide the hands around the chin, across the cheeks and onto the forehead. Repeat twice more.

Ending the massage: Hold the head for a moment with the thumbs together and the fingers towards the ear. Move to the side of your partner and squeeze their shoulders. Then place your hands on their hips and gently squeeze. Move down to your partner's knees and squeeze. Move to their feet and hold their feet for a moment.

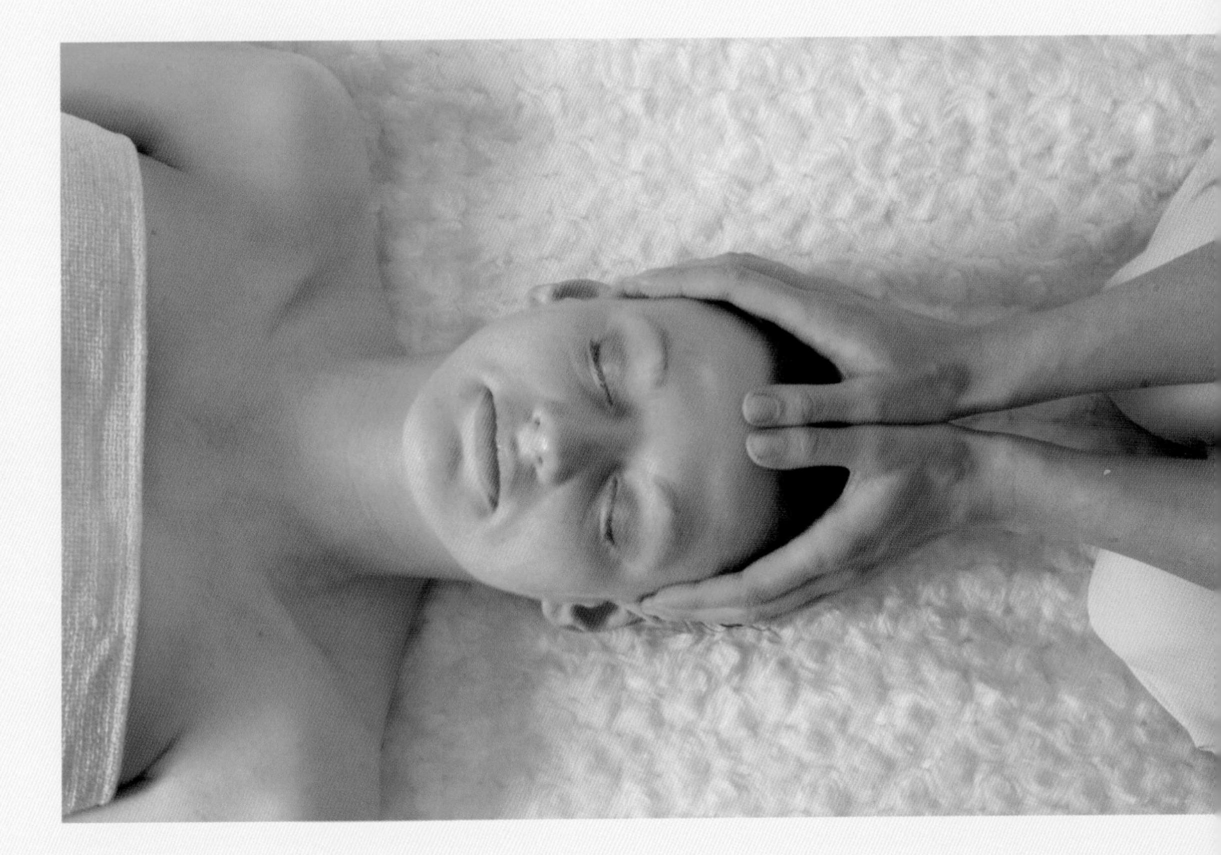

Quick guide – back

1. Softening

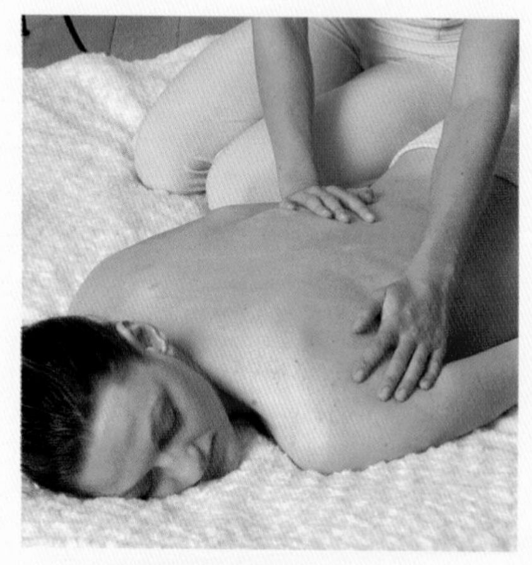

2. Spreading the oil

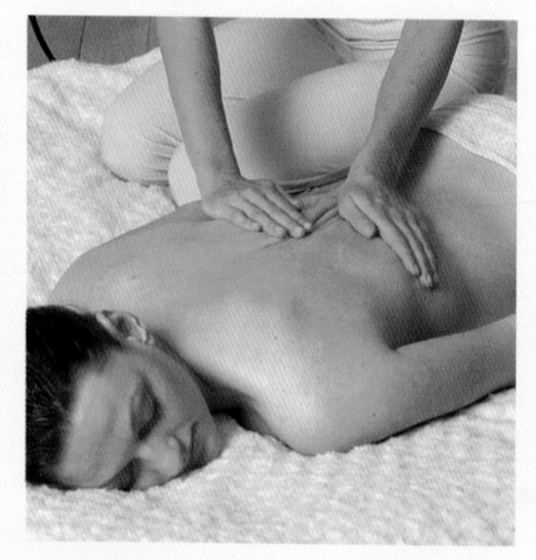

3. Effleurage figures-of-eight

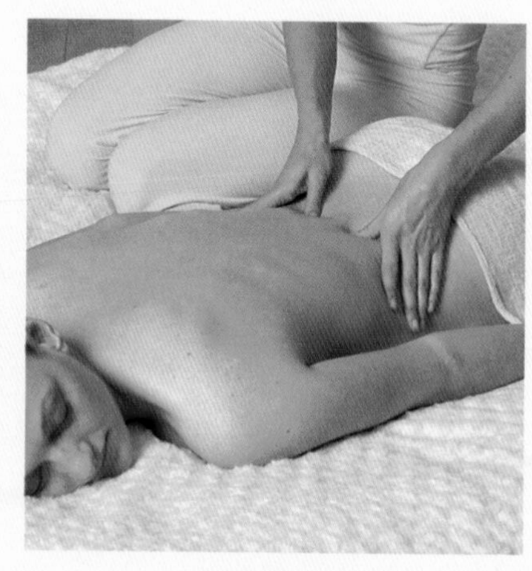

4. Friction

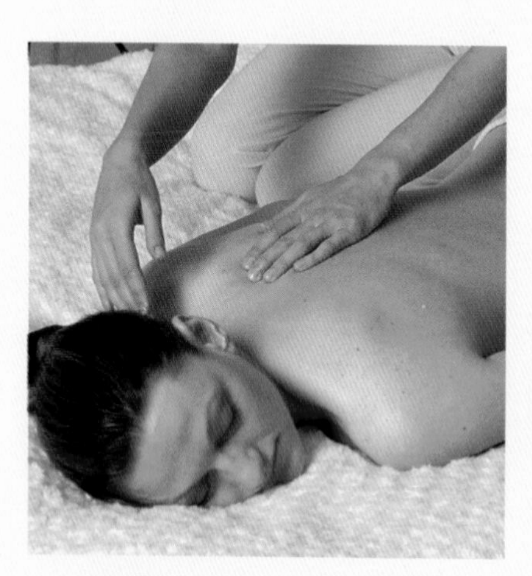

5. Pull-ups to shoulders

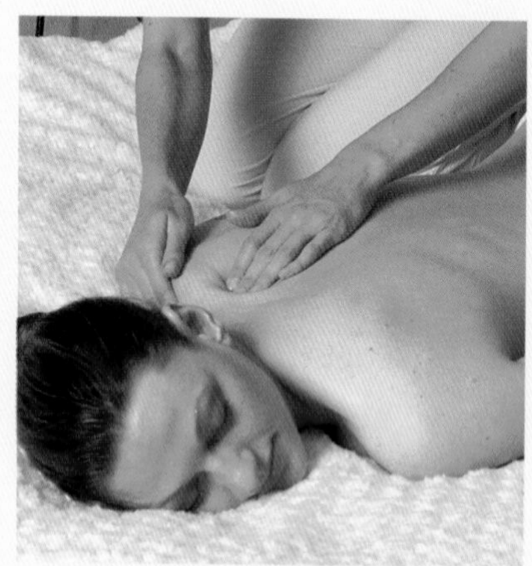

6. Kneading to shoulders and neck

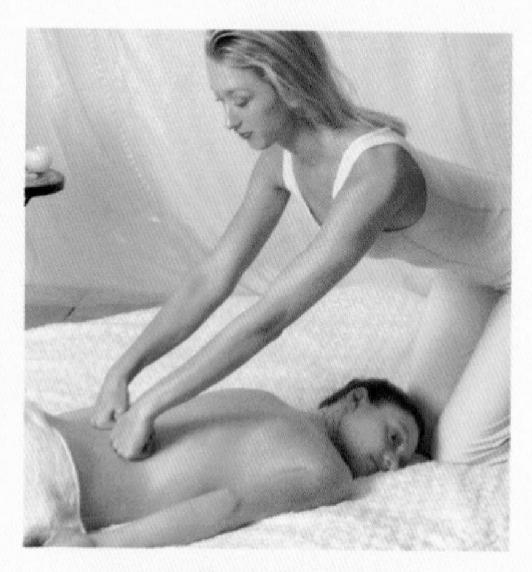

7. Knuckle slide

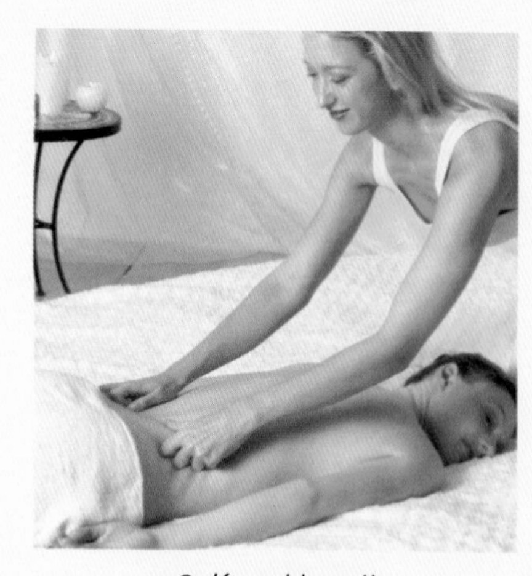

8. Knuckle roll

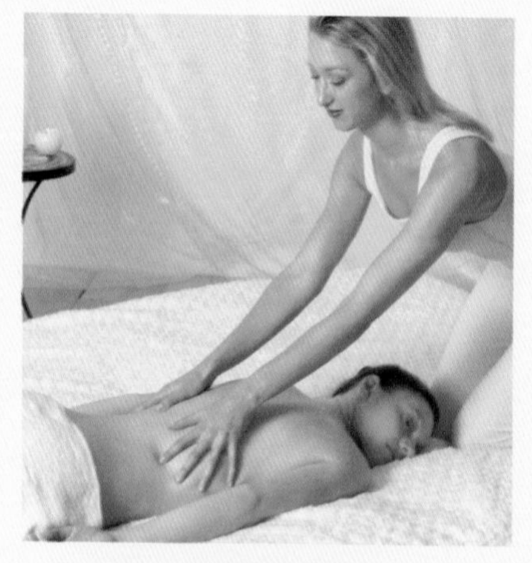

9. Fanning

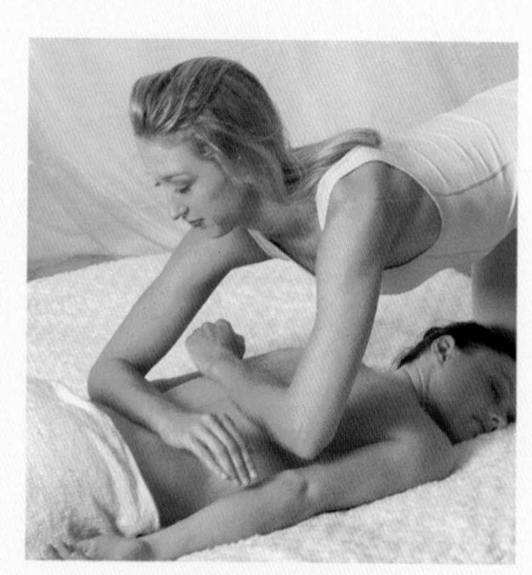

10. Forearms

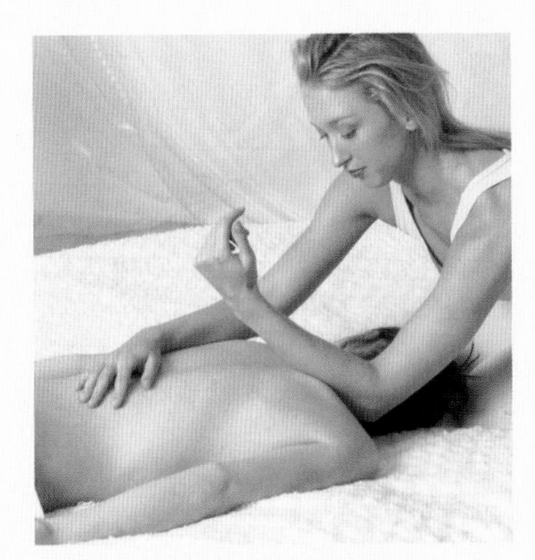

11. Forearm to the neck

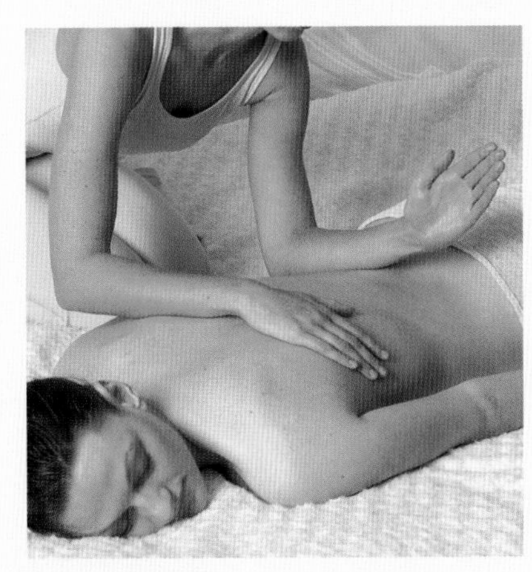

12. Forearm to the back

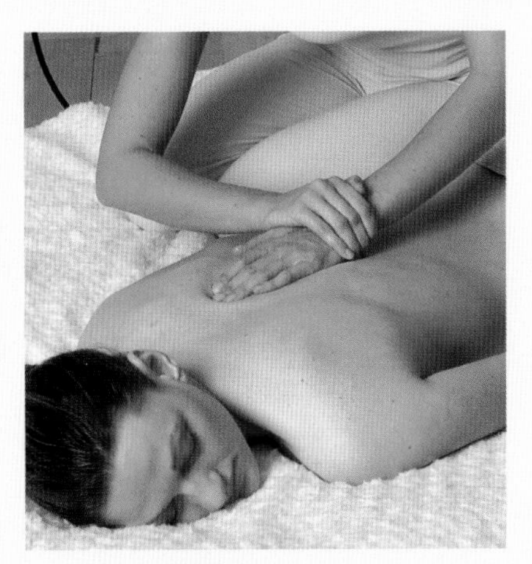

13. Digital pressure

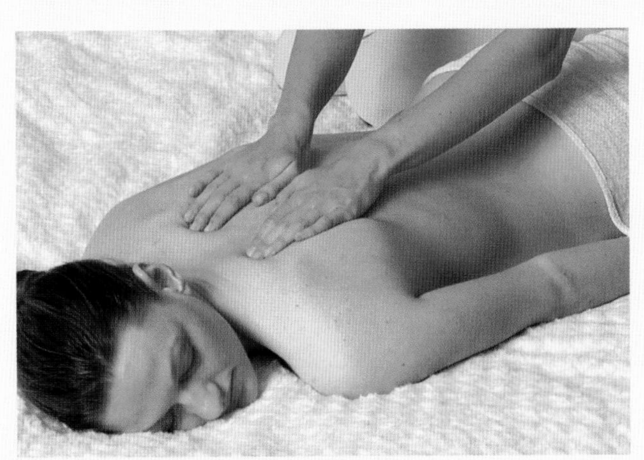

14. Basic effleurage

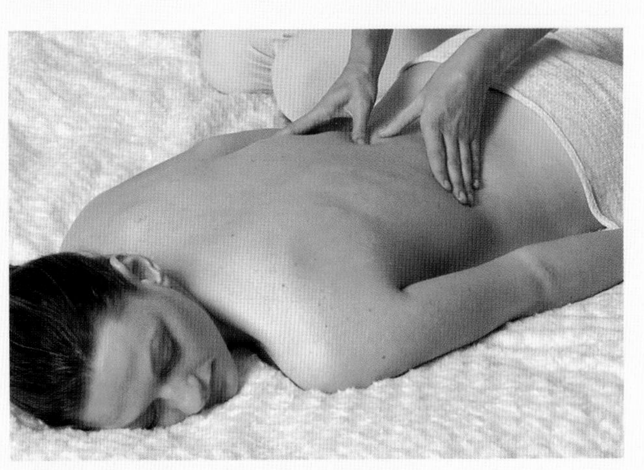

15. Thumb walking

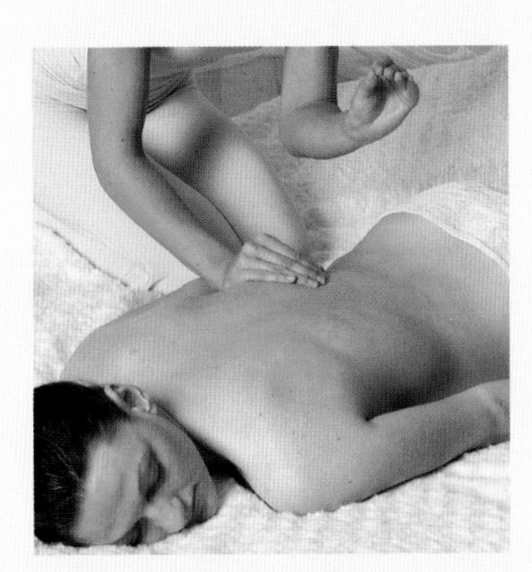

16. Cupping

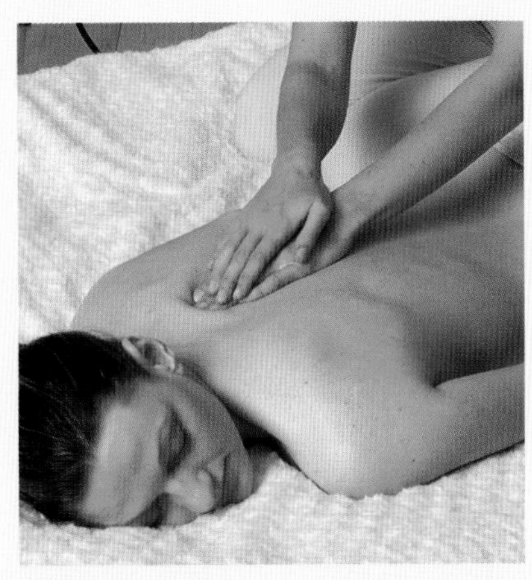

17. Hand-over-hand effleurage

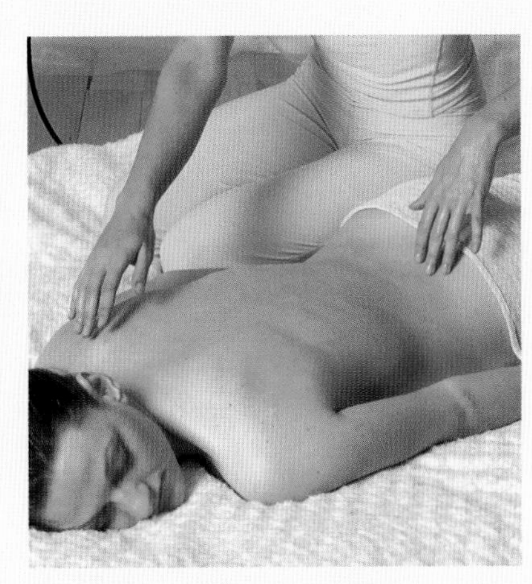

18. Feather stroking

Quick guide – buttocks

Fists

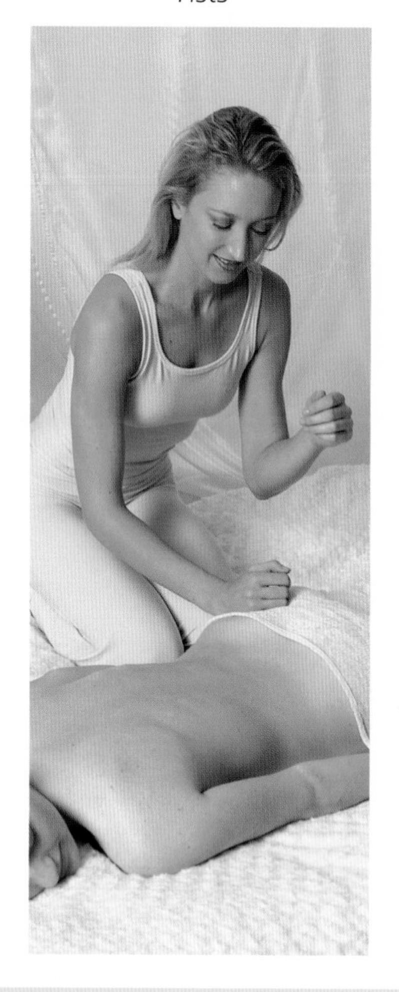

Quick guide – back of the leg

1. Softening

2. Spreading the oil

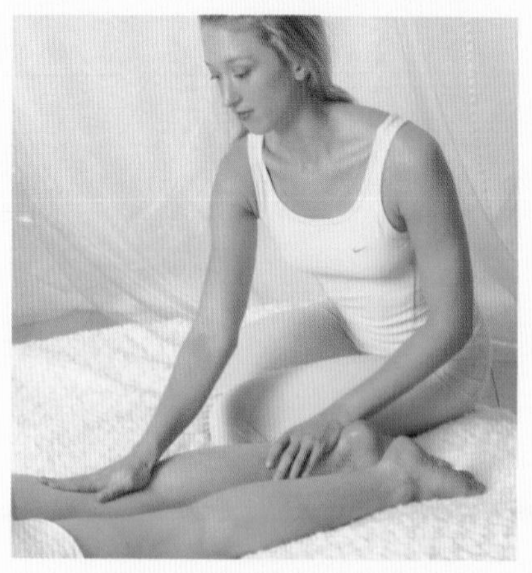

3. Alternating effleurage

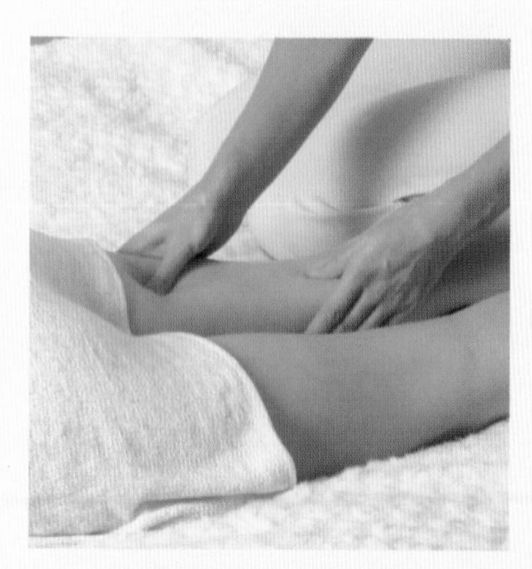

4. Friction to the thigh

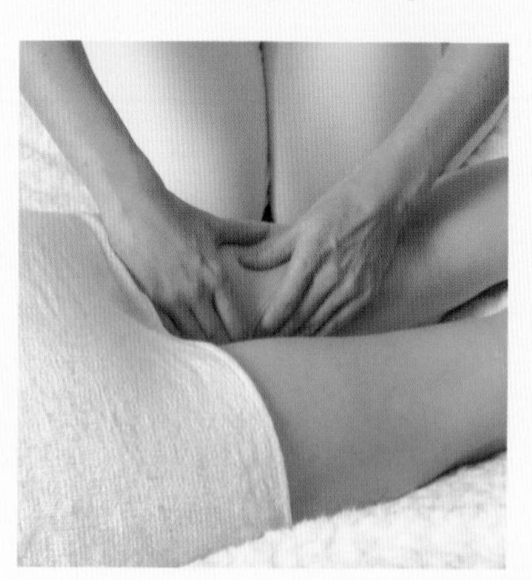

5. Kneading the inner thigh

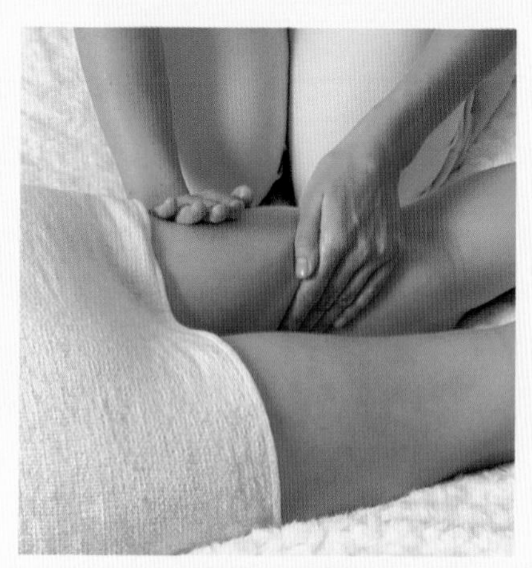

6. Wringing

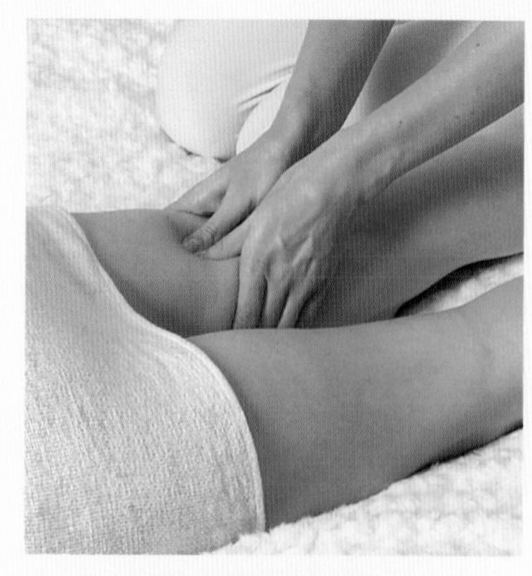

7. Train tracks up the thigh

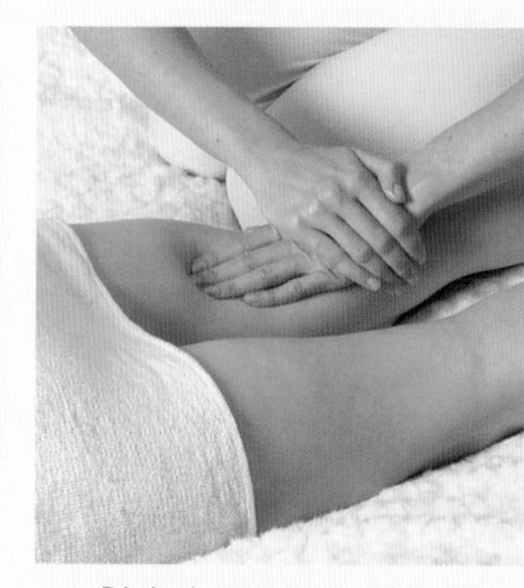

8. Digital pressure to the thigh

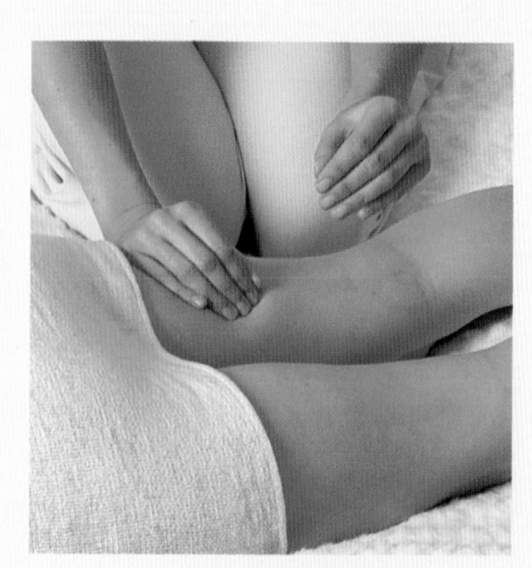

9. Cupping

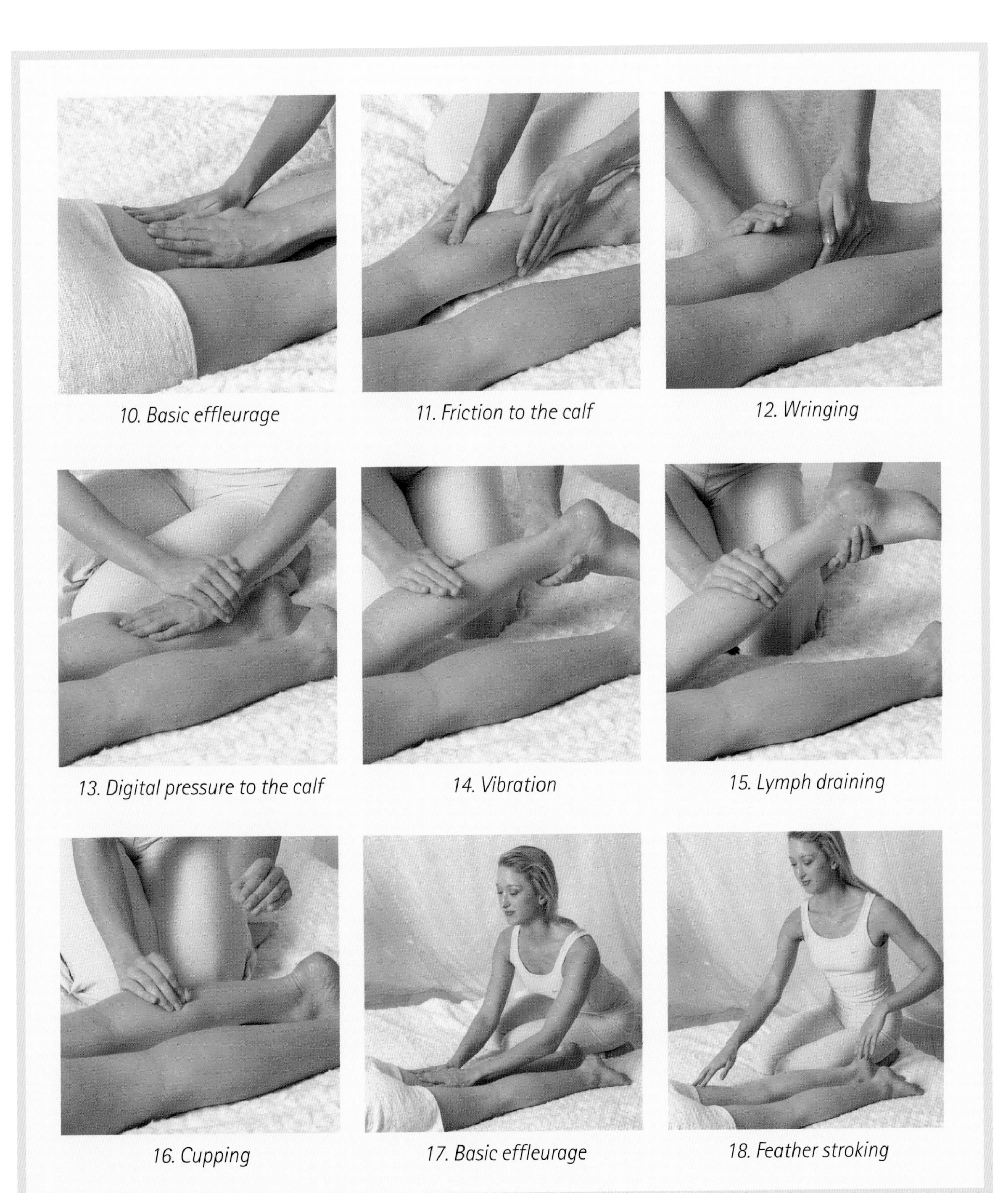

10. Basic effleurage

11. Friction to the calf

12. Wringing

13. Digital pressure to the calf

14. Vibration

15. Lymph draining

16. Cupping

17. Basic effleurage

18. Feather stroking

Quick guide – front of the leg

1. Softening

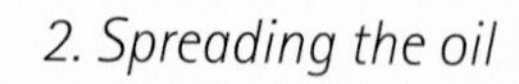

2. Spreading the oil

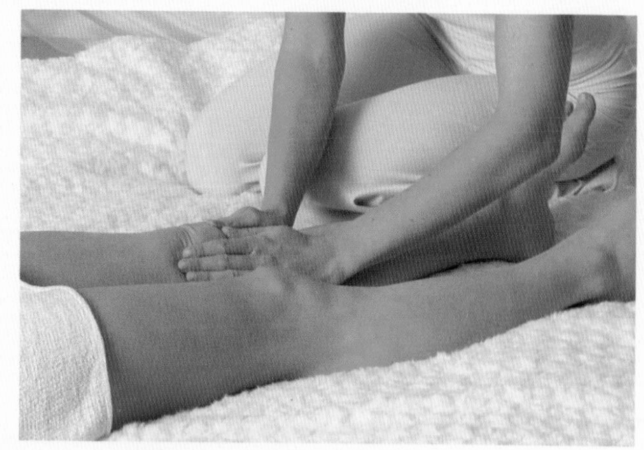

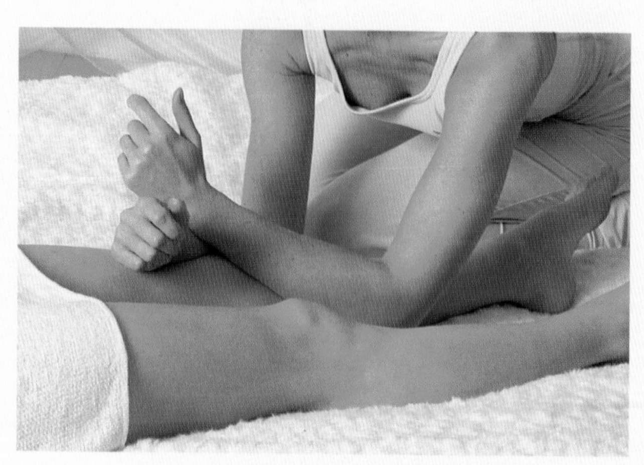

3. Basic effleurage

4. Forearms

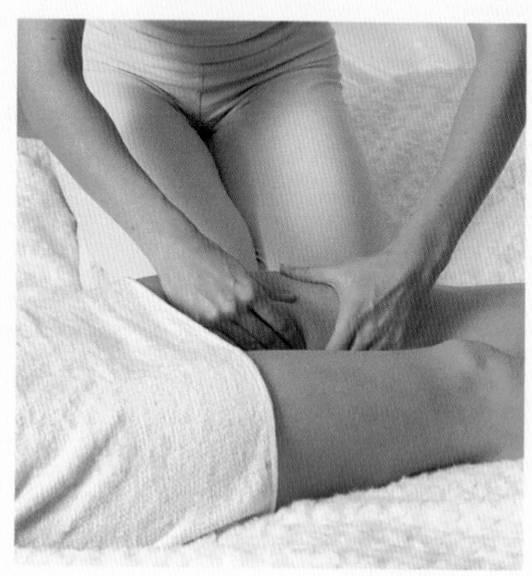

5. Kneading to the thigh

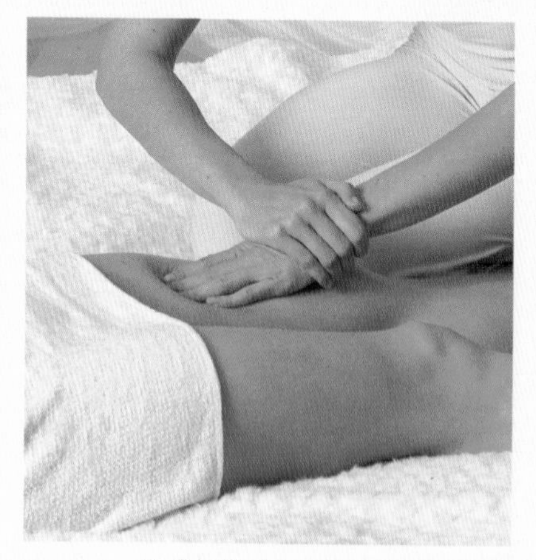

6. Digital pressure

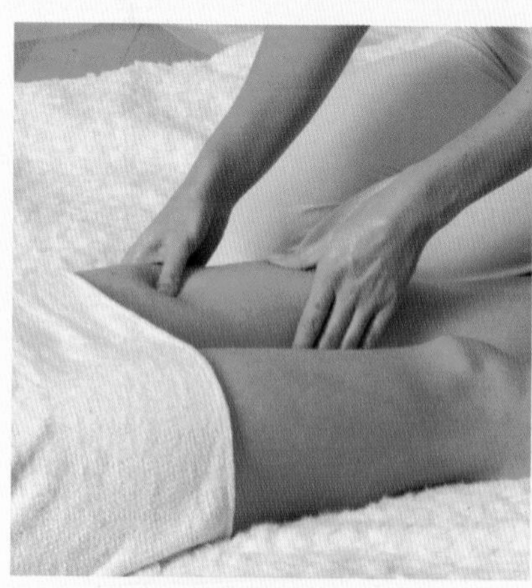

7. Friction to the thigh

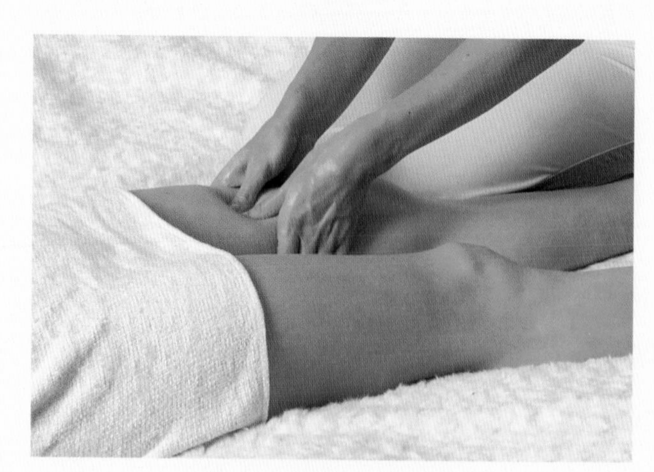

8. Train tracks to the thigh

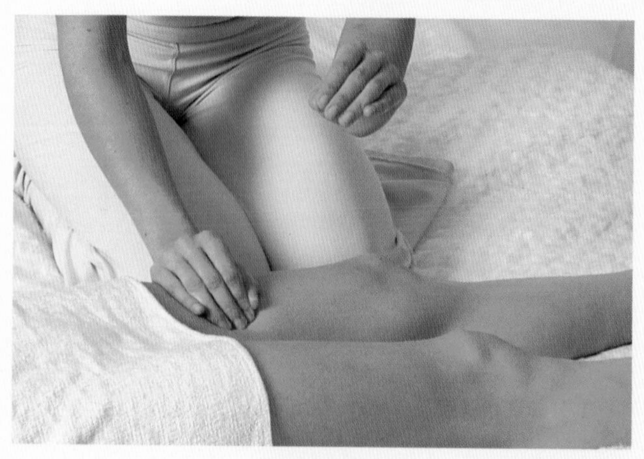

9. Cupping

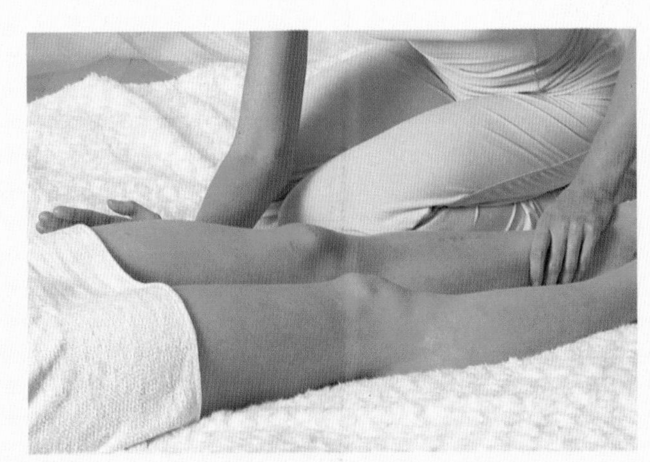

10. Heel of hand

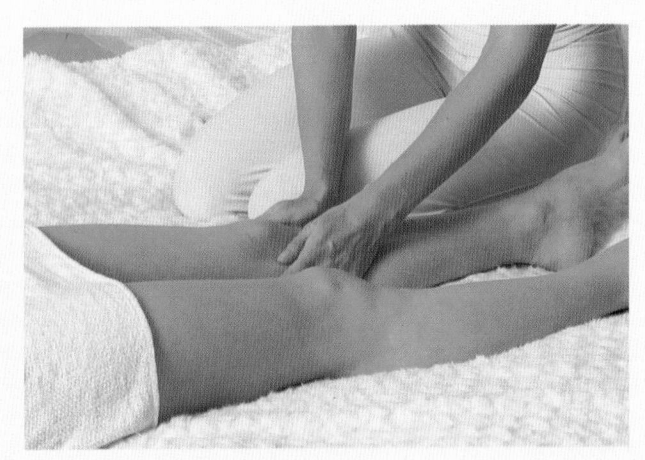

11. Opening

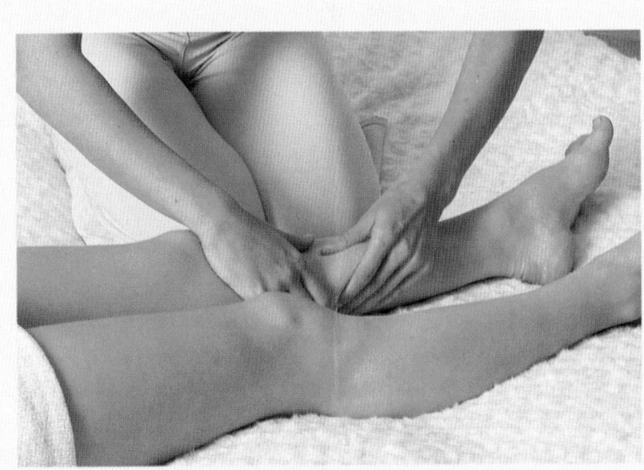

12. Kneading to the calf

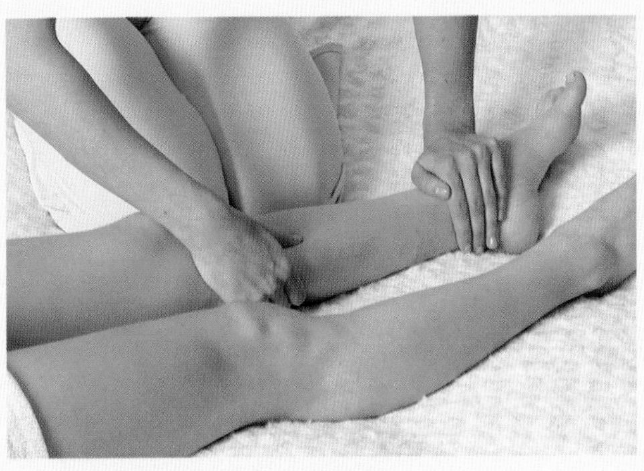

13. Friction

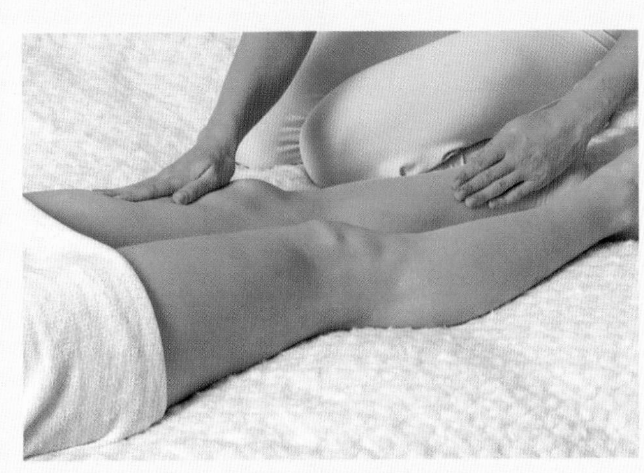

14. Alternating effleurage

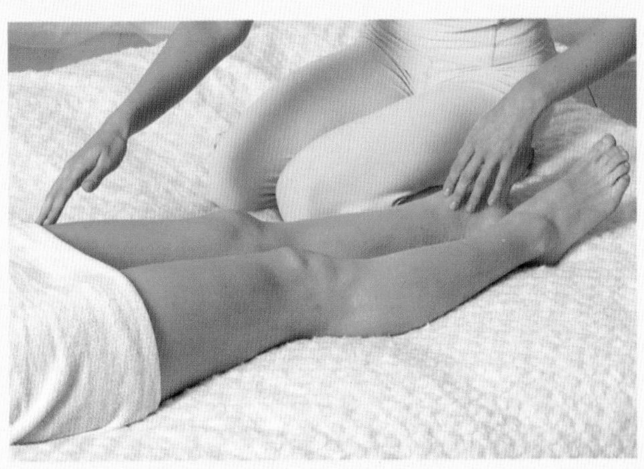

15. Feather stroking

Quick guide – foot

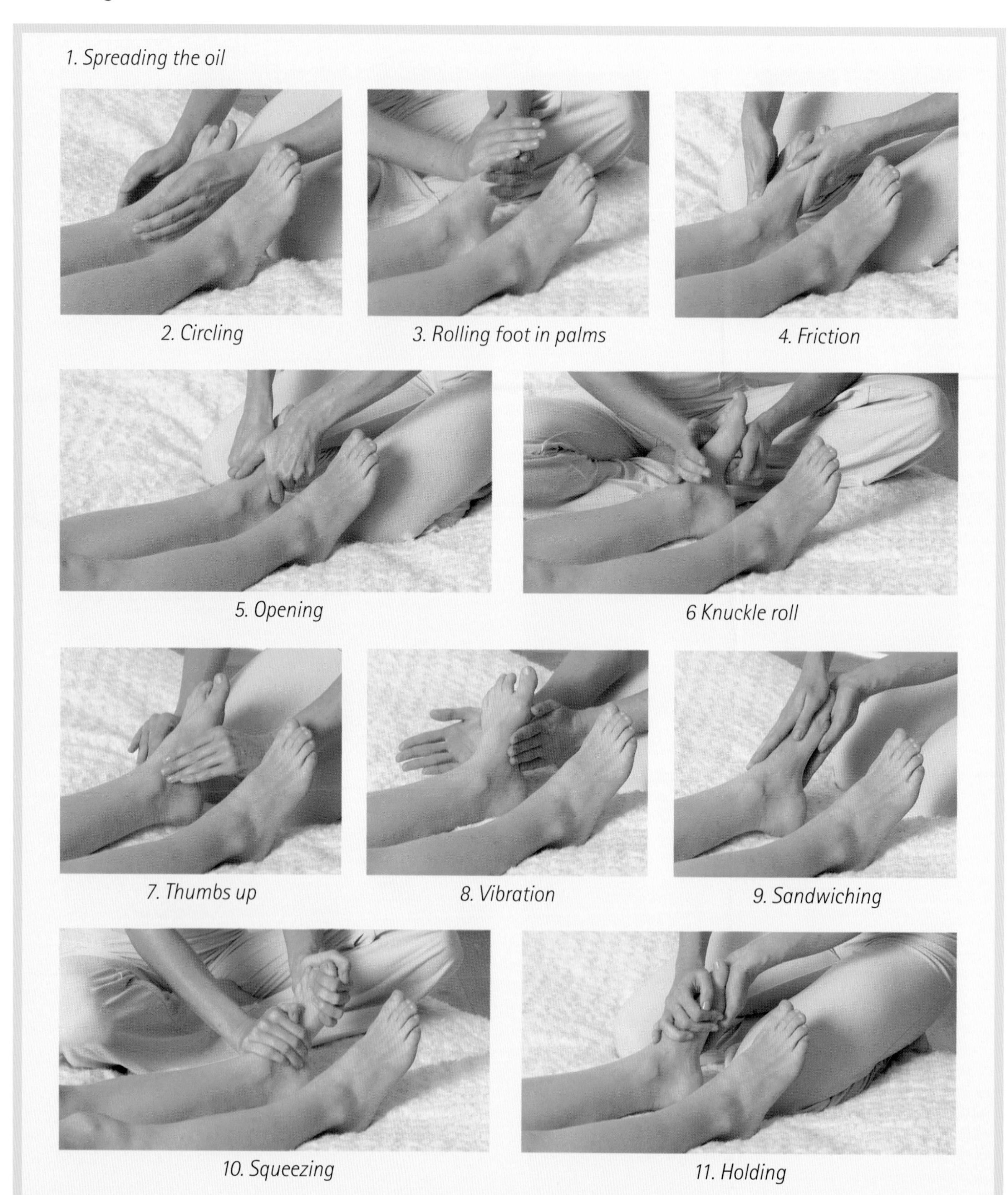

1. Spreading the oil

2. Circling

3. Rolling foot in palms

4. Friction

5. Opening

6 Knuckle roll

7. Thumbs up

8. Vibration

9. Sandwiching

10. Squeezing

11. Holding

Quick guide – stomach

1. Spreading the oil

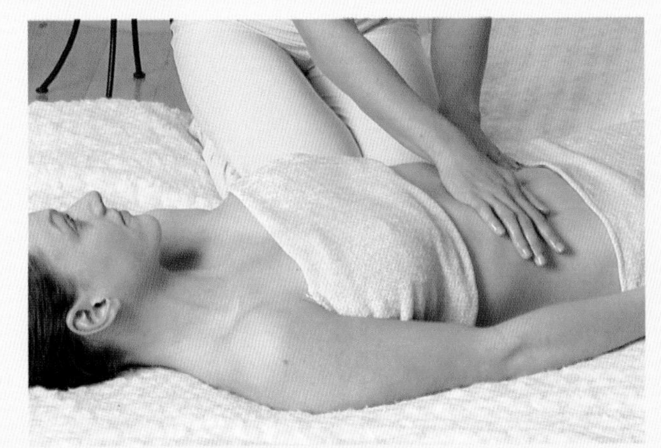

2. Circling

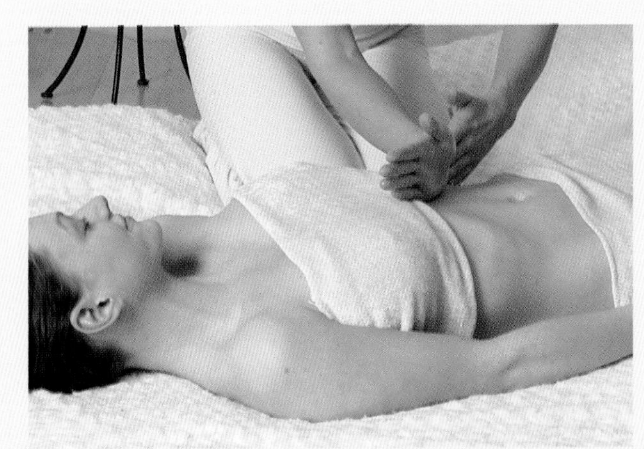

3. Flat hands along the rib

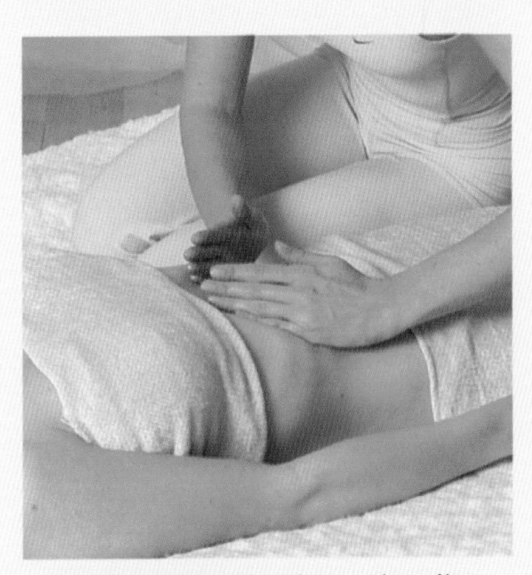

4. Both hands along the ribs

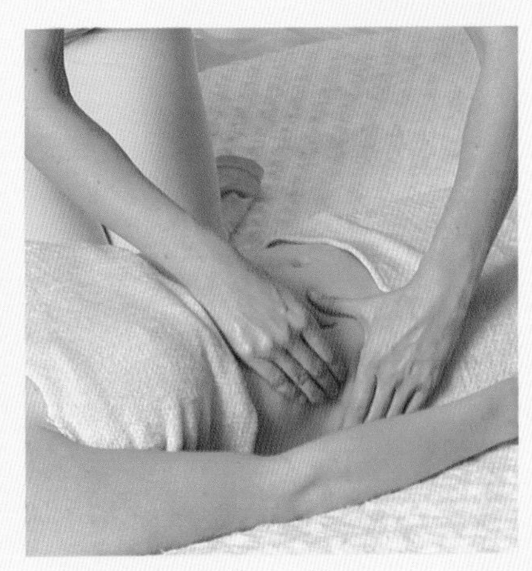

5. Kneading

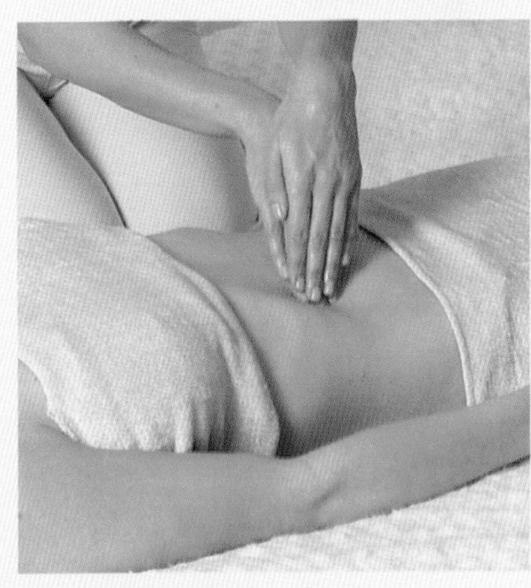

6. Double-handed circles

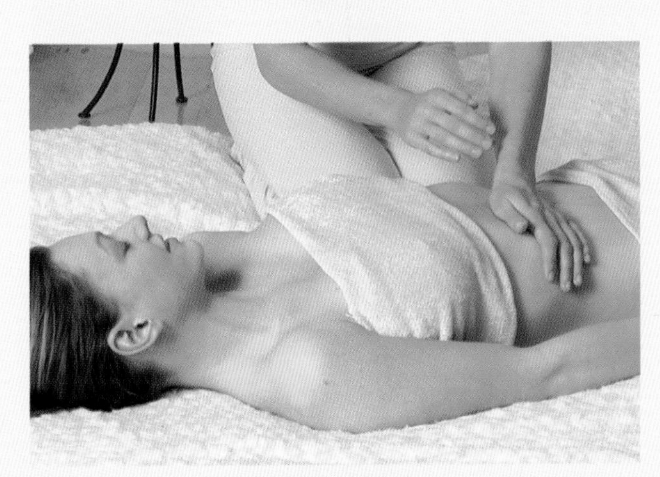

7. Circling

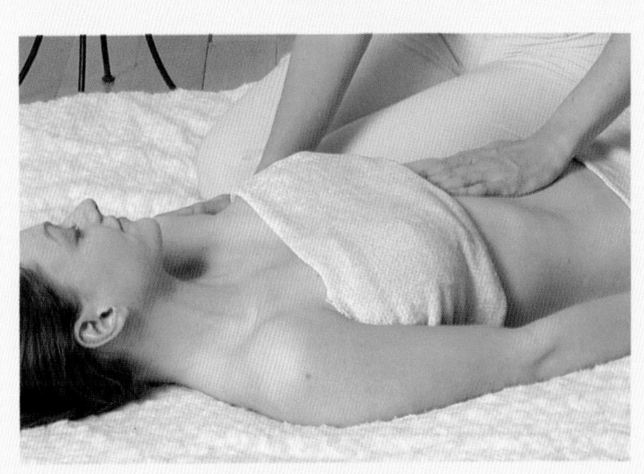

8. Rub solar plexus

Quick guide – arm

1. *Softening*

2. *Spreading the oil*

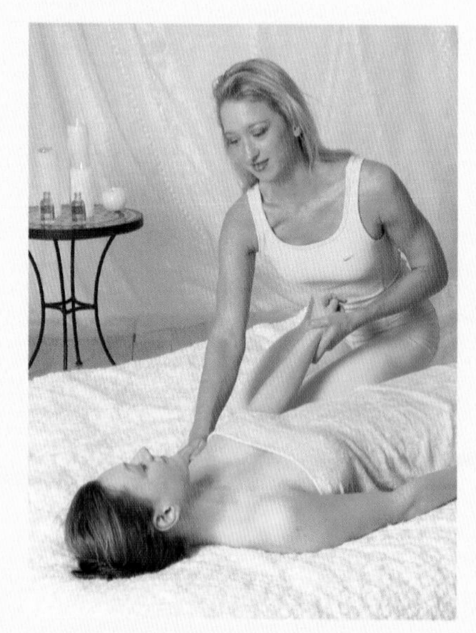

3. Alternating effleurage

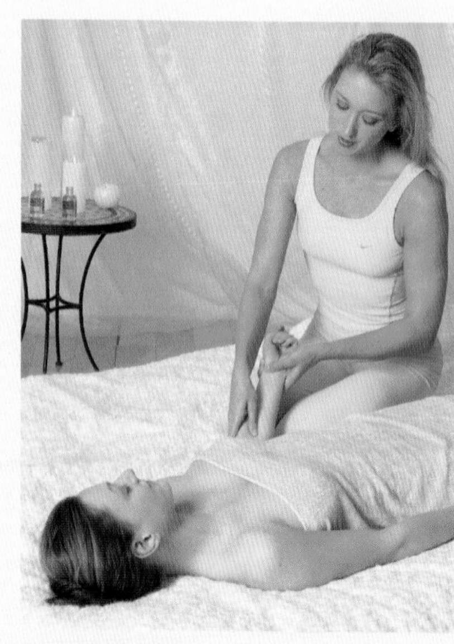

4. Friction to the lower arm

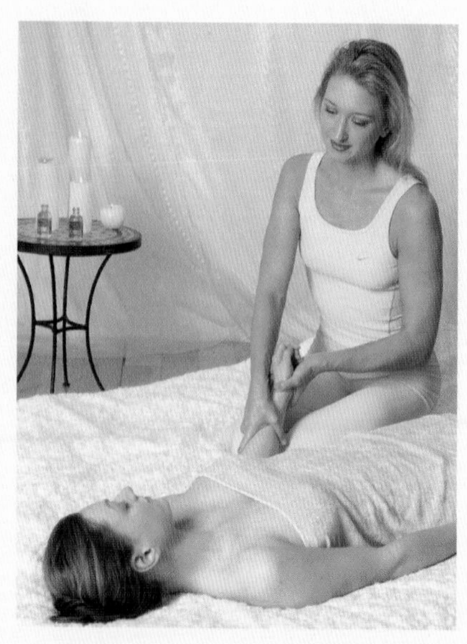

5. Draining to the lymph node

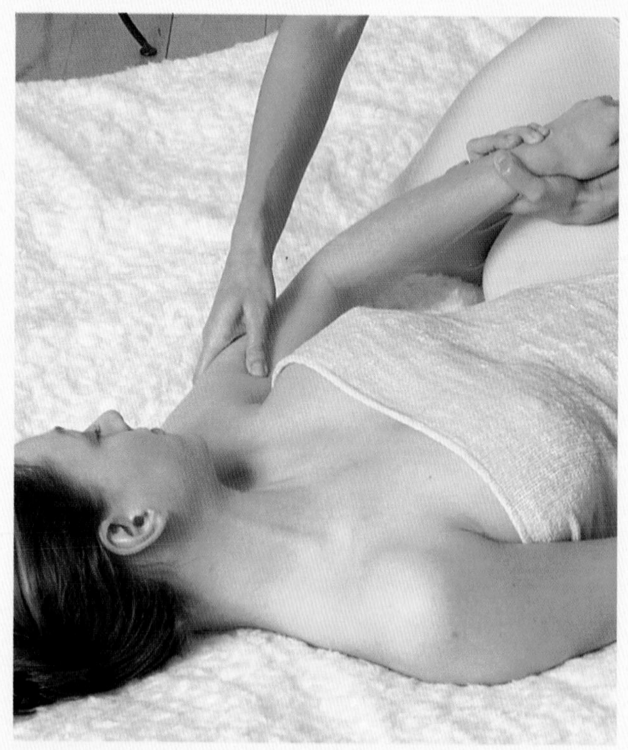

6. Friction to the upper arm

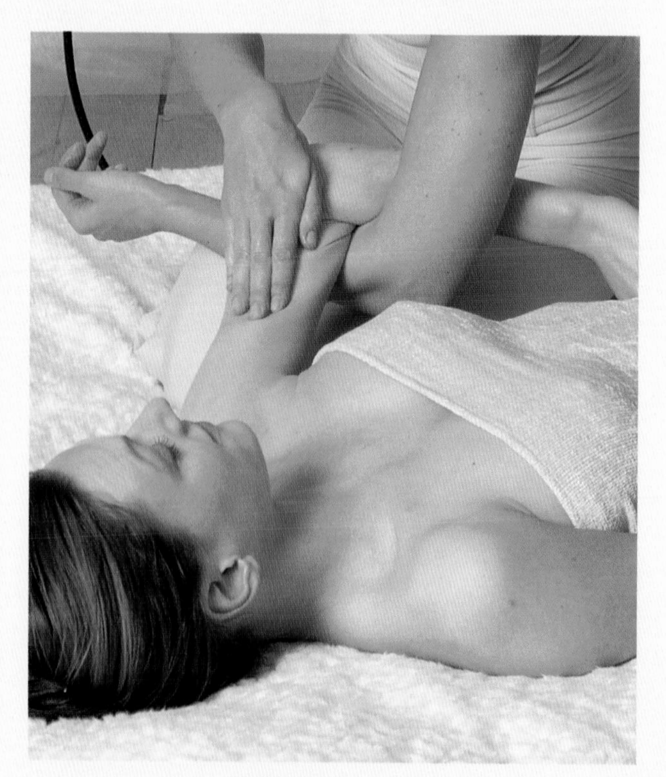

7. Digital pressure

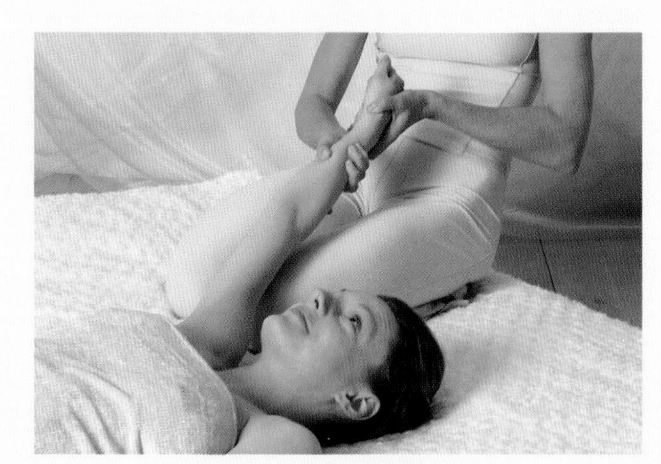

8. Arm stretch

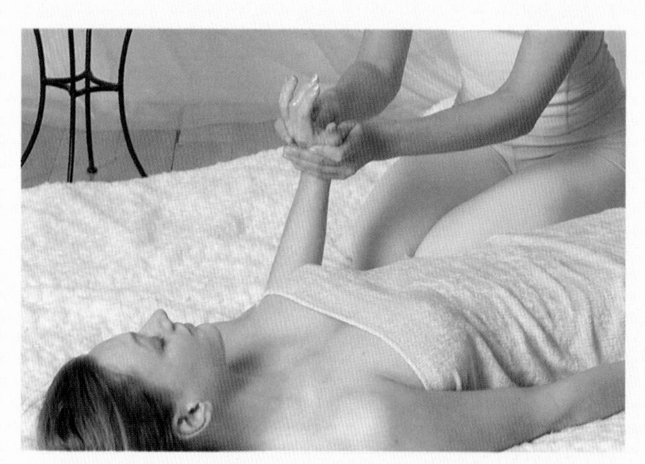

9. Friction to the hand and wrist

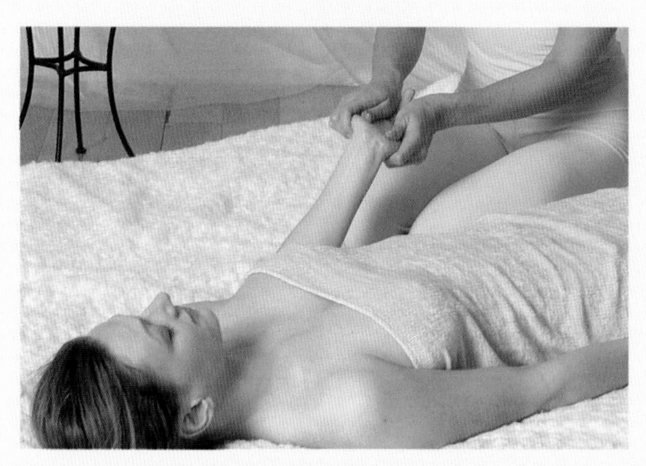

10. Opening

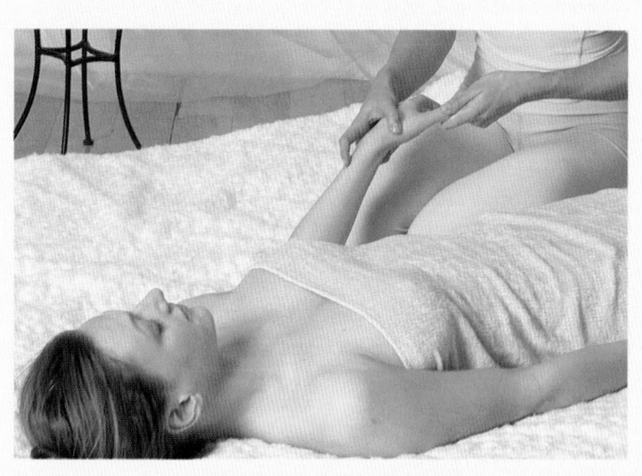

11. Finger massage

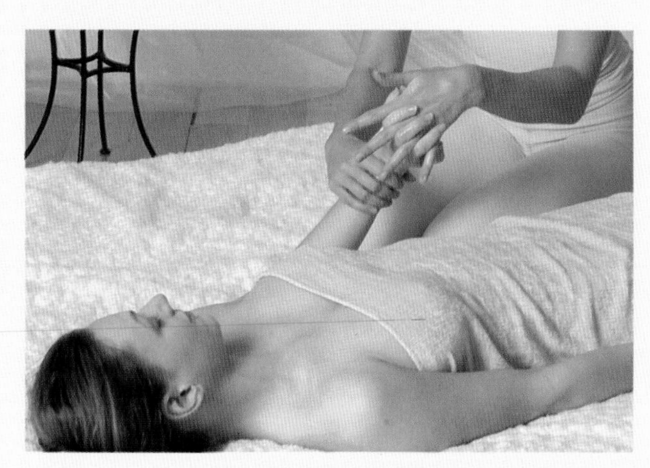

12. Fingers laced

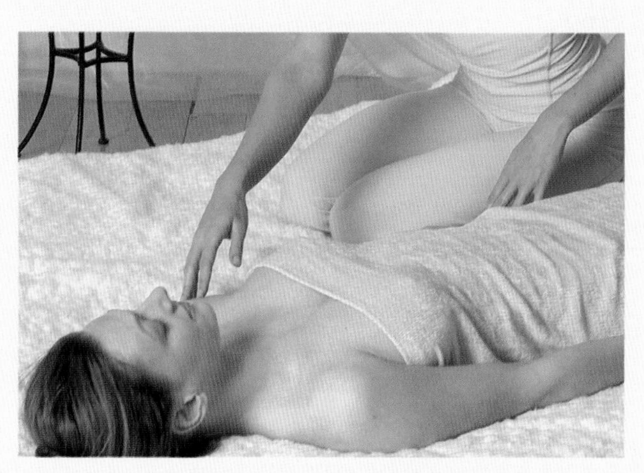

13. Feather stroking

Quick guide – chest

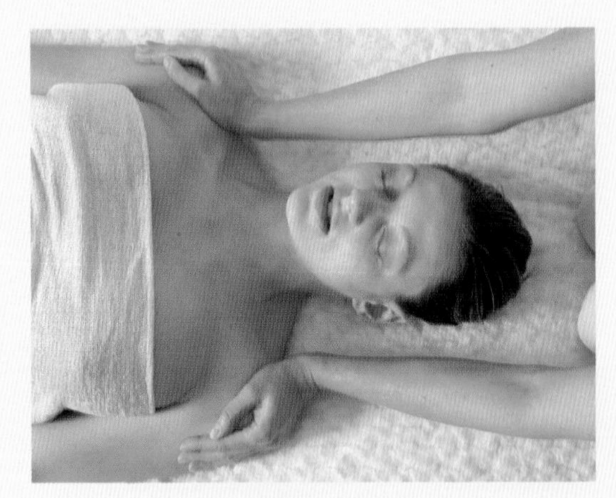

1. Rocking

2. Spreading the oil

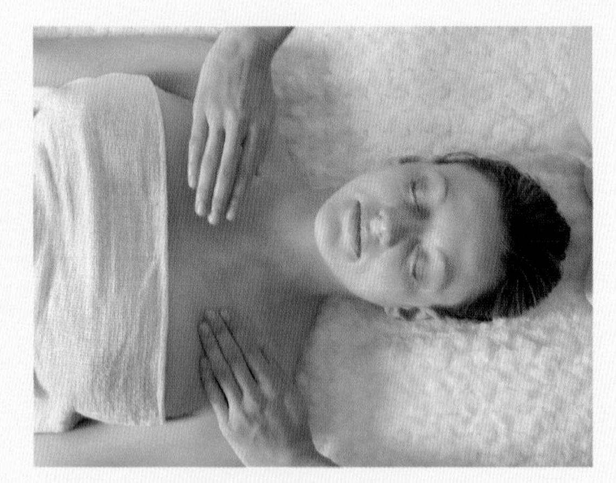

3. Alternating effleurage

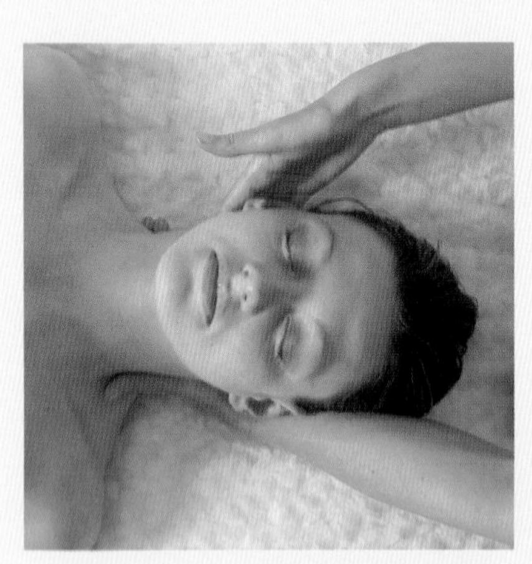

4. Hand-over-hand to the neck

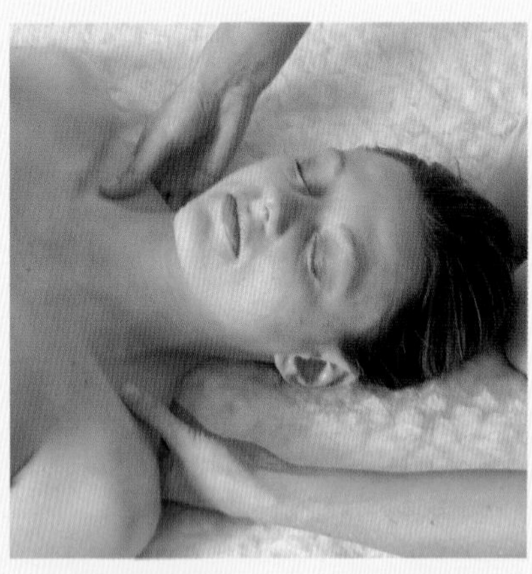

5. Friction to the shoulders

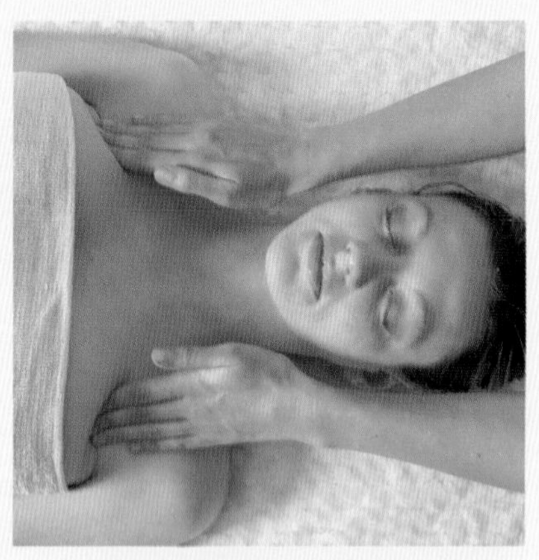

6. Friction to the pecs

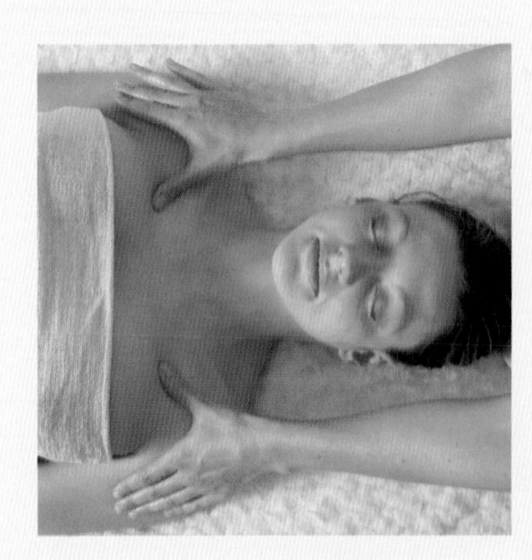

7. Lymph drainage

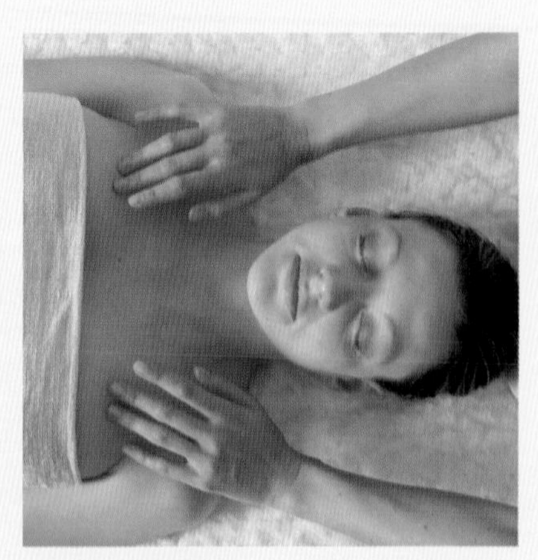

8. Tapoment

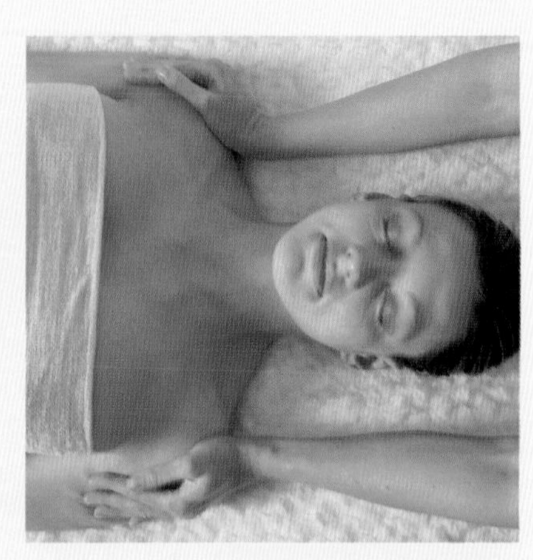

9. Circling

Quick guide – chest cont.

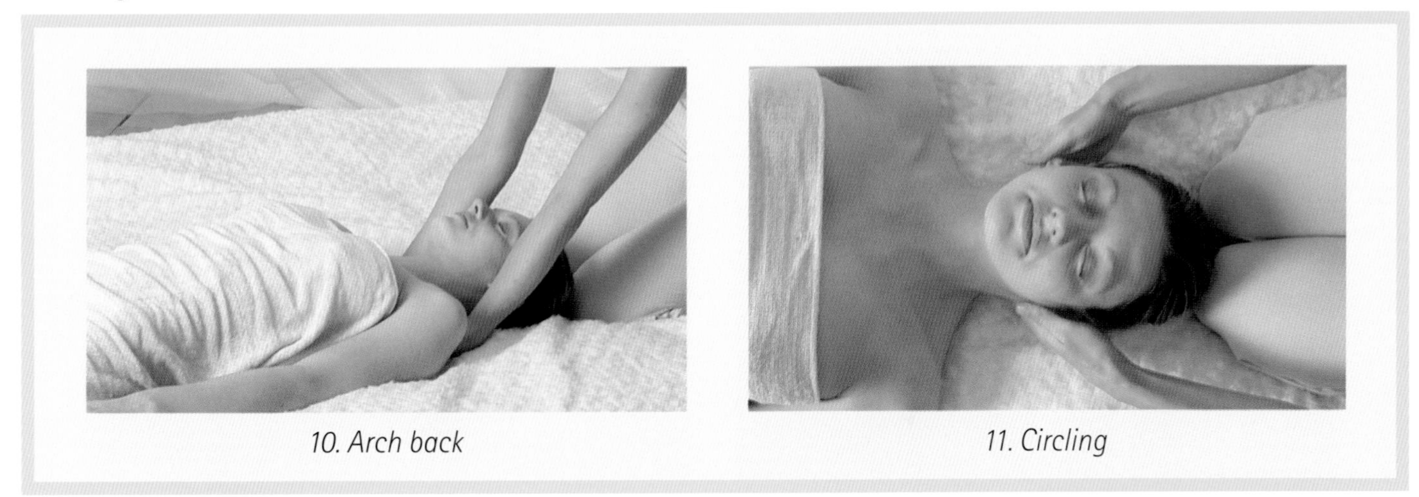

10. Arch back

11. Circling

Quick guide – neck, shoulders and head

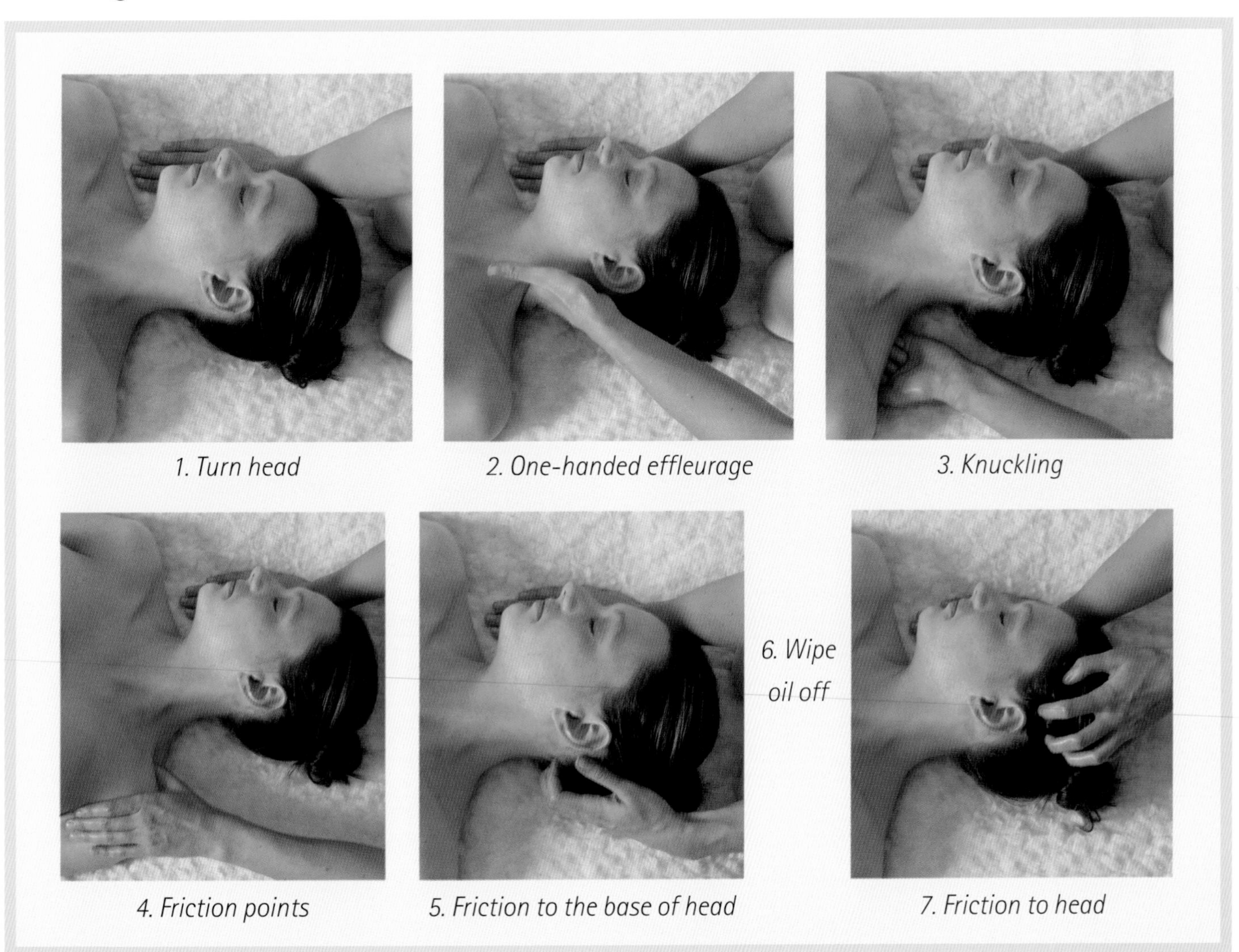

1. Turn head

2. One-handed effleurage

3. Knuckling

4. Friction points

5. Friction to the base of head

6. Wipe oil off

7. Friction to head

Quick guide – face

1. Spreading the oil

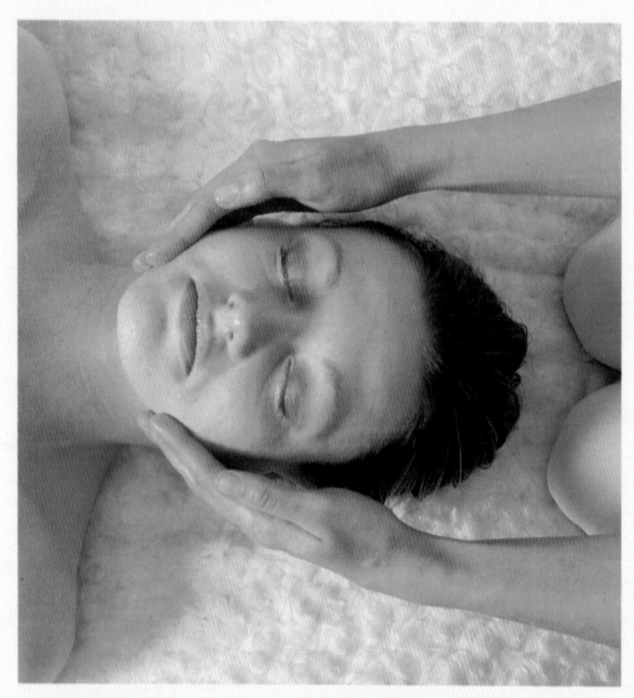

2. Effleurage to the chin

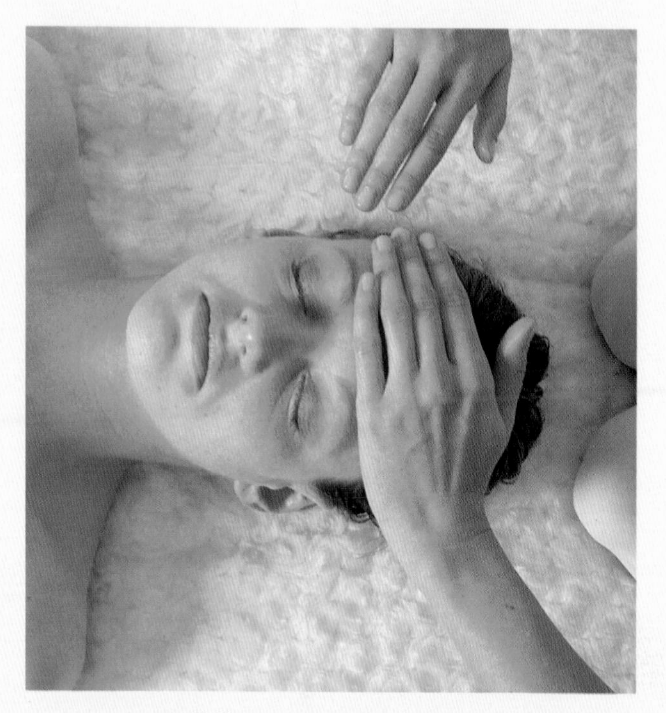

3. Effleurage to the forehead

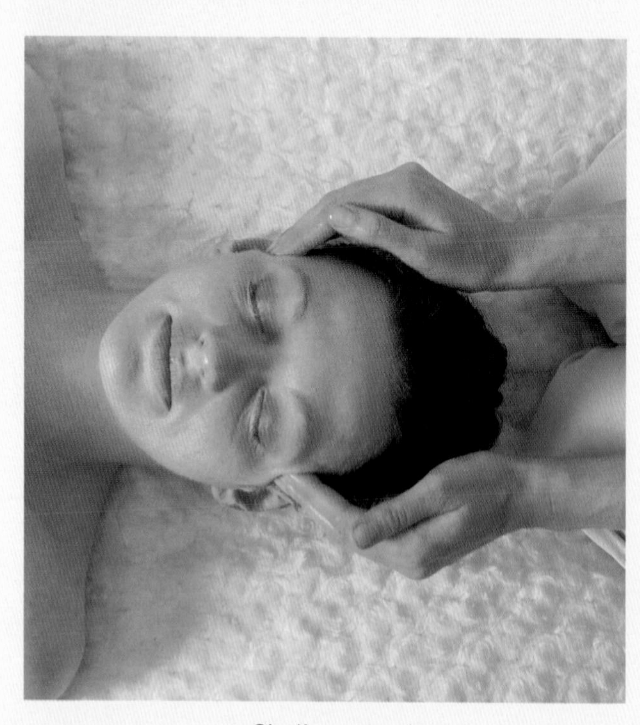

4. Circling temples

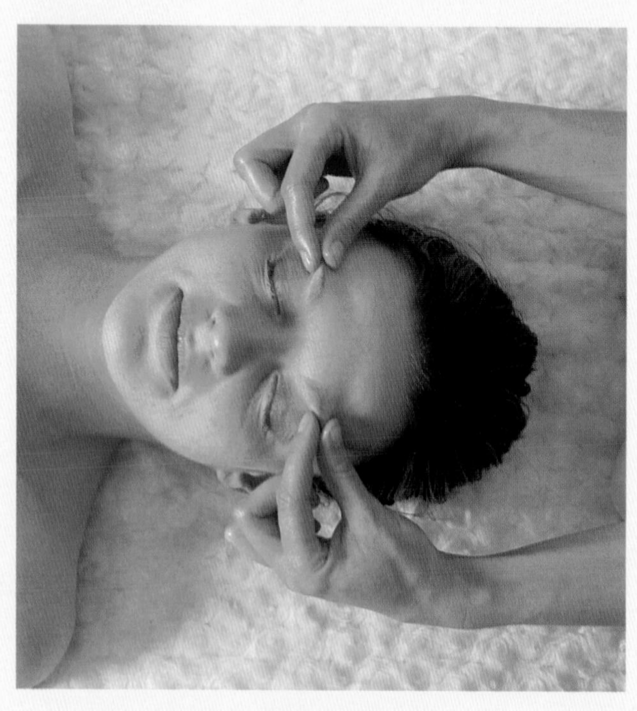

5. Squeeze eyebrows

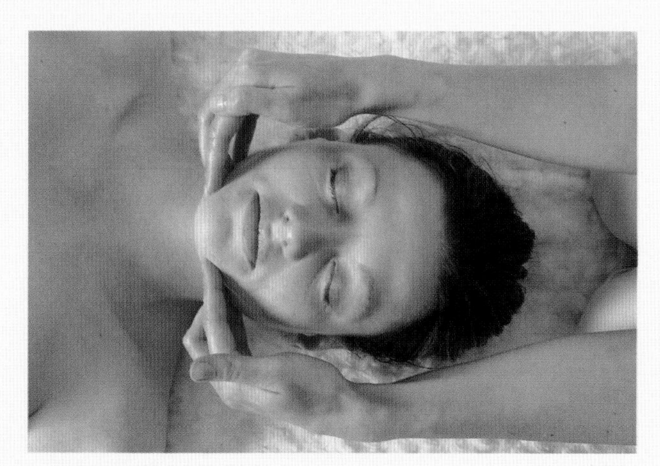

6. Friction

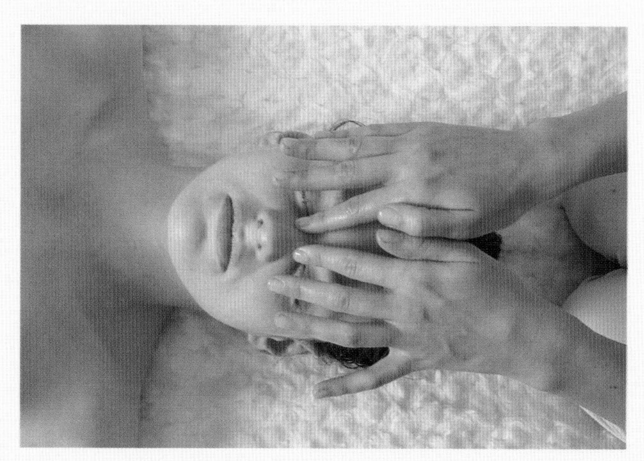

7. Circling the whole face

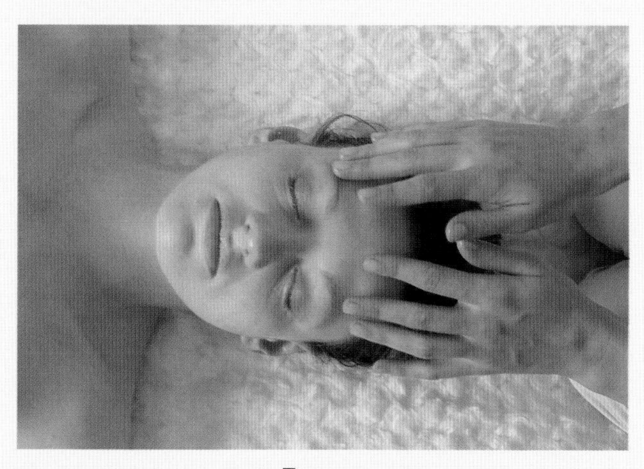

8. Tapoment

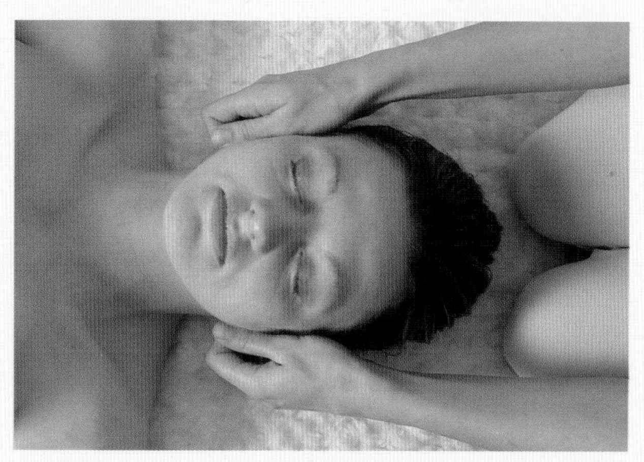

9. Circles to the ears

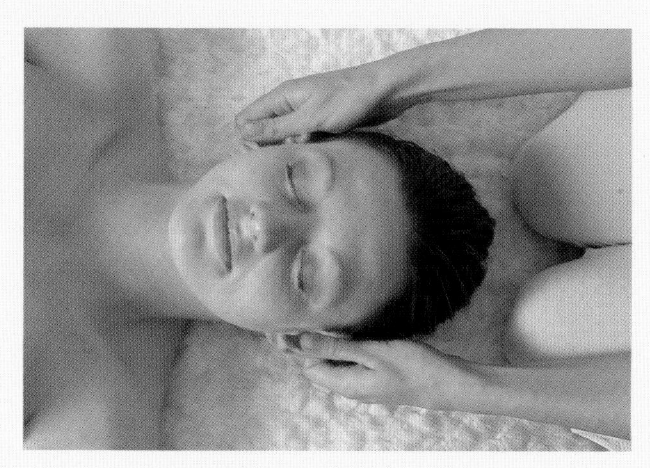

10. Massaging the ears

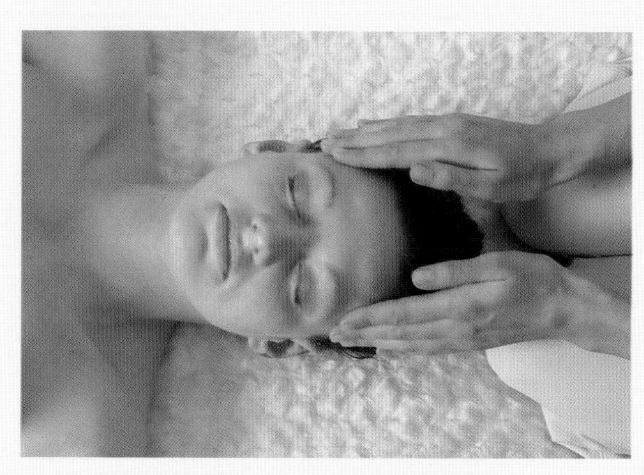

11. Effleurage the whole face

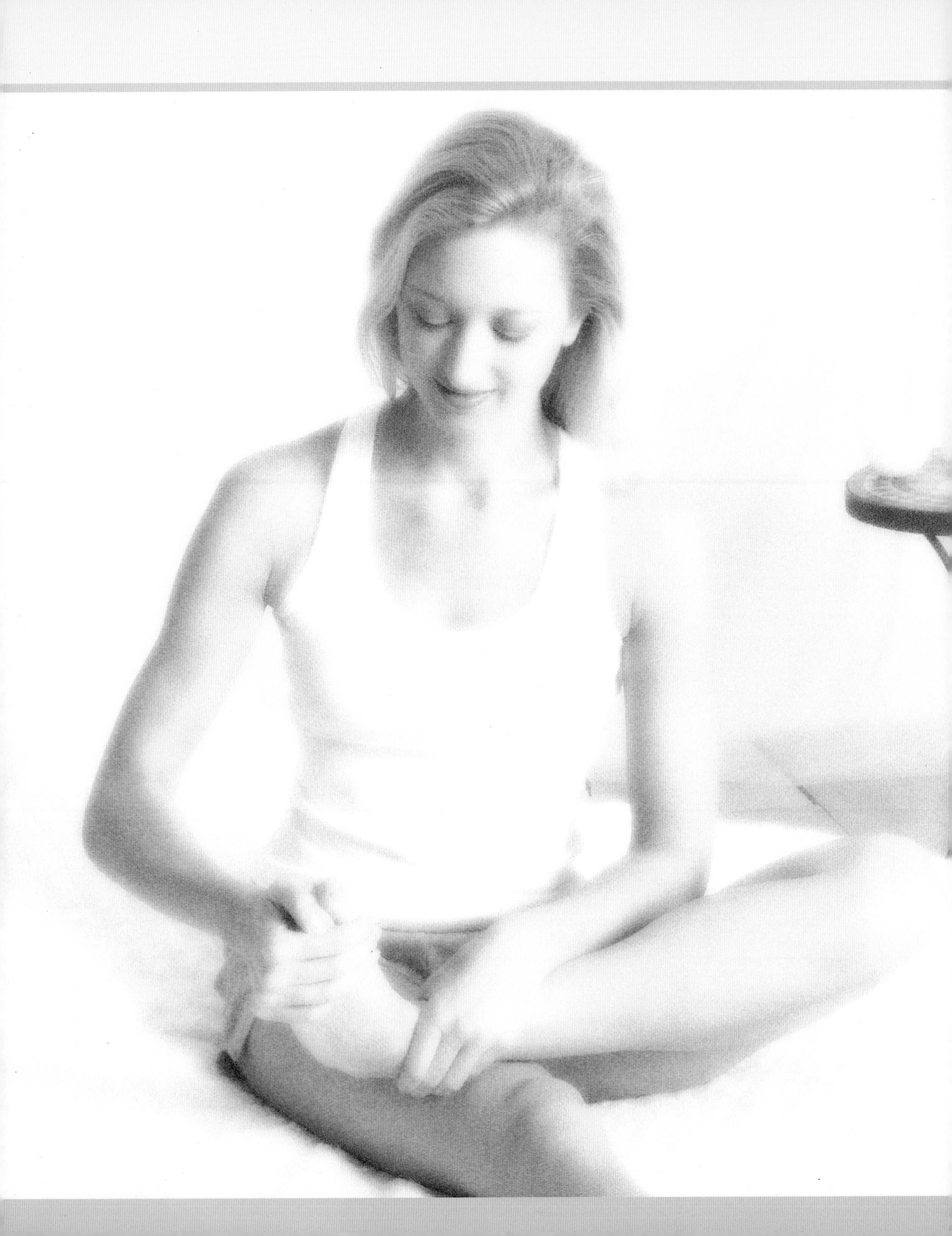

Self-massage

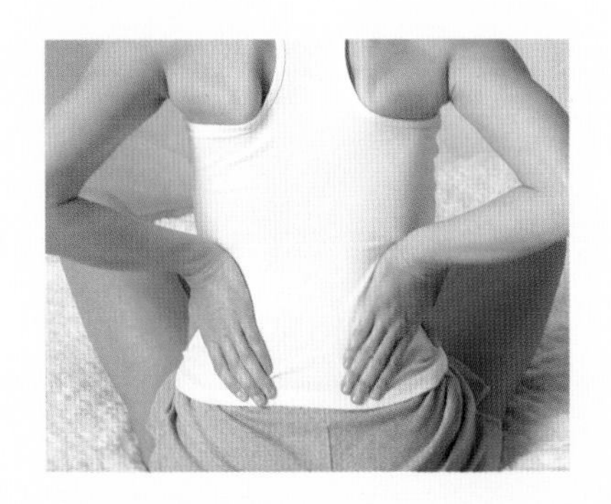

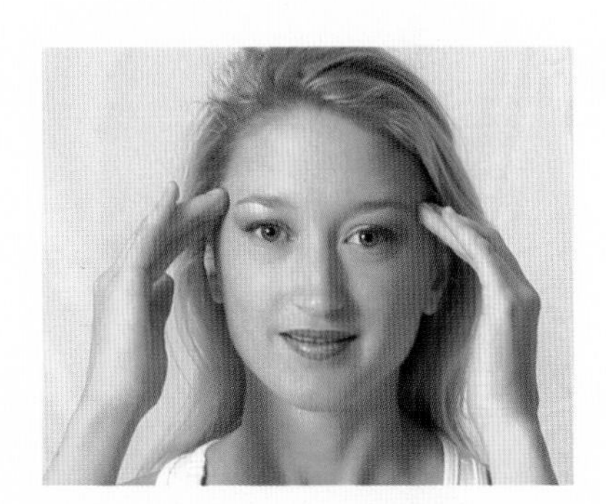

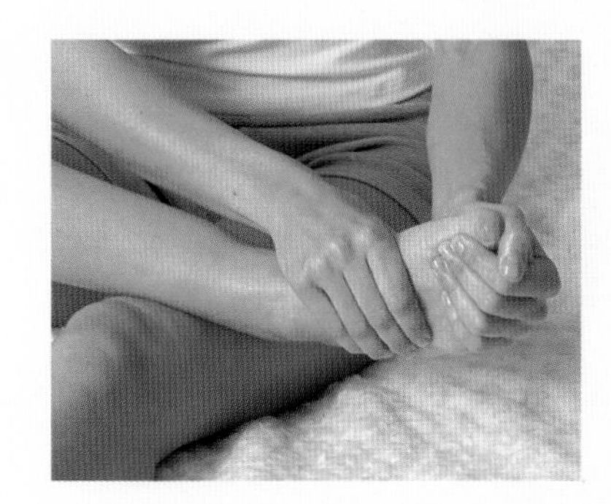

Self-massage has many benefits: you don't need to make an appointment, travel anywhere, or put aside several hours of your time. All you need is a few minutes to yourself and some oil or even lotion if you prefer. Self-massage can be extremely relaxing when you are feeling tired and achy. Here are some ideas to help you relax and unwind.

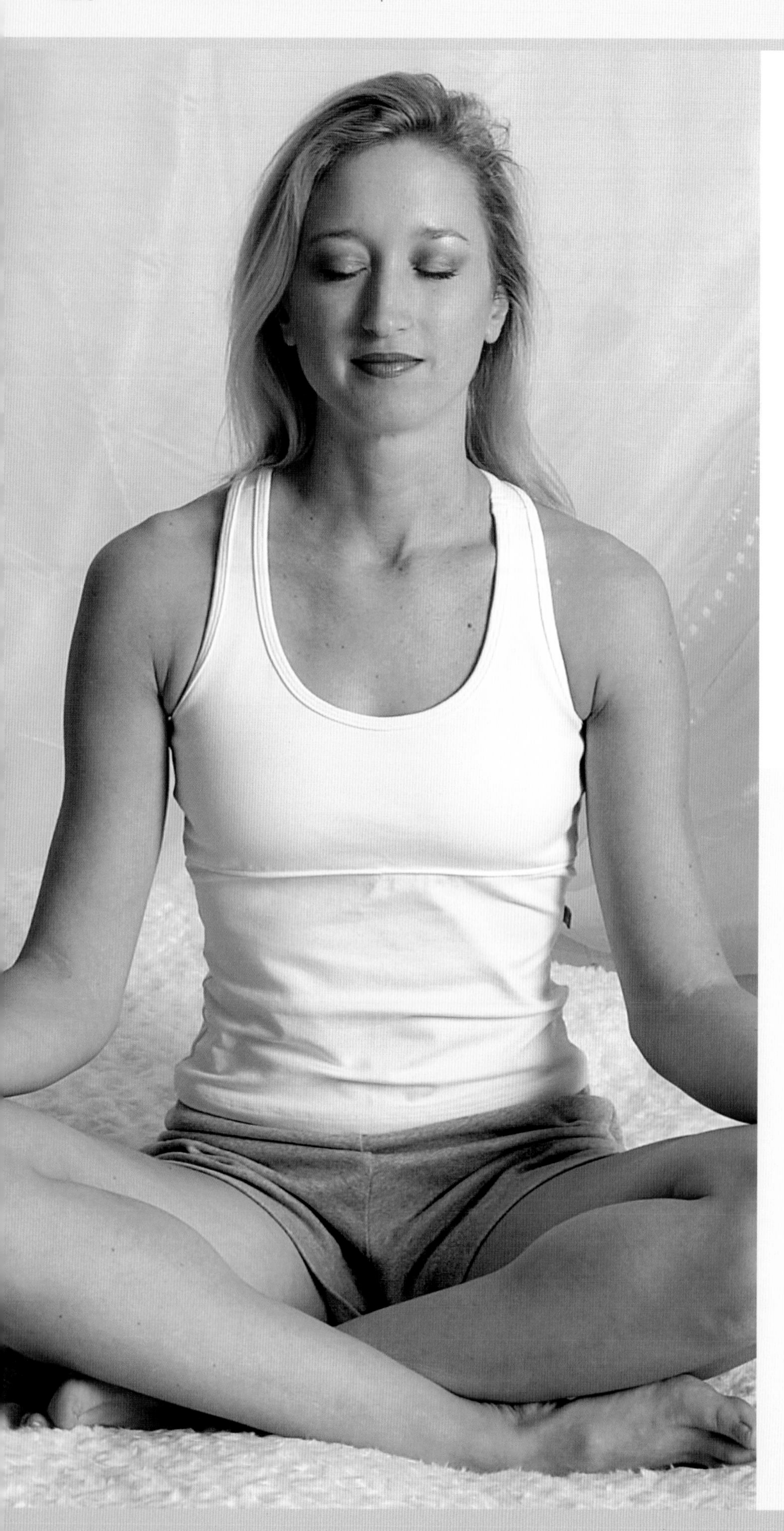

Preparation

Sit on the bed or floor with your legs crossed and your head lengthening up to the ceiling. If this position is uncomfortable, sit on a couple of pillows. Place your hands on your knees and close your eyes.

Relax and listen to your breathing. Try to clear your mind and focus on the rise and fall of your belly as you inhale and exhale.

Start to notice if you are feeling tension in any particular area of your body. Make a mental note of where it is and spend a few extra moments on that area when doing the self-massage.

Open your eyes.

You are now ready to begin!

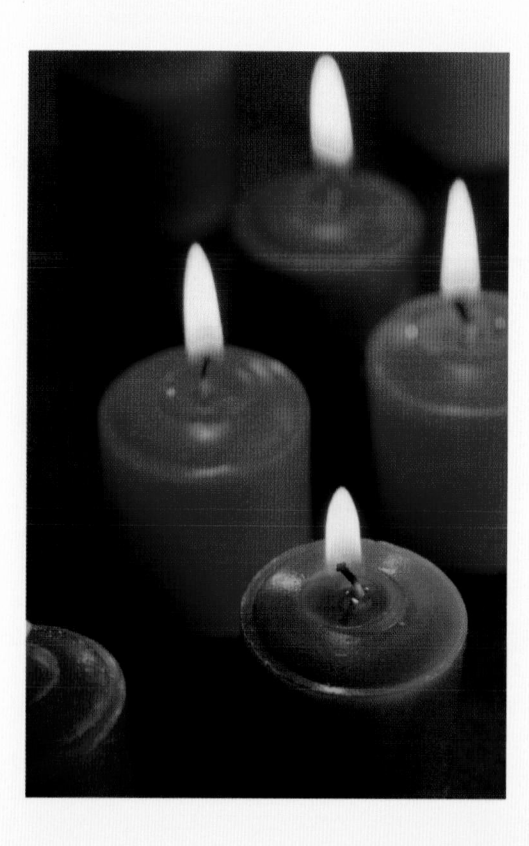

Foot

Spreading the oil: Sit on the floor or on a chair, and cross one ankle over your other knee. Place a small amount of oil or lotion in the palm of your hand. Spread it over the entire foot.

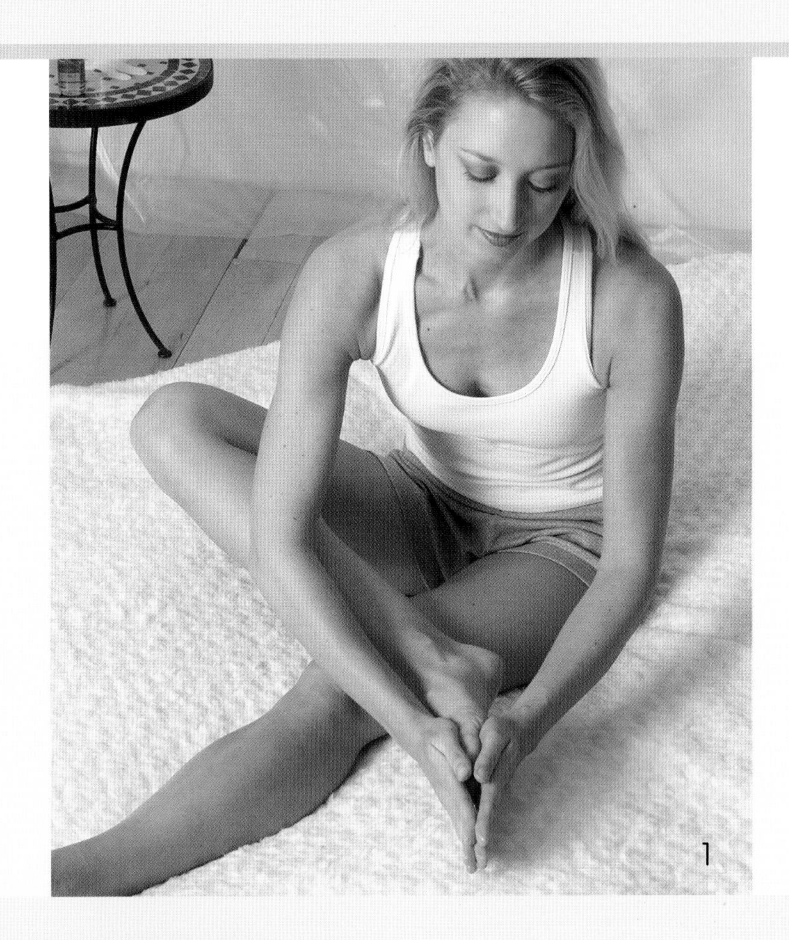

1

1 **Sandwiching:** Place one hand on the sole of the foot and one hand on the top of the foot with the fingers of both hands facing the toes. Squeeze the foot as you slide the hands up towards the toes until the palms are together. Repeat this action a few times.

2 **Friction:** Place the thumbs on the sole of the foot. Making circles with the thumbs, massage the entire sole of the foot.

3 Place the heel of the foot on the ground. Repeat to the top of the foot.

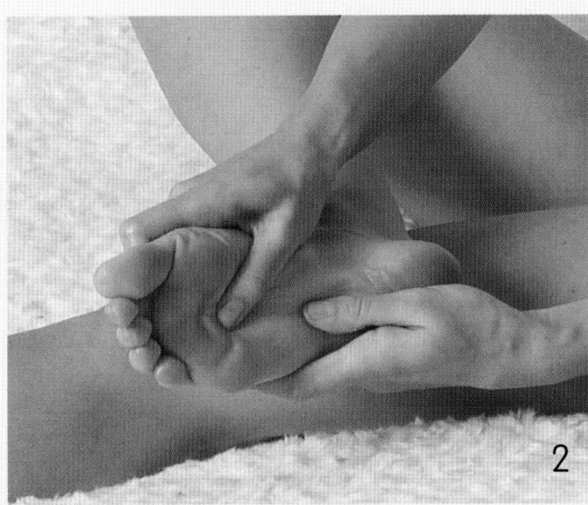

2

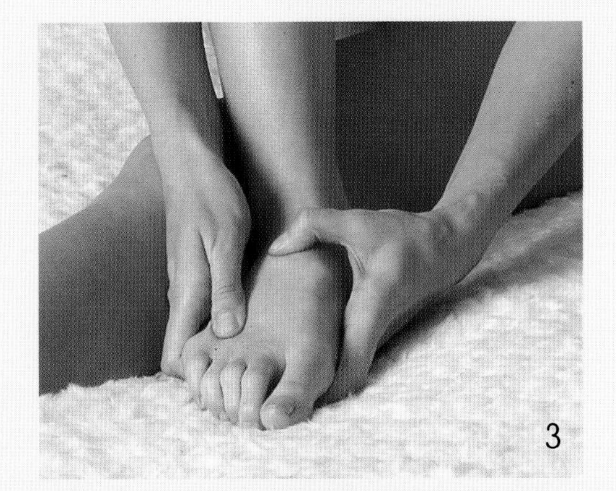

3

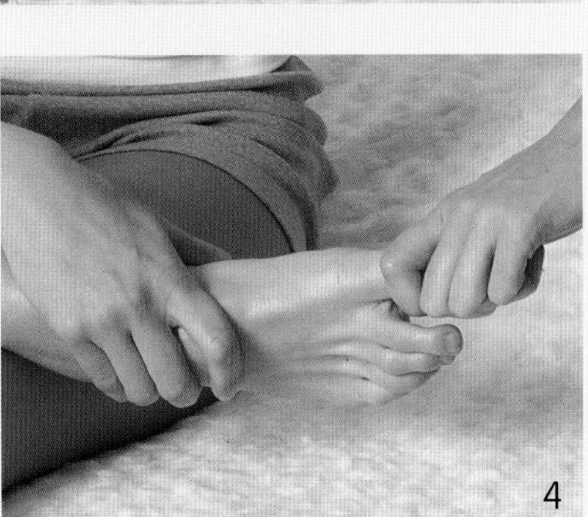

4

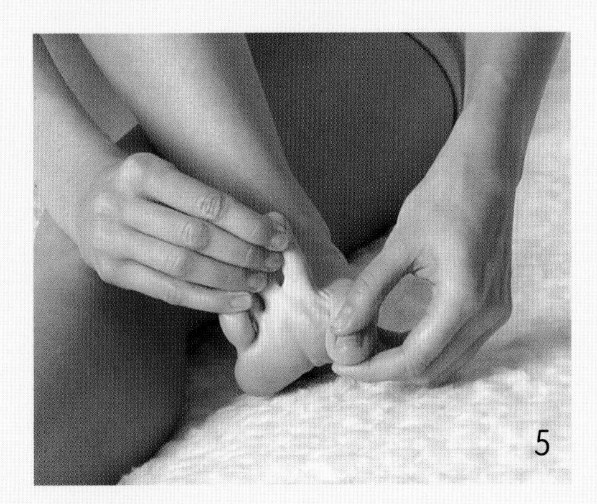

5

4 **Toe massaging:** With your thumb and forefinger hold onto one toe at the base. Make small circles up the toe and pinch the end as you release. Repeat to the next toe. Continue until all of the toes have been massaged.

5 **Toe walking:** Hold onto the big toe with the fingertips of one hand and the next toe with the fingertips of the other hand. Move one toe forwards and the other toe backwards, gently stretching them. Quickly move the toes in opposite directions, while thinking of the toes making fast walking steps. Shift your hands down one toe. Keep the same pace as you gradually walk all of the toes.

6 **Thumbs up:** Place your thumbs on the heel of the foot. Press into your foot as you slide the thumbs up the foot towards the toes. Repeat a few times.

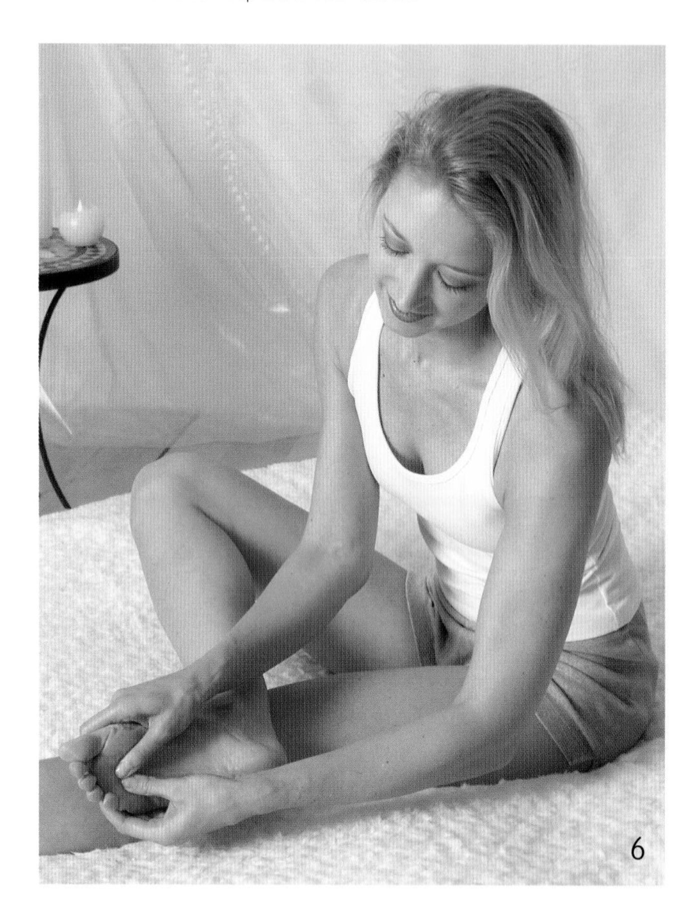

7 **Ankle circles:** Hold the foot with your outside hand. Circle the whole foot towards you, trying to stretch out the muscles. Circle a few times in this direction, and then reverse.

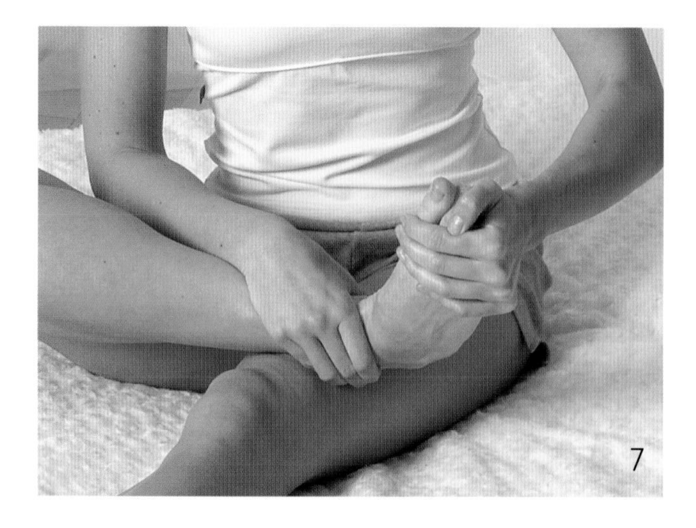

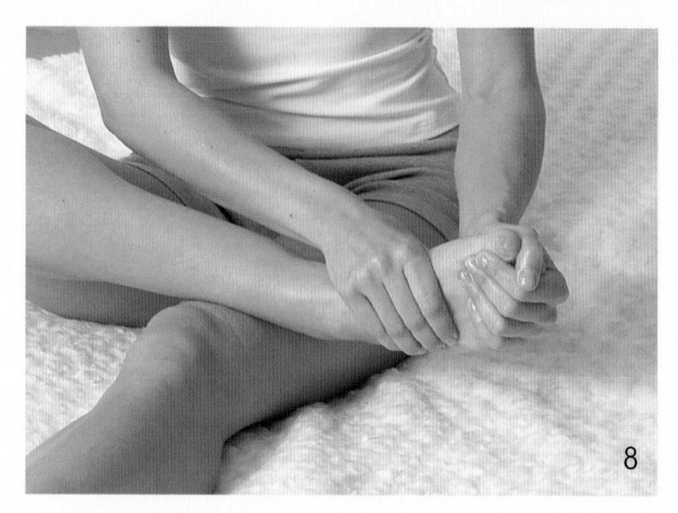

8 **Squeezing:** Hold the foot between the hands and squeeze. Change your hand position and repeat.

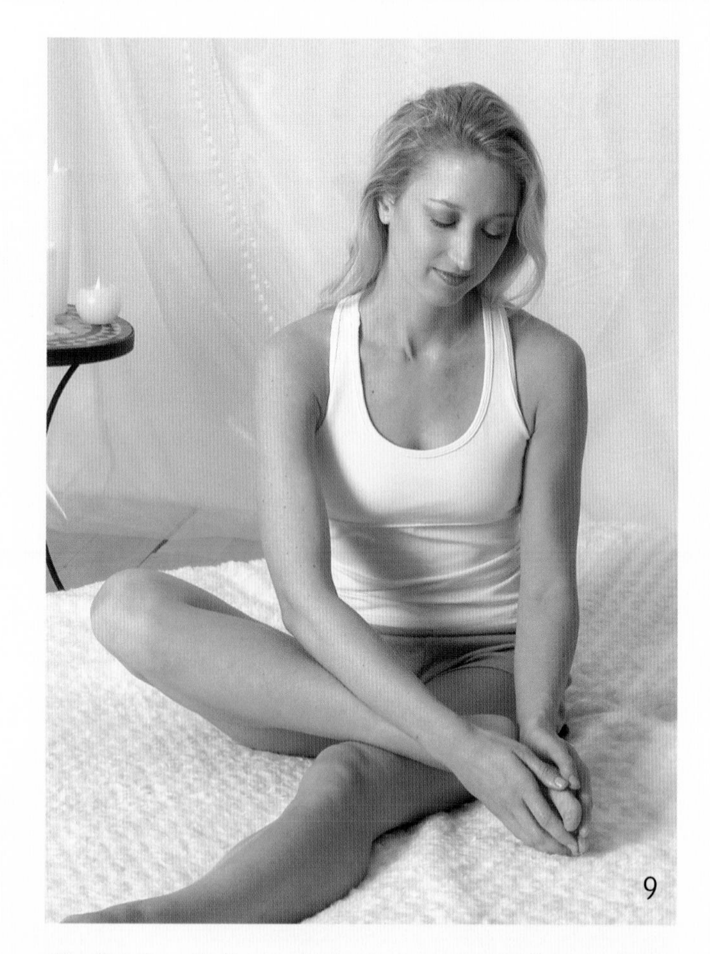

9 **Holding:** Hold your foot between your hands and relax. Feel the energy and heat from your hands penetrate through your foot.

Ending: Repeat to the other foot.

Calf

Spreading the oil: Place the foot flat on the ground with the knee bent. Pour a small amount of oil or cream onto your hand. Spread it out, starting at your ankle and working your way up to the knee.

1 **Friction with the palms:** Place the palms on the back of the ankle. Make small circles as you press the heel of the hand into your calf. Work all the way up to the knee. Slide the hands back down to the ankle and start again.

2 **Friction with the fingertips:** Place the fingertips on the ankle at the front. Making small circles, work your way up the entire shin to the knee. Repeat a few times, thinking of separating the muscle from the bone.

3 **Vibration:** Place the hands flat on either side of the calf. Move the hands quickly forwards and backwards so that the calf muscles shake back and forth. Move the hands up and down the leg, trying to keep the flow and rhythm of the movement.

4 **Thumbs up:** Place the thumbs at the ankle on the back of the leg with the fingertips touching in front of the ankle. Think of pressing the thumbs and fingers together as you slide the hands up towards the knee. Relax the hands as they glide back down to the ankle to start again. Repeat to the other side.

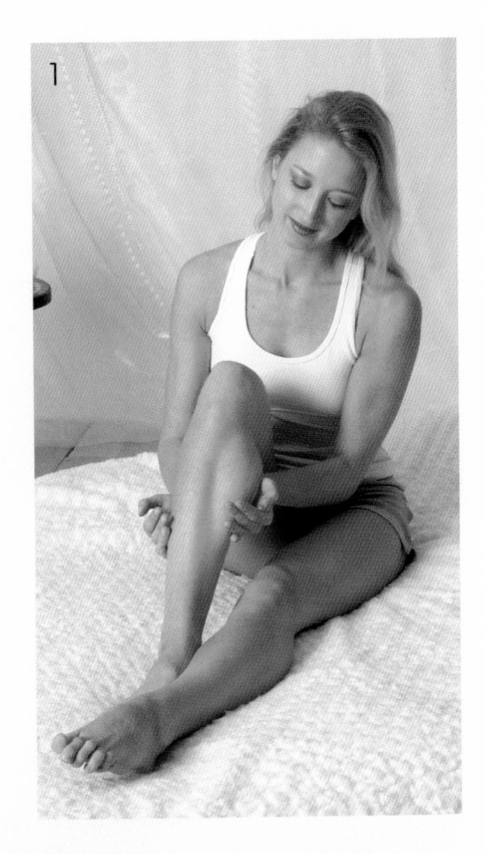

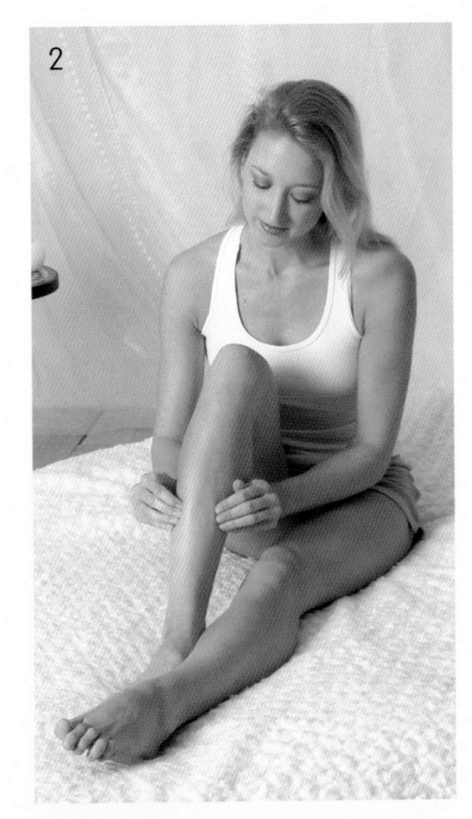

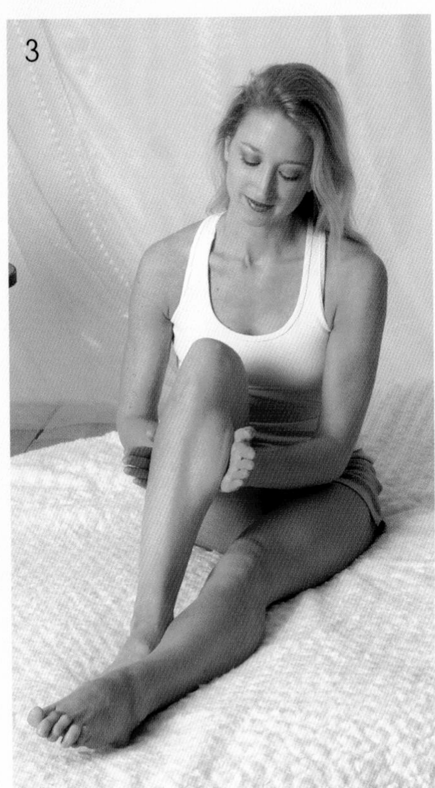

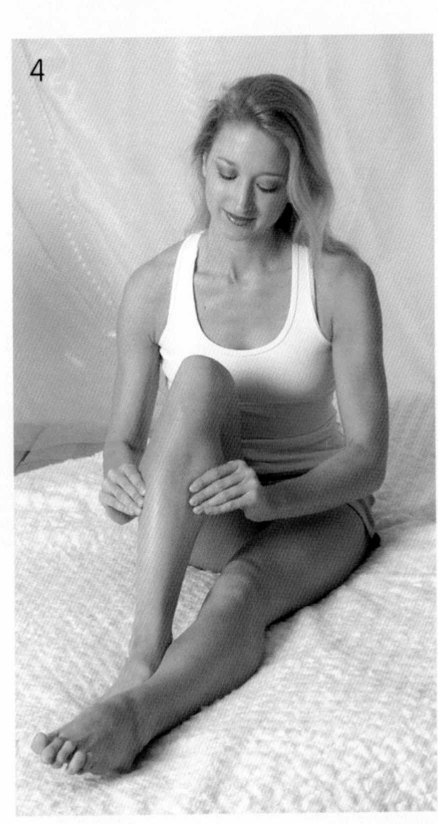

Thighs

Spreading the oil: Bend the knee and place the foot flat on the floor. Pour a small amount of oil or lotion into the palm of your hand. Rub your hands together and spread it over the entire thigh area.

1 **Friction:** Start with the thumbs on top of the thigh. Making small circles, cover the top of the thigh with your thumbs. Place the fingertips on the underneath of the thigh. Make small circles with the fingertips to massage the back of the thigh.

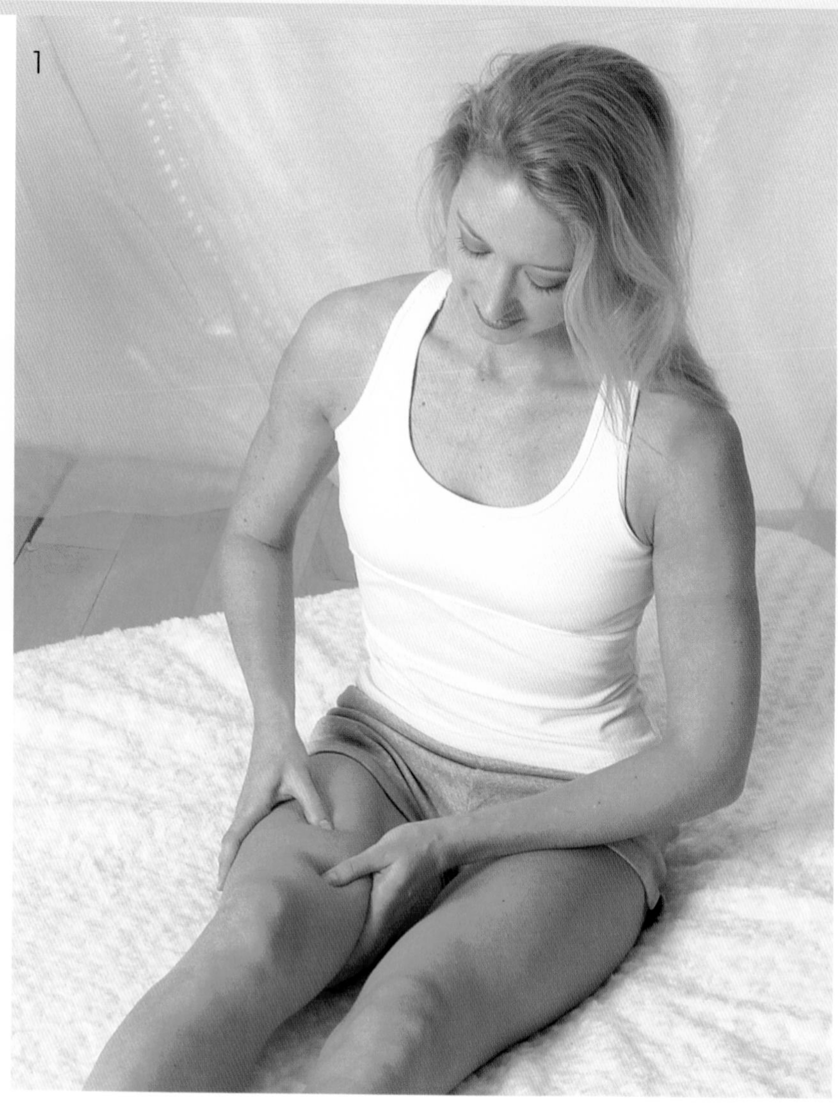
1

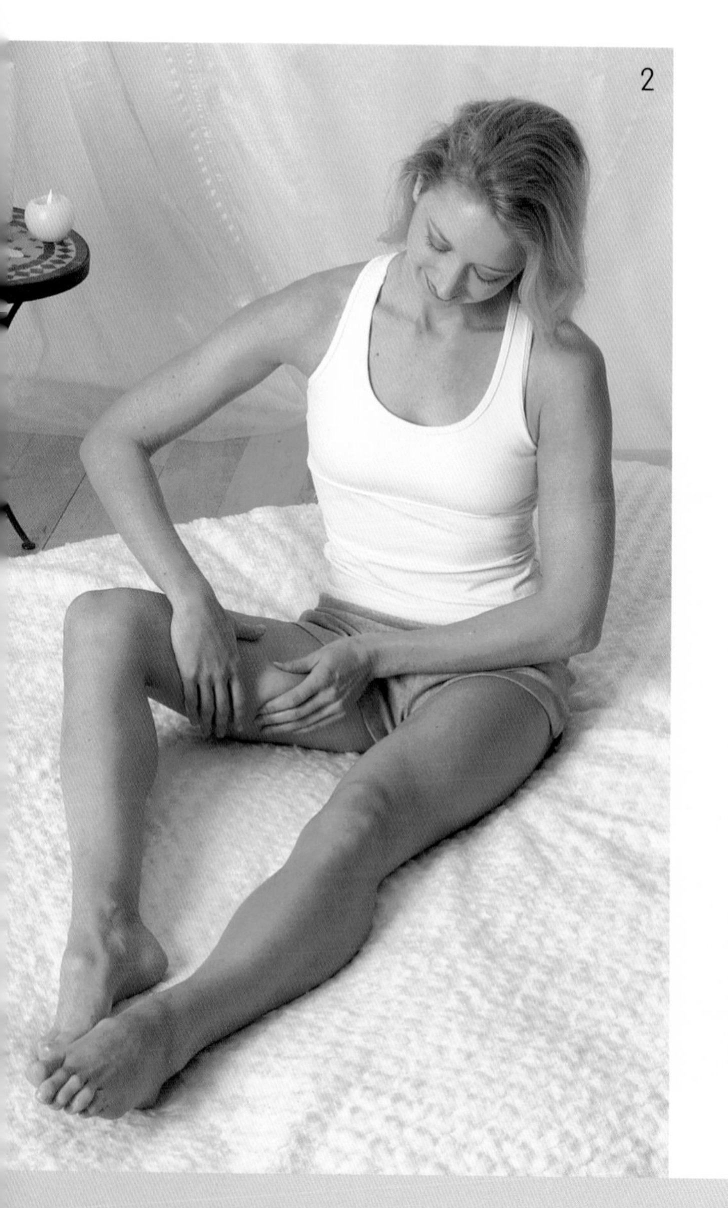
2

2 **Kneading the inner thigh:** Keep your knee bent and let it relax out to the side. Your inner thigh should be exposed so that you can place your hands on it with the fingers facing the floor. Pick up some of the flesh with one hand. Squeeze it as you slide the flesh towards the other hand. As you release the flesh, pick it up with the opposite hand. Repeat with a rhythmic motion, thinking of waves going back and forth between your hands.

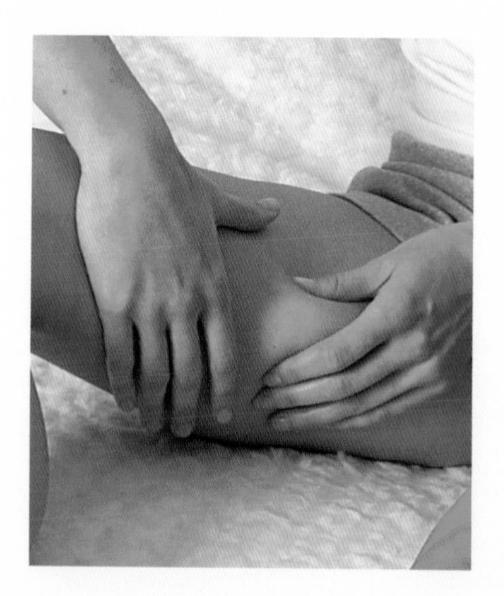

3 Shaking: Place the hands flat on either side of the thigh with your fingers facing away from you. Quickly move the hands back and forth, shaking the leg.

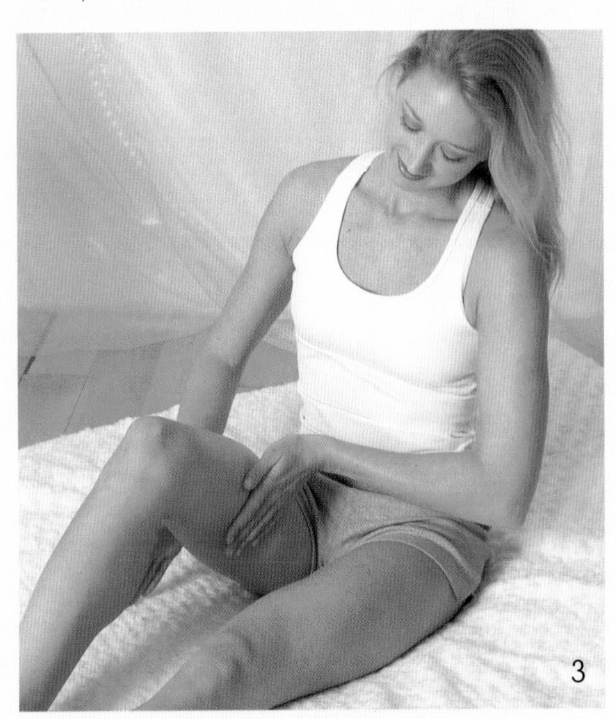
3

4 Hacking: Place the hands just above the thigh forming two parallel lines. The fingertips should be in opposite directions. Quickly strike the thigh with alternating hands. Try not to stay in the same place!

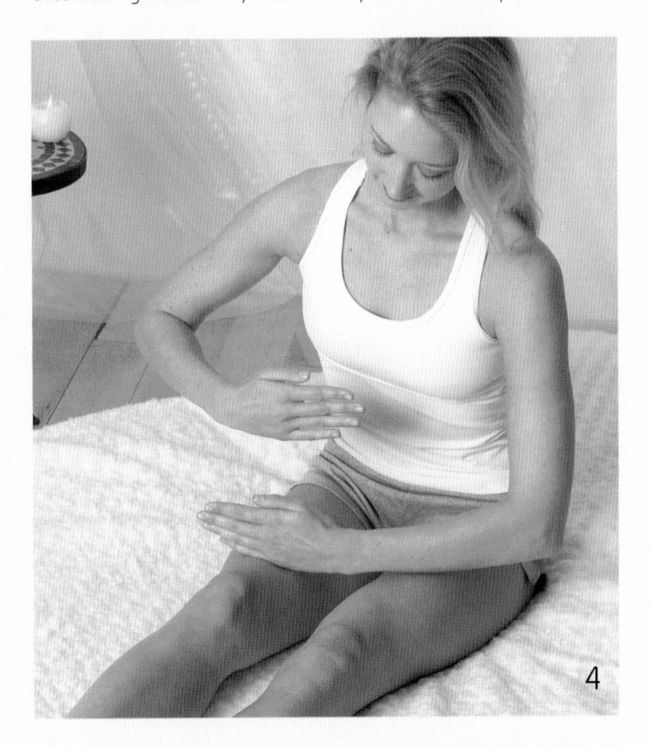
4

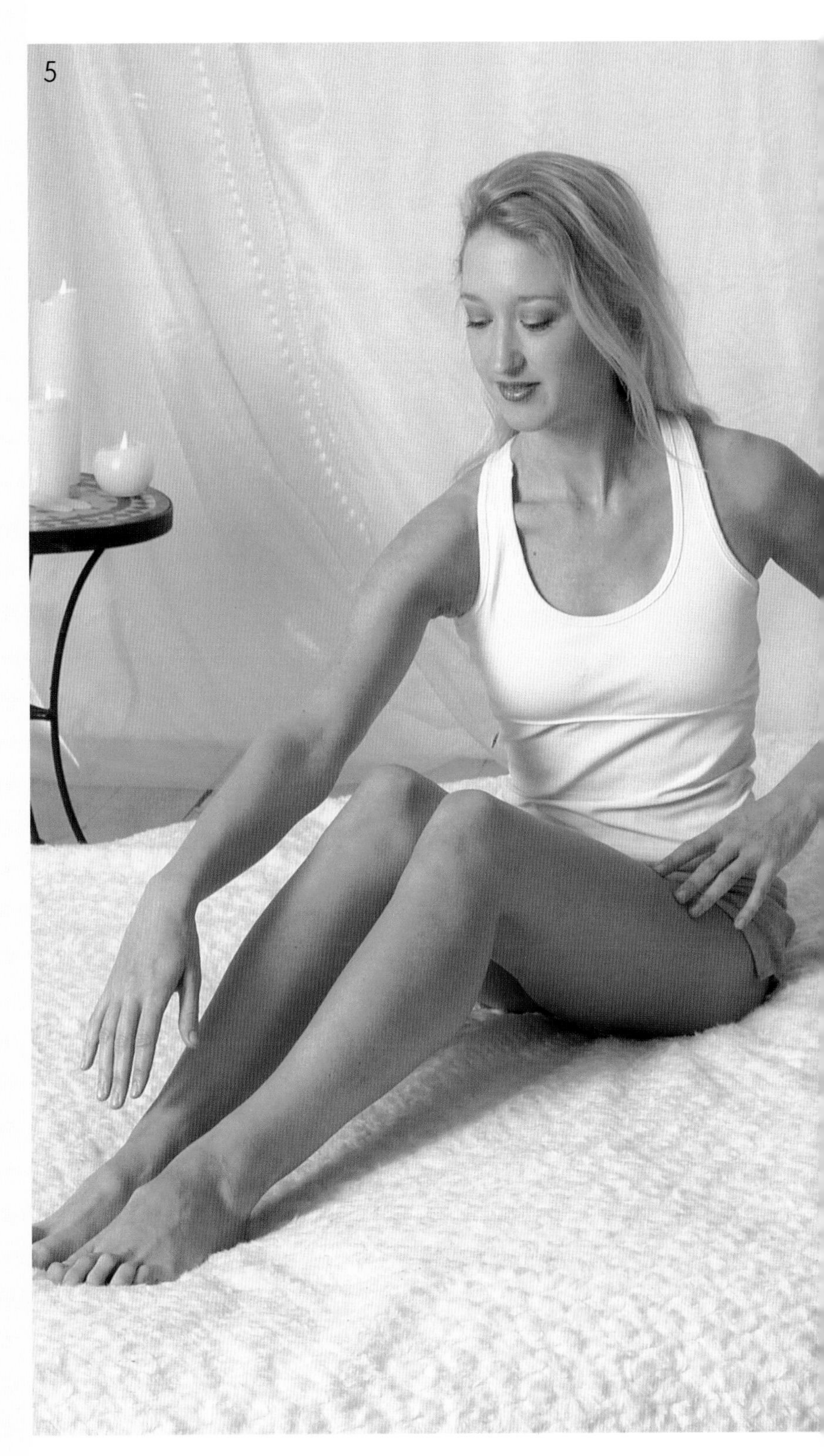
5

5 Ending: Bend both of your legs in front of you with the feet flat on the floor. Touch one ankle with the fingertips of one of your hands. Slide the fingertips over the contour of your leg to your hip. When your hand gets to your hip, repeat. Repeat the movement with the other hand. Repeat the whole sequence to the other side.

Knees

Opening: Place the thumbs lengthwise on the knee with the thumbs facing the ankle and the fingers out to the sides. Press out and away with the length of the thumb as you circle the knee with the pads of the thumb. Repeat three times.

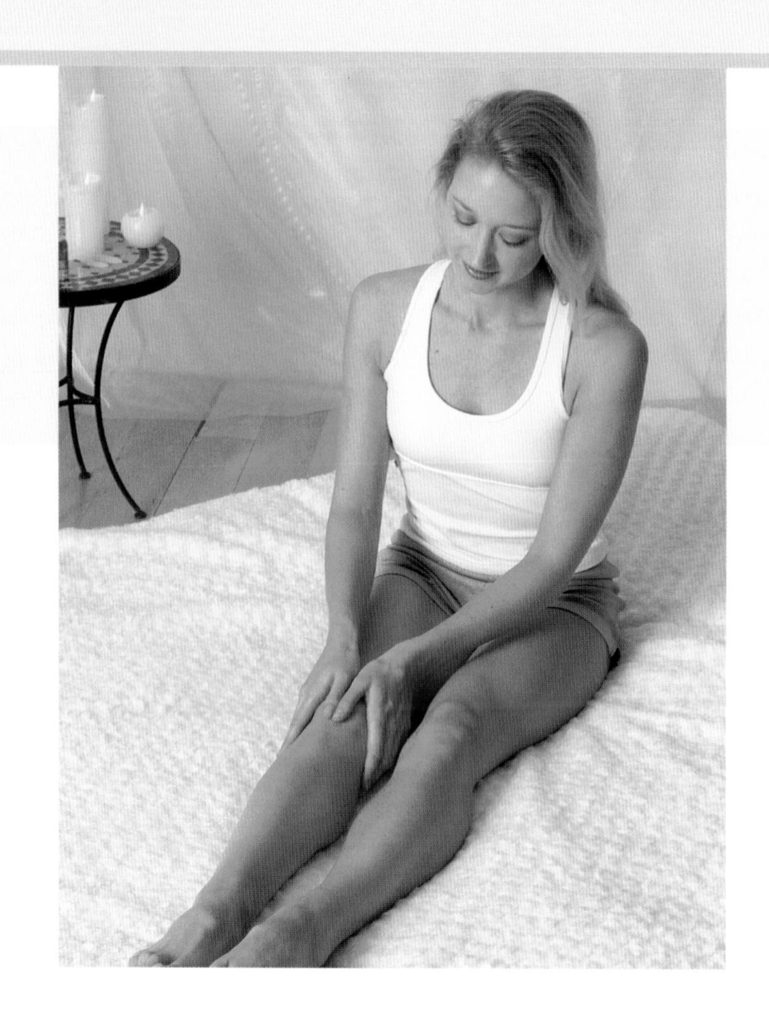

Stomach

Spreading the oil: If clothed, obviously do not apply oil! If stomach is bare, pour a small amount of oil or lotion onto your hand. Rub your hands together and place them flat on your stomach.

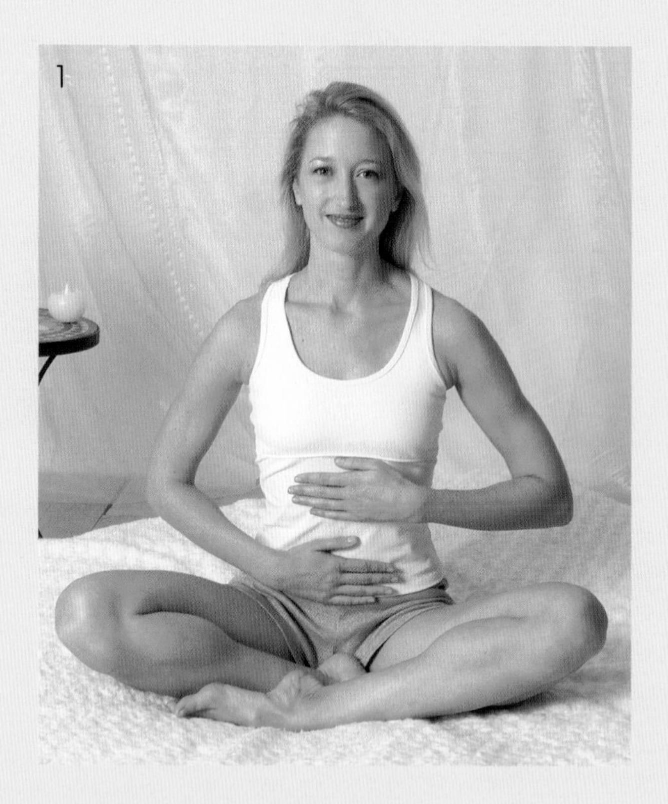
1

1 **Circling:** Circle your hands in a clockwise direction around your belly button.

2 **Kneading the waistline:** Place both hands on your hips with the fingertips facing down. Massage both hips at the same time by gently squeezing the fleshy area around the hip.

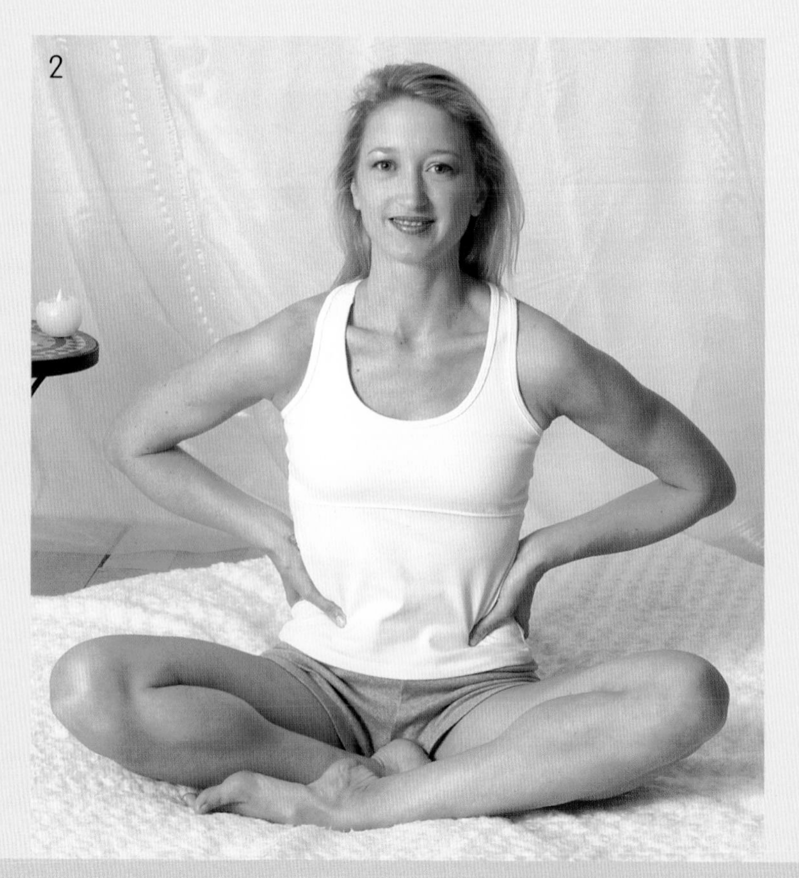
2

Back

Spreading the oil: Sit comfortably and pour a small amount of oil into your hand. Rub your hands together and spread it over your lower back.

1 **Friction:** Place your hands on your back with the fingertips facing down. Circle the fingers, covering the entire lower back.

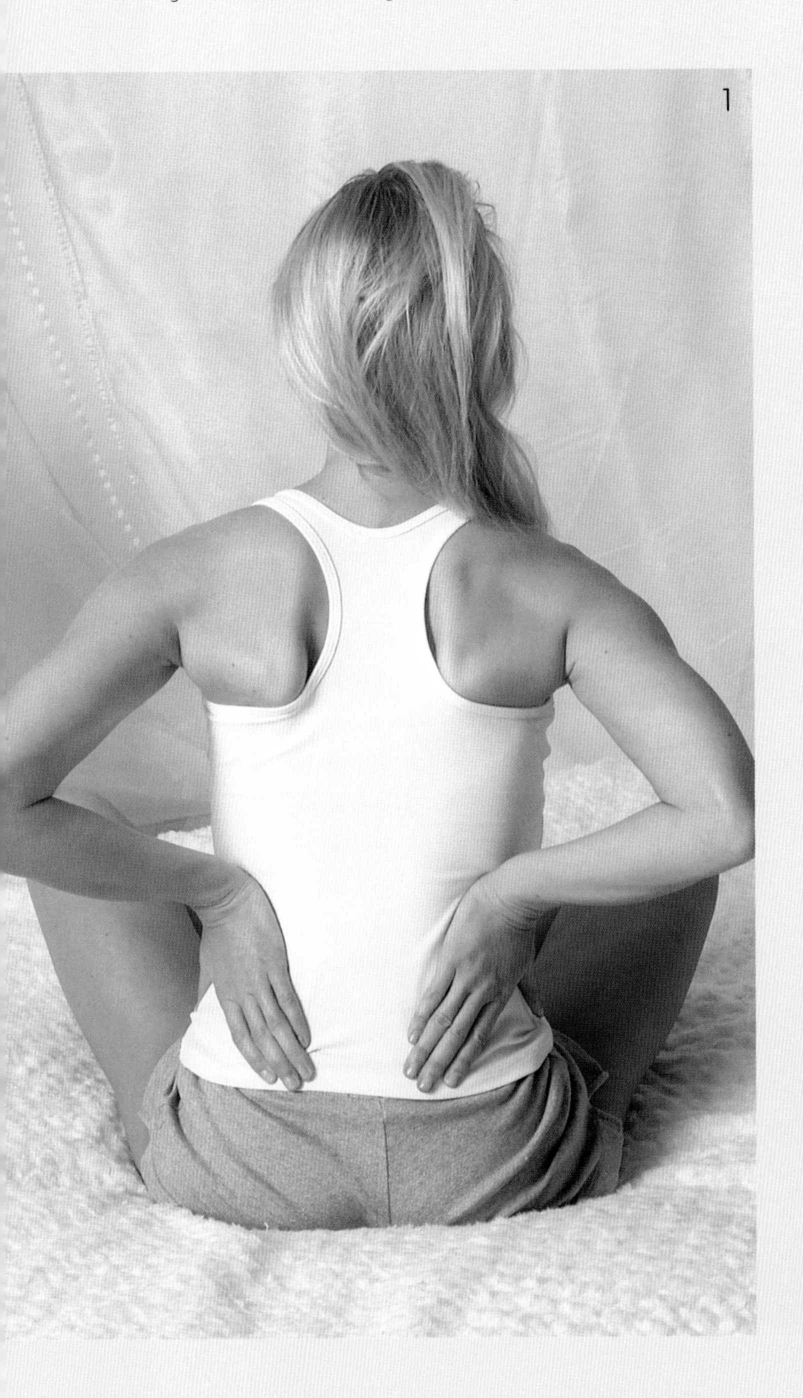
1

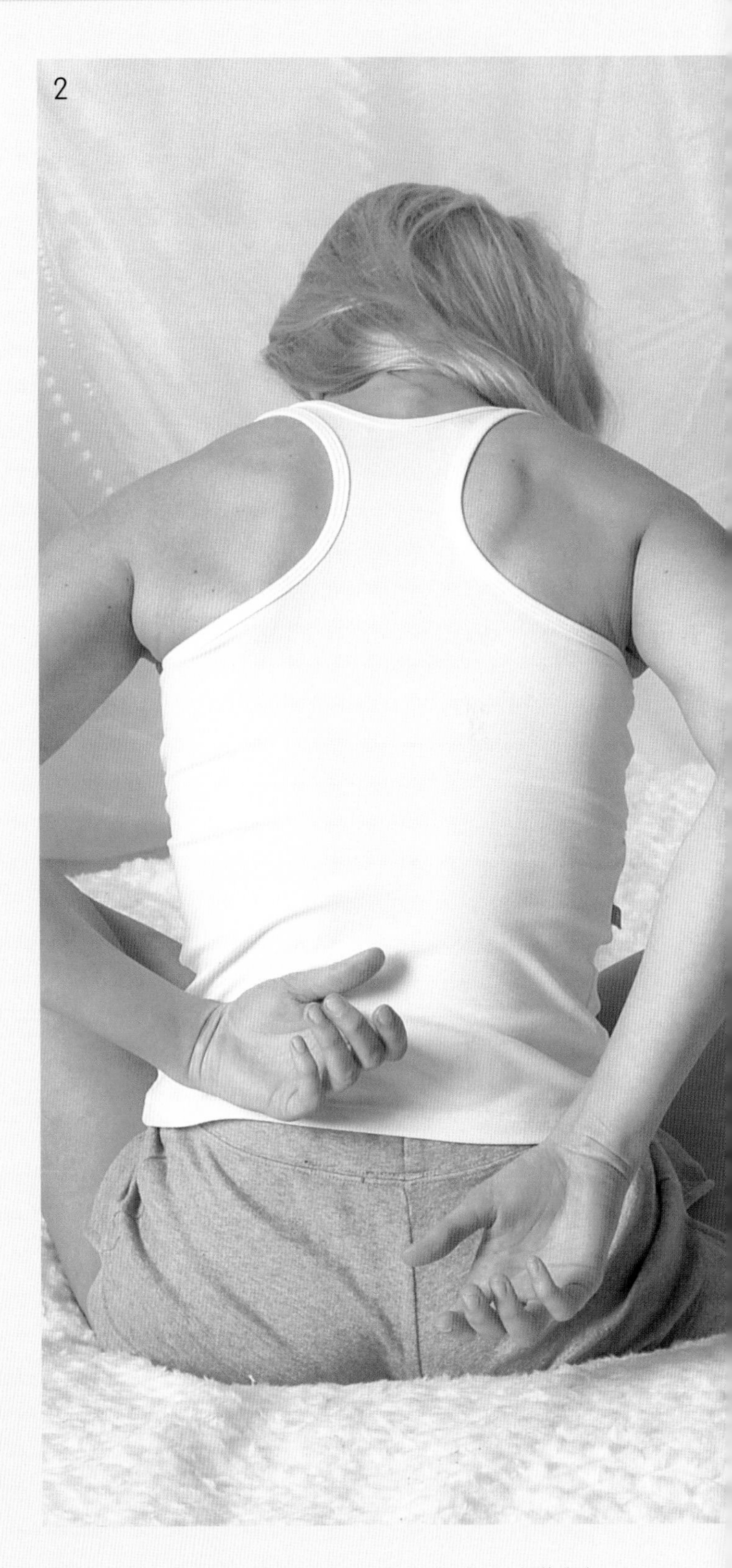
2

2 **Fists:** Make loose fists with the hands. Round slightly forward and gently hit the lower part of your back. Alternate your hands as you try to release the tension held in the back.

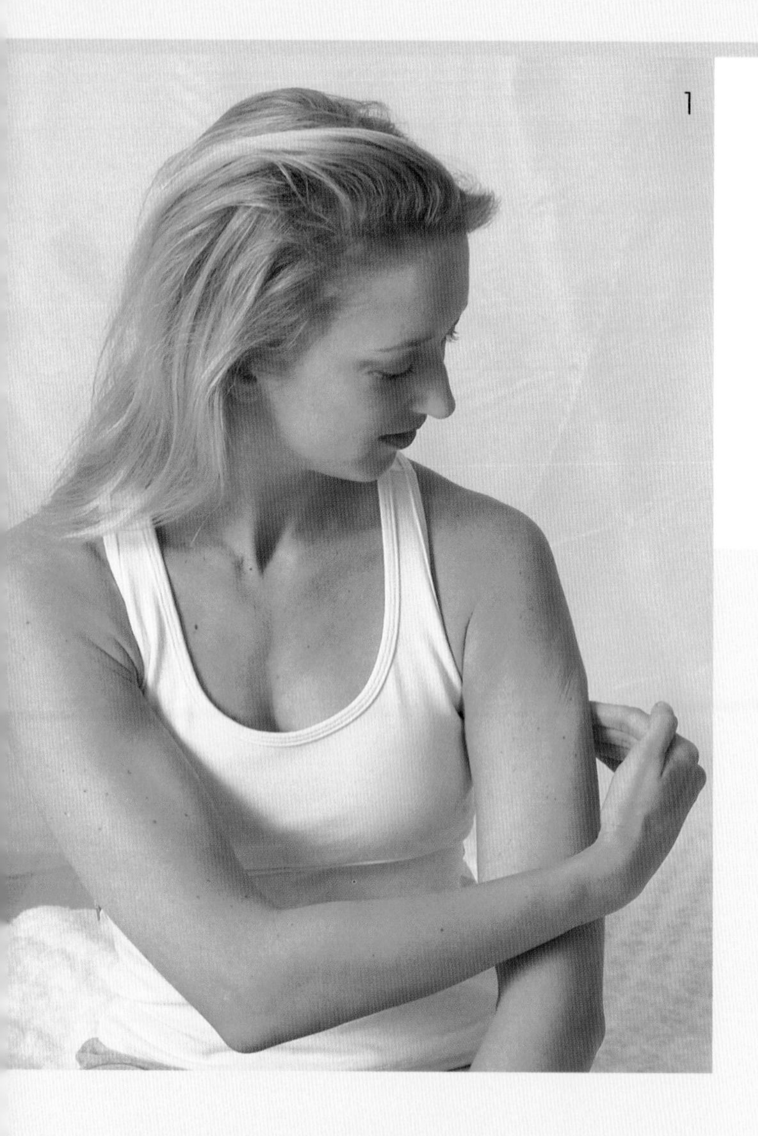

1

Arm

Spreading the oil: Pour a small amount of oil onto one hand. Spread the oil onto your opposite arm, starting at the wrist.

1 **Friction to upper arm:** Place your fingertips on the back of the arm you are working on. As you press into the muscle, make small circles with your fingertips. Work over the whole upper arm area.

2 **Squeezing:** Hold the flesh between the fingertips and the palm of your hand. Squeeze the flesh and release along the entire length of the arm.

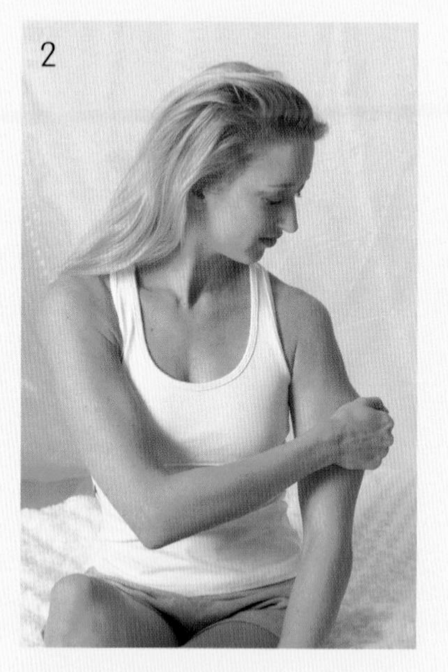

2

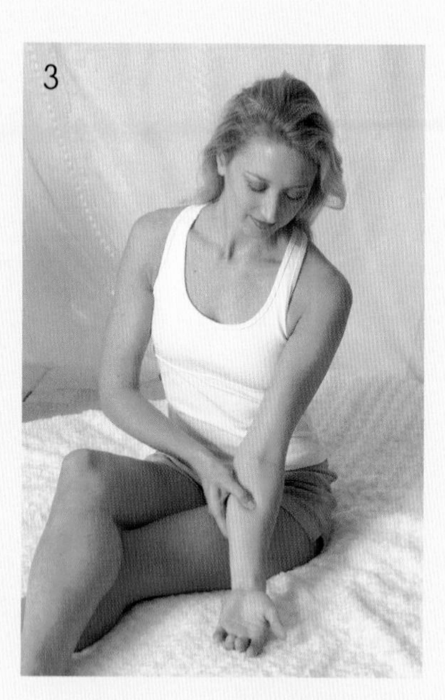

3

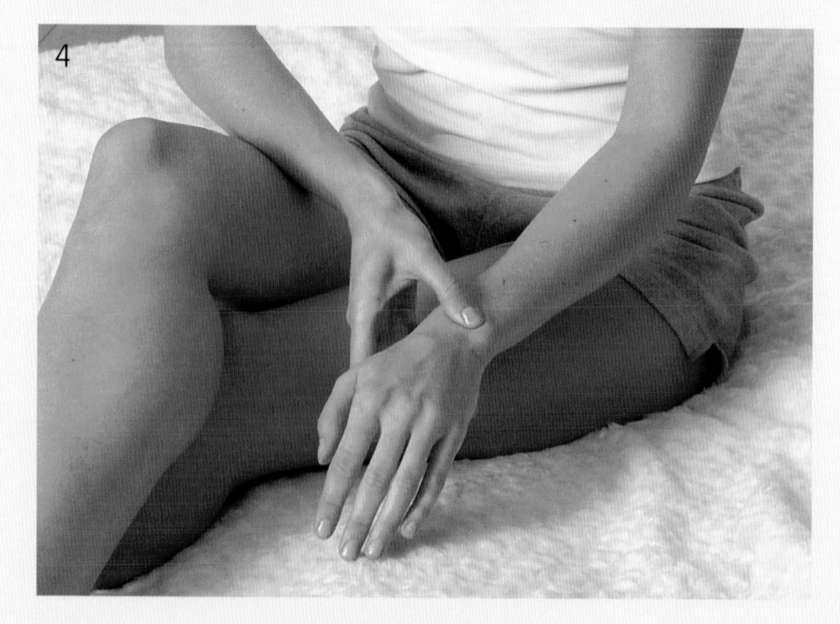

4

3 Turn your palm up and place the thumb of the opposite hand just below the elbow joint. Press and circle the thumb all the way up to the wrist. Repeat 2 more times. Turn the palm to face down. Place the thumb on top of the wrist and make circles going towards the elbow. Repeat 2 more times.

4 Friction: Place the thumb on top of the wrist with the fingertips holding your hand. Circle the thumb across the top of the hand and wrist. Turn the palm over. Massage the palm of the hand by making small circles with the thumb.

5 Finger massage: Start with the thumb and forefinger at the base of one of your fingers. Squeeze and circle the finger, working your way up to the tip. Repeat to the next finger until all of the fingers are done.

Ending: Repeat to the other side.

Shoulders and neck

1 Friction with one hand: Place one hand on the opposite shoulder. Place your fingertips directly on the fleshy area of the shoulder. Press firmly onto the shoulder as you do a circling motion with your fingers. Repeat to the other side.

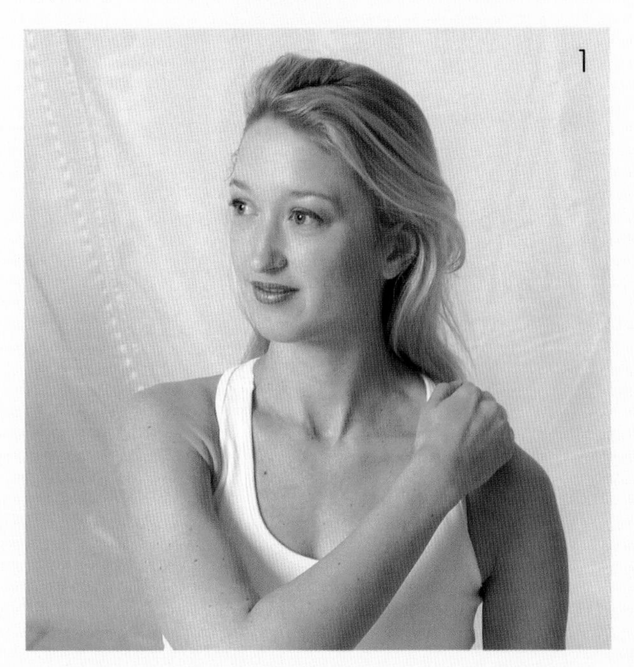

2 Friction with both hands: Place one hand on each shoulder. Press the fingertips into the belly of the muscle while making circles.

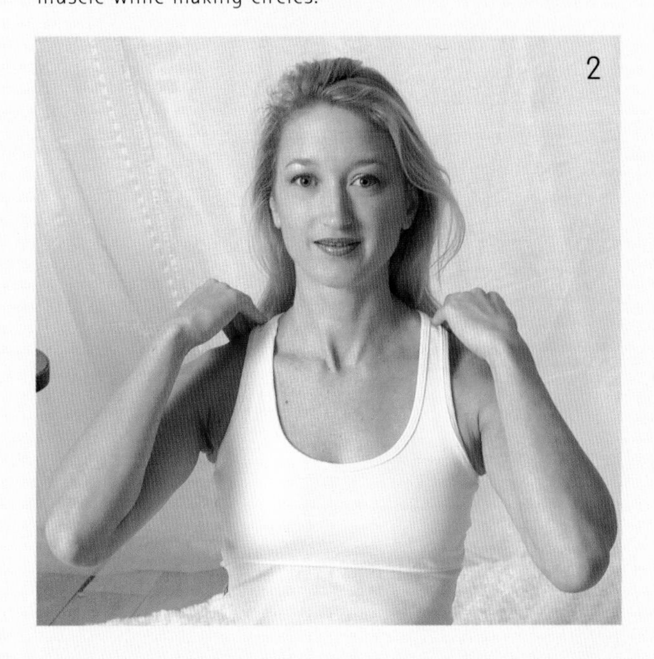

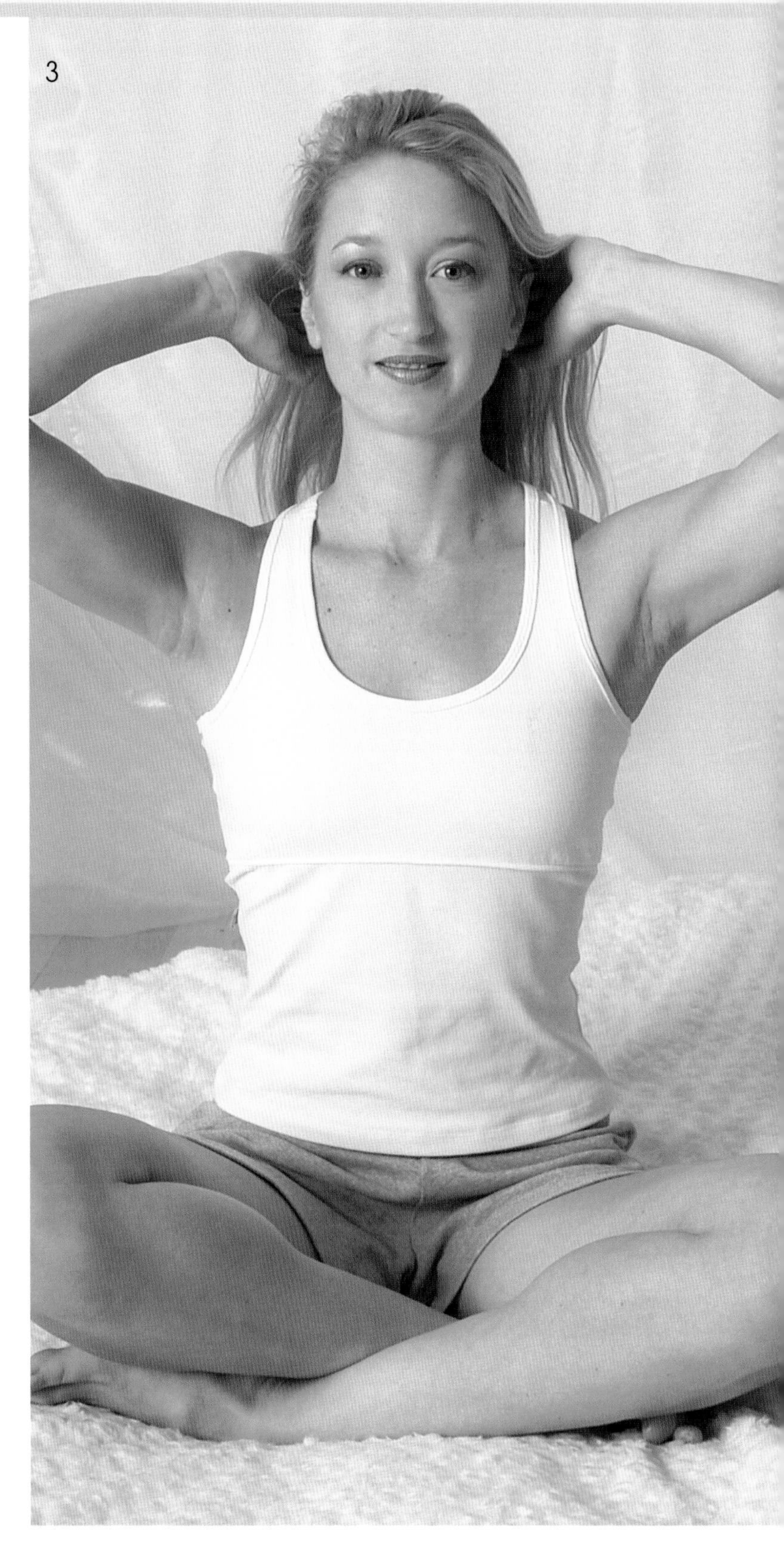

3 Friction to neck: Place the fingertips of both hands at the base of the neck. Making small circles, work your way up to the top of the neck.

Face

1 **Effleurage:** Start with the hands lightly touching the face at the chin. Circle your fingers around your mouth, up the sides of your nose, across the forehead, and back down the sides of the cheeks. This is very relaxing, so do not be afraid to spend some time on it.

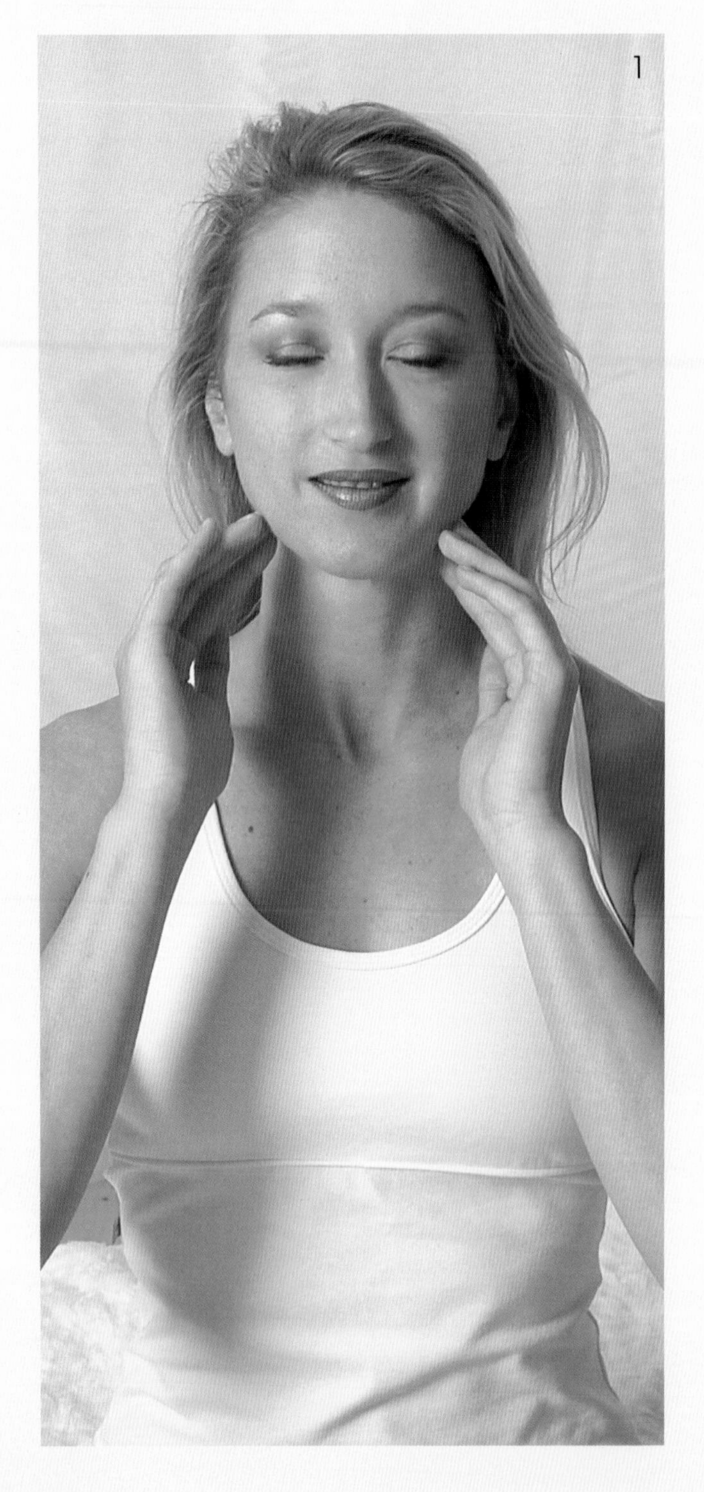

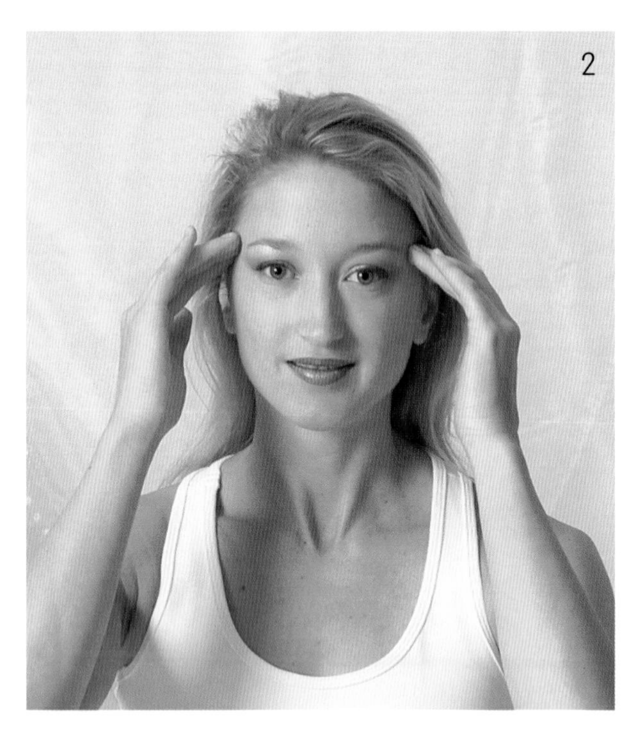

2 **Friction to temples:** Place the fingertips of both hands on the temples. Circle the temples with the fingers.

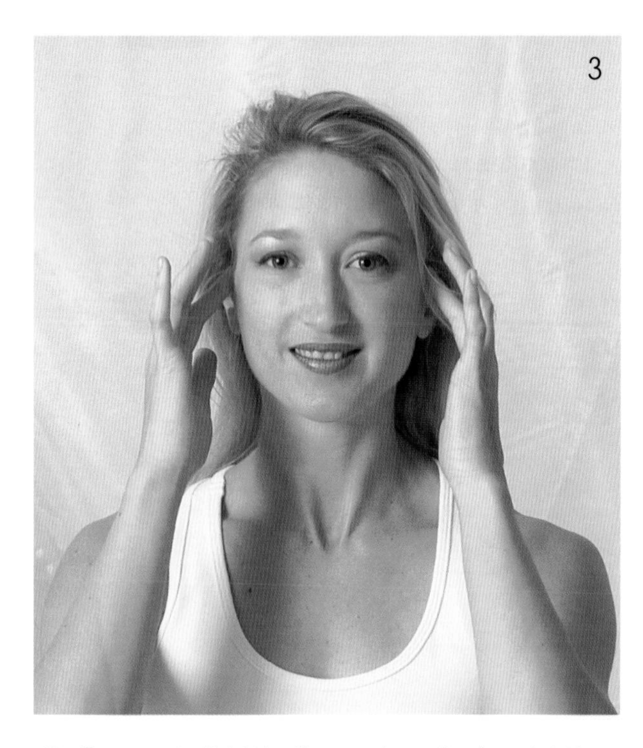

3 **Tapoment:** Hold the fingers above the face. Let the fingers fall separately like raindrops falling lightly on the surface of the skin.

4 Friction: Place the fingertips on the jaw. Massage the jaw with slow, rhythmic movements. Move up to the cheeks and repeat.

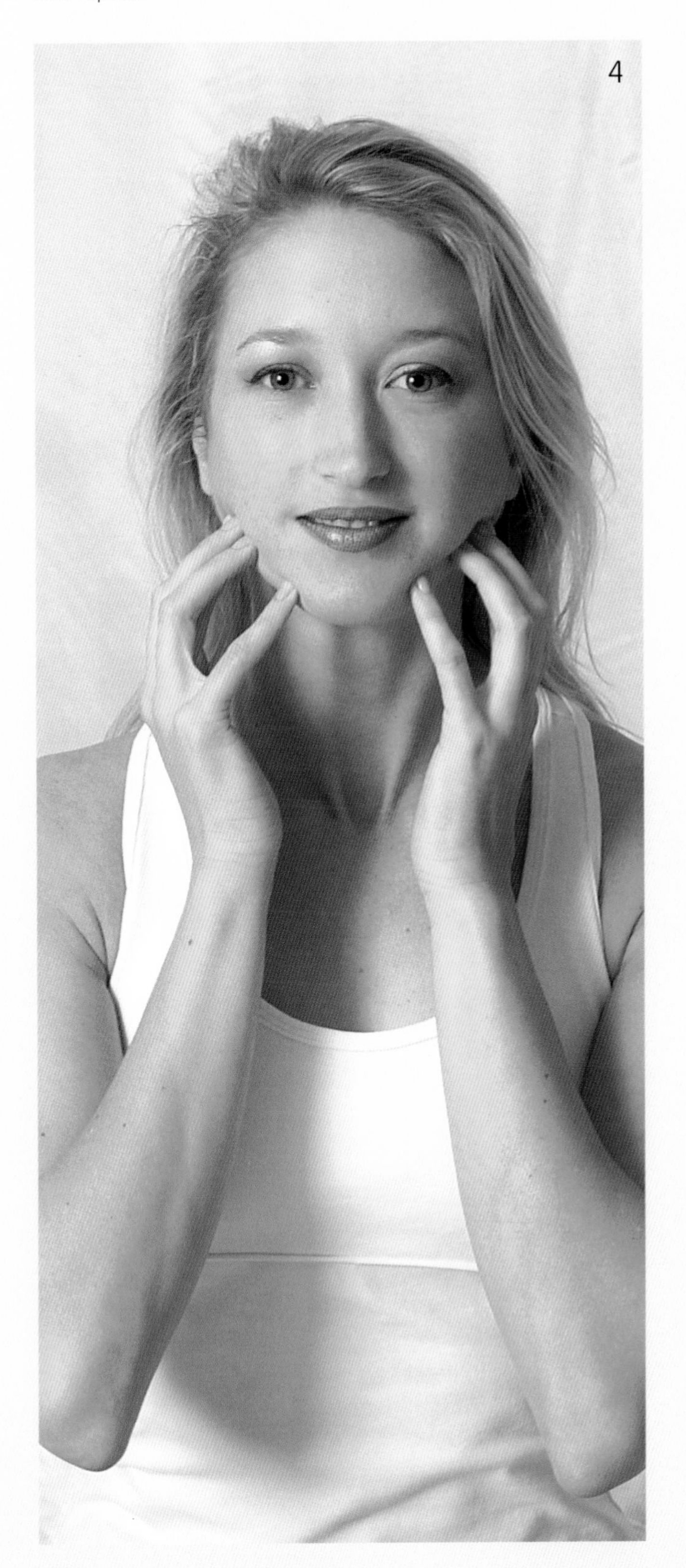

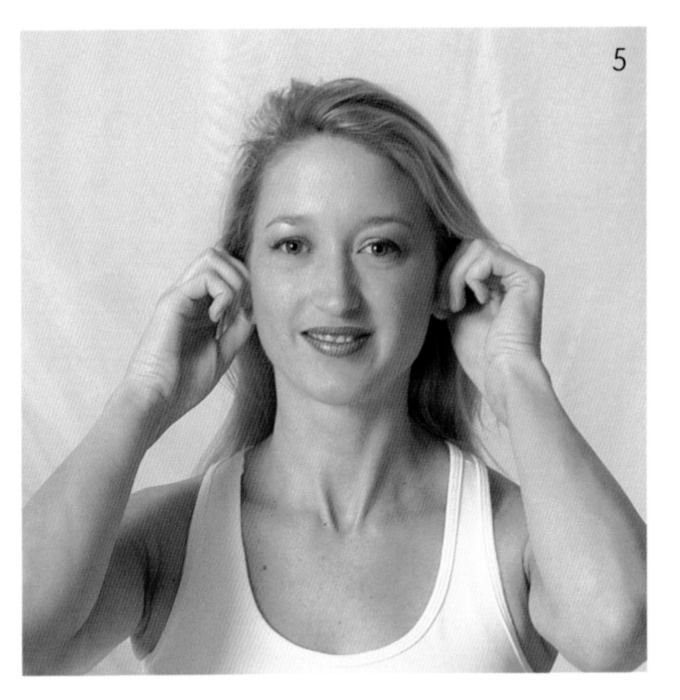

5 Massaging the ears: Place the thumb on the back of the ear and bend your forefinger in front of the ear. Circle the thumbs and forefingers, massaging the ears. Gently pull away as you do this.

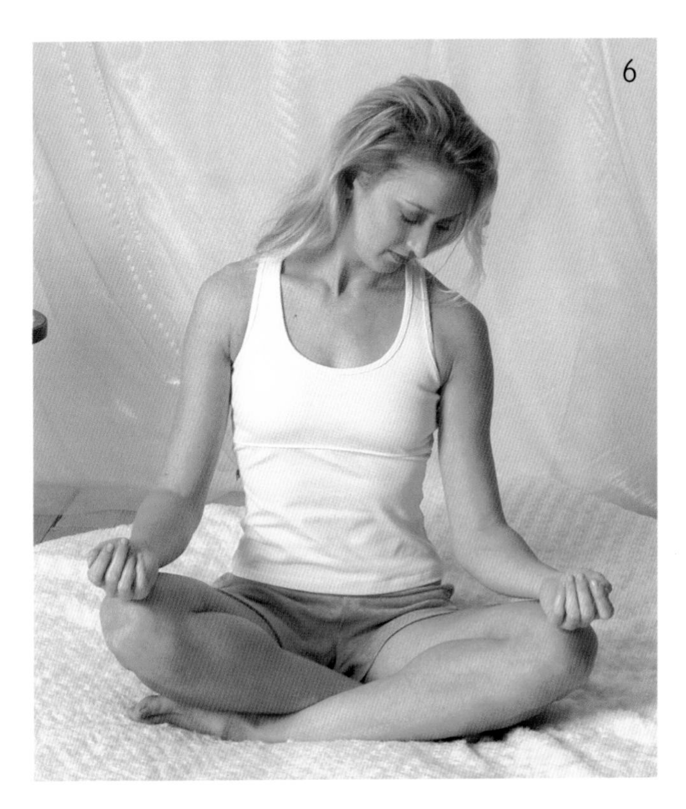

6 **Ending**: Try a couple of neck circles (see page 40).

Quick guide – foot

1. Spreading the oil

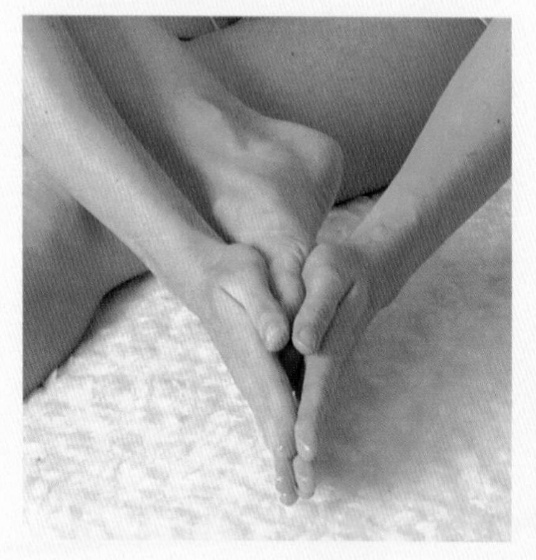

2. Sandwiching

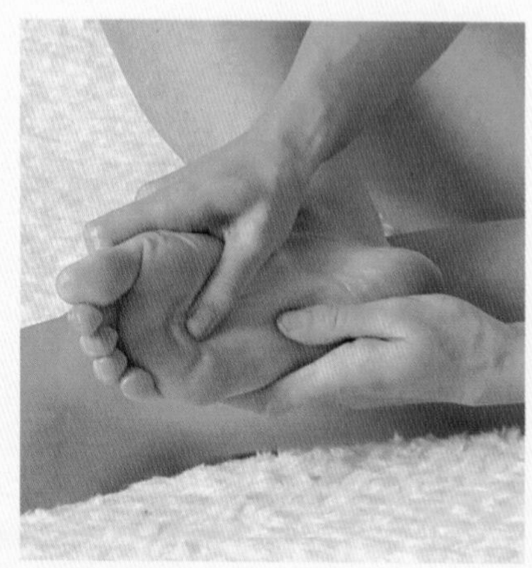

3. Friction

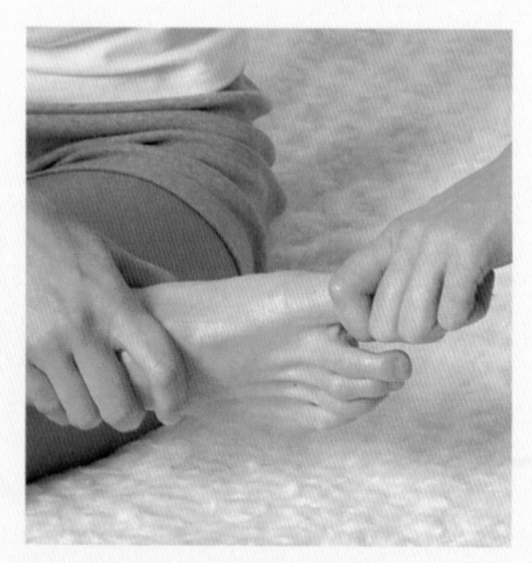

4. Toe massaging

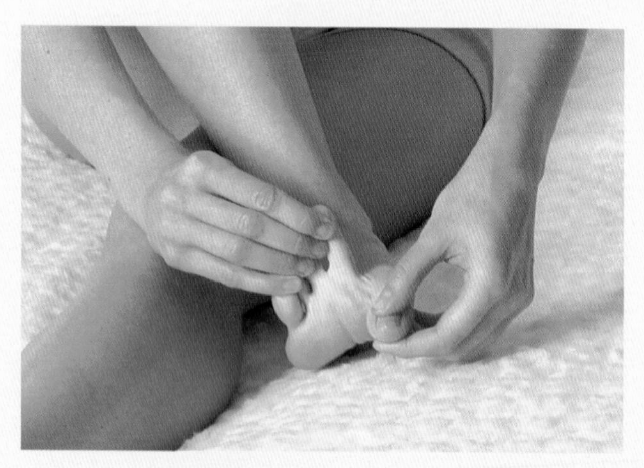

5. Toe walking

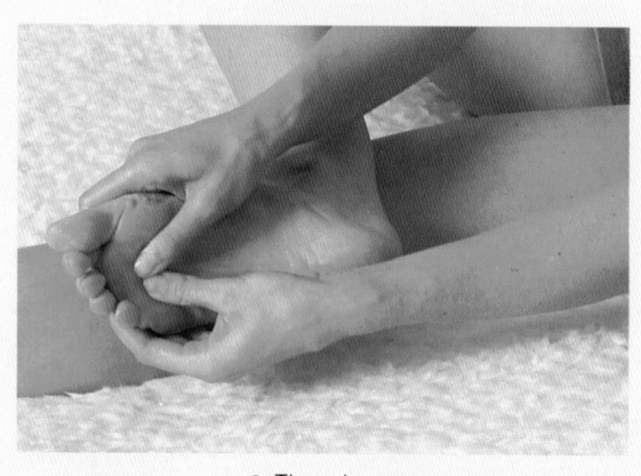

6. Thumbs up

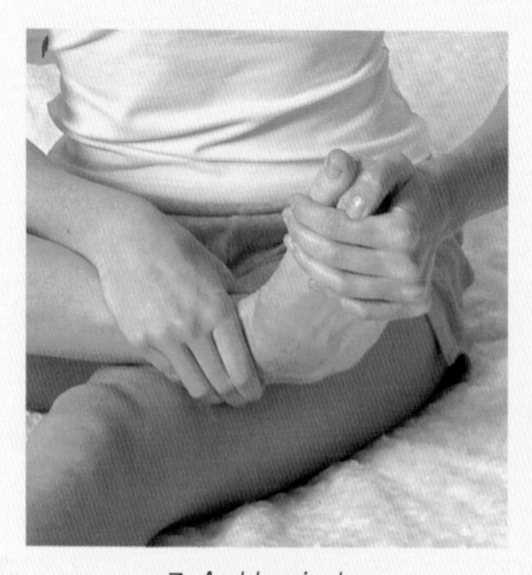

7. Ankle circles

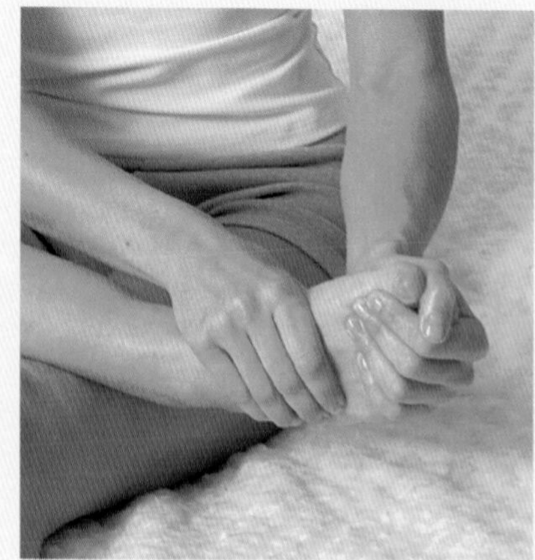

8. Squeezing

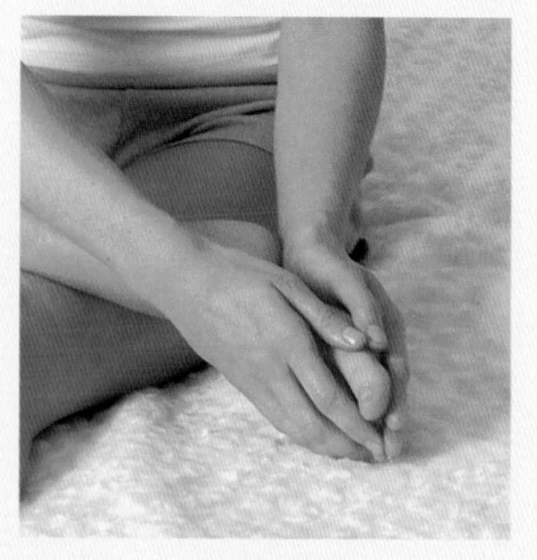

9. Holding

Quick guide – calf

1. Spreading the oil

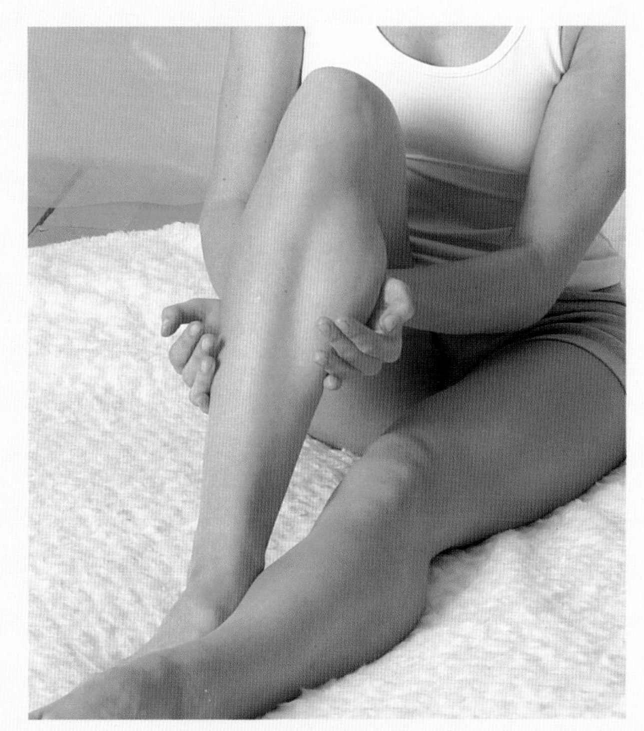

2. Friction with the palms

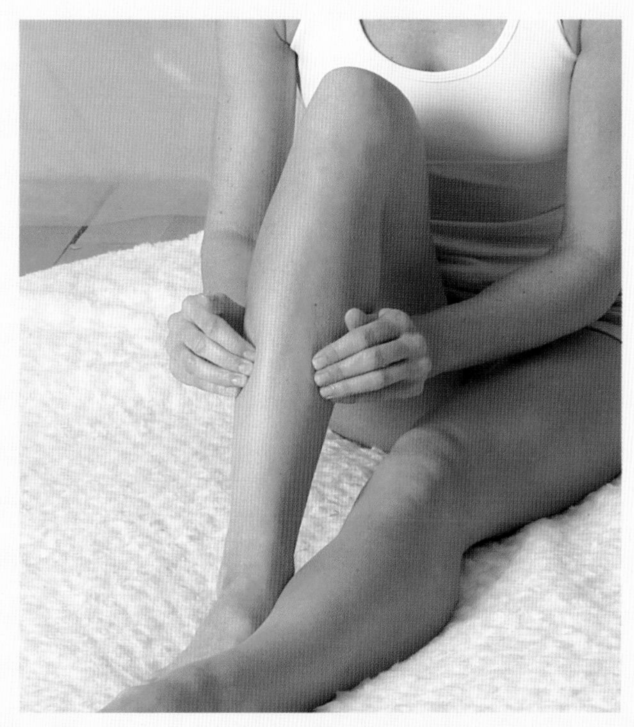

3. Friction with fingertips

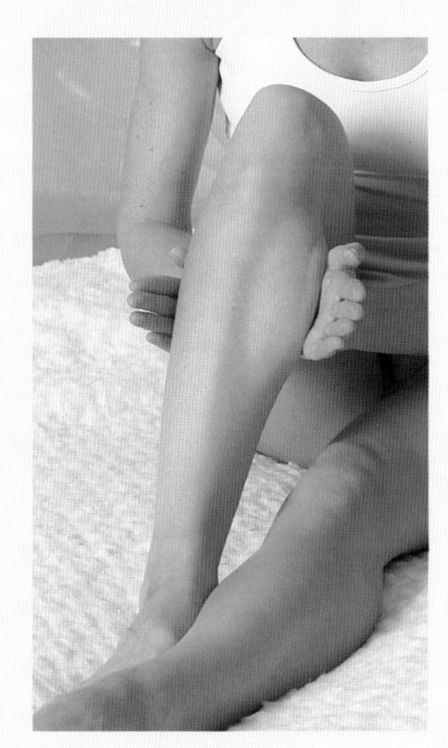

4. Vibration

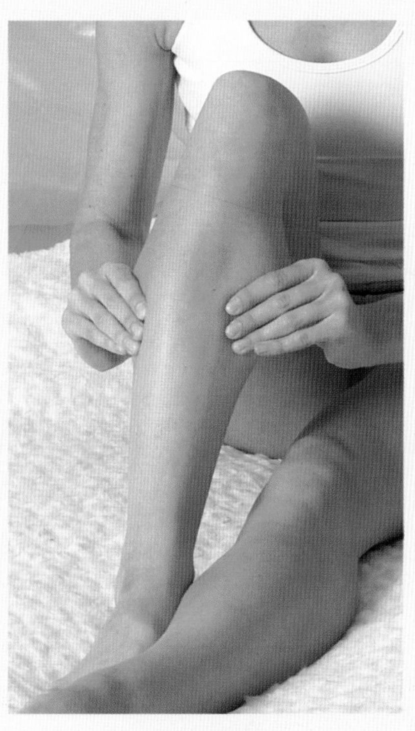

4. Thumbs up

Quick guide – knees

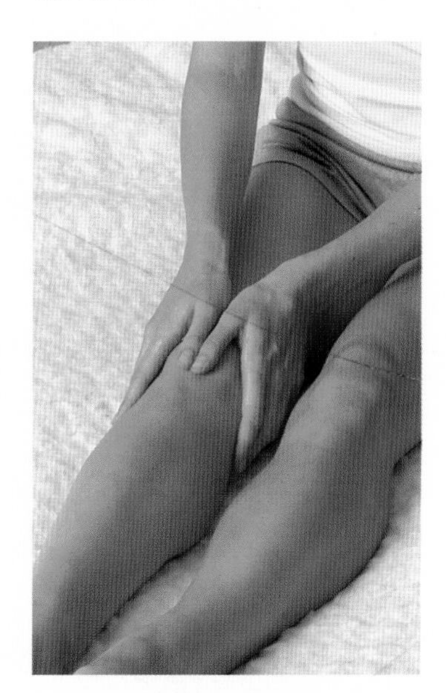

Opening

Quick guide – thigh

1. Spreading the oil

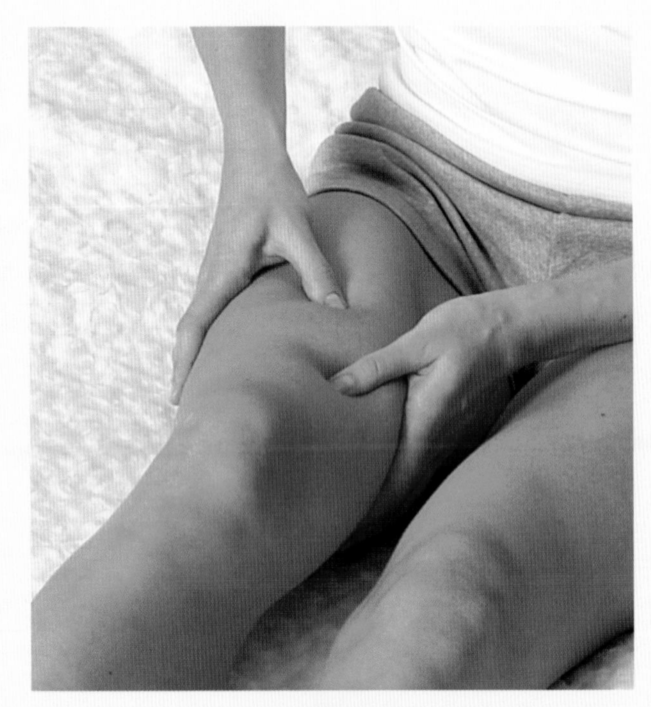

2. Friction

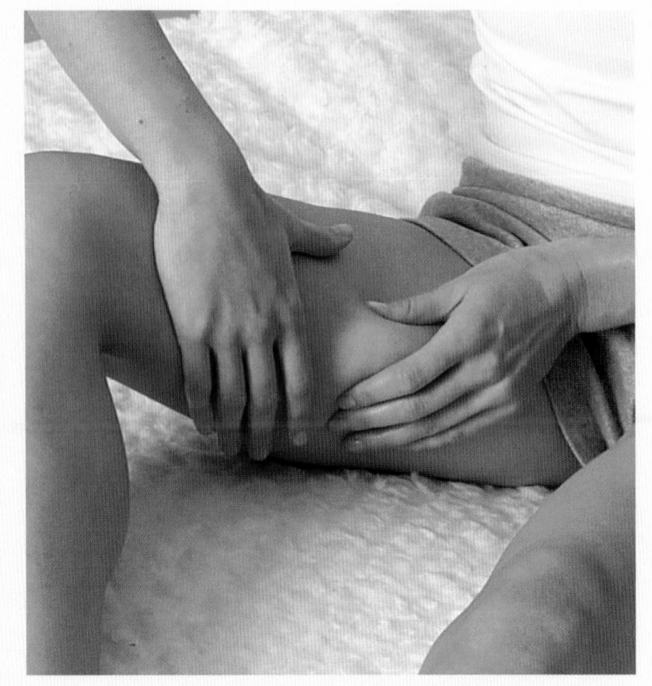

3. Kneading the inner thigh

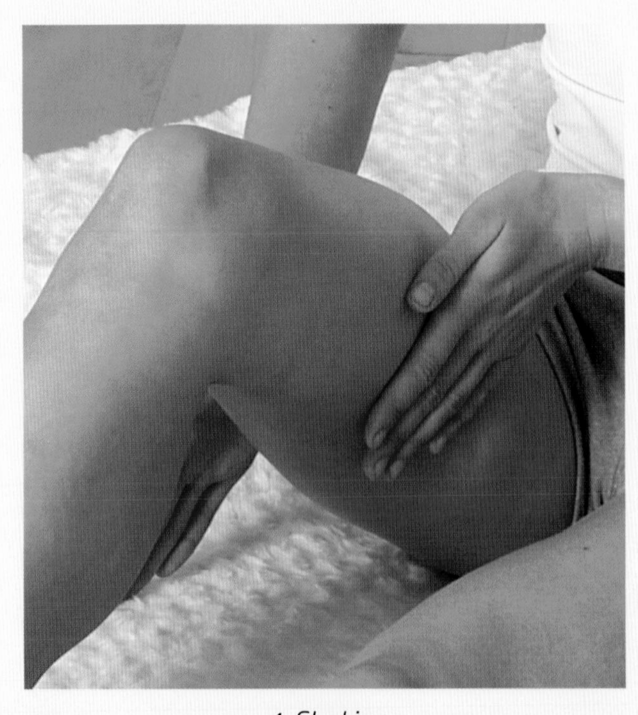

4. Shaking

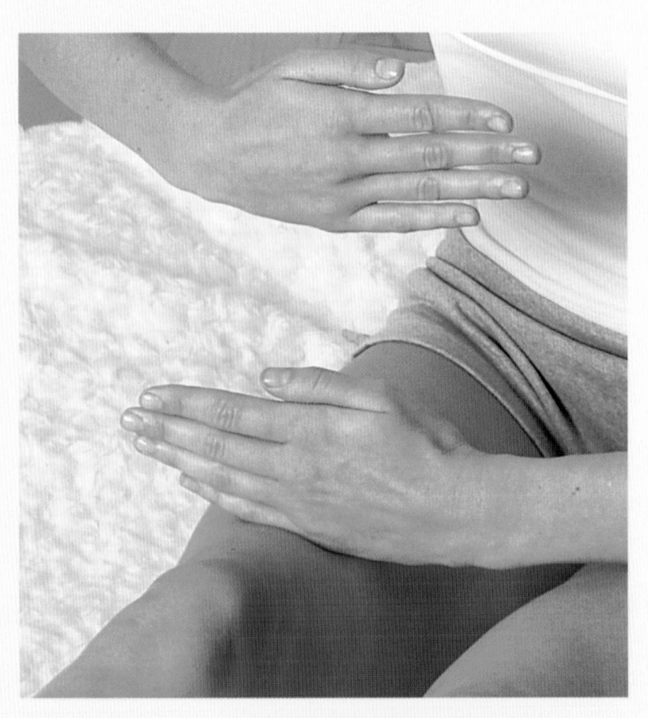

5. Hacking

Quick guide – stomach

1. *Spreading the oil if required*

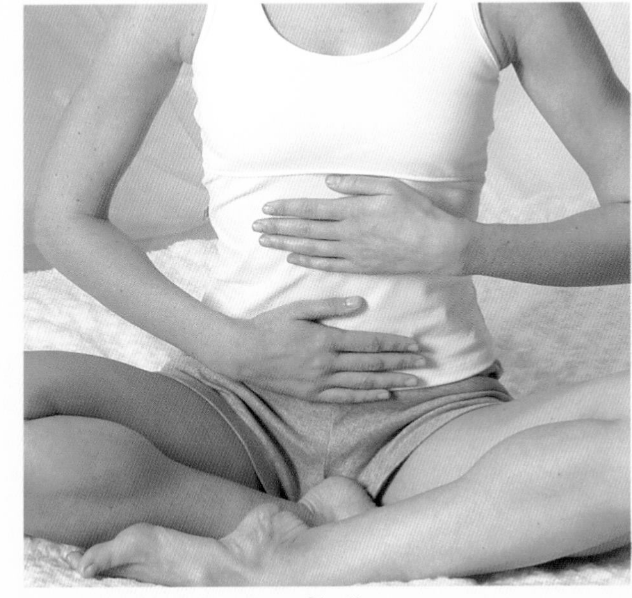

2. *Circling*

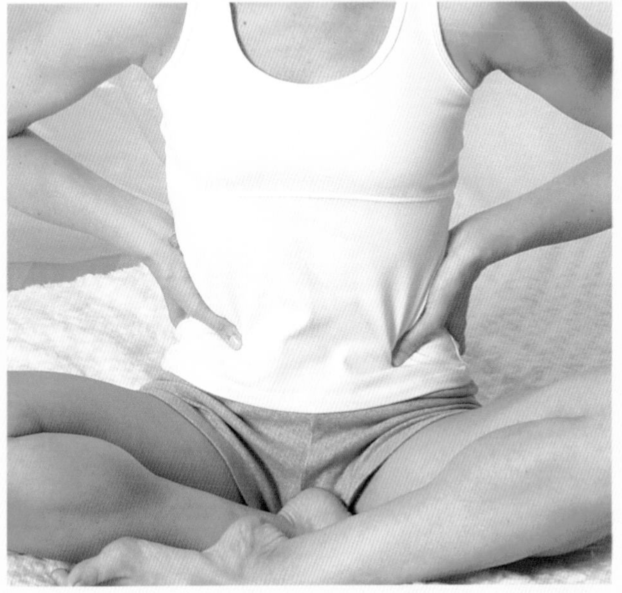

3. *Kneading the waistline*

Quick guide – back

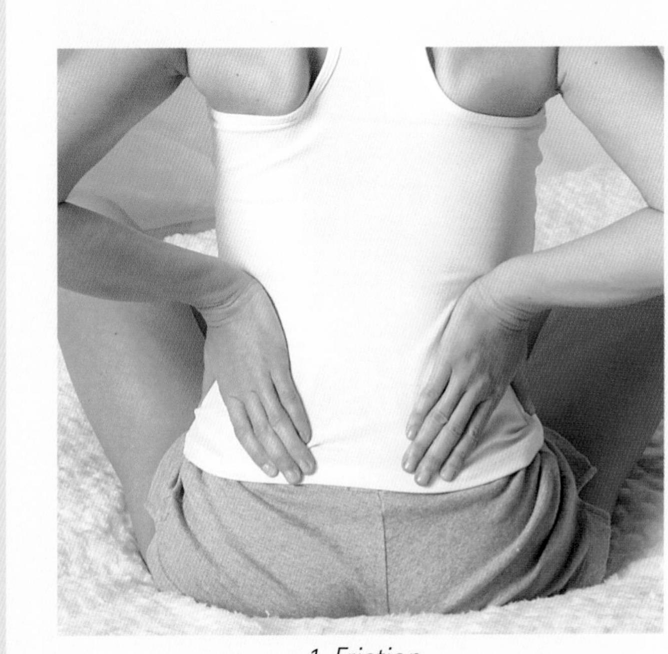

1. *Friction*

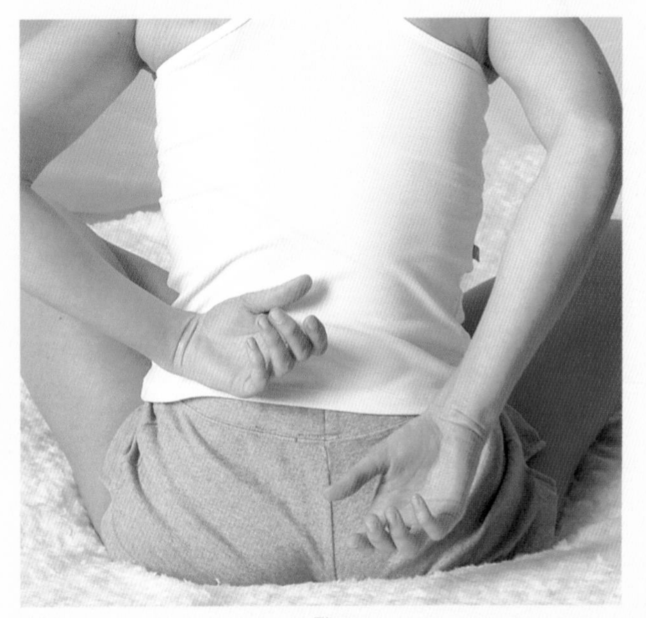

2. *Fists*

Quick guide – arm

1. Spreading the oil

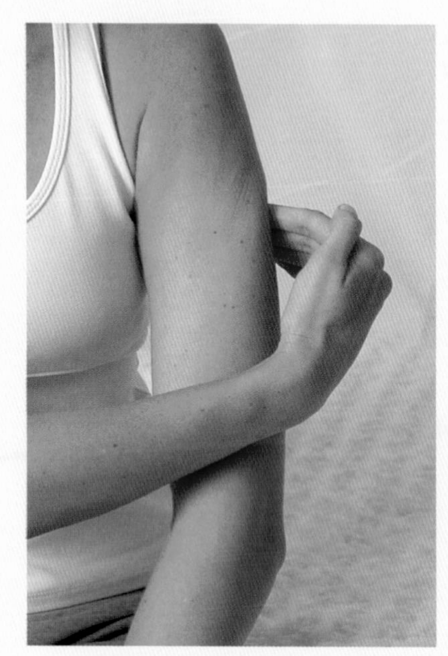

2. Friction to upper arm

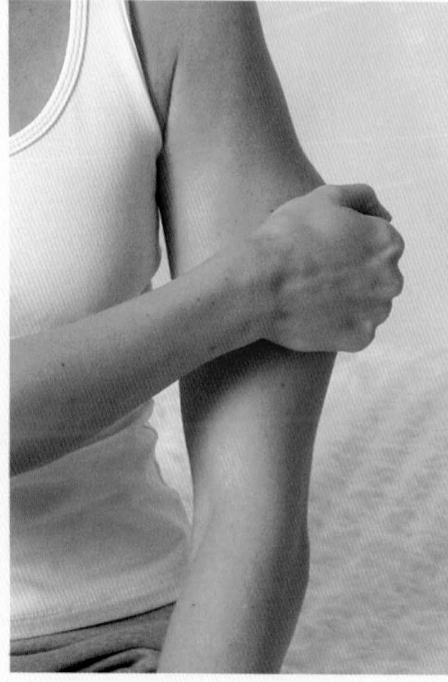

3. Squeezing

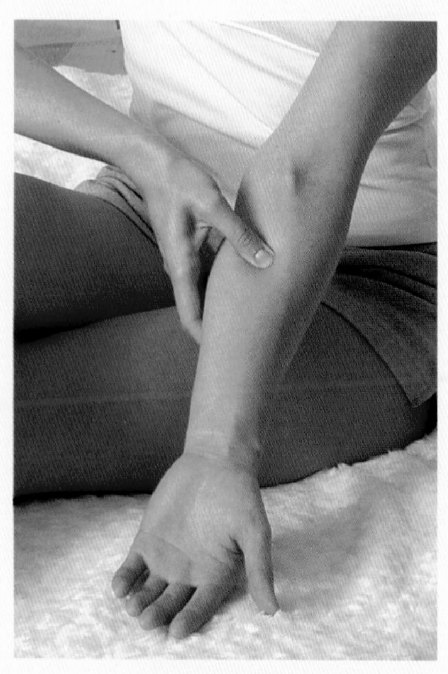

4. Circles

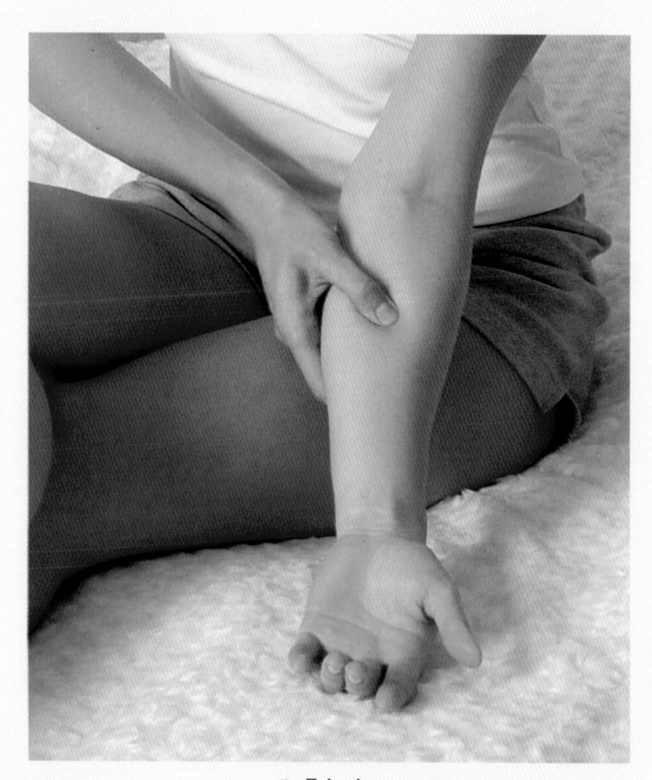

5. Friction

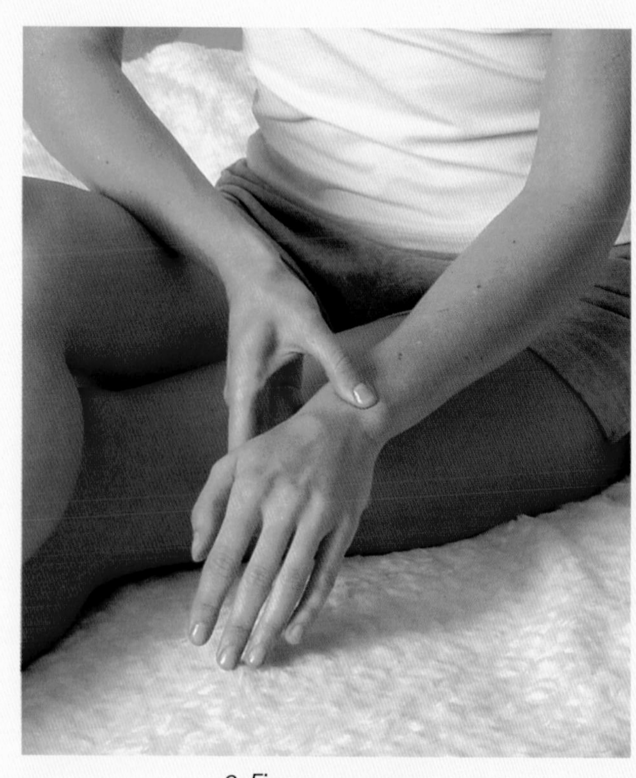

6. Finger massage

Quick guide – shoulders and neck

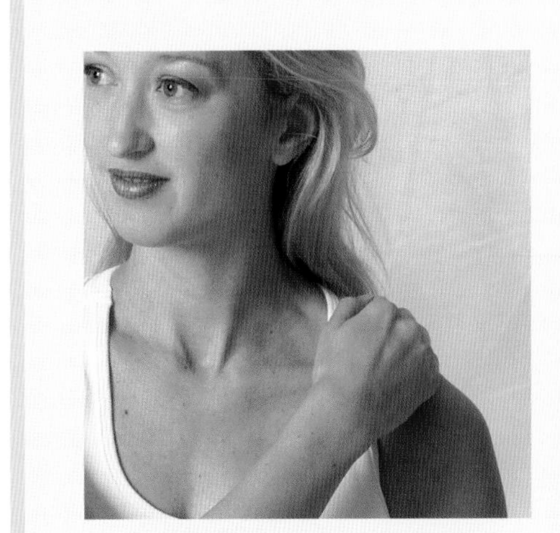

1. Friction with one hand

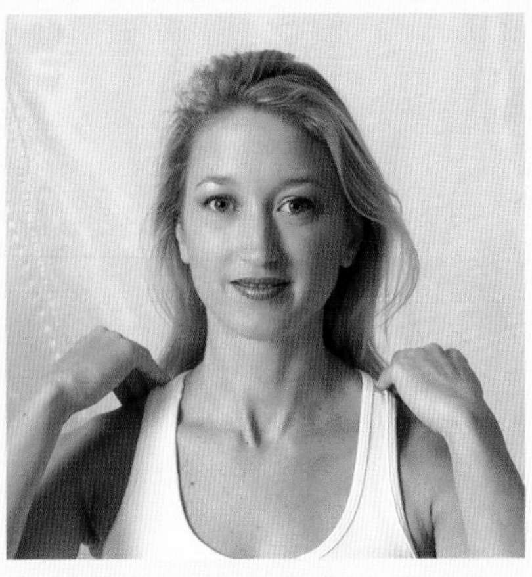

2. Friction with both hands

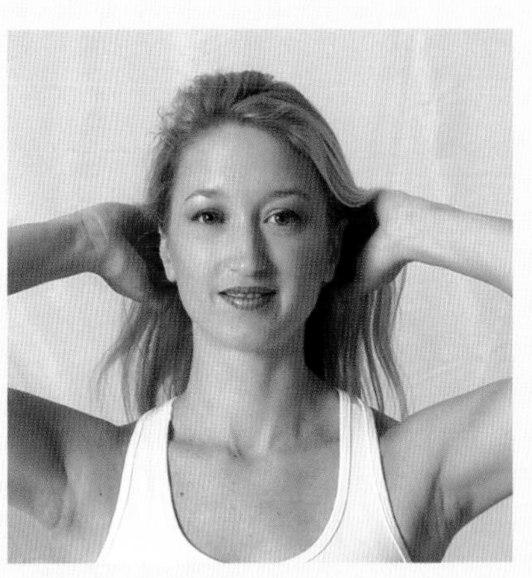

3. Friction to neck

Quick guide – face

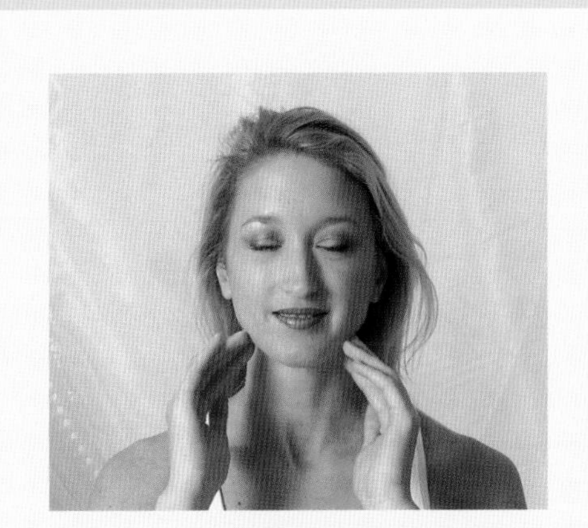

1. Effleurage

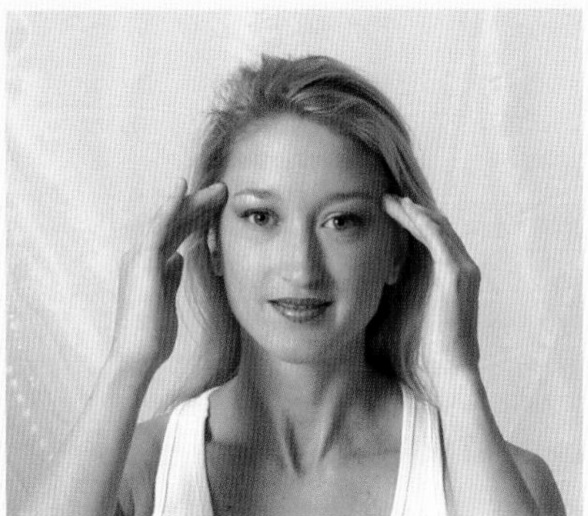

2. Friction to temples

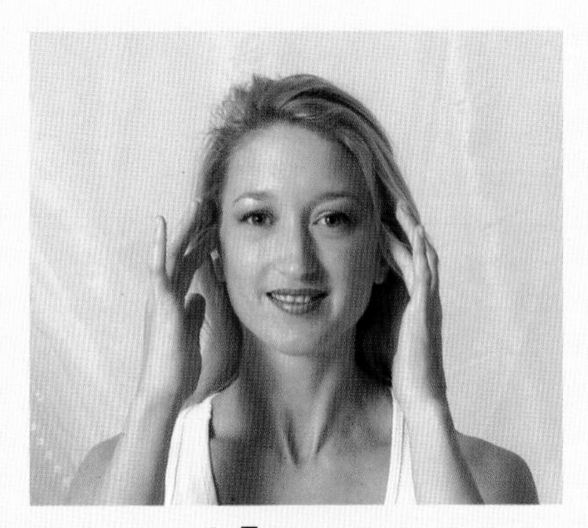

3. Tapoment

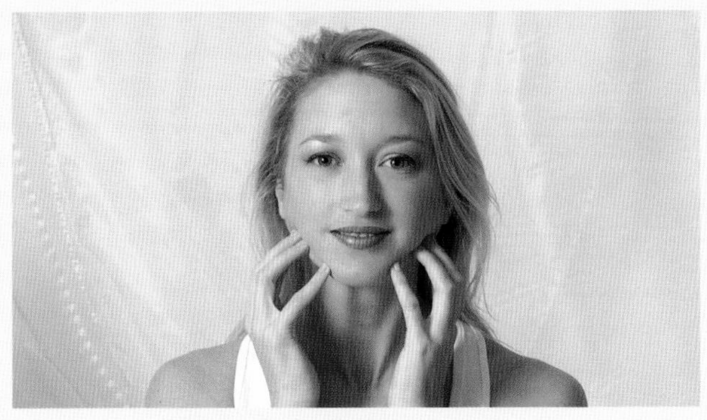

4. Friction

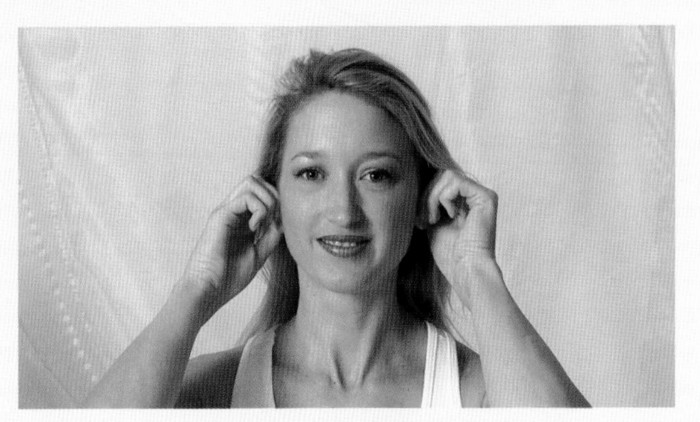

5. Massaging the ears

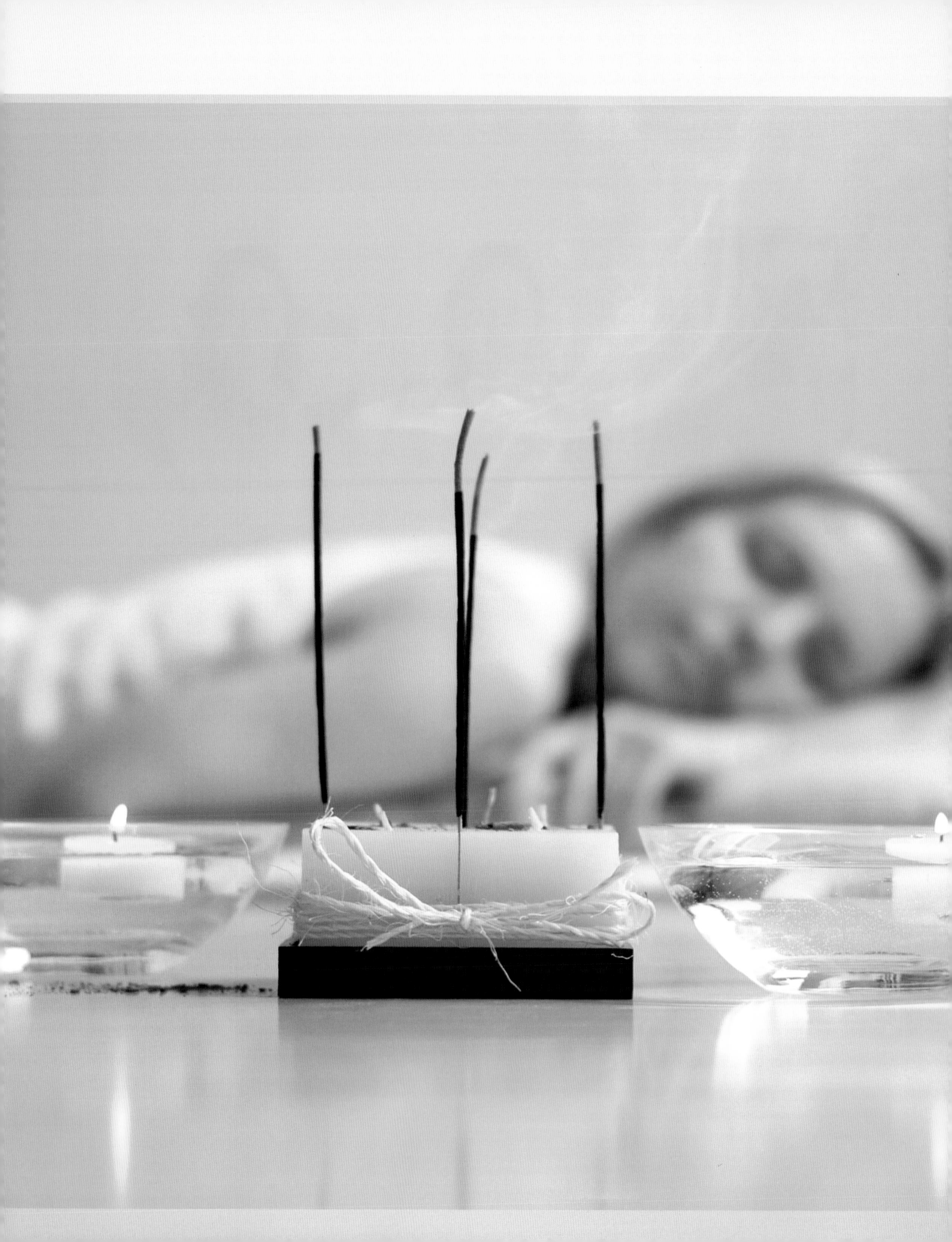

After a massage

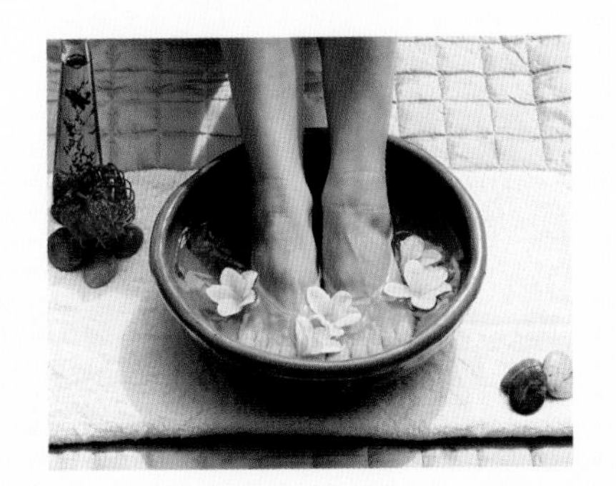

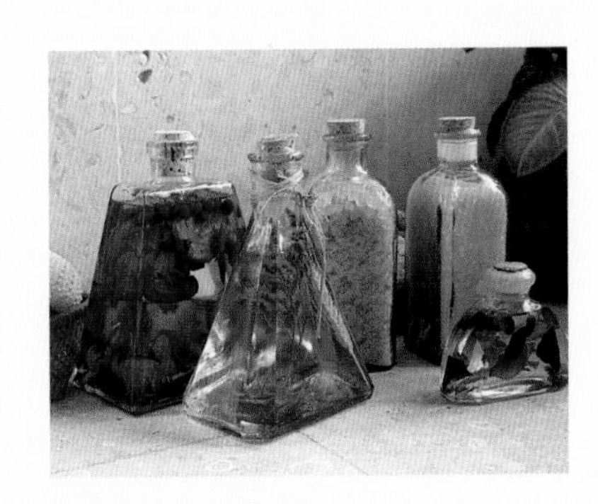

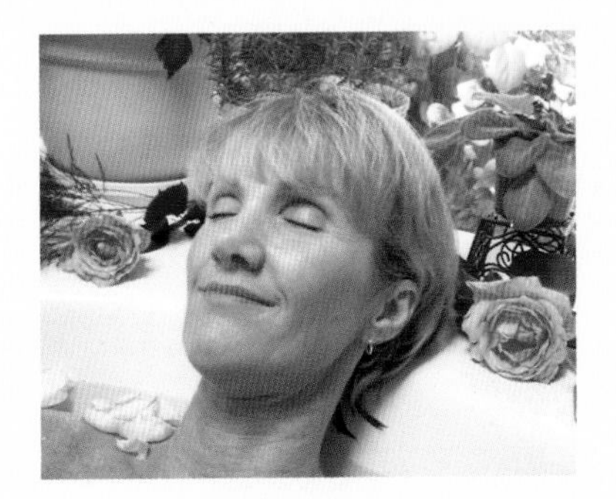

Giving a massage can be quite tiring. It is just as important for you to relax and unwind as your partner. Drink lots of water and set aside some time after a massage so that you can replenish your energy. You might want to take a bath or a relaxing walk.

Unwinding

Make sure that your partner has plenty of time to slowly get up, dress and talk about the experience. Your partner needs to drink water to flush out the toxins in the body. It is not advisable to drink alcohol before or after a massage. This is a special experience that you have both shared. Talk about what they really enjoyed and which strokes you felt were difficult. It is important to spend some time together. You could go for a walk or share a cup of herbal tea.

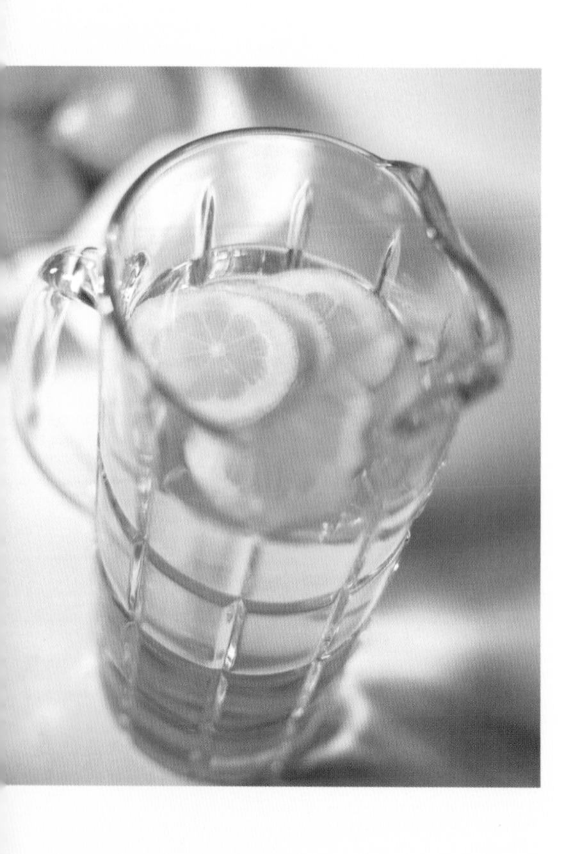

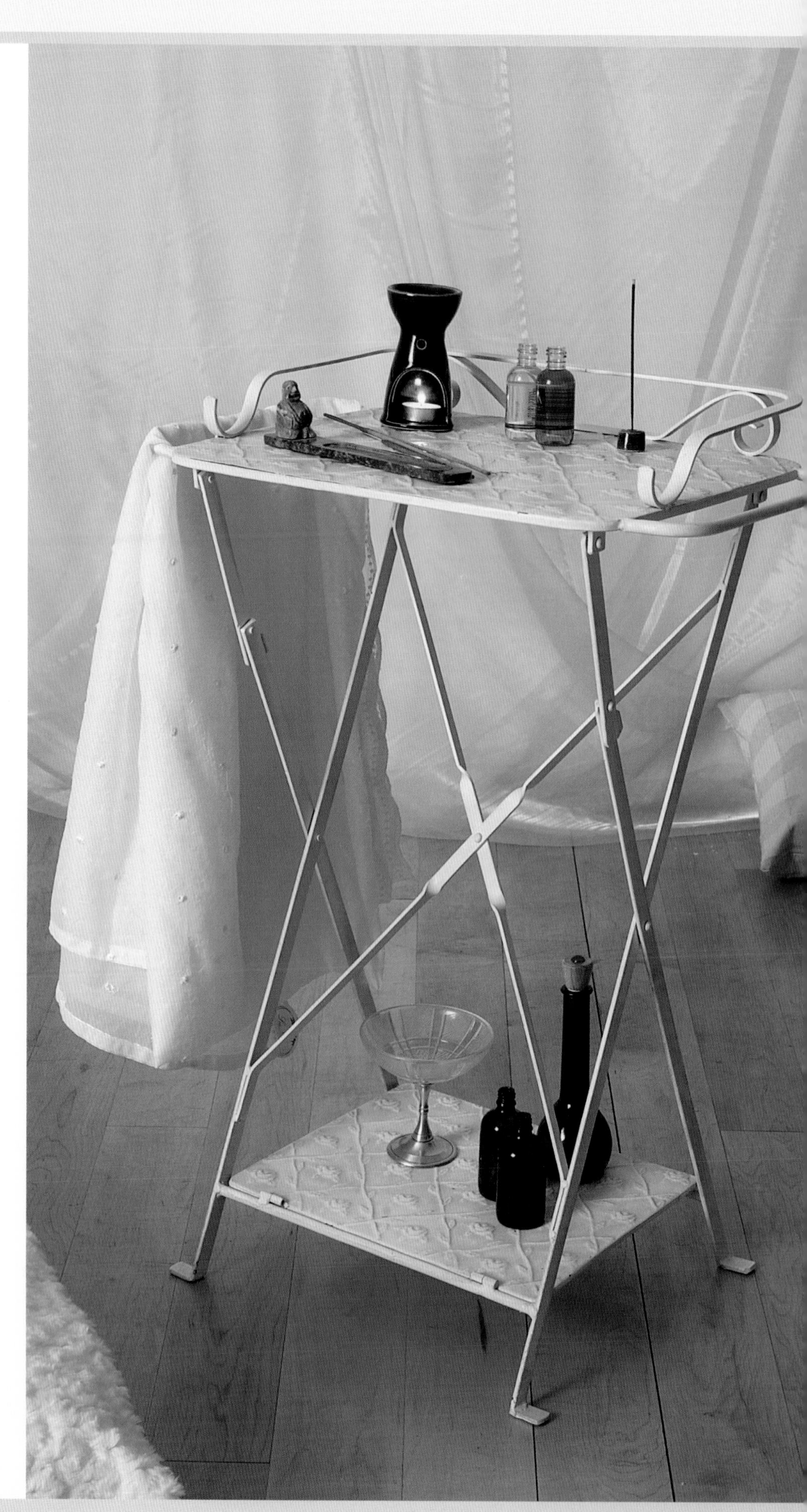

Baths

Baths are a great way to pamper yourself without a lot of fuss or preparation. Try adding eight drops of these essential oils to a base bath oil. Draw the bath first and add the mixture to the top before getting in.

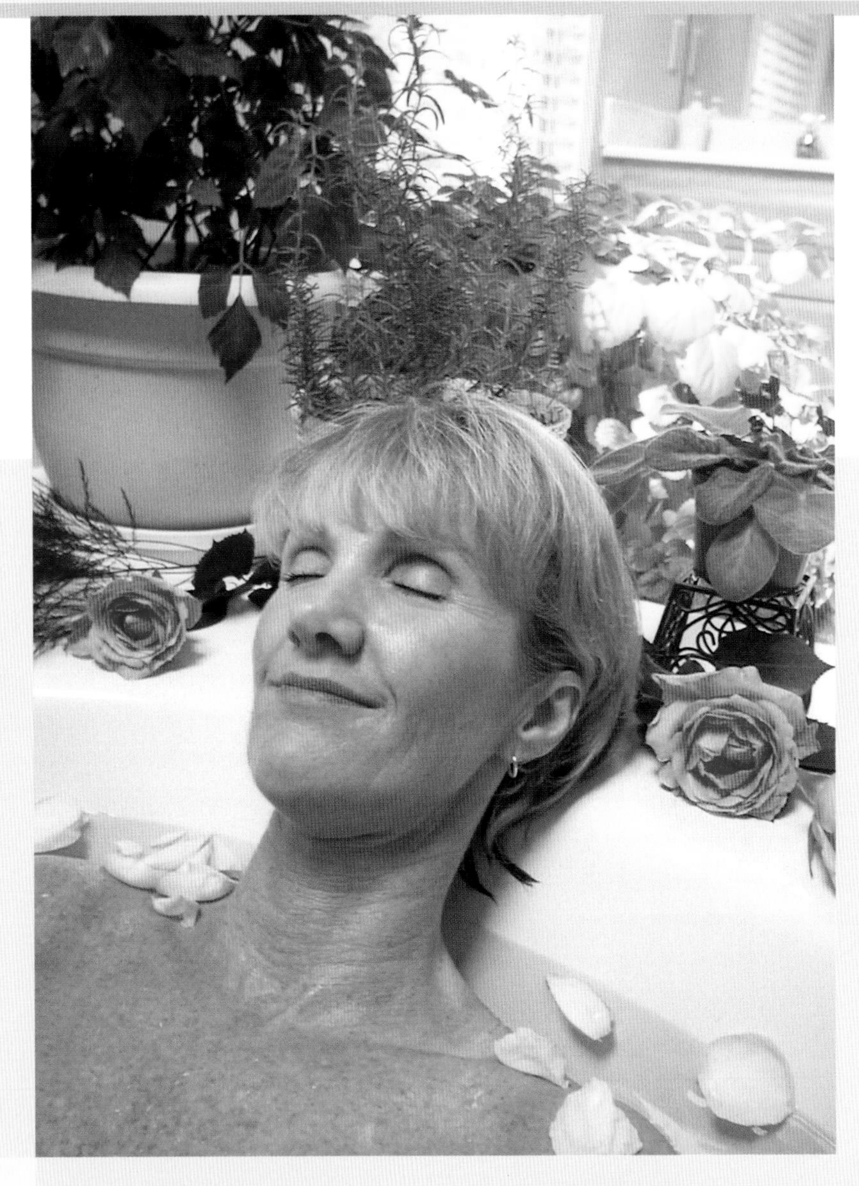

For aches and pains:
Juniper - 4 drops
Marjoram - 4 drops

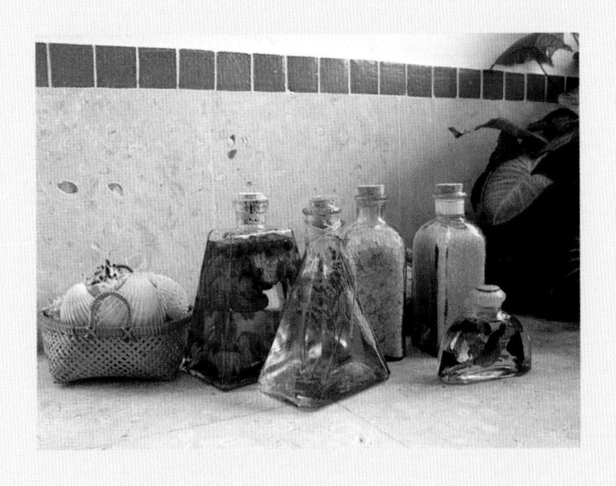

For relaxing:
Geranium - 4 drops
Bergamot - 4 drops

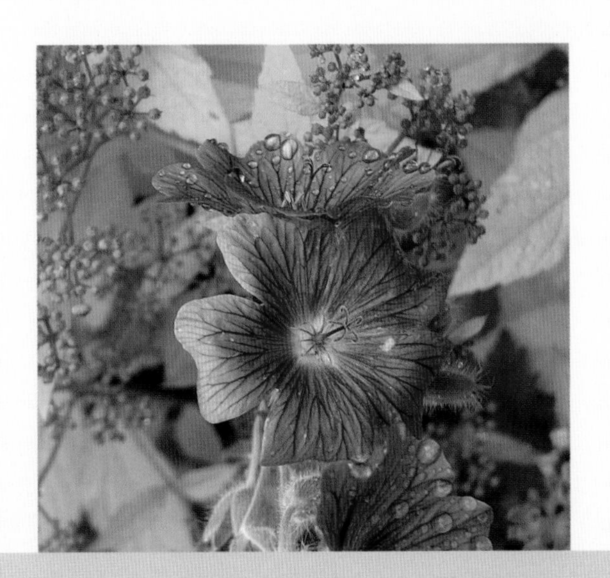

Sensual:
Rose - 4 drops
Jasmine - 4 drops

Uplifting:
Grapefruit - 4 drops
Lavender - 4 drops

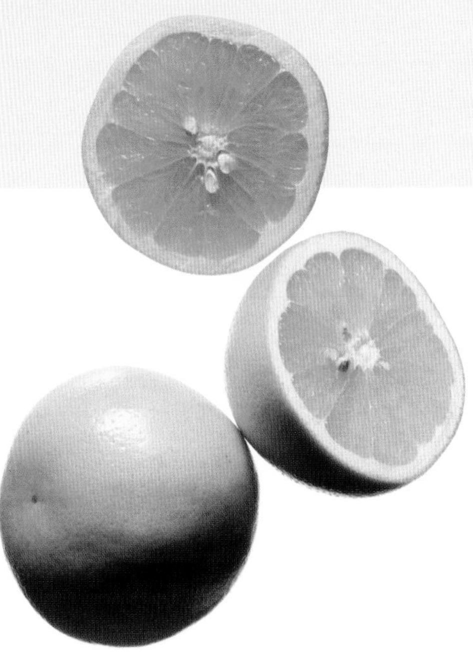

Oil burners

Oil burners diffuse essential oils into the air. They can change the energy in a room and create a relaxing atmosphere. Fill the top of the burner with water and add 13 drops of essential oil.

Hot compresses

These are great for aches and pains. Boil water and add 4 drops of essential oil. Place a small cloth in the water. Ring the cloth out and place on the area desired. Place a dry towel on top to keep the essential oil from evaporating into the air. Leave on for 5 minutes.

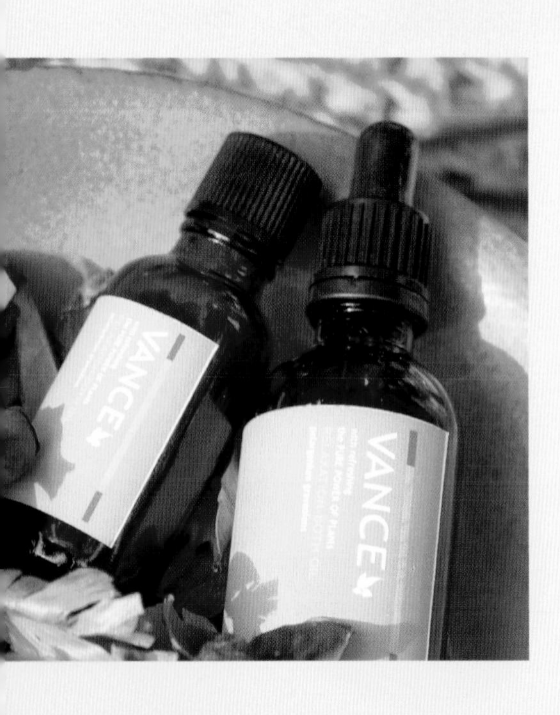

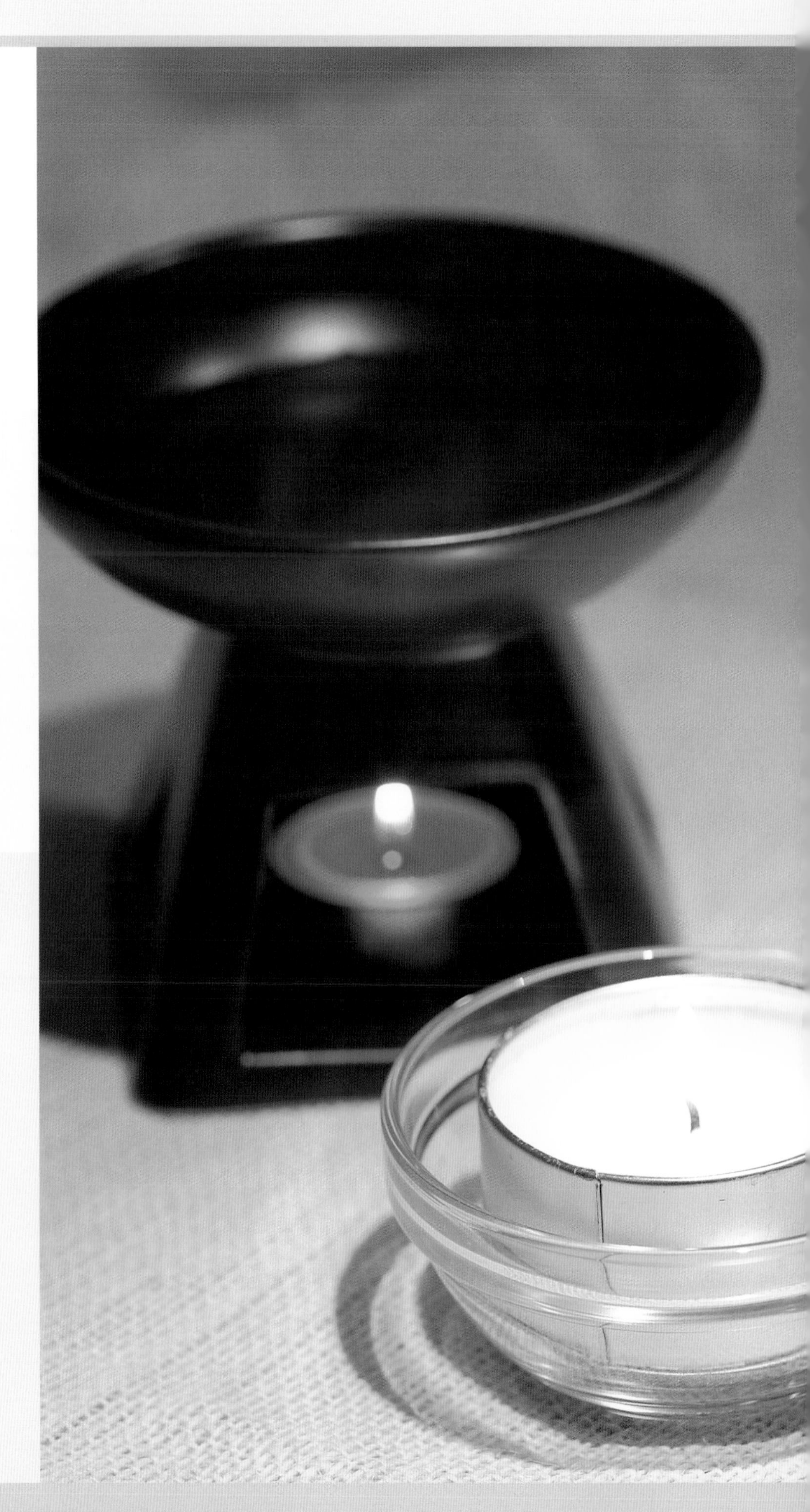

Face mask

Once you've treated your whole body to a massage, continue to look after yourself by pampering your skin. Keep these mixtures in the refrigerator and use within three days. Leave on the face for ten minutes.

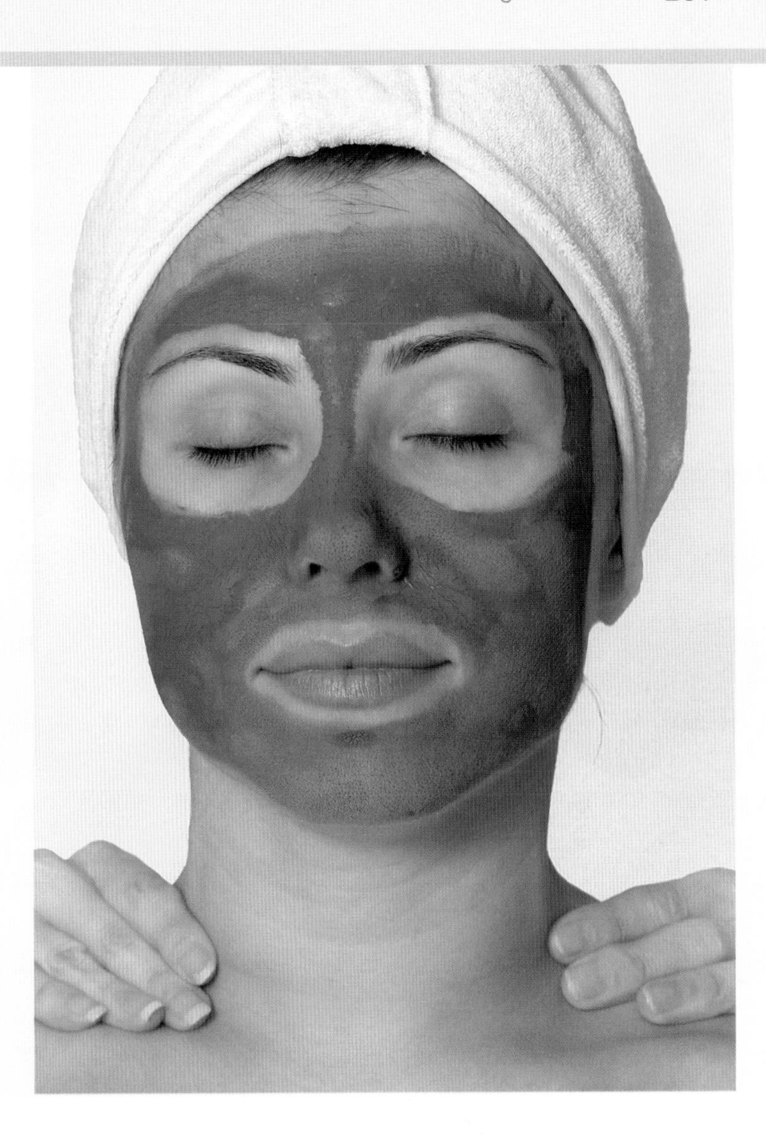

Avocado and honey – dry/sensitive skin
Half an avocado
1 dollop yoghurt
1 tbs honey
2 drops lavender essential oil

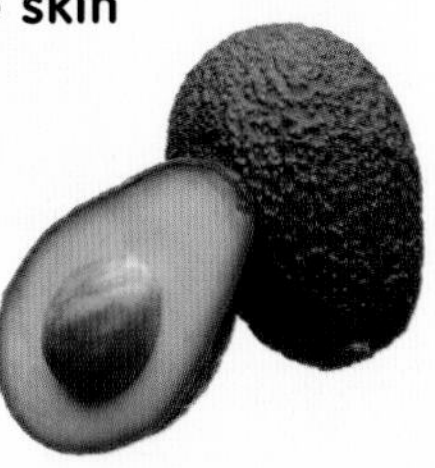

Strawberry – combination skin
3 parts strawberries
1 part sweet almond oil
2 drops ylang ylang essential oil

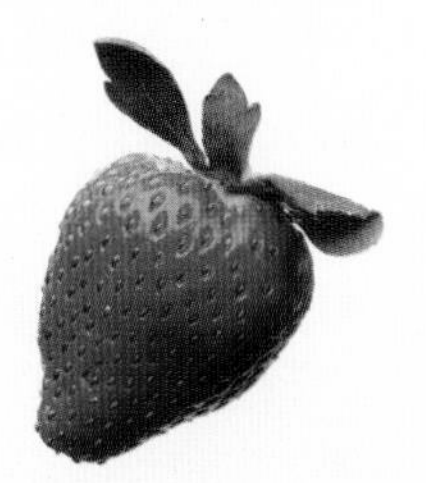

Face/body scrub

This mixture is a great exfoliator. Keep it in the refrigerator and use within three days.

Oatmeal
Enough sweet almond oil to bind ingredients
1 tbs honey
2 drops essential oil

Cream
Buy a base cream that is not scented. Add a few drops of the desired essential oil to make a luxurious moisturiser. Do not use the same essential oil for longer than three weeks.

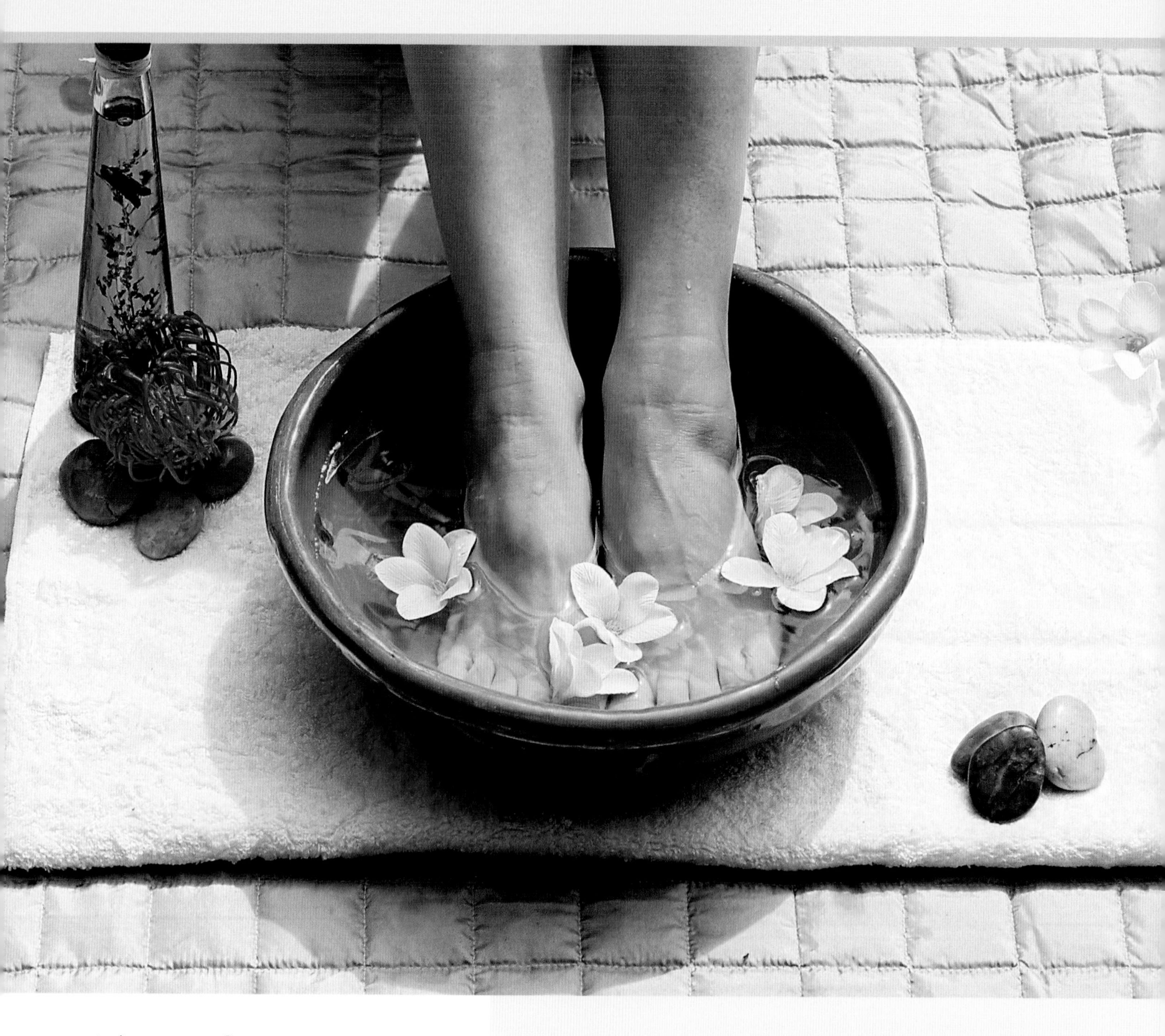

Ultimate foot pampering

You will need:

Large bowl

Hot water

Bath oil base

Lavender essential oil

Oatmeal

Sweet almond oil

1. Pour hot water into the large bowl.
2. Mix bath oil with 4 drops lavender essential oil.
3. Mix oatmeal and sweet almond oil in another bowl and set aside.
4. Add bath oil mixture to water.
5. Place feet in the bowl for 10 minutes.
6. Take feet out of water.
7. Rub a small amount of the oatmeal mixture over each foot.
8. Rinse both feet.

Bibliography

Brown, Denise Whichello,
A Complete Guide to Massage
(D&S Books Ltd, 2003)

Tucker, Louise,
An Introductory Guide to Aromatherapy
(Ruben Publishing Ltd, 2000)

Costa, Larry,
Massage, Mind and Body
(Dorling Kindersley Ltd, 2003)

Mumford, Susan,
A Complete Guide To Massage
(Hamlyn, 1995)

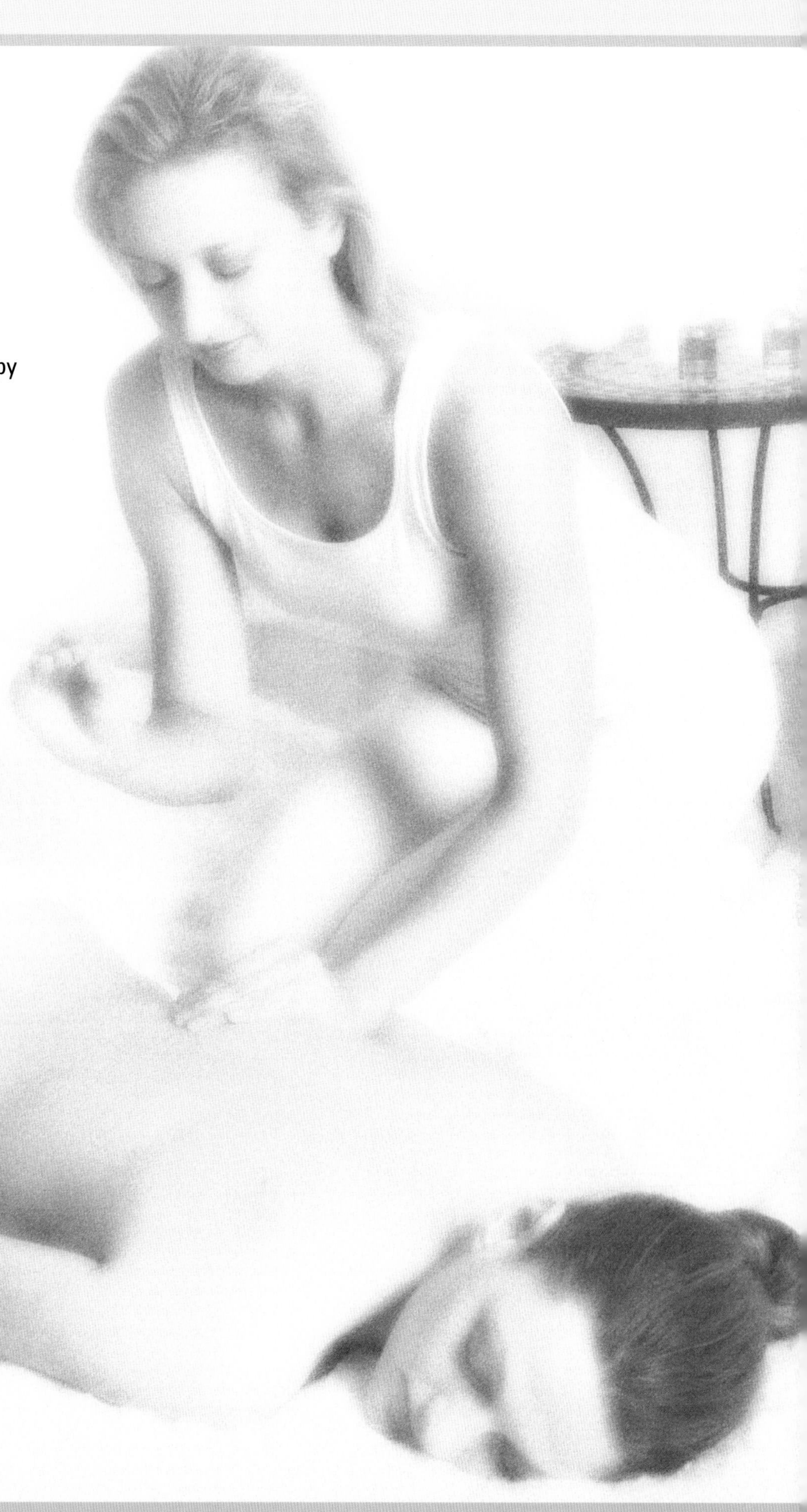

Index

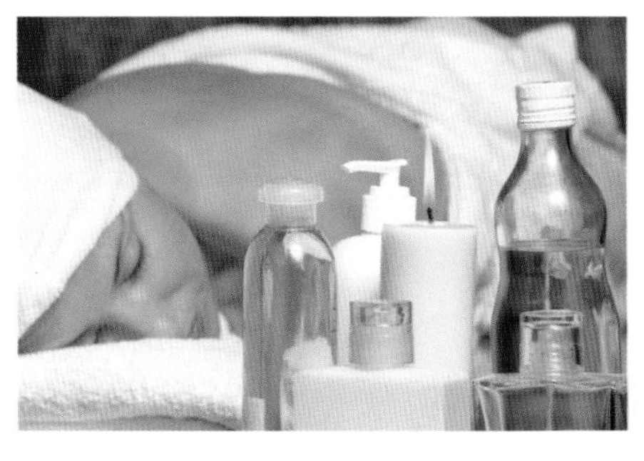

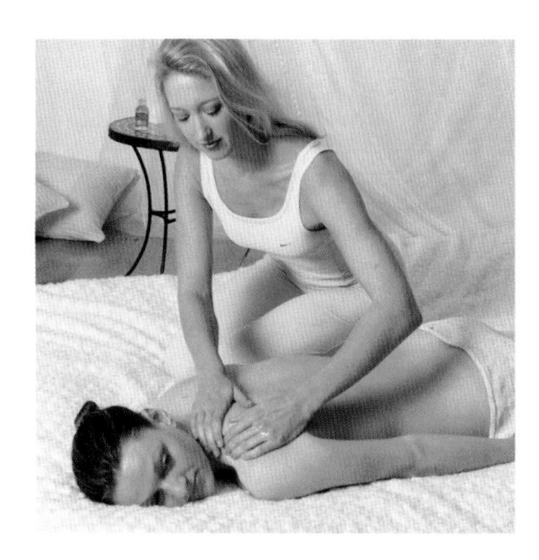

About the author

Caron Bosler received her Masters from The Laban Centre London. She became interested in holistic therapy in 1996 when she began studying Reiki. She received her Reiki Masters in 1998. From there she went on to get a diploma in Holistic Massage. She also has a certificate in Deep Tissue Massage.

Credits

I am grateful to David and Sarah for the opportunity to write this book. I would like to thank the following people for their support and encouragement: Paul Forrester, for the beautiful photographs and the hilarious banter you always bring to the photo shoots; my beautiful models, for their patience and understanding; Eduardo, for busting my chops whenever I take life too seriously; Elle for all the support and late night phone calls across the miles; Venetia and Foz for being the best friends a girl could ever hope for. And most of all to Nela for everything you ever taught me, and more.

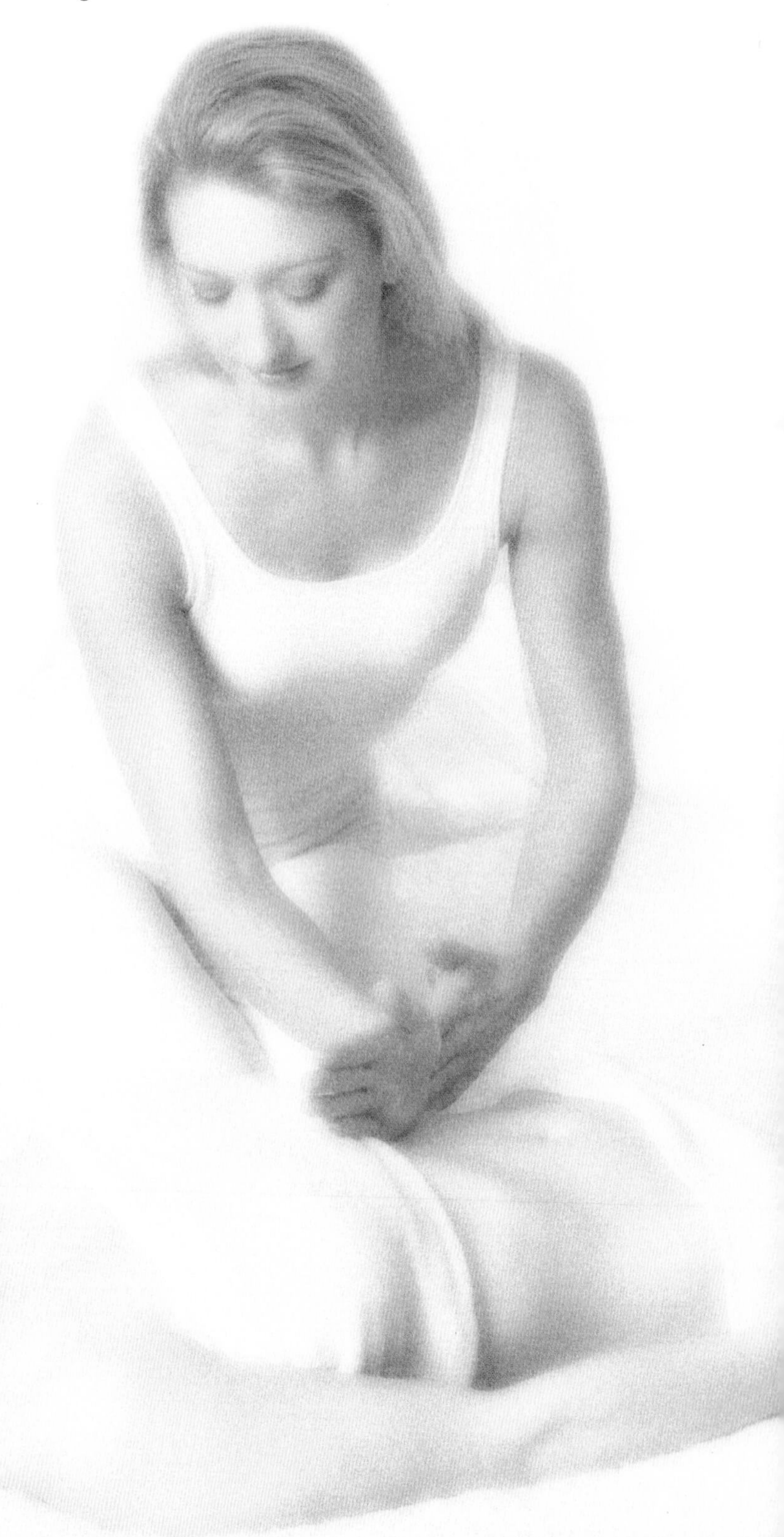